Systemic Disease Manifestations *in* the **Foot, Ankle,** *and* Lower Extremity

Systemic Disease Manifestations *in* the Foot, Ankle, *and* Lower Extremity

Rock G. Positano, DPM, MSc, MPH

Director
Non-surgical Foot and Ankle Service
Joe DiMaggio Sports Medicine Foot and Ankle
  Center
Sports Medicine Service
Hospital for Special Surgery
New York, New York

NewYork-Presbyterian Hospital/Weill Medical
  College of Cornell University
Department of Medicine
Department of Cardiothoracic Surgery
New York, New York

Professor and Chairman
Department of Academic Orthopedic Science
New York College of Podiatric Medicine
New York, New York

Christopher W. DiGiovanni, MD

Associate Professor and Vice Chairman
  (Academic Affairs), Harvard Medical School
Chief, Division of Foot & Ankle Surgery
Department of Orthopaedic Surgery
Massachusetts General Hospital & Newton
  Wellesley Hospital
Boston, Massachusetts

Jeffrey S. Borer, MD

Professor of Medicine, Cell Biology, Radiology,
  Surgery and Public Health
Director, The Howard Gilman Institute for
  Heart Valve Diseases and the Schiavone
  Cardiovascular Translational Research
  Institute
Formerly Chairman, Department of Medicine,
  and Chief, Division of Cardiovascular
  Medicine
State University of New York Downstate
  Medical Center
Adjunct Professor of Cardiovascular Medicine
  in Cardiothoracic Surgery
Weill Medical College of Cornell University
New York, New York

Michael J. Trepal, DPM, FACFAS

Professor of Surgery
Vice President for Academic Affairs
Dean
New York College of Podiatric Medicine
New York, New York

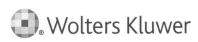 Wolters Kluwer

**Philadelphia • Baltimore • New York • London
Buenos Aires • Hong Kong • Sydney • Tokyo**

Acquisitions Editor: Brian Brown
Editorial Coordinator: Dave Murphy
Marketing Manager: Dan Dressler
Production Project Manager: Marian Bellus
Design Coordinator: Steve Druding
Manufacturing Coordinator: Beth Welsh
Prepress Vendor: S4Carlisle Publishing Services

9 8 7 6 5 4 3 2 1

Printed in China

Library of Congress Cataloging-in-Publication Data
ISBN-13: 978-1-4511-9264-3
ISBN-10: 1-4511-9264-9

Cataloging-in-Publication data available on request from the Publisher.

LWW.com

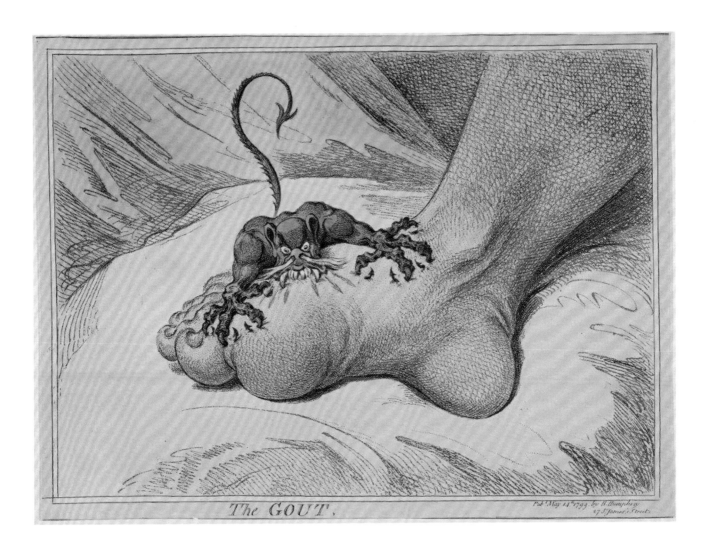

The GOUT.

Pub.d May 14.th 1799. by H. Humphrey
27 S.t James's Street.

CONTRIBUTORS

George S. Abdelmessieh, DPM, MD
PGY-2
Inova Fairfax Medical Campus
Falls Church, Virginia

Mostafa Abousayed, MD
Resident
Department of Orthopaedic Surgery
Albany Medical Center
Albany, New York

Jemima Akinsanya, DO
Resident Physician at Emory University Hospital
Emory University School of Medicine
Atlanta, Georgia

Todd J. Albert, MD
Surgeon-in-Chief and Medical Director
Korein-Wilson Professor of Orthopaedic Surgery
Weill Cornell Medical College
Hospital for Special Surgery
New York, New York

Maxwell C. Alley, BS
Medical Student
Department of Orthopaedic Surgery
Albany Medical Center
Albany, New York

Edward Amores, MD, MBA, CAQSM, FACEP
Clinical Instructor
Assistant Clinical Professor of Medicine
Department of Emergency Medicine
Weill Cornell Medical College
Attending Physician
Department of Emergency Medicine
New York-Presbyterian Hospital/Weill Cornell
    Medical Center
New York, New York

Panagiota Andreopoulou, MD
Assistant Professor of Clinical Medicine
Division of Endocrinology, Diabetes and Metabolism
Department of Medicine Weill Cornel Medical Center
New York Presbyterian Weill Cornell Medical College
New York, New York

Louis J. Aronne, MD, FACP, FTOS, DABOM
Sanford I. Weill Professor of Metabolic Research
Comprehensive Weight Control Center
Division of Endocrinology, Diabetes, & Metabolism
Weill Cornell Medical College
New York, New York

Sharon R. Barlizo, DPM
Assistant Professor
Division of Medical Sciences
New York College of Podiatric Medicine
New York, New York

Tara Blitz-Herbel, DPM, FACFAS
Attending Podiatric Surgeon
Metropolitan Hospital
Mount Sinai Medical Center
Assistant Professor
Medicine and Surgery
New York College of Podiatric Medicine
New York, New York

Karen Blitz-Shabbir, DO
Director
Rehabilitation Services
Holy Name Medical Center
Teaneck, New Jersey

John Boles, BS
Research Assistant
Hospital for Special Surgery
New York, New York

Jeffrey S. Borer, MD
Professor of Medicine, Cell Biology, Radiology, Surgery and
    Public Health
Director, The Howard Gilman Institute for Heart Valve Diseases and
    the Schiavone Cardiovascular Translational Research Institute
Formerly Chairman, Department of Medicine, and Chief,
    Division of Cardiovascular Medicine
State University of New York Downstate Medical Center
Adjunct Professor of Cardiovascular Medicine in Cardiothoracic
    Surgery
Weill Medical College of Cornell University
New York, New York

Brian P. Bosworth, MD, FACG
Professor of Medicine
Chief of Medicine
Tisch Hospital
NYU Langone Medical Center
New York, New York

Loretta Cacace, DPM, MPH
Resident Physician
New York Methodist Hospital
New York, New York

Anthony Casper, BS
Comprehensive Weight Control Center
Weill Cornell Medical College
New York, New York

Joseph C. D'Amico, DPM
Diplomate, American Board of Podiatric Medicine
Fellow, American College of Foot and Ankle Orthopedics &
    Medicine
Fellow, American Academy of Podiatric Sports Medicine
Fellow, American College of Foot and Ankle Pediatrics
Fellow, Emeritus National Academies of Practice
Professor and Past Chair Division of
    Orthopedics and Pediatrics
New York College of Podiatric Medicine
New York, New York

Henry DeGroot, MD, FAAOS
Associate Clinical Professor
University of Massachusetts Medical School
Staff Orthopedic Surgeon
Fishermen's Hospital
Marathon, Florida
Staff Orthopedic Surgeon
Southcoast Hospitals
New Bedford, Massachusetts

Thomas M. DeLauro, DPM
Professor, Divisions of Medical and Surgical Sciences
New York College of Podiatric Medicine
New York, New York

Christopher W. DiGiovanni
Associate Professor and Vice Chairman (Academic Affairs),
    Harvard Medical School
Chief, Division of Foot & Ankle Surgery
Department of Orthopaedic Surgery
Massachusetts General Hospital &
    Newton Wellesley Hospital
Boston, Massachusetts

Stephen J. DiMartino, MD, PhD, RhMSUS
Assistant Attending Rheumatologist
Hospital for Special Surgery
Instructor in Clinical Medicine
Weill Cornell Medical College
New York, New York

Joshua S. Dines, MD
Associate Attending
Sports Medicine and Shoulder Service
Department of Orthopaedic Surgery
Hospital for Special Surgery
New York, New York

Tyler A. Gonzalez, MD, MBA
Harvard Medical School
Harvard Combined Orthopaedic Residency Program
Department of Orthopaedic Surgery
Massachusetts General Hospital
Boston, Massachusetts

Daniel Guss, MD, MBA
Instructor, Harvard Medical School
Foot and Ankle Service
Department of Orthopaedic Surgery
Massachusetts General Hospital
Boston, Massachusetts
Newton-Wellesley Hospital
Newton, Massachusetts

Raymond Hsu, MD
Orthopedic Fellow
Department of Orthopedics
Brown University
Providence, Rhode Island

Leon Igel, MD
Assistant Professor of Clinical Medicine
Weill Cornell Medical College
Attending Endocrinologist
New York-Presbyterian Hospital/Weill Cornell Medical Center
New York, New York

Sravisht Iyer, MD
Resident
Department of Orthopaedic Surgery
Hospital for Special Surgery
New York, New York

Sachin Kumar Amruthlal Jain, MD
Endovascular Interventional Cardiology Fellow
Mount Sinai Heart
New York, New York

Khurram H. Khan, DPM
Associate Professor
Department of Podiatric Medicine
Temple University School of Podiatric Medicine
Philadelphia, Pennsylvania

Mark Kosinski, DPM, FIDSA
Professor
Division of Medical Sciences
New York College of Podiatric Medicine
Attending
Department of Surgery/Podiatry
Metropolitan Hospital Center
New York, New York

Prakash Krishnan, MD, FACC
Director of Endovascular Services
Cardiac Catheterization Laboratory
Assistant Director of Mount Sinai Heart Network
Mount Sinai Heart
Assistant Professor of Medicine
Mount Sinai School of Medicine
New York, New York

Rekha Kumar, MD
Assistant Professor of Medicine
Attending Endocrinologist
Comprehensive Weight Control Center
Weill Cornell Medical College
New York, New York

Mark Lebwohl, MD
Professor and Chairman
Department of Dermatology
Mount Sinai School of Medicine
New York, New York

Leonard A. Levy, DPM, MPH
Associate Dean for Research and Innovation
Director, Institute for Disaster and Emergency Preparedness
Professor of Family Medicine/Public Health/Biomedical
    Informatics
Nova Southeastern University College of Osteopathic Medicine
Fort Lauderdale, Florida

Steven K. Magid, MD
Professor, Clinical Medicine
Weill Cornell Medical College
Attending Physician
Hospital for Special Surgery
New York-Presbyterian Hospital
New York, New York

Bella Mehta, MD
Rheumatology Fellow
Hospital for Special Surgery
New York, New York

Caroline Miranda, MD
Resident
Department of Neurology
New York-Presbyterian/Weill Cornell Medical Center
New York, New York

Jeffrey Y.F. Ngeow, MD
Associate Attending Anesthesiologist
Hospital for Special Surgery
Clinical Associate Professor of Anesthesiology
Weill Cornell Medical College
New York, New York

Helene Pavlov, MD, FACR
Professor of Radiology
Professor of Radiology in Orthopaedic Surgery
Weill Cornell Medical College
Attending Radiologist
New York, New York

Mary Ann Picone, MD
Medical Director
Multiple Sclerosis Comprehensive Care Center at Holy Name
    Hospital
Teaneck, New Jersey

Rock C. J. Positano, BA
New York College of Podiatric Medicine
Joe DiMaggio Sports Medicine Foot and Ankle Center
Hospital for Special Surgery
New York, New York

Rock G. Positano, DPM, MSc, MPH
Director
Non-surgical Foot and Ankle Service
Joe DiMaggio Sports Medicine Foot and Ankle Center
Sports Medicine Service
Hospital for Special Surgery
New York, New York

NewYork-Presbyterian Hospital/Weill Medical College of Cornell
    University
Department of Medicine
Department of Cardiothoracic Surgery
New York, New York

Professor and Chairman
Department of Academic Orthopedic Science
New York College of Podiatric Medicine
New York, New York

Bhaskar Purushottam, MD
Fellow
Endovascular & Structural Interventional Cardiology
Mount Sinai Medical Center
New York, New York

Alyssa G. Rehm, MD
Resident
Department of Neurology
New York-Presbyterian Hospital
New York, New York

Satinder S. Rekhi Jr., MD
Radiology Fellow
Department of Radiology
Hospital for Special Surgery
Fellow
Department of Radiology
Weill Cornell Medical College
New York, New York

Andrew J. Rosenbaum, MD
Fellow
Foot and Ankle Service
Department of Orthopaedic Surgery
Hospital for Special Surgery
New York, New York

Yecheskel Schneider, MD
Clinical and Research Fellow
Division of Gastroenterology and Hepatology
NewYork-Presbyterian/Weill Cornell Medical Center
New York, New York

Brian Shaffer
Associate Professor
Department of Obstetrics & Gynecology - Maternal Fetal
    Medicine
Oregon Health & Science University
Portland, Oregon

Rahul Sharma, MD, MBA, CPE, FACEP
Executive Vice Chief
Associate Professor of Clinical Medicine
Division of Emergency Medicine
Weill Cornell Medical College
New York, New York

Alpana Shukla, MD, MRCP(UK)
Assistant Professor of Research in Medicine
Comprehensive Weight Control Center
Division of Endocrinology, Diabetes, & Metabolism
Weill Cornell Medical College
New York, New York

Carolyn M. Sofka, MD, FACR
Associate Professor of Radiology
Department of Radiology
Weill Cornell Medical College
Associate Attending Radiologist
Department of Radiology
Hospital for Special Surgery
New York, New York

Jessica R. Spivey, MD
Radiology Resident
Department of Radiology
New York-Presbyterian/Weill Cornell Medical Center
New York, New York

Dexter Y. Sun, MD, PhD
Clinical Professor of Neurology
Weill Cornell Medical College
New York-Presbyterian Hospital/Weill Cornell Medicine
Hospital for Special Surgery
New York, New York

Mark H. Swartz, MD
Professor
Department of Medical Science
Vice President, Medical and Professional Affairs
New York College of Podiatric Medicine
Professor of Medicine
SUNY Downstate College of Medicine
Adjunct Clinical Professor of Medicine
Albert Einstein College of Medicine
Adjunct Professor of Medicine
New York Medical College
New York, New York

Ishaan Swarup, MD
Resident
Department of Orthopaedic Surgery
Hospital for Special Surgery
New York, New York

Minyi Tan, MD
Assistant Professor
Department of Anesthesiology
Stony Brook University School of Medicine
Stony Brook, New York

Arthur Tarricone, MPH
Mount Sinai Heart
Mount Sinai Medical Center
New York, New York

Jason P. Tartaglione MD
Resident
Department of Orthopaedic Surgery
Albany Medical Center
Albany, New York

Michael J. Trepal, DPM, FACFAS
Professor of Surgery
Vice President for Academic Affairs
Dean
New York College of Podiatric Medicine
New York, New York

Hunter Vincent, DO
Resident Physician
Department of Physical Medicine and Rehabilitation
University of California, Davis
Sacramento, California

Riham M. Wahba, MD
Research Assistant
Johns Hopkins University School of Medicine
Baltimore, Maryland

Clover Youn West, DO
Resident
Neurology
Mount Sinai Beth Israel
New York, New York

Geoffrey H. Westrich, MD
Associate Professor
Department of Orthopaedic Surgery
Hospital for Special Surgery
New York, New York

Peter Z. Yan, MD
Chief Resident
Clinical Operations
Department of Neurology
Weill Cornell Medical Center
New York-Presbyterian Hospital
New York, New York

FOREWORD

*M*edicine has needed a cutting-edge, authoritative textbook on how systemic disease can manifest in the foot, ankle, and overall lower extremity. It is with great pleasure, and from the personal point of view of a satisfied consumer, that I write the foreword for this fascinating book.

Podiatric problems provide vital insights into the health care system as a window to systemic disease, covering all the body systems such as nerves, vascular, skin, endocrine, and musculoskeletal.

Foot and ankle pain will often bring a person into the health care system because of how it threatens their lifestyle. It happens quite often that a podiatric evaluation will point to other pathologies that can then be identified and treated by the appropriate specialist.

Therefore, while a patient may present with seemingly minor maladies, it is critical that the medical professional has the knowledge and insight to identify those lower extremity pathologies as markers for more systemic disease. From quality-of-life issues to a more serious examination of overall health, the Doctor of Podiatric Medicine (DPM)

in conjunction with the Doctor of Medicine (MD) has the opportunity to open a portal to an integrated science–based health care approach that seeks to heal the whole body.

As Dr. Positano and I have discussed, there has been no significant research in Western medicine that "maps" out the foot and the many meridians that Eastern medicine has always recognized as critical to well-being. For the first time, there is an authoritative book, clearly, compellingly, and eloquently written, that provides a benchmark for the practicing medical professional.

It is rare that I recommend a medical textbook as both sage and illuminating. But I do so herein with no reservation.

Paul Greengard, PhD
Nobel Laureate (2000) Physiology or Medicine
Vincent Astor Professor
Laboratory of Molecular and Cellular Neuroscience
The Rockefeller University
New York, New York

PREFACE

The foot, ankle, and lower extremity *is often referred to by those health care providers who specialize in these areas as a* mirror of systemic disease *because* many systemic diseases, including heart disease, diabetes, skin disease, and neurologic disease, first present in *this anatomic region of* the body. *Although all too frequently ignored,* examination of the lower extremity can reflect a person's general health, *both physical and psychological,* and the overall condition of the body's functional systems such as cardiovascular, neurologic, dermatologic, musculoskeletal, and endocrinologic. Yet, when patients visit their internists, they are usually instructed to "Take off everything but your shoes and socks." By not examining the foot and ankle, the physician can miss the early warning system of disease that the lower extremity can provide.

The foot is unique because it contains all the systems of the body, *including musculoskeletal, vascular, neurologic, dermatologic, and immune.*

A painful foot, heel, bunion, tendon, knee, hip, or lower back will bring a patient into the health care system, because the pain interferes with mobility. The ability to do everyday tasks, such as exercise, walking, shopping, playing sports, is often limited. Foot, ankle, and lower extremity *pathologic* conditions may not be life threatening *in most cases,* but they do restrict lifestyle *both directly and indirectly and also the physical and mental health.* This disruption in the quality of life will bring the patient into the health care system, which can result in early identification of many more serious medical problems and can lead to referral to the appropriate medical specialist. *Significant life-threatening pathologies including malignant neoplasms, cardiovascular disorders, immunosuppressive syndromes, and progressive neuromuscular disease may initially manifest with subtle lower extremity signs and symptoms.*

Health professionals with the MD, DPM, DO, DC, DPT, and PA titles, who specialize in musculoskeletal care, can often recognize systemic disease in its infancy or more advanced stages. Clinical medical studies could be derived from the thorough examination of the foot, ankle, and lower extremity in relation to systemic disease. Internal medicine and musculoskeletal disciplines potentially could meet, explore, and produce a new area of specialization.

For these reasons, practitioners of internal medicine, orthopedics, and podiatric medicine need to make the examination of the foot, ankle, and lower extremity an important and integral part of their physical examination. Residents, fellows, medical students, and musculoskeletal practitioners should be instructed in the thorough examination of the foot, ankle, and lower extremity. It is a powerful diagnostic tool that is too often ignored.

Rock G. Positano, DPM, MSc, MPH
Christopher W. DiGiovanni, MD
Jeffrey S. Borer, MD
Michael J. Trepal, DPM

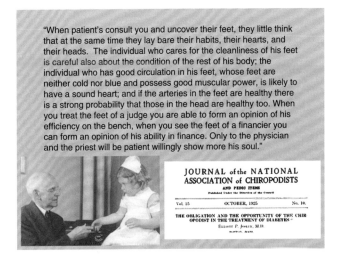

"When patient's consult you and uncover their feet, they little think that at the same time they lay bare their habits, their hearts, and their heads. The individual who cares for the cleanliness of his feet is careful also about the condition of the rest of his body; the individual who has good circulation in his feet, whose feet are neither cold nor blue and possess good muscular power, is likely to have a sound heart; and if the arteries in the feet are healthy there is a strong probability that those in the head are healthy too. When you treat the feet of a judge you are able to form an opinion of his efficiency on the bench, when you see the feet of a financier you can form an opinion of his ability in finance. Only to the physician and the priest will be patient willingly show more his soul."

JOURNAL of the NATIONAL
ASSOCIATION of CHIROPODISTS
AND PEDIC ITEMS

Vol. 15   OCTOBER, 1925   No. 10.

THE OBLIGATION AND THE OPPORTUNITY OF THE CHIROPODIST IN THE TREATMENT OF DIABETES

CONTENTS

xv

Systemic Disease Manifestations *in* the **Foot, Ankle,** *and* **Lower Extremity**

CHAPTER 1

Presentation of Systemic Disease When Imaging the Lower Extremity

HELENE PAVLOV • CAROLYN M. SOFKA • SATINDER S. REKHI JR. • JESSICA R. SPIVEY

The foot and ankle are constantly being stepped on and stressed by both normal and extraordinary forces. Feet are taken for granted, until they are hurt, limit ambulation, make wearing shoes difficult, cause gait disturbances, or some other malady forces the foot and/or ankle to take on a new level of importance. Most of the time, foot conditions are localized to a bunion, flat foot, or Achilles tendon injury that can be treated with orthotics, change of footwear, exercises, local injection, or a combination of these therapies and/or surgery. On other occasions, foot and/or ankle pain and abnormalities of the lower extremity may result from an underlying systemic condition. When reviewing imaging examinations, for example, radiographs (X-ray), magnetic resonance imaging (MRI), ultrasound, or computerized tomography (CT) examinations of the lower extremity, possible underlying systemic conditions must be considered. Familiarity with systemic conditions that can be identified on an imaging examination facilitates early diagnosis and intervention. These conditions fall into the classic categories of arthritis, infection, tumor, vascular, developmental, metabolic, and other. In this chapter, the imaging findings of various systemic conditions that can present with changes in the lower extremity are organized alphabetically.

FIBROUS DYSPLASIA

Fibrous dysplasia is a sporadic bone disease in which benign fibro-osseous lesions develop during skeletal formation.[1] Occasionally, fibrous dysplasia can arise as a component of McCune–Albright syndrome or Mazabraud syndrome.[2] Lesions can occur anywhere on the skeleton, with the craniofacial bones, ribs, and long bones most commonly involved.[1] In the lower extremity, the femur and tibia are most often affected.[1] Fibrous dysplasia occurs in both monostotic and polyostotic forms, with the former accounting for approximately 80% of all cases.[2] Often asymptomatic, fibrous dysplasia is diagnosed incidentally on radiographs obtained for unrelated reasons.[1] In such cases, no treatment is needed.[1] The polyostotic form is more likely to produce symptoms including pain, limp, and deformity, and large lesions are prone to pathologic fracture.[1] Rarely, fibrous dysplasia is complicated by malignant degeneration, particularly in previously irradiated areas.[1]

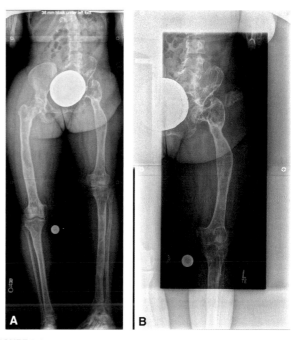

FIGURE 1-1. Radiographic pattern of fibrous dysplasia. Frontal X-ray of the lower extremities **(A)** and left femur **(B)** demonstrates expansile lesions with characteristic ground glass matrix, thin cortices, and bowing deformities. Not atypically, polyostotic fibrous dysplasia affects one side more than the other.

Fibrous dysplasia demonstrates a characteristic radiographic appearance of intramedullary, well-defined, and expansile lesions with a radiolucent "ground glass" matrix.[1,2] Shepherd's crook deformity of the proximal femur is a lateral bowing deformity and coxa vara.[2] Saber shin deformity is an anterior bowing deformity of the tibia commonly associated with fibrous dysplasia (**Fig. 1-1**).

GOUT

Gout, an inflammatory arthritis, is a crystal arthropathy characterized by hyperuricemia and subsequent deposition of monosodium urate (MSU) crystals in joints and soft tissues.[3] Gout is a common and potentially debilitating condition, disproportionately affecting men.[3] Affected individuals experience recurrent acute inflammatory flares as well as chronic destructive changes secondary to MSU crystal deposition. Gout can involve any joint but most frequently affects the feet, demonstrating a predilection for the 1st metatarsophalangeal (MTP) joint.[4] Gout can be associated with metabolic syndromes, myocardial infarction, and diabetes mellitus.

Radiographs of involved joints may reveal marginal "punched out" erosions, sclerotic margins, and overhanging edges, with relative preservation of the joint space; however, X-ray changes typically occur late in the course of the disease.[3,4] Radiographs may also demonstrate macroscopic

depositions of MSU crystals, or tophi, which are a hallmark feature of chronic gout.[4] Tophi may be periarticular or intra-articular; CT is particularly useful in detecting intra-articular depositions.[4] Tophi display intermediate or low signal on T1-weighted MRI sequences, with variable appearance on T2-weighted sequences.[3] Postcontrast sequences generally demonstrate enhancement, and there is often associated synovial thickening and adjacent marrow edema.[3,4] MRI can also reveal erosions before they become visible on radiographs (**Fig. 1-2**).[4]

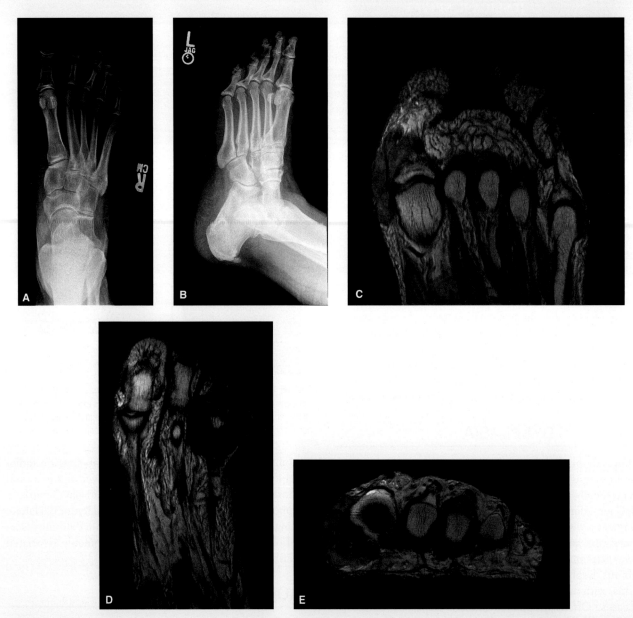

FIGURE 1-2. Radiographic and MR patterns of gout. A and **B:** Frontal and oblique radiographs of the foot in different patients with gout. **A:** Frontal X-ray of the foot demonstrates medial soft tissue prominence of gouty tophus adjacent to the metatarsal head of the great toe without underlying bone or joint abnormalities. **B:** Oblique X-ray view demonstrates classic "overhanging edge" of gout at the medial and lateral aspects of the metatarsal head of the great toe. **C to E:** MR demonstration of gout. **C:** Coronal fast spin echo MR image of the 1st MTP joint demonstrates the heterogeneously hyperintense soft tissue mass of gouty tophus medial to the 1st MTP joint. **D:** Coronal fast spin echo proton density-weighted image demonstrates a heterogeneous expansile hyperintense mass of gouty typhus circumferentially about the 3rd PIP joint. **E:** Axial fast spin echo proton density-weighted image through the forefoot demonstrates focal heterogeneously hyperintense soft tissue tophus within the plantar margins of both the 1st and 3rd MTP joints. The soft tissue tophus about the 3rd MTP joint extends dorsally.

HYPERTROPHIC PULMONARY OSTEOARTHROPATHY

Hypertrophic pulmonary osteoarthropathy (HPO) or Pierre Marie–Bamberger syndrome is a syndrome of unknown etiology characterized by the triad of periosteal bone deposition, clubbing of the digits, and arthralgia, which occurs in association with pulmonary pathology.[5,6] HPO can develop in many chronic pulmonary conditions, but in the majority of cases is associated with primary lung malignancies.[5] Rarely, patients with extrathoracic diseases such as inflammatory bowel disease can develop HPO.[5] Patients typically present with pain, tenderness, and swelling. Radiographs demonstrate generalized periosteal reaction along the diaphyses and metaphyses of long bones sparing the epiphyses.[6] MRI can be helpful in demonstrating adjacent soft tissue swelling and muscular edema (**Fig. 1-3**).[6]

INFARCT AND OSTEONECROSIS

Osteonecrosis and bone infarct define bone death. Osteonecrosis is typically used to describe ischemic bone death in a subchondral location, and bone infarct is used when the lesion is not in a subchondral location. Systemic causes of bone death are corticosteroids, sickle cell anemia, collagen vascular disease, alcoholism, and idiopathic.[7] The most common cause of osteonecrosis in a subchondral location is trauma that presents as mixed lytic and sclerotic areas on radiographs and that can progress to microfractures in articular collapse if left untreated.[8]

Infarcts in the lower extremity occur primarily in the medullary cavity of the long bones.[8] On radiographs, infarcts present as an elongated serpiginous rim of sclerosis with a central lucency. MRI is the most sensitive test for suspected bone infarct and demonstrates characteristic findings.[7] The lesions contain a center of devitalized marrow surrounded by a rim of granulation tissue and sclerosis, which gives these lesions a central high signal from adipose marrow with a surrounding ring of hyperintense inner granulation tissue and hypointense outer ring of sclerosis and is classically referred to as the "double-line" sign (**Fig. 1-4**).

MAFFUCCI SYNDROME

Maffucci syndrome is a nonhereditary and rare dyschondroplasia of unknown origin characterized by multiple enchondromas combined with soft tissue venous malformations.[9] Enchondromas are benign cartilaginous lesions within the metadiaphysis of tubular bones that typically present as osteolytic expansile lesions with central stippled calcifications characteristic of a chondroid matrix (**Fig. 1-5**).[10]

MELORHEOSTOSIS

Melorheostosis is an uncommon sclerosing bone dysplasia of unknown etiology.[11,12] Patients are usually asymptomatic but can present with limb stiffness or pain.[11] The typical appearance on radiographs is of flowing hyperostosis along the outer cortical surface of the long bones of the lower extremity, which usually has an undulating appearance, referred to as "dripping candle wax sign" (**Fig. 1-6**).[11]

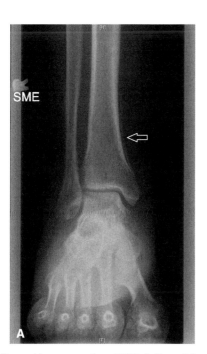
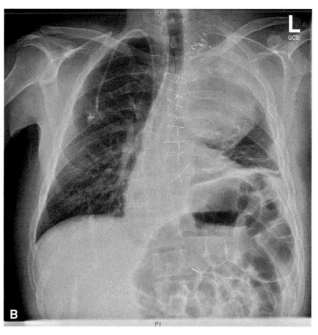

FIGURE 1-3. Radiographic presentation of HPO. A: X-ray of the right ankle demonstrates thick periosteal reaction at the distal aspect of the long bone, sparing the epiphysis (*arrow*) without underlying bone pathology. Posteroanterior (PA) radiograph of the chest (**B**) in the same patient demonstrates a large, left upper lobe lesion.

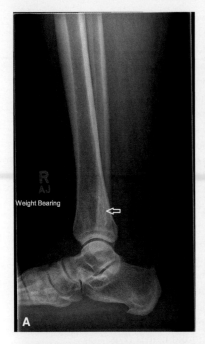

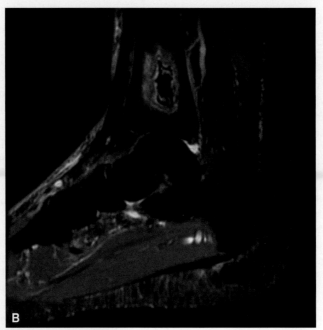

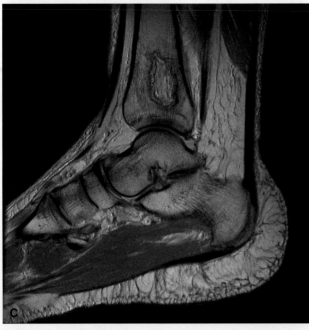

FIGURE 1-4. X-ray and MR findings of bone infarct. A: Lateral X-ray of the ankle demonstrates a classic bone infarct with an irregular serpiginous elongated lucency in the distal tibia without periosteal or endosteal reaction (*arrow*). Sagittal inversion recovery **(B)** and proton density-weighted images **(C)** demonstrate the characteristic heterogeneously hyperintense serpiginous pattern of bone infarct on MRI.

METASTATIC DISEASE

Bone is a common site of metastatic involvement in malignancy.[13] Many primary malignancies can metastasize to the skeleton; however, breast, prostate, and lung carcinoma are most frequently associated with osseous involvement.[13] Less frequently, kidney and thyroid cancers metastasize to the bone. Metastatic lesions can be painful and may lead to pathologic fracture if extensive cortical destruction is present.[14] The axial skeleton and proximal long bones are disproportionately affected in metastatic disease, in part because of the higher relative content of vascularized red marrow.[14]

The radiographic appearance of osseous metastases depends on the primary malignancy and the bone response elicited by the metastatic deposit.[13] Breast and lung carcinoma typically produce mixed lytic and blastic lesions.[13] Lytic lesions are characterized by excessive bone resorption and are often seen with thyroid and renal carcinoma, whereas blastic (sclerotic) lesions, characterized by excessive bone formation, are often seen with prostate carcinoma.[13] Radiographic features associated with osseous metastases include poorly defined margins, endosteal scalloping, cortical destruction, and periosteal reaction. An extraosseous soft tissue component may occasionally be associated (**Fig. 1-7**).[14]

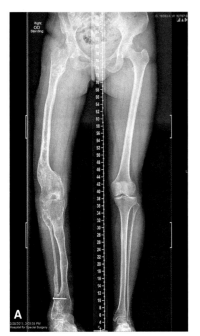
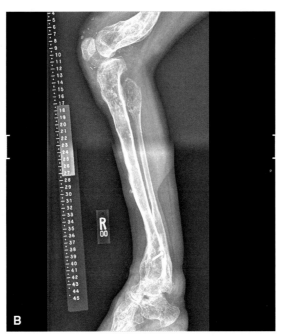
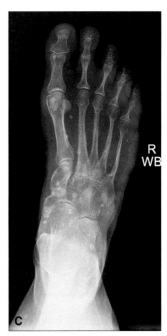

FIGURE 1-5. Radiographic manifestations of Maffucci syndrome in two separate patients. A: Standing anteroposterior (AP) examination of the lower extremities demonstrates numerous deforming enchondromas throughout the right lower extremity involving the tibia, fibula, femur, and the pelvis. Asymmetric distribution is common, with up to 50% of lesions being unilateral.[9] **B:** Lateral view of the right tibia and fibula demonstrates soft tissue calcifications representative of venous malformation anterior to the knee and tibia. **C:** AP of the foot demonstrates classic calcified venous malformations in the soft tissues and scalloping of the metatarsals. The enchondromas are less evident in the foot of this patient.

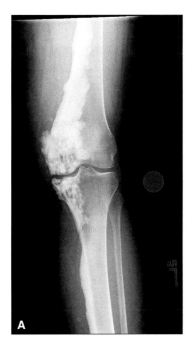
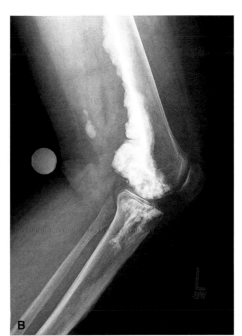
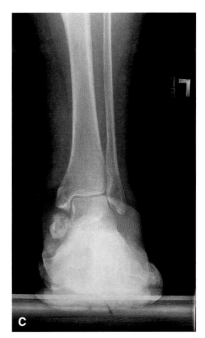

FIGURE 1-6. Radiographic and CT presentation of melorheostosis. AP **(A)** and lateral **(B)** X-rays of the left knee demonstrate the classic "dripping candle wax" appearance of melorheostosis with cortical hyperostosis along the posteromedial aspect of the distal femur and the medial cortex of the tibia. Small extraosseous soft tissue ossification in the posterior muscle is seen on the lateral radiograph. **C:** Frontal radiograph of the left ankle in the same patient demonstrates a large ossification in the soft tissues inferior to the medial malleolus, representing an uncommon extraosseous manifestation of melorheostosis. **D:** Coronal reformatted CT image of the left hip demonstrates a heterogeneous ossific mass contiguous with the lesser trochanter in this patient with melorheostosis.

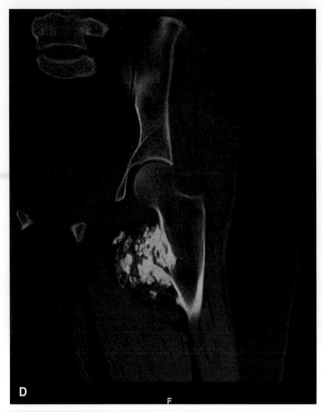

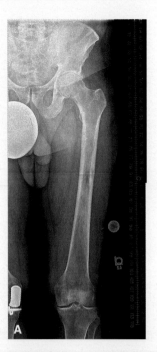

FIGURE 1-6. (*continued*)

MULTIPLE HEREDITARY EXOSTOSIS

Multiple hereditary exostosis (MHE), also known as familial osteochondromatosis or diaphyseal aclasis, is an autosomal dominant inherited disease presenting with multiple osteo-chondromas (exostoses).[15,16] Osteochondromas are classically sessile or pedunculated lesions with cortical and medullary continuity with the underlying bone, capped by cartilage.[15] Most patients are diagnosed by 5 years of age. The lesions commonly occur in the metaphysis of long bones with a predilection for the distal femur as well as the proximal and distal tibia and fibula. Larger osteochondromas can result in significant skeletal deformity.[15] The exostosis should cease growth when the closest physis is closed, and continued growth suggests malignant transformation (**Fig. 1-8**).

NAIL–PATELLA SYNDROME (FONG DISEASE)

Nail–Patella syndrome, also known as Fong disease, is a rare autosomal dominant condition classically characterized by a tetrad of nail, elbow, and pelvic and knee abnormalities.[17] Affected individuals have a distinct lean body habitus, and may also present with eye abnormalities and renal dysfunction.[17] Radiographs of the pelvis reveal bony processes arising from the posterior aspect of the iliac bones in more than 80% of

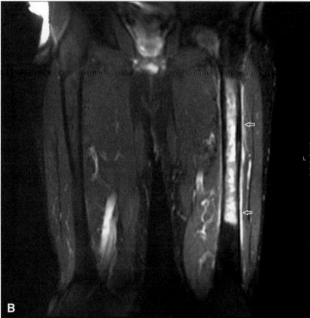

FIGURE 1-7. X-ray and MR findings of metastatic disease in the left femur and in the left foot. A: Frontal radiograph of the left femur demonstrates classic mottled bone marrow in left femur. **B:** Coronal inversion recovery image of both femora demonstrates diffuse infiltrative hyperintensity in the femoral head and in the medullary cavity of the left femoral diaphysis with surrounding periosteal reaction (*arrows*). **C:** Coronal T1-weighted image of both femora demonstrates diffuse low-signal-intensity marrow replacement throughout the left femoral diaphysis and femoral head. **D:** Axial inversion recovery image demonstrates diffuse hyperintense marrow replacement in the left femur with near circumferential periosteal reaction (*arrows*). **E to G:** MR demonstrates metastatic disease in the medial cuneiform. Coronal inversion recovery image **(E)** demonstrates diffuse infiltrative hyperintensity throughout the medial cuneiform. Axial **(F)** and sagittal **(G)** fast spin echo proton density-weighted images demonstrate a geographic hypointense marrow replacement process largely localized to the plantar aspect of the medial cuneiform.

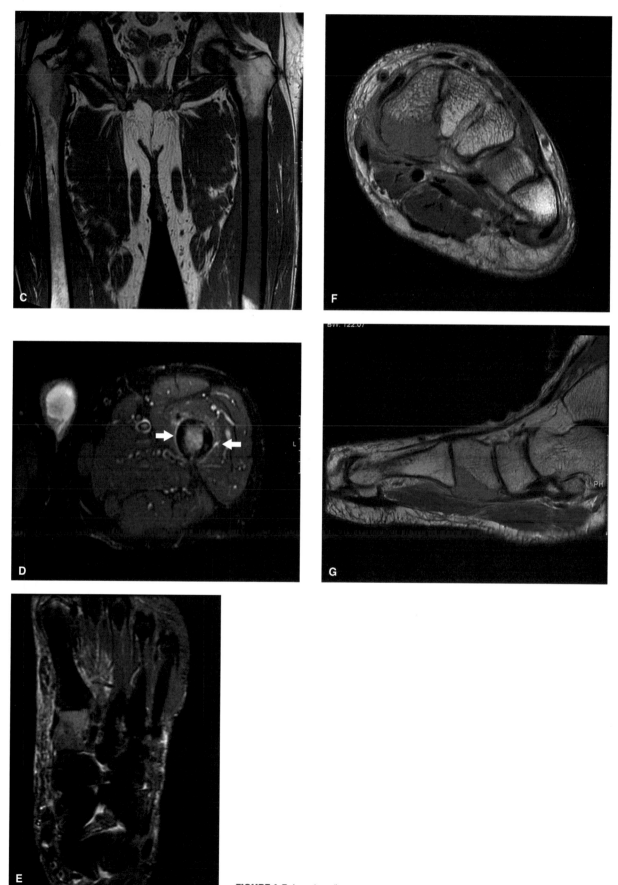

FIGURE 1-7. (*continued*)

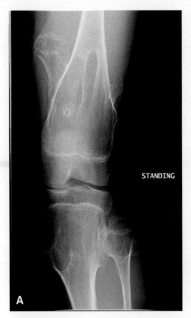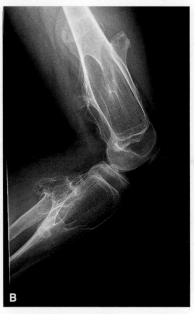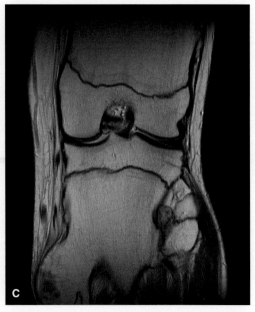

FIGURE 1-8. X-ray and MR demonstration of MHE. AP **(A)** and lateral **(B)** radiographs in this skeletally immature patient with MHE demonstrate both sessile and pedunculated exostosis of the distal femur and proximal tibia and fibula. The sessile-type lesions usually deform and expand the medullary metaphyseal regions of the involved bones. A large pedunculated exostosis extends superiorly from the medial cortex of the femur and terminates with a typical cauliflower-like tuft. **C:** MR coronal proton density-weighted image demonstrates multiple broad-based and pedunculated exostoses about the knee, with the largest localized medially, arising from the proximal tibial metaphysis. Note the continuity with the medullary cavity of the proximal tibia.

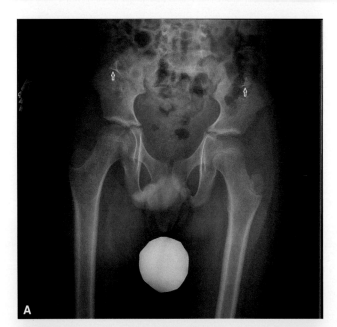

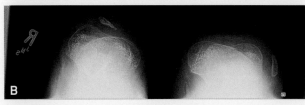

FIGURE 1-9. Radiographic presentation of Nail-Patella Syndrome. Frontal view of the pelvis **(A)** demonstrates the classic iliac horns (*arrows*) characteristic of Nail–Patella syndrome. Merchant view of the knees **(B)** demonstrates the bilateral hypoplastic patellae, shallow femoral sulci and dislocation of the left patella.

patients, which are known as "iliac horns".[18] These protuberances may be palpable and are characteristically bilateral. Knee and elbow involvement can be asymmetric. Radiographs of the knee may reveal dysplasia, hypoplasia, or absence of the patella, often with superolateral displacement.[17] Elbow radiographs may demonstrate hypoplasia or absence of the radial head with or without radial head dislocation, as well as epicondylar and capitellar abnormalities (**Fig. 1-9**).[17]

NEUROFIBROMATOSIS TYPE 1

Neurofibromatosis type 1 (NF1), also known as von Recklinghausen disease, is an autosomal dominant neuroectodermal disorder that is characterized by the formation of neurofibromas and mesodermal dysplasias affecting numerous organs, with skeletal involvement in up to 50% of patients.[19,20] The lower extremity manifestations of dysplasia usually result in tibia and/or fibula bowing, which presents within the first year of life in these patients and often is evident before the other signs of NF1.[19,20] The bowing commonly results in fractures and pseudarthrosis (**Fig. 1-10**).[19,20]

NEUROPATHIC (CHARCOT) FOOT

Neuropathic foot, also known as Charcot foot, is an osteoarthropathy caused by a variety of conditions, the most common being diabetes.[21] The neuropathic foot can be separated into both acute and chronic phases. In the acute phase, the disease can present with clinical manifestations of warmth, swelling, and erythema that can mimic osteomyelitis.[22] X-ray

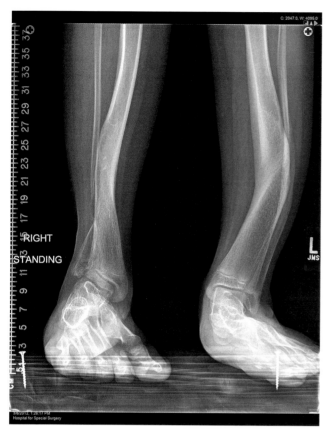

FIGURE 1-10. Radiographic presentation of Neurofibromatosis. Standing AP radiograph of both tibias and fibulas in this patient with NF1 demonstrates severe bowing. There is secondary deformity of the ankle joints, right greater than left, where there is marked medial slanting of the tibial plafond and ankle joint.

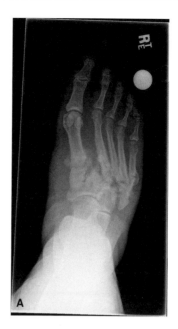

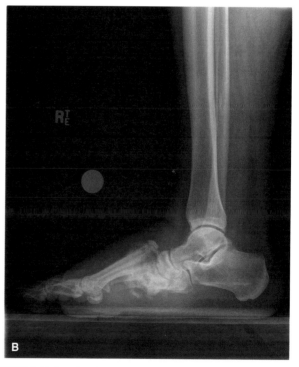

changes may be subtle, with the earliest finding being focal demineralization and flattening of the metatarsal heads.[23] In the early stages, MRI examination may demonstrate bone marrow edema, joint effusions, fluid collections, and marrow enhancement, which mimics osteomyelitis, complicating the accurate diagnosis.[22]

In the chronic phase, neuropathic joint involvement assumes a more specific and identifiable pattern, with classic findings commonly classified by the "6Ds": dense bones (absence of osteopenia), degeneration, destruction of cartilage, deformity, debris (loose bodies), and dislocation. In the foot, the midfoot and invariably the tarsometatarsal (Lisfranc) joints are most typically affected, which can lead to collapse of the longitudinal arch.[21,23] A common term for a Charcot joint is "a bag of bones" (**Fig. 1-11**).

OLLIER DISEASE (MULTIPLE ENCHONDROMAS)

Ollier disease is a benign rare nonhereditary chondroid dysplasia involving multiple asymmetrically distributed enchondromas.[24] Enchondromas usually involve the small bones of the hands and feet or occur centrally within the

FIGURE 1-11. Imaging demonstration of neuropathic (Charcot) foot on radiographs and of the ankle on radiograph, CT, and MR. AP **(A)**, lateral **(B)**, and oblique **(C)** X-ray views of the right foot demonstrate extensive Charcot-type arthropathic changes at the tarsometatarsal joints with bone destruction, fractures, fragmentation, and dislocations. Owing to sensory deficiencies associated with the underlying diabetic neuropathy, pain is not always present, so the patient keeps ambulating, hence the lack of osteopenia or dense bones. X-ray **(D)**, CT **(E)**, and MR **(F)** findings in a neuropathic ankle. **D:** Lateral X-ray demonstrates fragmentation and collapse of the talus and distal tibia. There is a healing fracture of the distal fibula. **E:** Sagittal reformatted CT image of the ankle demonstrates marked destructive arthropathy with multifocal articular surface loss and subchondral cysts. **F:** Sagittal fast spin echo proton density–weighted MR image demonstrates a marked multifocal destructive arthropathy throughout the articulations of the midfoot and hindfoot with collapse and fragmentation of the talus and disorganization of the ankle joint.

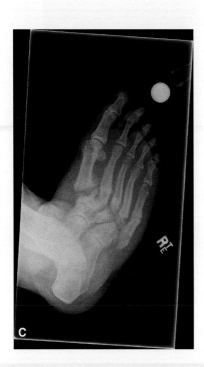

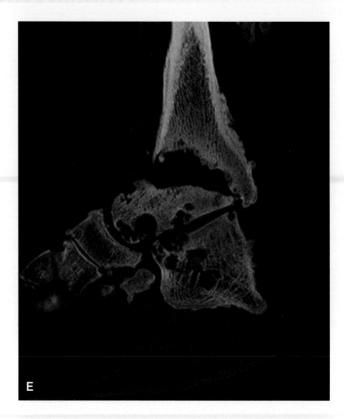

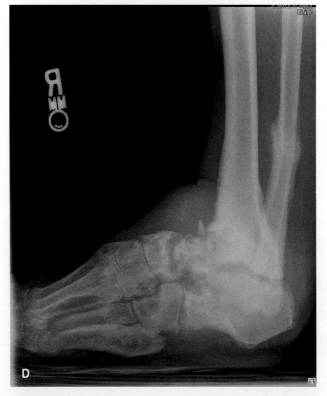

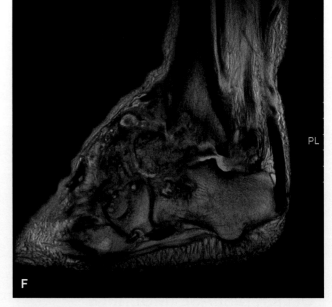

FIGURE 1-11. (*continued*)

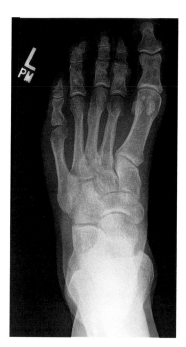

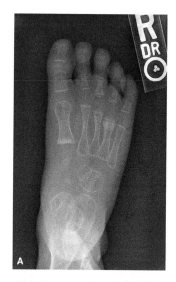

FIGURE 1-12. Radiographic presentation of multiple Enchondromas. AP radiograph of the left foot demonstrates multiple intramedullary, expansive, osteolytic lesions within the metatarsals and phalanges, most evident in the 2nd to 4th proximal phalanges. A more eccentric lesion is seen along the lateral distal cortex of the 3rd metatarsal. The 2nd and 5th metatarsals are short secondary to growth disturbance from the enchondromas.

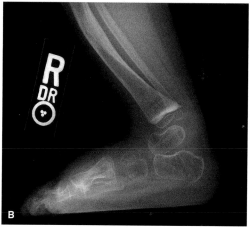

metadiaphysis of tubular bones.[10,24] They are benign cartilaginous lesions that are typically osteolytic with chondroid matrix calcifications. Although enchondromas are considered benign, patients with Ollier disease are at a 5% to 50% risk for malignant transformation of the enchondroma to chondrosarcoma (Fig. 1-12).[24]

OSTEOGENESIS IMPERFECTA

Osteogenesis imperfecta (OI) is a congenital, non–sex-linked hereditary disorder of the connective tissue. The disease is commonly separated into four distinct subtypes (I to IV) based on severity and clinical findings, with type II resulting in perinatal demise.[25] The usual musculoskeletal presentation is frequent fractures from excessive bone malleability secondary to the inherent lack or abnormality of type 1 collagen.[26] The radiographic features include osteopenia, multiple fractures, and bony deformities including gracile bones and bowing.[26] The fractures most commonly occur in the diaphysis of long bones and the spine.[26] The mainstay of treatment is with bisphosphonates, which can result in dense metaphyseal bands (Fig. 1-13).[26]

OSTEOPETROSIS

Osteopetrosis (Albers-Schönberg disease) is a rare hereditary disorder in which there is a genetic defect of osteoclast function.[27] There are both autosomal dominant (adult type)

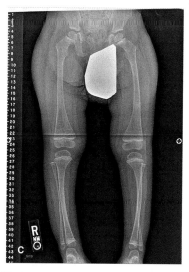

FIGURE 1-13. Two examples of OI in different patients. A: Lateral view of the ankle demonstrates anterior bowing of tibia and a healing fracture in the posterior tibial cortex. **B:** AP radiograph of the lower extremities in this 3-year-old child with OI demonstrates diffuse osteopenia, gracile bones, bowing deformities, and multiple healing fractures of the mid- to distal diaphysis of the left femur and the midshaft of the right fibula. Note the dense metaphyseal bands at the distal tibia and at the proximal and distal tibia compatible with bisphosphonate treatment. **C:** Frontal view of the foot demonstrates severe osteopenia and healing fracture of the distal 4th metatarsal.

and autosomal recessive (infantile type) forms of the disease, with the latter often resulting in intrauterine or early demise.[28] The typical radiographic appearance is that of dense medullary cavity sclerosis that is classically described to have a "bone within bone appearance." Other typical findings are Erlenmeyer flask deformities of tubular bones and "sandwich vertebra," where there is dense sclerosis of the endplates. Many patients are completely asymptomatic, with a minority presenting with anemia and pathologic fractures owing to the fragile nature of the abnormal bone (**Fig. 1-14**).[28]

PAGET DISEASE

Paget disease (osteitis deformans) is a common bone disorder characterized by disorganized bone turnover and remodeling resulting from osteoclast overactivity.[29,30] The disease affects up to 5% of the Caucasian population over 50, and can increase in up to 10% of the population over the age of 70.[30] The etiology of the disease remains unknown, with some postulating a viral origin.[30] Although the majority of patients are asymptomatic, some present with pain, tenderness, and

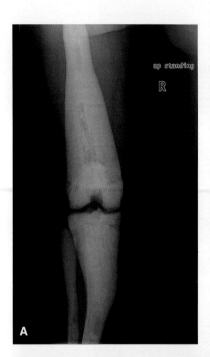
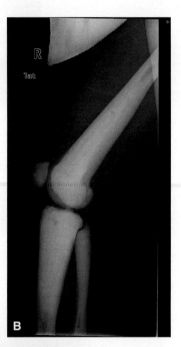
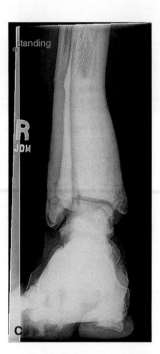
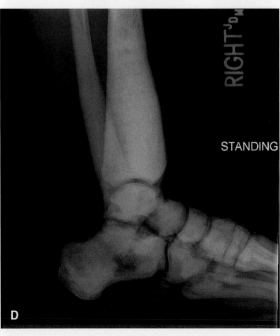

FIGURE 1-14. Radiographic presentation of Osteopetrosis. AP **(A)** and lateral **(B)** radiographs of the right knee and ankle **(C and D)** in this adult with autosomal dominant osteopetrosis demonstrate dense "bone within bone" sclerosis of the femur, tibia, and fibula with Erlenmeyer flask deformity of the ends of the bones. The metadiaphyseal bowing of the distal tibia is likely attributable to fracture remodeling.

deformity.[29] Paget disease classically is described as having three phases: lytic, mixed, and late. The disease often presents with polyostotic osseous involvement and with different phases presenting in the same patient.[29] The overall, almost pathognomonic finding is that of disorganized, thickened trabeculae, cortical thickening, and bony enlargement.[29] Paget disease is commonly seen in the pelvis and long bones of the lower extremity (**Fig. 1-15**).

PSORIATIC ARTHRITIS

Psoriatic arthritis is an inflammatory arthritis in patients with skin lesions of psoriasis, classified as a seronegative spondyloarthropathy owing to the lack of serum rheumatoid factor. Approximately 10% to 15% of patients with skin manifestation of psoriasis will develop psoriatic arthritis.[31] The disease most commonly involves the hands, with the feet being the second most common site. In the feet, similar to the hands, the findings may be bilateral or unilateral, symmetric or asymmetric.[32] Classically, the inflammation results in swelling of an entire digit, resulting in the classic findings of "sausage digit." Although the disease predominates in the interphalangeal joints, it can also affect the metacarpophalangeal joints, presenting with joint erosion, articular surface irregularity, and, in later stages, bony ankylosis.[32] The radiographic findings include periostitis, articular marginal bone erosion ("pencil-in-cup" deformities), bony proliferation, and in rare cases dense sclerosis of the distal phalanx that can affect the great toe, a condition termed "ivory phalanx" (**Fig. 1-16**).[31,32]

RHEUMATOID ARTHRITIS

Rheumatoid arthritis (RA) is a systemic inflammatory disease of unknown origin that predominantly affects joint synovial tissues.[33] RA is two to three times more common in women, and onset generally peaks in the fourth and fifth decades. Clinically, patients may present early with fatigue and generalized aches, with arthritis then developing in the proximal joints of hands and wrists. Involvement in the feet may occur, concurrently. Bilateral symmetric marginal erosions, joint space loss, juxta-articular osteopenia, and soft tissue swelling around the

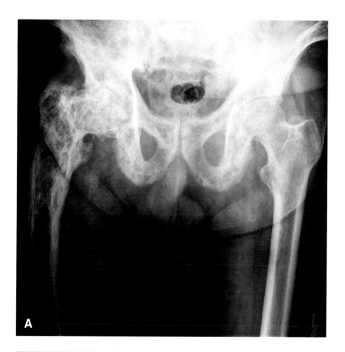

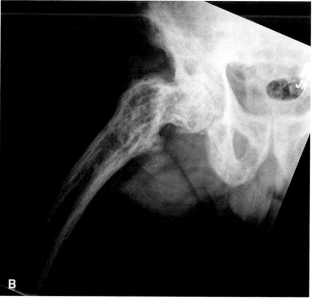

FIGURE 1-15. Radiographic presentation Paget's. AP radiograph of the pelvis (**A**) and frog leg lateral view of the right femur (**B**) demonstrate diffuse involvement of the pelvis and right femur with Paget disease. There is bilateral thickening of the iliopectineal and ischiopubic lines, diffuse trabecular thickening in the affected areas, most apparent in the proximal right femur, where there is a classic coxa vara deformity and diaphyseal bowing.

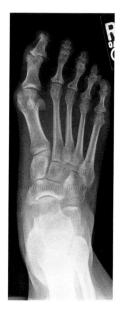

FIGURE 1-16. Radiographic presentation Psoriasis. AP radiograph of the right foot in this patient with a history of psoriasis demonstrates erosions of the bases of proximal phalanges of 2nd to 4th digits, and of the interphalangeal joints of all digits, consistent with an inflammatory arthritis such as psoriatic arthritis.

joints are the most common radiographic hallmarks of RA.[33,32] In the feet, as in the hands, there is a predilection for proximal joint involvement (e.g., proximal interphalangeal [PIP] and MTP joints), commonly at the 4th and 5th MTP joints.[33,32] The lateral margin of the 5th metatarsal head is often the 1st site of a bone erosion in the foot and may occur before hand or wrist involvement.[32] Inflammatory retrocalcaneal bursitis with adjacent calcaneal erosions can also occur in the early stages of the disease (**Fig. 1-17**).

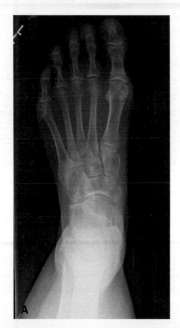

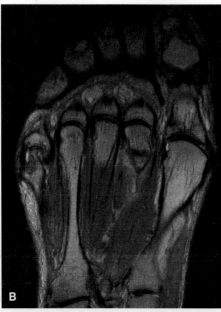

FIGURE 1-17. X-ray and MR demonstration of RA. A: Frontal radiograph of the left foot in a patient with RA demonstrates periarticular osteoporosis and the classic erosions of the metatarsal head of the 5th digit and bony destruction of the proximal articular surface of the proximal phalanx of the 5th digit, representative of RA. **B:** Coronal fast spin echo MR images of the left forefoot demonstrate uniform cartilage wear in the 5th MTP joint with characteristic erosions at the head of the 5th metatarsal and subchondral cysts.

RICKETS

Rickets is a disorder of childhood characterized by decreased physeal mineralization and delayed endochondral ossification, resulting in disordered growth at the growth plates.[34] Although many conditions can cause rickets, nutritional rickets accounts for the majority of cases and arises from vitamin D deficiency.[34] Rickets may not be radiographically evident early in the disease course, or may be associated with only subtle diffuse demineralization of the osseous structures.[35] Classic rachitic findings appear later in the course of the disease and are most evident in rapidly growing bones.[35] In the lower extremity, the distal femur and proximal and distal tibia are most affected.[35] Findings include bowing of the long bones, commonly resulting in genu varus, metaphyseal flaring and cupping, and physeal widening.[35] The edges of the metaphyses may appear frayed.[35] Insufficiency fractures can occur in mobile children with radiographically evident rickets (**Fig. 1-18**).[36]

SARCOIDOSIS

Sarcoidosis is a systemic inflammatory disorder of unknown etiology characterized by noncaseating granuloma formation. Although sarcoidosis most commonly manifests with thoracic involvement, any organ system can be affected, and skeletal involvement is reported in 5% to 10% of patients.[37] Skeletal involvement is variable and often asymptomatic.[38] When symptomatic, patients most frequently present with inflammatory arthralgia.[37] Sarcoidosis can affect long and small bones throughout the body, with the phalanges of the hands and feet most commonly involved, usually in a bilateral distribution.[38] Radiographs of the affected joints are often unremarkable.[37] X-ray findings are a lacelike pattern of osteolysis, classically seen in the digits of the

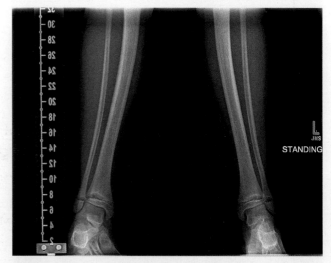

FIGURE 1-18. Radiographic presentation Rickets. Frontal view of the ankles demonstrates symmetric widening of the tibial and fibular physis with irregular fraying of the physeal margins.

hand,[37,38] and with similar manifestations when the foot is involved. Radiolucent cystic lesions and osteoporosis may also occur.[37,39] Pathologic fractures can occur in regions of extensive cortical destruction.[38] When arthralgia, erythema nodosum, and mediastinal lymphadenopathy are present together, they form the triad known as Löfgren syndrome, a manifestation of sarcoidosis that generally resolves spontaneously **(Fig. 1-19)**.[38]

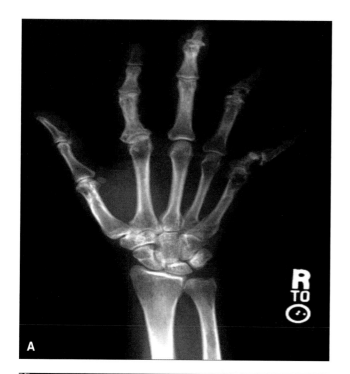

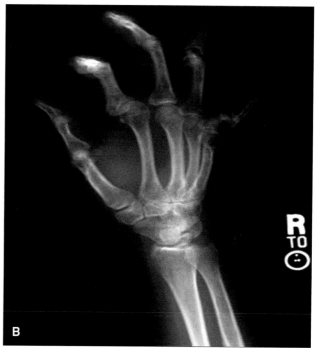

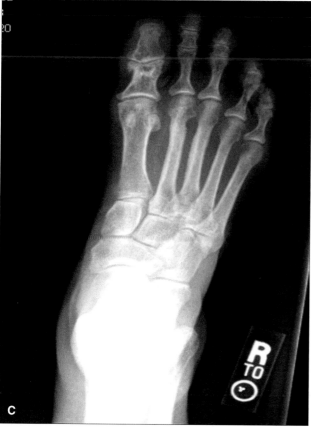

FIGURE 1-19. Radiographic presentation Sarcoid. AP **(A)** and oblique **(B)** radiographs of the right hand and right foot **(C)** demonstrate lacelike lesions in the phalanges, metacarpals, and metatarsals with bony destruction, cortical scalloping, joint destruction, and dislocation.

REFERENCES

Fibrous Dysplasia

1. DiCaprio MR, Enneking WF. Fibrous dysplasia. Pathophysiology, evaluation, and treatment. *J Bone Joint Surg Am.* 2005;87(8):1848–1864.
2. Fitzpatrick KA, Taljanovic MS, Speer DP, et al. Imaging findings of fibrous dysplasia with histopathologic and intraoperative correlation. *Am J Roentgenol.* 2004;182(6):1389–1398.

Gout

3. Girish G, Glazebrook KN, Jacobson JA. Advanced imaging in gout. *Am J Roentgenol.* 2013;201(3):515–525.
4. Dalbeth N, McQueen FM. Use of imaging to evaluate gout and other crystal deposition disorders. *Curr Opin Rheumatol.* 2009;21(2):124–131.

Hypertrophic Pulmonary Osteoarthropathy

5. Rana RS, Wu JS, Eisenberg RL. Periosteal reaction. *Am J Roentgenol.* 2009;193(4):W259–W272.
6. Capelastegui A, Astigarraga W, García-Iturraspe C. MR findings in pulmonary hypertrophic osteoarthropathy: case reports. *Clin Radiol.* 2000;55(1):72–75.

Infarct and Osteonecrosis

7. Murphey MD, Foreman KL, Klassen-Fische MK, et al. From the radiologic pathology archives imaging of osteonecrosis: radiologic-pathologic correlation. *Radiographics.* 2014;34(4):1003–1028.
8. Pearce DH, Mongiardi CN, Fornaiser VL, et al. Avascular necrosis of the talus: a pictorial essay. *Radiographics.* 2005;25(2):399–410.

Maffucci Syndrome

9. Zwenneke FH, Ginai AZ, Wolter OJ. Best cases from the AFIP. Maffucci syndrome: radiologic and pathologic findings. Armed Forces Institutes of Pathology. *Radiographics.* 2001;21(5):1311–1316.
10. An YY, Kim JY, Ahn MI, et-al. Enchondroma protuberans of the hand. *Am J Roentgenol.* 2008;190(1):40–44.

Melorheostosis

11. Bansal A. The dripping candle wax sign. *Radiology.* 2008;246(2):638–640.
12. Greenspan A, Azouz EM. Bone dysplasia series. Melorheostosis: review and update. *Can Assoc Radiol J.* 1999;50(5):324–330.

Metastatic Disease

13. Rubenstein J. Imaging of skeletal metastases. *Tech Orthop.* 2004;19(1):2–8.
14. Rybak LD, Rosenthal DI. Radiological imaging for the diagnosis of bone metastases. *Q J Nucl Med.* 2001;45(1):53–64.

Multiple Hereditary Exostosis

15. Murphey MD, Choi JJ, Kransforf MJ, et-al. Imaging of osteochondroma: variants and complications with radiologic-pathologic correlation. *Radiographics.* 2000;20(5):1407–1434.
16. Sandell LJ. Multiple hereditary exostosis, EXT Genes, and skeletal development. *J Bone Joint Surg Am.* 2009;91(suppl 4):58–62.

Nail–Patella Syndrome (Fong Disease)

17. Sweeney E, Fryer A, Mountford R, et al. Nail patella syndrome: a review of the phenotype aided by developmental biology. *J Med Genet.* 2003;40(3):153–162.
18. Karabulut N, Ariyurek M, Erol C, et al. Imaging of "iliac horns" in nail-patella syndrome. *J Comput Assist Tomogr.* 1996;20(4):530–531.

Neurofibromatosis Type I

19. Patel NB, Stacy GS. Musculoskeletal manifestations of neurofibromatosis type 1. *Am J Roentgenol.* 2012;199(1):W99–W106.
20. Van Meerbeeck SF, Verstraete KL, Janssens S, et al. Whole body MR imaging in neurofibromatosis type 1. *Eur J Radiol.* 2009;69(2):236–242.

Neuropathic (Charcot) Foot

21. Egren BF, Sanverdi ES, Oznur A. Charcot foot in diabetes and an update on imaging. *Diabet Foot Ankle.* 2013;4:21884. doi:10.3402/dfa.v4i0.21884.
22. Ahmadi ME, Morrison WB, Carrino JA, et al. Neuropathic arthropathy of the foot with and without superimposed osteomyelitis: MR imaging characteristics. *Radiology.* 2006;238(2):622–631.
23. Rogers LC, Bevilacqua NJ. Imaging of the Charcot foot. *Clin Podiatr Med Surg.* 2008;25(2):263–274.

Ollier Disease

24. Melamud K. Diagnostic imaging of being and malignant osseous tumors of the fingers. *Radiographics.* 2014;34(7):1954–1976.

Osteogenesis Imperfecta

25. Renaud A, Aucourt J, Weill J, et al. Radiographic features of osteogenesis imperfecta. *Insights Imaging.* 2013;4(4):417–429.
26. Burnei G, Vlad C, Georgescu I, et al. Osteogenesis imperfecta: diagnosis and treatment. *J Am Acad Orthop Surg.* 2008;16(6):356–366.

Osteopetrosis

27. Tolar J, Teitelbaum SL, Orchard PJ. Ostepetrosis. *N Engl J Med.* 2004;351:2839–2849.
28. Ihde LL, Forrester DM, Gottsegen CL, et al. Sclerosing bone dysplasias: review and differentiation from other causes of otosclerosis. *Radiographics.* 2011;31:1865–1882.

Paget Disease

29. Smith SE, Murphy MD, Motamedi K, et al. Radiologic spectrum of Paget disease of bone and its complications with pathologic correlation. *Radiographics.* 2002;22:1191–1216.
30. Whitehouse RW. Paget's disease of bone. *Semin Musculoskelet Radiol.* 2002;6(4):313–322.

Psoriatic Arthritis

31. Klecker RJ, Weissman BN. Imaging features of psoriatic arthritis and Reiter's syndrome. *Semin Musculoskelet Radiol.* 2003;7:115–126.
32. Jacobson JA, Girish G, Jiang Y, et al. Radiographic evaluation of arthritis: inflammatory conditions. *Radiology.* 2008;248(2):378–389.

Rheumatoid Arthritis

33. Sommer OJ, Kladosek A, Weiler V, et al. Rheumatoid arthritis: a practical guide to state-of-the-art imaging, image interpretation, and clinical implications. *Radiographics*. 2005;25(2):381–398.

Rickets

34. Shore RM, Chesney RW. Rickets: part I. *Pediatr Radiol*. 2013;43:140–151.
35. Shore RM, Chesney RW. Rickets: part II. *Pediatr Radiol*. 2013;43:152–172.

36. Chapman T, Sugar N, Done S, et al. Fractures in infants and toddlers with rickets. *Pediatr Radiol*. 2010;40:1184–1189.

Sarcoidosis

37. Koyama T, Ueda H, Togashi K, et al. Radiologic manifestations of sarcoidosis in various organs. *Radiographics*. 2004;24(1):87–104.
38. Vardhanabhuti V, Venkatanarasimha N, Bhatnagar G, et al. Extrapulmonary manifestations of sarcoidosis. *Clin Radiol*. 2012; 67:263–276.
39. Wilcox A, Bharadwaj P, Sharma OP. Bone sarcoidosis. *Curr Opin Rheumatol*. 2000;12:321–330.

CHAPTER 2

Seronegative and Seropositive Rheumatologic Disorders Affecting the Lower Extremity

STEPHEN J. DIMARTINO

Rheumatic diseases and other inflammatory disorders of the lower extremity are seen less commonly than mechanical conditions and local injuries. But because all inflammatory disorders may present in a similar fashion and because some have the potential to cause permanent damage without appropriate therapy, one must always be on the alert for their presence. Inflammatory disorders can be grouped into several categories: autoimmune, crystalline, and infectious (**Table 2-1**). In general, these conditions are systemic and, therefore, may involve the upper extremities and spine as well as organ systems outside of the musculoskeletal. Indeed, the pattern of joint involvement combined with associated symptoms (e.g., rash, oral ulcers, inflammation of the eye, interstitial lung disease) may be the most important clues to identify a systemic illness. Some systemic illnesses tend to favor the lower extremities such as gout, spondyloarthropathy, Lyme disease, and sarcoidosis (Lofgren syndrome), but they all will often involve other body regions. Therefore, it is important to always perform a careful history and physical examination when inflammatory disease is suspected.

SPECIAL CONSIDERATIONS IN THE APPROACH TO POTENTIAL INFLAMMATORY DISEASE

Urgent and Emergent Conditions

Failure to recognize certain conditions may lead to irreversible morbidity or mortality. These include septic monoarthritis, systemic sepsis, osteomyelitis, compartment syndrome, cellulitis, deep venous thrombosis (DVT), ischemia or infarction due to embolus, thrombosis or vasospasm, fracture, spinal cord compression, mononeuritis multiplex, and vasculitis (**Table 2-2**). The following features of the history and exam, though frequently nonspecific, can be helpful to direct one toward more urgent testing.[1,2]

Inability to Bear Weight

The inability to bear weight on a joint raises suspicion of fracture, a septic joint/prosthesis, or gout. Usually, a history of trauma will prompt workup for fracture; however, in patients

Table 2-1. List of Inflammatory Disorders of the Lower Extremity
Autoimmune
Rheumatoid arthritis
Spondyloarthropathy
Ankylosing spondylitis
Psoriatic arthritis
Reactive arthritis
Enteropathic arthritis (associated with inflammatory bowel disease)
SAPHO (*s*ynovitis, *a*cne, *p*ustulosis, *h*yperostosis, *o*steitis)
Sarcoidosis
Systemic lupus erythematosus
Inflammatory myopathy: especially antisynthetase syndrome
Crystalline
Gout (monosodium urate)
Pseudogout (calcium pyrophosphate)
Basic calcium phosphate deposition
Infectious
Lyme disease
Parvovirus
Gonococcus
Poststreptococcal reactive arthritis and rheumatic fever
Alfa viruses such as chikungunya
Tuberculosis (direct seeding of joints or reactive)
Fungal

with osteoporosis, fractures may occur with minimal trauma. Risk factors for osteoporosis include being postmenopausal, prior or current use of corticosteroids, smoking, low body mass, a personal history of fracture, a family history of hip fracture, inflammatory disease such as rheumatoid arthritis, excessive alcohol intake, and low vitamin D.[3] Furthermore, spontaneous fractures may occur in patients with an underlying tumor or, in rare instances, in patients taking bisphosphonates.[4]

Table 2-2. Urgent/Emergent Conditions

Septic monoarthritis
Systemic sepsis
Osteomyelitis
Compartment syndrome
Cellulitis
Deep venous thrombosis
Ischemia/infarction due to thrombus
Raynaud phenomenon associated with gangrene
Fracture
Spinal cord compression
Mononeuritis multiplex
Vasculitis

Erythema

Erythema of a joint is rarely seen in patients with systemic inflammatory disorders such as rheumatoid arthritis or spondyloarthropathy. The presence of erythema raises suspicion for a septic joint, gout, or cellulitis. When a cellulitis lies over a joint, it can be a challenge to distinguish it from gout or septic arthritis because it may also limit range of motion of the joint owing to pain caused by stretching of the skin and subcutaneous tissues. An obvious portal of entry or an off-center distribution of erythema (relative to the joint space) can be helpful clues to cellulitis, if present. Although gout is often thought of as a condition isolated to joints, tenosynovium and subcutaneous tissue are commonly involved, and when this occurs it can also cause an off-center distribution of erythema on the joint. Point-of-care musculoskeletal ultrasound (MSKUS) can be valuable in these situations, as it will show edema in the subcutaneous fat in the case of cellulitis or can show joint/tendon involvement in the cases of gout or septic arthritis.

Constitutional Symptoms

Although many systemic autoimmune conditions and even crystalline arthropathy can present with constitutional symptoms, the presence of fever, malaise, weight loss, and/or an elevated leukocyte count should prompt the clinician to rule out infection. Blood cultures, synovial fluid cultures, and culture of other distant symptomatic sites are necessary. Patients with known underlying conditions that can cause fever such as systemic lupus erythematosus (SLE) or systemic vasculitis often take immunosuppressive drugs, increasing the risk of infection. Therefore, when these patients present with a fever, it is difficult to discern whether there is a flare of disease, an infection, or both. Also, it is important to note that corticosteroids will often cause an elevation in the WBC count, confounding a situation where infection needs to be ruled out. Moreover, patients who are on corticosteroids, especially doses greater than 30 mg of prednisone daily (or the

equivalent), may not mount a fever even when septic, or they may have reduced symptoms in the setting of an infection. In a patient taking high doses of corticosteroids, any infection has likely been present longer than one might suspect based on their symptoms; therefore, one must have a low threshold to initiate antibiotic therapy as soon as is possible.

Neurologic Symptoms

Weakness, numbness, paresthesia, and a burning quality of pain can all be clues to neurologic involvement such as radiculopathy, myelopathy, compartment syndrome, or mononeuritis multiplex/vasculitis. It is important to keep in mind that pain in a joint will often result in weakness, making assessment of strength challenging. Furthermore, inflammation in a region in which a peripheral nerve passes through (such as the tarsal tunnel or volar wrist) can lead to compression of the nerve and resultant paresthesia or numbness.

Diffuse Edema

Diffuse edema, especially when unilateral, may raise suspicion for the presence of a DVT. The typical presentation of a DVT is that of pain, swelling, and erythema on the lower extremity; however, all of these symptoms need not be present, and there are many other conditions such as venous insufficiency, popliteal cysts, cellulitis, and muscle injury that may present in a similar fashion. Furthermore, arthritis or periarthritis of the ankle, which may be seen in any type of systemic inflammatory arthritis, may present this way. Risk factors for DVT include states that promote hypercoagulability such as recent surgery or injury, pregnancy, malignancy, genetic hypercoagulable states such as Factor V Leiden, and autoimmune conditions such as the antiphospholipid antibody symptoms and granulomatous angiitis.[5] A personal or family history of DVT is also a risk factor. Diagnosis can be made with ultrasound of the lower extremity; the location of the clot often does not correlate with the location of symptoms. Treatment of DVT with anticoagulation is critical to reduce the risk of pulmonary embolus.

Articular versus Periarticular Disorders

Patients who present with a complaint of joint pain often find it difficult to distinguish between a true articular problem and a periarticular disorder. In general, an articular disorder will be associated with pain throughout the range of motion of the joint involved, whereas a periarticular disorder (e.g., tendonitis, bursitis) will be associated with pain through only a segment of the full range of motion. Well-localized tenderness over a tendon or bursa further supports the conclusion of a periarticular disorder. It is not only possible, but rather common for both processes to occur simultaneously during an inflammatory illness. Therefore, the presence of periarticular pain does exclude the existence of a systemic inflammatory disorder. For example, rheumatoid arthritis frequently affects tendons in addition to joints[6] and may in fact be common in early presentation of the disease. In gout, uric acid crystals may not only deposit in joints and tendons but also disperse to surrounding soft tissue. In spondyloarthropathy, the major target of the autoimmune attack is the enthesis: the attachment of tendons and ligaments to bone.[7] Therefore, patients will often present with both clear synovitis manifested by tenderness and swelling of a joint with pain throughout the range of motion and also localized tenderness over a nearby tendon such as the Achilles, quadriceps, or patellar tendons.

Monoarticular Arthritis versus Oligo-/Polyarticular Arthritis

Septic arthritis, traumatic arthritis, and crystalline arthritis (i.e., gout, pseudogout) are the main entities to consider when a patient presents with monoarticular joint pain. However, it is important to keep in mind that gout and pseudogout can involve more joints in a significant proportion of patients, and can even present, albeit rarely, as a symmetric polyarthritis of the small joints of the hands and feet, mimicking rheumatoid arthritis. Furthermore, any typically polyarticular process such as rheumatoid arthritis and spondyloarthropathy can present as monoarticular disease, especially early in the disease course and especially with onset in the elderly. After working up a monoarticular arthritis for infection, injury, and crystalline disease, it is important to give consideration to systemic inflammatory disease. The failure to recognize a systemic condition that has manifested atypically as a monoarticular arthritis may result in multiple unnecessary procedures, including surgery. Increasingly, MSKUS has been found to be useful in distinguishing between mono- and oligo-/polyarticular disorders and articular versus periarticular disorders.

Use of Ultrasound in Rheumatology

Over the last 10 to 15 years, MSKUS has become an established technique for evaluation and follow-up of patients with rheumatic diseases. Technologic advances, including faster computers and probes that can see greater detail, allow even today's low-budget machines to detect tiny fluid collections within joints, resolve small defects in bone and cartilage, and provide color maps of the joint, indicating where inflammation is taking place. The advantages of ultrasound over other imaging modalities include the following: portability due to the small size of the machines, noninvasiveness, lack of radiation (allowing for frequent repeat imaging), relative inexpensiveness, the ability to scan multiple joints in a brief period, and the ability to look at the joint while it is in motion (i.e., dynamic imaging). These features make ultrasound particularly well suited not only for the diagnosis of rheumatic disease but also for monitoring the progress of therapy. Therefore, a rheumatologist with a clinical understanding of the patient's problem can scan and interpret images at the bedside, rather than sending the patient for a second appointment. Treatment decisions can be made immediately, thereby greatly improving the efficiency of medical care. Finally, ultrasound at the bedside

has tremendous educational value for the patient as they struggle to understand their own disease process. With only brief explanations, the patients can see real-time images of the inflammatory process damaging their joint, making a concrete notion of what was previously only abstract. This is of great utility to the practitioner when discussing the reasons for medical therapy, which are often immunosuppressive or chemotherapeutic drugs with numerous toxicities.

Indeed, a large body of literature supports the above assertions. For example, studies examining the utility of ultrasound in the rheumatology clinic have shown that ultrasound is more accurate than clinical examination at detecting joint fluid and inflammation.[8,9] In a study of 100 consecutive patients, Karim et al.[10] have shown that use of ultrasound in a busy outpatient rheumatology clinic changed the management plan that was made prior to the performance of ultrasound 56% of the time and that overall diagnosis was changed 5% of the time. Several studies[11–13] have shown that, in rheumatoid arthritis, baseline power Doppler signal is a strong predictor of joint damage 1 year later.

For several types of inflammatory arthritis, studies have examined the role of performing ultrasound in rheumatic disease patients with the following aims: clarifying the differential diagnosis in early, undifferentiated rheumatic disease, defining the number of joints inflamed and/or damaged, monitoring the success of therapy in established disease, guidance of joint aspirations and injections. Indeed, there have been a growing number of rheumatologists using point-of-care ultrasound to enhance patient care in recent years.[14]

WHEN AND WHY TO REFER A PATIENT WITH SUSPECTED INFLAMMATORY ARTHRITIS

In the past several decades, studies in cohorts of patients with early inflammatory arthritis (not fulfilling the American College of Rheumatology criteria of rheumatoid arthritis at onset) have shown that while many of these patients have a self-limited illness, a significant proportion of these patients go on to develop rheumatoid arthritis (RA).[15,16] Several observations have led to the conclusion that RA patients should be identified early and treated aggressively. Machold and colleagues[15] have shown in a study of patients with inflammatory joint disease of less than 3 months' duration that 61.1% of patients went on to develop rheumatoid arthritis, 12.8% had erosions on their first X-rays, and 27.6% had erosions by their first year. This highlights the fact that permanent joint damage can begin very early in the disease process. In addition, many patients with RA are forced to leave work within 5 to 10 years of disease onset, and life spans of RA patients are significantly shortened. The persistent inflammatory burden associated with RA can lead to premature atherosclerosis and death due to cardiac events. Data such as these have led investigators to compare treatment strategies in patients with early inflammatory arthritis.

There is now clear evidence that patients who have early rheumatoid arthritis have significantly better outcomes when they are treated within the first few weeks to months of their illness. For example, Lard and colleagues[17] have shown (utilizing medications that are now considered relatively weak disease-modifying antirheumatic drugs (DMARDs)) that treatment initiated within a few weeks of symptom onset resulted in less radiographic damage (as measured by Sharp score) and less overall disease activity (as measured by the disease activity score).

Furthermore, over the last 15 years, the introduction of biologic medications, especially those that block tumor necrosis factor α (TNF-α), has revolutionized the practice of rheumatology, allowing for greater control of the inflammation of RA than was previously possible. The TNF-α blockers, which include etanercept, infliximab, adalimumab, golimumab, and certolizumab pegol, not only greatly reduce disease activity but also can slow the progression of joint destruction. Because early treatment results in better outcomes and because we now have very effective agents for doing so, early inflammatory arthritis should be treated with a sense of urgency. While RA is the classic inflammatory arthritis, there are many other conditions that are virtually indistinguishable from RA early in their course, some of which can be equally destructive, but may require different or additional therapies. These diseases include (but are certainly not limited to) the following: SLE, psoriatic arthritis (PsA), ankylosing spondylitis, systemic sclerosis, relapsing polychondritis, inflammatory myositis, granulomatous angiitis, adult-onset Still disease, polymyalgia rheumatica, and giant cell arteritis.

Emery and colleagues[18] suggest the following guidelines for referral of a patient with arthritis and any of the following to a rheumatologist: (a) ≥3 swollen joints; (b) a positive "squeeze test" (transverse compression of the metatarsophalangeal (MTP) or metacarpophalangeal (MCP) joints); (c) morning stiffness lasting greater than 30 minutes; (d) elevated acute-phase reactants including erythrocyte sedimentation rate (ESR) or C-reactive protein (CRP); (e) positive serologies including rheumatoid factor (RF) or anti-cyclic citrullinated protein (anti-CCP); (f) joint symptoms lasting greater than 6 weeks.

COMMONLY OBSERVED RHEUMATIC DISEASES OF THE LOWER EXTREMITY

Rheumatoid Arthritis

Rheumatoid arthritis is a systemic inflammatory disease affecting approximately 1% of the population. It is primarily characterized by an immune-mediated attack on the joints; indeed, tissue taken from the joints of RA patients shows that leukocytes have migrated from the blood to the synovial tissue and synovial space. Although joints and tendons are the primary site of inflammation, other organs such as the eye, lungs, skin, and blood vessels can also be affected. Peak incidence is between 25 and 50 years of age, but any age can

be affected. The condition affects women more than men at a ratio of approximately 3:1.

Rheumatoid arthritis is a disease of unknown cause; however, both genetic and environmental influences have been suggested. In the case of monozygotic twins, where one of the twin pair has rheumatoid arthritis, the incidence of the second twin developing rheumatoid arthritis is 15% to 30%. Because the incidence of RA in the general population is only 1%, this suggests a strong genetic influence on disease; however, the incidence of the second twin developing RA is not 100%, suggesting an environmental component as well. In addition, there is a genetic association with an allele of the major histocompatibility complex (MHC) class II receptor, HLA-DR4. Suggestions of environmental influences include an association with periodontal disease and the association of more aggressive disease in patients who have the anti-CCP antibody and who concomitantly smoke.[19]

At the cellular level, the synovial lining of the joints of patients with rheumatoid arthritis becomes infiltrated with immune cells such as T lymphocytes, B lymphocytes, plasma cells, and macrophages (**Fig. 2-1**). Immune complexes and neutrophils are found within the synovial fluid. Furthermore, proinflammatory cytokines have been shown to be upregulated in the synovium of patients with rheumatoid arthritis, and these include TNF-α, interleukin-6 (IL-6), IL-1, and IL-17. The thickened synovial lining containing inflammatory cells and mediators is known as a pannus. The chronic, unregulated inflammatory response of the pannus has the ability to degrade both bone and cartilage, leading to the destructive arthropathy seen in rheumatoid arthritis. When bone and cartilage of the joint are destroyed, this can be visualized on X-ray, ultrasound, or MRI as an erosion (**Fig. 2-2**).

Many laboratory tests may be abnormal in patients with rheumatoid arthritis. The ESR and CRP are both nonspecific markers of inflammation that may be elevated but can also be normal; thus, their absence cannot be taken as the absence of disease. In addition, the patient may have an anemia of chronic disease that may improve as the disease is controlled. Synovial fluid aspirated from a clinically swollen or tender joint often will be inflammatory and contain numerous neutrophils, but will be negative for culture and crystals. RF and anti-CCP are autoantibodies that are highly associated with rheumatoid arthritis. RF recognizes the Fc region of immunoglobulin G, while anti-CCP antibodies recognize citrullinated proteins usually present within connective tissue. Patients may have one of these autoantibodies, both, or neither. Anti-CCP antibodies are present in 50% to 70% of patients with rheumatoid arthritis, but are only present in less than 2% of the population. In contrast, RF is much more widely seen in the general population, with a prevalence of about 10%. Interestingly, anti-CCP antibodies may appear years before the patient displays symptoms,[20] suggesting that the abnormality which is autoimmunity exists long before the patient can even sense the first symptom.

The classic clinical presentation of rheumatoid arthritis is a symmetric polyarthritis involving the small joints of the

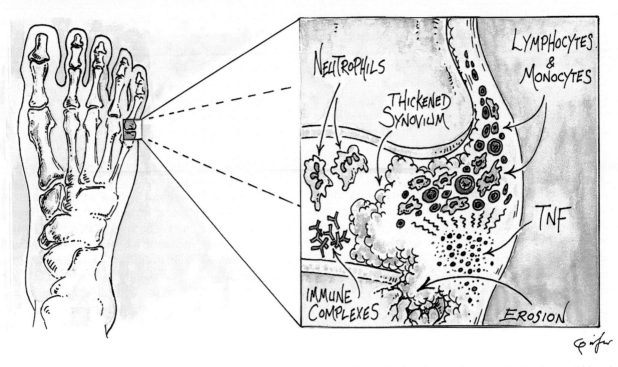

FIGURE 2-1. Rheumatoid arthritis. Lymphocytes and monocytes migrate into the rheumatoid synovium from the vasculature, causing it to become thickened. Neutrophils migrate into the synovial space, and immune complexes can be found here as well. The proinflammatory mediators produced by these cells, including cytokines such as TNF-α and degradative enzymes, can cause destruction of the bone and cartilage, which can be seen on imaging as an erosion.

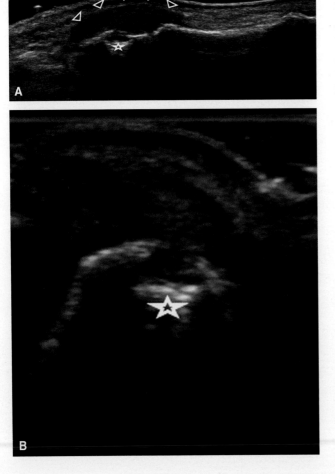

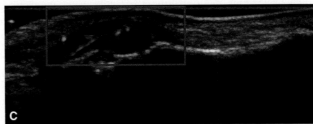

FIGURE 2-2. Typical ultrasound findings in rheumatoid arthritis. Gray scale (**A and B**) and power Doppler (**C**) images of the proximal interphalangeal joint of a patient with rheumatoid arthritis in longitudinal (**A and C**) and short axis views (**B**). The left side of the image is proximal in (**A and C**); medial in (**B**). A dark region emanating from the joint (**A**; *arrowheads*) indicates synovial thickening, and an erosion is also seen (*star*). The synovium demonstrates power Doppler signal (*red color*), indicating inflammation.

hands and feet, but about 25% of patients may have oligo- or monoarticular arthritis. The hands and feet will be involved in the vast majority of patients at some point in the disease course. When a patient presents with monoarticular arthritis, the knee will be involved approximately 50% of the time. Older patients have a tendency to present with a nonclassic presentation such as monoarticular arthritis or episodic disease. In the hands, the usual involved joints are the MCP joints and the proximal interphalangeal joints. In the feet, the MTP joints and intertarsal joints are most often affected; however, any joint of the foot can be involved. The cervical spine may also be affected in severe cases and may present as weakness of the legs due to atlantoaxial subluxation or basilar invagination, causing impingement on the cervical spinal cord. These patients may not present with neck pain but rather weakness (such as difficulty arising from a chair or ascending steps) or difficulty with ambulating. Therefore, in rheumatoid arthritis patients scheduled to undergo general anesthesia, it is reasonable to first obtain lateral view X-rays of the cervical spine in both flexion and extension to assess for instability of the second cervical vertebrae relative to the first cervical vertebrae. Rheumatoid arthritis, if untreated, has a high likelihood of causing joint damage or destruction. Many patients, if untreated, will accumulate disability within the first 1 to 3 years of disease onset. It has become clear over the last decade that early aggressive therapy is important for the prevention of long-term joint destruction and patient disability.

Because it is a systemic disease, rheumatoid arthritis can affect other organs in addition to the joints. Systemic disease manifestations are seen less frequently today because over the last decade and a half, improved therapies, which have been deliberately engineered to target different components of the inflammatory response, have revolutionized the treatment of rheumatoid arthritis. These improved therapies have made the extraarticular manifestations of rheumatoid arthritis rare. When present, many potential organ systems can be affected by the autoimmune process. Pulmonary involvement may include effusions, nodules, interstitial lung disease, and vasculitis. Cardiac involvement may include pericarditis or amyloidosis. The patient may develop rheumatoid nodules, which are usually found over the extensor surface of the forearm but can also be present in the lung. Eye involvement may take the form of either scleritis or uveitis. The presence of scleritis is an emergency because, if untreated, it can rapidly lead to melting of the sclera. Neurologic involvement may include an entrapment syndrome such as carpal tunnel syndrome or ulnar nerve entrapment, or mononeuritis multiplex: a vasculitis of the vasa nervorum in which the patient may present with a hand drop or foot drop. Of note, patients may also present with a drop of the fourth and fifth fingers not related to neurologic cause but rather secondary to rupture of the fourth and fifth extensor tendons on a jaggedly eroded ulnar styloid. Felty syndrome is a presentation of RA in which the patient has leukopenia, splenomegaly, and lower extremity ulcerations.

Patients with rheumatoid arthritis, similar to patients with other systemic inflammatory diseases such as SLE, have a higher incidence of atherosclerosis and coronary events, and this leads to earlier mortality in this population. When compared with age-matched controls, coronary artery disease occurs in patients with rheumatoid arthritis at younger ages. Furthermore, the control of rheumatoid arthritis with disease-modifying agents such as methotrexate leads to a decreased incidence of coronary artery disease, linking the inflammation caused by rheumatoid arthritis to the presence of atherosclerosis.[21] This suggests that the inflammatory burden of RA impacts on the vasculature in ways that promote atherosclerosis; therefore, lowering the inflammatory burden of the disease with medical therapy significantly reduces the burden of atherosclerosis as well.

The differential diagnosis for rheumatoid arthritis, especially early in the disease course, is quite broad because many inflammatory conditions can present in a similar fashion. Other conditions to consider include polymyalgia rheumatica, PsA and other spondyloarthropathies, crystalline arthropathy such as gout and pseudogout, SLE, Sjögren syndrome, systemic sclerosis, and sarcoidosis. Infections such as Lyme disease, parvovirus infection, and a poststreptococcal reactive arthritis can present similarly to rheumatoid arthritis as well.

X-ray findings that may be suggestive of inflammatory arthritis include soft tissue swelling, periarticular osteopenia, and joint space narrowing. The presence of erosions in characteristic locations such as the ulnar styloid and lateral 5th MTP joint can be a clue to the presence of rheumatoid arthritis. Ultrasound findings may include synovial hypertrophy, effusions, erosions, and power Doppler signal (**Fig. 2-2**). In early rheumatoid arthritis, power Doppler signal at baseline is predictive of damage at 1 year.[12] In addition, it is clear that many patients who are felt to be in clinical remission still have power Doppler signal on ultrasound, and this is associated with joint damage.[13]

Many years ago, standard of care for treatment of rheumatoid arthritis included the initiation of nonsteroidal anti-inflammatory drugs (NSAIDs). Since then, it has been shown that even though NSAIDs have the ability to reduce pain, the destructive process of RA is not altered: patients may have less joint pain but will continue to undergo joint destruction. Therefore, the treatment paradigm has shifted to early initiation of DMARDs and biologic agents. Early aggressive therapy with these drugs results in a slowing of disease progression in addition to reduction in daily pain and disability. Furthermore, there is a reduction in atherosclerosis, which leads to an improvement in mortality of patients. The general approach to treating patients with rheumatoid arthritis has recently been outlined, and guidelines were published in 2015.[22] The general treatment approach is to start with a DMARD as soon as possible once the diagnosis of rheumatoid arthritis is made. Adding a biologic agent or switching to a biologic agent is then considered if the patient does not have a great enough response to the DMARD. Combinations of two or three DMARDs and combinations of a DMARD and biologic are routinely employed.

DMARDs include the following agents: hydroxychloroquine, sulfasalazine, methotrexate, leflunomide, and cyclosporine. These are small molecules that work, in part, by suppressing the immune system by interfering with the activation and proliferation of the cells of the adaptive immune response. They are typically given by mouth, although methotrexate can be injected subcutaneously. They tend to work slowly, usually requiring 6 to 12 weeks before seeing a response. Patients must be monitored frequently with blood tests for hepatotoxicity and marrow suppression.

Biologic agents are molecules that have been engineered to specifically target molecules or cells that have been shown to play a crucial role in dysregulated inflammatory response that takes place in rheumatoid arthritis. One of the first biologic agents introduced includes the group of molecules that block TNF-α (infliximab, adalimumab, etanercept, golimumab, and certolizumab), a critical proinflammatory molecule found to be elevated in patients with rheumatoid arthritis. Abatacept is a molecule that blocks the costimulatory pathway between antigen-presenting cells and T lymphocytes. The purpose of this molecule is to prevent the propagation of an adaptive immune response by interfering with this signal. Rituximab is a chimeric monoclonal antibody that recognizes and rapidly depletes B lymphocytes, the cells responsible for antibody production, and thus autoantibody production. Tocilizumab is a humanized monoclonal antibody that binds to the IL-6 receptor and prevents signaling by this potent proinflammatory molecule through its receptor. Tofacitinib is a small molecule that blocks signaling of immune cells through the Janus kinase pathway. This is an important pathway for proinflammatory cytokine signaling. All of the biologic agents described above have been studied in patients with rheumatoid arthritis (usually in combination with methotrexate) and have been shown to be extremely effective at not only controlling the day-to-day symptoms but also in preventing the destructive process of the disease.

Patients taking DMARDs or biologics or both will require regular blood tests to assess for hematologic and hepatic toxicities. Patients who are about to start biologics may need to be tested for hepatitis B, hepatitis C, and/or tuberculosis infection as these medications can worsen or activate these conditions. All patients on immunosuppressive drugs have a higher susceptibility to infection, and the symptoms of infection may be masked by the drug. It is common practice to stop these medications when an infection is suspected and have a low threshold for the initiation of antibiotics. Finally, vaccinations against influenza, pneumonia, and zoster are frequently suggested to patients taking DMARDs and biologic agents to partly counteract their higher risk of infections. Influenza and pneumonia vaccines can be given to patients who are concomitantly taking either DMARDs or biologic agents, and these patients will generate an immune response to the vaccine.

Spondyloarthropathy

Spondyloarthropathy is a group of inflammatory arthritides that include the following entities: ankylosing spondylitis, PsA, enteropathic arthritis (the arthritis associated with inflammatory bowel disease), reactive arthritis (an arthritis that follows an episode of dysentery or a sexually transmitted disease), and SAPHO (synovitis, acne, pustulosis, hyperostosis, and osteitis; the arthritis associated with pustular acne and hidradenitis suppurativa). These entities are tied together by the following features: a genetic association with HLA-B27, spine involvement (a region usually not targeted in rheumatoid arthritis), and involvement of the enthesis—the region where a tendon or ligament inserts into bone.

HLA-B27 is an MHC class I molecule that is suspected to play a role in presenting antigens that can trigger autoimmunity. Although HLA-B27 is present in approximately 8% of the general population, it is present in greater than 90% of patients with ankylosing spondylitis, 30% to 70% of patients with either reactive arthritis or inflammatory bowel disease, 40% to 50% of patients with PsA, and 70% of patients with undifferentiated spondyloarthropathy.[23] However, because the incidence of spondyloarthropathy is approximately 1% in the general population, it is important to remember that less than 10% of people with HLA-B27 develop spondyloarthropathy.

In general, the pattern of arthritis in spondyloarthropathy tends to be asymmetric, involving medium and large joints, and involving four or less joints (oligoarthritis). Making the diagnosis is difficult because there are no reliable blood tests for the conditions and because the radiologic findings may take decades to develop. Because these patients tend to present in their second through fifth decades of life, many patients are active and will often attribute their joint pains to whatever physical activity they have recently been performing. They may report that their injury has taken longer than expected to heal, or they may report that they have been repeatedly getting injured. Joint swelling, morning stiffness, the involvement of multiple joints, a family history of psoriasis or inflammatory bowel disease, and a history of a favorable response of the joint pain to oral corticosteroids may all be clues to the presence of a spondyloarthropathy. The spondyloarthropathies may present with systemic symptoms, but this is not a prevalent feature as it is in rheumatoid arthritis and lupus.

Enthesitis (**Fig. 2-3**) is a common feature in all spondyloarthropathies, as several studies have demonstrated. For example, in the study of D'Agostino et al.,[24] 164 patients with spondyloarthropathy were compared with 34 controls (mechanical low back pain, and 30 rheumatoid arthritis patients). For each patient, the following regions were scanned using gray scale and power Doppler ultrasound: greater trochanter of the hip, plantar fascia, patellar ligament, quadriceps tendon, pubis, Achilles tendon, medial and lateral epicondyles of the elbow, and tibialis anterior insertion. The presence of erosions at the tendon insertion and the presence of power Doppler signal within the tendon allowed significant discrimination of spondyloarthropathy (SpA) patients from

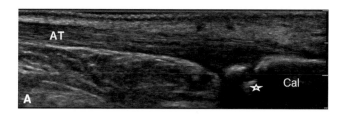
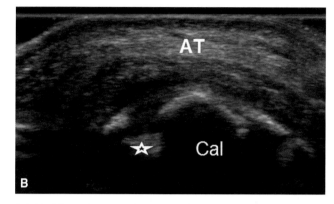
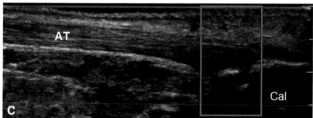
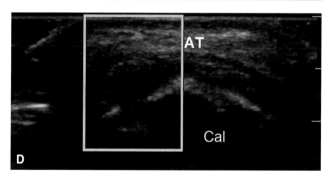

FIGURE 2-3. Enthesitis. Longitudinal **(A and C)** and short axis **(B and D)** views of the distal Achilles tendon (AT) as it inserts in the calcaneus (Cal). Left side is proximal and medial. There is slight thickening of the tendon as it inserts into the calcaneus, and an erosion is seen (*star*). Power Doppler signal, indicating inflammation, is seen within the erosion.

controls; 81% of SpA patients had power doppler (PD) signal in at least one enthesis, whereas zero controls had PD signal; 19% of SpA patients had erosions compared with no controls that had erosions. In the study of D'Agostino et al.,[25] power Doppler signal at baseline in at least one enthesis was the best predictor of SpA at 2 years. Dactylitis is another clinical finding that tends to be associated with spondyloarthropathy. Patients who have this phenotype develop swelling of either a toe or a finger throughout the entire length of the digit such that it appears to resemble a sausage.

Ankylosing Spondylitis

This is a condition that is characterized by sacroiliitis and fusion of the sacroiliac joints as well as the spine, which usually takes place after many years of disease (**Fig. 2-4**). Patients present with inflammatory back pain that is worst in the morning and improves as the day goes on. Often, peripheral symptoms in an asymmetric distribution of larger median joints are also present. Previous classification criteria have focused on X-ray findings, which may take decades to develop. Therefore, new classification criteria have been developed[26] that focus on a combination of imaging by X-ray or MRI, the presence of HLA-B27, and clinical features. In contrast to rheumatoid arthritis, initiation of therapy begins with NSAIDs, but the recommendation is to change to TNF blockers if symptoms

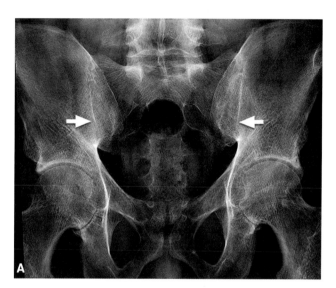
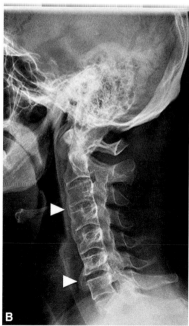

FIGURE 2-4. Ankylosing spondylitis. Frontal view of the pelvis **(A)** demonstrating fusion of the sacroiliac joints bilaterally (*arrows*). In **(B)**, syndesmophytes (*arrowheads*) bridge the anterior portions of the cervical spine.

are not controlled after a few months. Furthermore, the IL-23/IL-17 cytokine pathway has been recently implicated in ankylosing spondylitis and other spondyloarthropathies. Elevated levels of the cytokines have been found in the blood and joints of these patients. Agents that block this pathway are now available for therapy.

Psoriatic Arthritis

About 30% of patients with psoriasis will develop PsA, and 50% of these patients may go on to develop some joint deformities. PsA differs from other spondyloarthropathies in that there are five clinical patterns of arthritis that may occur in isolation or in overlap with other phenotypes: an asymmetric oligoarthritis (the typical spondyloarthropathy pattern); a rheumatoid arthritis–like presentation with symmetric polyarthritis of the small joints of the hands and feet; distal interphalangeal joint involvement (often with dactylitis), axial involvement; severe destructive involvement also known as arthritis mutilans. PsA may coexist with either gout or osteoarthritis, so it is important to rule out these conditions prior to making the diagnosis.

In about 15% of patients, the arthritis may precede the joint symptoms. In addition, psoriasis may be located in regions that the patient may fail to appreciate or mention such as the scalp, behind the ears, the umbilicus, the penis, and the gluteal fold. Psoriatic nail changes including pitting, ridging, and onycholysis may or may not be present. Classification criteria for PsA[27] include the presence of an inflammatory arthritis plus two or more of the following: evidence of current psoriasis, history of psoriasis or a first- or second-degree family now with psoriasis; nail dystrophy; negative RF; dactylitis or history of dactylitis; X-ray showing juxta-articular new bone formation. Occasionally, patients will have an elevated ESR or CRP, but not frequently. X-ray findings might include sacroiliitis, pencil and cup deformity of the fingers or toes (a whittling down to a point of the distal aspect of the proximal phalanx paired with a flaring of the proximal portion of the more distal phalanx such that the appearance is that of a pencil going into a cup), and erosions. On ultrasound, one may see synovial thickening, effusion, synovitis or tenosynovitis, erosion, or enthesitis.

Treatment of the skin disease depends on the location and severity and may be limited to topical therapy or light therapy, with systemic therapy reserved for extensive disease. Treatment of the arthritis again depends on the severity of symptoms. NSAIDs may be reserved for mild disease, but more aggressive arthritis is usually treated with a first line of DMARD such as methotrexate, followed by addition or switching to biologic agents including the TNF blockers, a blocker of the IL-12/23 pathway (ustekinumab), or a phosphodiesterase 4 inhibitor (apremilast).

Crystalline Arthritis

The most common crystalline arthropathies that present in the lower extremity are gout and pseudogout. Both entities share the theme of a salt precipitating within a joint and/or surrounding tissues and triggering a robust inflammatory response. In gout, the salt is monosodium urate, whereas in pseudogout the salt is calcium pyrophosphate. On occasion, both crystals may be found within the joint. In addition, the crystals may be found within the joint even in the absence of a flare of arthritis. When the joint is traumatized or if there is a septic process within the joint, there may be release of the crystals, which then may be observed in the synovial fluid. Therefore, the presence of crystals in a synovial aspirate does not rule out the presence of infection.

Gout

Gout is one of the most painful arthropathies and, if untreated, has the potential to be destructive to affected joints (**Fig. 2-5**). One of the more commonly involved joints is the 1st MTP; however, it is important to remember that spondyloarthropathy and rheumatoid arthritis may also affect this joint. The onset of pain during a flare of gout is usually rapid; sometimes, within hours the pain level can crescendo: often people cannot bear weight on the affected joint. Erythema and swelling are frequently observed. Fever and elevated white count, although not common, can be associated with severe flares. If gout is untreated, it may progress to tophaceous gout in which large deposits of uric acid grow to be palpable beneath the skin and may erode into adjacent bone. The dorsum of the hands and feet, the extensor surface of the elbows, and the ears are commonly affected locations.

Gout is caused by elevated uric acid in the blood and tissue. When the concentration of uric acid exceeds the limits of solubility, it tends to precipitate as sodium-urate salt in the extracellular tissues. The presence of a high uric acid does not guarantee gout; indeed, there are many patients with very high uric acids who have never had a gout flare. Therefore, asymptomatic hyperuricemia does not need to be treated prophylactically. When uric acid crystals precipitate with the joint, they cause acute inflammation as they are ingested by neutrophils. The crystals may activate complement directly or may stimulate leukocytes to produce proinflammatory mediators such as IL-1. Gout crystals may be identified within the synovial fluid as needle-shaped crystals that are either yellow or blue under a polarizing filter. When the polarizing filter is oriented parallel to the direction of the crystal, it will appear yellow; when the polarizer filter is oriented perpendicular to the direction of the crystal, it will appear blue. Uric acid is a waste product of nucleic acid metabolism, and the sources of uric acid in patients with gout are both foods that are high in purines and also from breakdown of the DNA from one's own cells. In addition, 80% of patients with elevated uric acid have decreased excretion through the kidneys. Alcohol and some medications such as aspirin and diuretics can also decrease uric acid excretion in the kidney, precipitating a flare of gout.

Typical X-ray findings of gout include punched out erosions with overhanging edges and the appearance of tophi or collections of uric acid crystals. These findings may also be seen in ultrasound associated with synovial thickening,

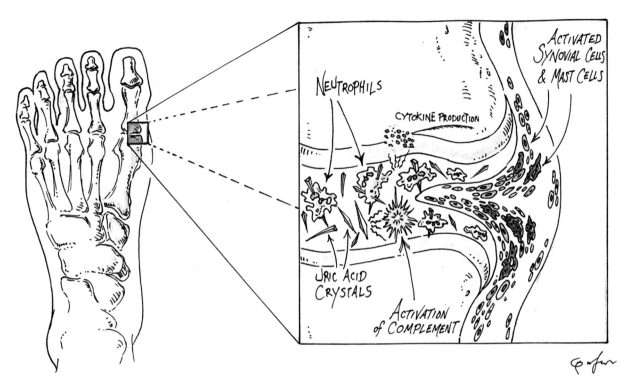

FIGURE 2-5. Gout. Crystals of uric acid precipitate within the joint or periarticular structures, leading to activation of complement and production of cytokines such as interleukin-1, causing a robust acute inflammatory response.

effusions, and increased power Doppler signal (**Fig. 2-6**). In an article published by Thiele and Schlesinger,[28] 37 joints from 23 patients with crystal-proven gout were examined by gray scale ultrasound and compared with 23 controls. The "double contour sign" (**Fig. 2-7**) was seen in 92% of the gout patients and none of the controls. Tophi were observed

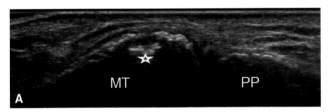

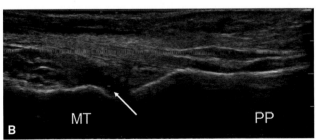

FIGURE 2-6. Examples of ultrasound findings in gout. Two longitudinal views of the 1st metatarsal-phalangeal gout over the medial (**A**) and dorsal (**B**) regions of the joint in a patient with known gout. Left side is proximal. A punched out erosion with overhanging edges is demonstrated (**A**) in the 1st metatarsal head (*star*). In (**B**), a dark region emanating from the joint, suggesting synovial thickening, contains a bright punctate spot suggestive of a uric acid deposit (*arrow*). MT, metatarsal head; PP, proximal phalanx.

in all 1st MTPs of gout patients and none of the controls. Erosions were seen in 65% of the 1st MTPs of gout patients and one control patient.

Most NSAIDs are effective at treating acute gout, but often their use may be in conflict with one of the many comorbidities that are associated with gout. Colchicine is an old drug that inhibits microtubule formation in leukocytes and interferes with cell migration. It is often used at a dose of 1.2 mg once followed by 0.6 mg shortly thereafter. Colchicine is then continued at 0.6 mg once or twice daily until symptoms resolve. In addition, it may be used on an ongoing basis at 0.6 mg once or twice daily as a prophylactic agent to prevent flares. Intravenous colchicine has the potential to cause severe marrow suppression and so is rarely used. Corticosteroids such as prednisone and methylprednisone are very effective at controlling gout flares both in oral forms and when injected into a symptomatic joint. In patients with chronic gout symptoms, tophi, or urate nephropathy, uric acid lowering therapy may be initiated with either allopurinol or febuxostat. The target uric acid in patients with chronic gout is less than 6.0 mg/dL or less than 5.0 mg/dL in patients with tophi. Uric acid levels equilibrate approximately 2 weeks after changing the dose of a urate-lowering agent; therefore, frequent follow-up is required to titrate the dose to that which achieves the desired level of uric acid.

Pseudogout (Calcium Pyrophosphate Deposition)

Pseudogout is similar to gout in that symptoms are also caused by a salt, calcium pyrophosphate, which has deposited within joints and surrounding tissues. Like gout crystals, pseudogout

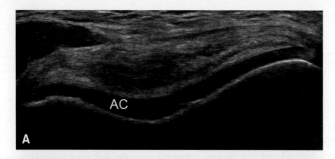

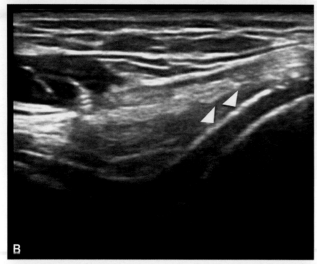

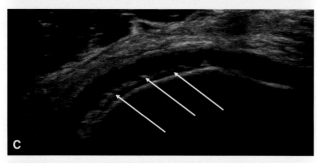

FIGURE 2-7. Ultrasound findings in crystalline arthropathy: Axial **(A and B)** and sagittal **(C)** views of the anterior knee in full flexion to expose the articular cartilage (AC). Left side is medial **(A and B)** or proximal **(C)**. A normal knee is shown in **(A)**. Image **(B)** demonstrates the double contour sign observed in gout, a bright band superficial to the articular cartilage (*arrowheads*). Image **(C)** demonstrates deposition of calcium pyrophosphate crystals within articular cartilage (*arrows*). (Images kindly provided by Dr. Lisa Vasanth and Dr. Jonathan Samuels.)

crystals may also be observed within joint aspirates; however, the crystals appear rhomboid shaped and have a blue appearance when they are oriented parallel to the polarizing filter. Pseudogout can take either an acute or a chronic form. When patients have an acute pseudogout flare, the common joints involved are the knees and wrists. Because pseudogout crystals contain calcium, they are more easily seen on X-rays than gout crystals and often may be observed in the knees and wrist. In the study of Filippou et al.,[29] 42 crystal-proven calcium pyrophosphate dihydrate (CPPD) patients were examined by gray scale ultrasound. The most frequently observed sites for CPPD were the femoral condyle of the knee (**Fig. 2-7**), the menisci, and

the triangular fibrocartilage complex of the wrist. Occasionally, calcium pyrophosphate may be seen surrounding the dens of the 2nd cervical vertebrae. This may cause headaches and/or neck pain and is called crowded dens syndrome—diagnosis is made by computerized axial tomography scan of the cervical spine. Risk factors for pseudogout include ochronosis, hyperparathyroidism, thyroid abnormalities, hemochromatosis, Wilson disease, hypophosphatemia, and hypomagnesemia. Treatment of pseudogout is more challenging than gout because there are no agents to reduce the crystal burden. Therapy is usually limited to NSAIDs, corticosteroids, and colchicine.

CONCLUSIONS

Rheumatic diseases of the lower extremity may present in a similar fashion to mechanical problems. It is important to identify these conditions early because some have the potential to cause permanent damage without appropriate therapy. New therapies have revolutionized the treatments of these conditions. Clues to a systemic illness may be found in associated symptoms or on the physical examination; therefore, it is important to always perform a careful history and physical examination when inflammatory disease is suspected. In addition, the growing use of MSKUS is making early and more accurate diagnosis possible. Some of the more common rheumatic diseases that may be observed in the lower extremity include rheumatoid arthritis, spondyloarthropathies, and crystalline arthropathies.

REFERENCES

1. Guidelines for the initial evaluation of the adult patient with acute musculoskeletal symptoms. American College of Rheumatology Ad Hoc Committee on Clinical Guidelines. *Arthritis Rheum.* 1996;39:1–8.
2. Baker DG, Schumacher HR Jr. Acute monoarthritis. *N Engl J Med.* 1993;329:1013–1020.
3. Kanis JA, Borgstrom F, De Laet C, et al. Assessment of fracture risk. *Osteoporos Int.* 2005;16(6):581–589.
4. Puhaindran ME, Farooki A, Steensma MR, et al. Atypical subtrochanteric femoral fractures in patients with skeletal malignant involvement treated with intravenous bisphosphonates. *J Bone Joint Surg Am.* 2011;93(13):1235–1242.
5. Qaseem A, Snow V, Barry P, et al; Joint American Academy of Family Physicians/American College of Physicians Panel on Deep Venous Thrombosis/Pulmonary Embolism. Current diagnosis of venous thromboembolism in primary care: a clinical practice guideline from the American Academy of Family Physicians and the American College of Physicians. *Ann Intern Med.* 2007;146(6): 454–458.
6. Lillegraven S, Bøyesen P, Hammer HB, et al. Tenosynovitis of the extensor carpi ulnaris tendon predicts erosive progression in early rheumatoid arthritis. *Ann Rheum Dis.* 2011;70(11):2049–2050. doi:10.1136/ard.2011.151316.
7. McGonagle D, Marzo-Ortega H, O'Connor P, et al. Histological assessment of the early enthesitis lesion in spondyloarthropathy. *Ann Rheum Dis.* 2002;61(6):534–537.
8. Backhaus M, Kamradt T, Sandrock D, et al. Arthritis of the finger joints: a comprehensive approach comparing conventional radiography, scintigraphy, ultrasound, and contrast-enhanced magnetic resonance imaging. *Arthritis Rheum.* 1999;42(6):1232–1245.

9. Szkudlarek M, Klarlund M, Narvestad E, et al. Ultrasonography of the metacarpophalangeal and proximal interphalangeal joints in rheumatoid arthritis: a comparison with magnetic resonance imaging, conventional radiography and clinical examination. *Arthritis Res Ther*. 2006;8(2):R52.

10. Karim Z, Wakefield RJ, Conaghan PG, et al. The impact of ultrasonography on diagnosis and management of patients with musculoskeletal conditions. *Arthritis Rheum*. 2001;44(12):2932–2933.

11. Taylor PC, Steuer A, Gruber J, et al. Comparison of ultrasonographic assessment of synovitis and joint vascularity with radiographic evaluation in a randomized, placebo-controlled study of infliximab therapy in early rheumatoid arthritis. *Arthritis Rheum*. 2004;50(4):1107–1116.

12. Naredo E, Collado P, Cruz A, et al. Longitudinal power Doppler ultrasonographic assessment of joint inflammatory activity in early rheumatoid arthritis: predictive value in disease activity and radiologic progression. *Arthritis Rheum*. 2007;57(1):116–124.

13. Brown AK, Conaghan PG, Karim Z, et al. An explanation for the apparent dissociation between clinical remission and continued structural deterioration in rheumatoid arthritis. *Arthritis Rheum*. 2008;58(10):2958–2967.

14. Samuels J, Abramson SB, Kaeley GS. The use of musculoskeletal ultrasound by rheumatologists in the United States. *Bull NYU Hosp Jt Dis*. 2010;68(4):292–298.

15. Machold KP, Stamm TA, Eberl GJ, et al. Very recent onset arthritis. Clinical, laboratory, and radiological findings during the first year of disease. *J Rheumatol*. 2002;29:2278–2287.

16. Verpoort KN, van Dongen H, Allaart CF, et al. Undifferentiated arthritis disease course assessed in several inception cohorts. *Clin Exp Rheumatol*. 2004;22:S12–S17.

17. Lard LR, Visser H, Speyer I, et al. Early versus delayed treatment in patients with recent-onset rheumatoid arthritis: comparison of two cohorts who received different treatment strategies. *Am J Med*. 2001;111:446–451.

18. Emery P, Breedveld FC, Dougados M, et al. Early referral recommendation for newly diagnosed rheumatoid arthritis: evidence based development of a clinical guide. *Ann Rheum Dis*. 2002;61:290–297.

19. Mahdi H, Fisher BA, Källberg H, et al. Specific interaction between genotype, smoking and autoimmunity to citrullinated alpha-enolase in the etiology of rheumatoid arthritis. *Nat Genet*. 2009;41(12):1319–1324.

20. Rantapää-Dahlqvist S, de Jong BA, Berglin E, et al. Antibodies against cyclic citrullinated peptide and IgA rheumatoid factor predict the development of rheumatoid arthritis. *Arthritis Rheum*. 2003;48(10):2741–2749.

21. Atzeni F, Turiel M, Caporali R, et al. The effect of pharmacological therapy on the cardiovascular system of patients with systemic rheumatic diseases. *Autoimmun Rev*. 2010;9(12):835–930.

22. Singh JA, Saag KG, Bridges SL Jr, et al. 2015 American College of Rheumatology Guideline for the treatment of rheumatoid arthritis. *Arthritis Care Res (Hoboken)*. 2016;68:1–25.

23. Khan MA. HLA-B27 and its pathogenic role. *J Clin Rheumatol*. 2008;14(1):50–52.

24. D'Agostino MA, Said-Nahal R, Hacquard-Bouder C, et al. Assessment of peripheral enthesitis in the spondylarthropathies by ultrasonography combined with power Doppler: a cross-sectional study. *Arthritis Rheum*. 2003;48(2):523–533.

25. D'Agostino MA, Aegerter P, Bechara K, et al. How to diagnose spondyloarthritis early? Accuracy of peripheral enthesitis detection by power Doppler ultrasonography. *Ann Rheum Dis*. 2011;70(8):1433–1440.

26. Sieper J, Rudwaleit M, Baraliakos X, et al. The Assessment of SpondyloArthritis international Society (ASAS) handbook: a guide to assess spondyloarthritis. *Ann Rheum Dis*. 2009;68 Suppl 2:ii1–ii44.

27. Taylor W, Gladman D, Helliwell P, et al; CASPAR Study Group. Classification criteria for psoriatic arthritis: development of new criteria from a large international study. *Arthritis Rheum*. 2006;54(8):2665–2673.

28. Thiele RG, Schlesinger N. Diagnosis of gout by ultrasound. *Rheumatology (Oxford)*. 2007;46(7):1116–1121.

29. Filippou G, Filippucci E, Tardella M, et al. Extent and distribution of CPP deposits in patients affected by calcium pyrophosphate dihydrate deposition disease: an ultrasonographic study. *Ann Rheum Dis*. 2013;72(11):1836–1839.

CHAPTER 3

Pedal Manifestations of Cardiac Disease

MICHAEL J. TREPAL • MARK H. SWARTZ • ROCK G. POSITANO • LORETTA CACACE

The feet contain approximately one quarter of the body's total bones, with each foot having more than 30 joints; 100 tendons, muscles, and ligaments; and countless nerves, arteries, and veins. Our feet and lower extremity can, in addition, serve as a window to the rest of the body and tell us a great deal about the presence or status of concomitant known or occult systemic disease. Such systemic pathologies include neurologic, rheumatologic, orthopedic, diabetic, and other endocrine, dermatologic, neoplastic, gastrointestinal, renal, and psychological disorders. Many cardiovascular pathologies are closely related to those involving the lower extremity including generalized atherosclerosis, coronary artery disease (CAD), arrhythmias, valvular heart disease, pulmonary disease, cardiac neoplasms, and cardiomyopathies. Each of them has unique pedal signs and symptoms that may initially bring the condition to the attention of a health care provider and must in turn be comanaged.

PERIPHERAL ARTERY DISEASE

Peripheral artery disease (PAD) refers to varied pathologies such as atherosclerosis and vasculitis involving the peripheral circulation separate from cardiac and cranial arteries and affects more than 8.5 million Americans and 200 million people worldwide.[1] It occurs commonly in conjunction with CAD. Unfortunately, it is all too frequently underdiagnosed and untreated,[2] resulting in potentially avoidable lower limb amputations, myocardial infarctions, and cerebral vascular accidents. Individuals with symptoms and signs of PAD have an increased risk for heart disease and stroke[3] and must be encouraged to seek medical attention for evaluation and ruling out of associated cardiovascular disease. According to the American Heart Association, individuals with PAD have four to five times' greater risk for myocardial infarction and a cerebral vascular accident because atherosclerosis is a disease of the entire cardiovascular system. Nearly a quarter of individuals with claudication due to PAD will die within 5 years because of a myocardial infarction or stroke. Interestingly, patients with documented PAD have a 1 year higher incidence of fatal myocardial infarction than those with preexisting CAD.[4]

Appropriately, the patient diagnosed with PAD should be screened for CAD, and, conversely, the patient diagnosed with CAD should be screened for PAD. Kowantor et al.[5] reported that 26% of 1,340 patients with documented CAD presented with undiagnosed PAD. Arterial fatty plaque buildup in vessels of patients with atherosclerosis reduces the flow of blood in the lower extremities and feet, and at a critical threshold, ischemic-related signs and symptoms will begin to manifest. Progression of untreated disease may ultimately reach a point of critical limb ischemia, which all too frequently results in loss of limb or ultimately life. The lower extremity signs and symptoms are generally subtle at first but eventually become obvious and ultimately debilitating. Unfortunately, the underlying systemic atherosclerotic disease may be previously unrecognized, resulting in serious comorbidities in the heart, brain, kidney, and other internal organs. Well established risk factors for CAD and stroke such as family history, hyperlipidemia, hypertension, diabetes, and smoking likewise increase one's risk for PAD.

The main symptoms of PAD may include, in proportion to disease severity, claudication, fatigue, achiness, burning, and discomfort in the buttocks, thighs, and calves. Erectile dysfunction may also result. These symptoms first appear during extensive walking or exercise, and disappear after several minutes of rest. As the PAD progresses, symptoms will occur with less exercise or activity and with an earlier onset. Claudication pain may be likened to symptoms of angina seen in patients with CAD. The most commonly utilized system to classify intermittent claudication and lower extremity ischemia is the Rutherford classification, which is divided into seven stages (see **Table 3-1**).[6] Lower extremity ischemia leading to extremity numbness or intense pain at rest with ultimate tissue necrosis has been informally referred to as a heart attack of the foot. These symptoms frequently intensify with elevation of the limb, and it is not uncommon to observe the patient maintain the affected limb(s) in a position of dependency. The presence of pain at rest can be classified as a situation of critical limb ischemia where some type of intervention is urgently or emergently necessary to prevent necrosis of tissue and potential loss of limb.

Clinical findings consistent with PAD include decreased posterior tibial (PT) and/or dorsalis pedis (DP) blood pressure, weak or nonpalpable pulses, arterial bruits, increased capillary fill time, dermal atrophy, coolness of the skin, increase in temperature gradient, lower extremity hair loss, pallor on elevation, or cyanosis. The end-stage critically ischemia limb will frequently manifest dependent edema and a ruborous-like

Table 3-1. Rutherford Classification Listing Stages of Peripheral Arterial Disease

Stage	Findings
0	Asymptomatic
1	Mild claudication
2	Moderate claudication—The distance that delineates mild, moderate, and severe claudication is not specified
3	Severe claudication
4	Rest pain
5	Ischemic ulceration not exceeding ulcer of the digits of the foot
6	Severe ischemic ulcers or frank gangrene

hue resulting from the chronically dilated microvascular structures. The development of nonhealing ulcers or frank gangrene is further evidence of critical limb ischemia requiring urgent or emergent intervention (**Fig. 3-1**).

Noninvasive testing for PAD includes the ankle-brachial index (ABI), which is a painless office-based examination that compares the ratio of blood pressure in the distal lower extremity to that in the upper extremity. This inexpensive test takes only a few minutes and can easily be performed by the health care professional. Guidelines of the American College of Cardiology and American Heart Association recommend its use for screening individuals at high risk such as those over 65 years old or over 50 years old in diabetics or smokers.[4] The appropriate method to measure ABI is to have the patient lying flat, with Doppler measurements obtained following 5 to 10 minutes of rest.[7] Cuff width should be at least 40% of limb circumference. Systolic blood pressure (SBP) is measured in each arm and ankle including the DP and PT arteries. ABI of each leg is then calculated by dividing the higher of the PT or DP pressure by the higher of the right or left arm SBP (**Fig. 3-2**).

Normally, the ankle blood pressure is at least 90% of the upper extremity pressure; with severe arterial narrowing, the ankle pressure may be reduced to less than 50%. Low ABI has been established as an independent risk factor of CAD.[8–10] Conversely, Allison et al.[11] showed that an abnormally high ABI (which is due to inelasticity of the arterial wall secondary to plaque buildup) is also associated with increased risk of CAD. The test can also be performed postexercise on a treadmill to better detect milder disease.

If the ABI is abnormal in the presence of symptoms, further testing is generally indicated to better evaluate the magnitude and precise location of the disease. Segmental pressures, pulse volume recording, ultrasonography in conjunction with Doppler imaging (duplex scan), and transcutaneous oximetry are other noninvasive techniques that evaluate arterial flow and/or tissue perfusion. Segmental pressures or sound waves measuring the blood flow in an artery can indirectly indicate the extent and location of a blockage. Computed Tomography and magnetic resonance angiography are additional noninvasive techniques demonstrating the extent of the disease. Invasive testing including angiography is the most specific test for determining the specific location and severity of occlusive lesions. Intravascular ultrasound is a newer technique that can image directly a blockage without subjecting the patient to radiographic dyes. This is beneficial in patients with allergies or renal disease.

The management of early PAD is centered on goals of reducing risks of further progression of atherosclerosis and most notably lessening the incidence of acute coronary syndromes and cerebral vascular accidents. With respect to the

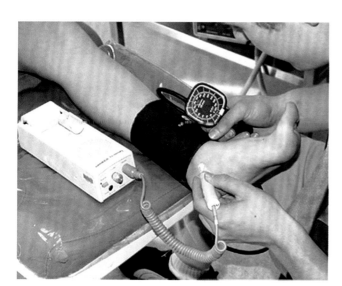

FIGURE 3-1. Technique to measure ankle-brachial index.

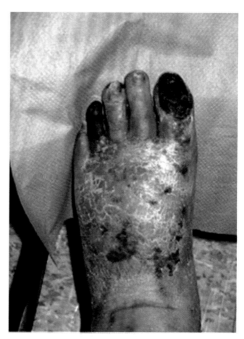

FIGURE 3-2. Critical limb ischemia manifesting rubor and gangrene.

lower extremity disease, the goal is to improve function and preserve the limb itself. Accordingly, cardiovascular risk factors such as hypertension, hyperlipidemia, and hyperglycemia must be controlled. Lifestyle modifications including smoking cessation and supervised exercise programs are also essential. The use of antiplatelet agents must be weighed against the risk of increased bleeding. Revascularization procedures are indicated for limb salvage in patients with activity-altering claudication, ulcerations, or gangrene. They are also indicated in patients who have failed medical management and lifestyle modifications where the procedure can reasonably be expected to result in increased functionality. In addition to classic open surgical bypass procedures, the trend has been decidedly toward endovascular interventions including angioplasties, atherectomy, bare metal and drug-eluting stents, and, most recently, drug-eluting balloons. Appropriate cardiac interventions are also frequently required where indicated.

Although generalized atherosclerosis is associated with poor long-term prognosis, the early identification and intervention can improve both quality of life and longevity.

DIABETES

Diabetes affects more than 24 million Americans. It has been estimated that 6 million people do not even know that they have the disease. Risk factors in addition to familial history include those associated with classic metabolic syndrome such as hypertension, hyperlipidemia, and central obesity. The obesity component also potentiates unrelated musculoskeletal injuries and overuse syndromes that will cause the patient to present for medical evaluation. It is not uncommon that specific diabetic foot–related disease is the precipitating factor that stimulates individuals to seek medical attention and the subsequent diagnoses of other systemic diabetic complications including cardiovascular disease, nephropathy, and retinopathy. Most common pedal signs and symptoms of diabetes include diminished circulation and peripheral neuropathies.[12]

In addition to classic signs and symptoms of PAD affecting the large vessels and discussed previously, diabetics can manifest disorders of the microcirculation resulting from altered permeability of capillary membranes and arteriovenous shunting in the midfoot area. Consequently and paradoxically, it is possible for a patient to have distal digital ischemia in the presence of palpable pedal pulses. Neuropathy is a very common and potentially serious complication of diabetes and may be hyposensory or hypersensory in nature. It can be painful, disabling, and even fatal. Patients with diabetic neuropathy often experience paresthesias and reduced ability to experience changes in temperature. Sharp lancinating pain that worsens at night is frequently experienced. Increased sensitivity to the lightest touch can be agonizing. Muscle weakness, difficulty in waking, and joint contractures may also occur and lead to increased pressure points and ulcerations. Autonomic neuropathy may dull the senses and result in lack of awareness that blood glucose is low. Frequent urinary

tract infections, incontinence, erectile dysfunction, as well as vaginal dryness and other sexual dysfunction may occur.

Diabetic mononeuropathy may also develop, affecting specific nerves in the face, torso, or leg. The signs and symptoms depend upon which nerve is involved. Visual changes may result when one of the extraocular muscles is involved; paralysis of one side of the face may occur with facial nerve involvement; and pain in the shin, thigh, or foot when other nerves are affected.

ARTERIAL EMBOLISM

Arterial embolism is a sudden interruption of blood supply to an organ or body part caused by a migrated blood clot, resulting in damage or necrosis of the area supplied by the native artery (**Fig. 3-3**). Arterial emboli often become lodged in the distal circulation of the legs and feet. Emboli that migrate to the cerebral circulation result in a cerebral vascular accident. One of the most common etiologies and sources of emboli is the result of abnormal cardiac dysrhythmias, often being atrial fibrillation. Atrial fibrillation, which is estimated to affect slightly over 4% of the population over 60 years of age, can be classified into paroxysmal (intermittent/temporary) and chronic. Paroxysmal atrial fibrillation is defined as

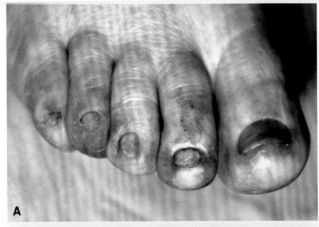

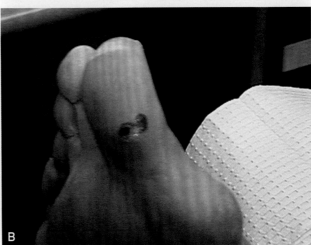

FIGURE 3-3. (A and B) Microemboli in a patient with atrial fibrillation.

at least two separate episodes of atrial fibrillation that terminate spontaneously in less than 7 days. Both paroxysmal and chronic atrial fibrillation have the same rate of cardioembolic events.[13] Symptoms of atrial fibrillation include an irregular, rapid pulse; weakness and shortness of breath; chest pain; and decreased blood pressure. Causes of atrial fibrillation include mitral stenosis with resultant left atrial enlargement that often results in thrombus and emboli formation. Other causes of arterial embolism include damage to an arterial wall and blood clotting abnormalities such as thrombocytosis.

Some of the more common early symptoms of arterial embolization to the lower extremity include a cold extremity, decreased or absent pulses in the involved limb (although the contralateral pulse remains normal), lack of ability to move the extremity, severe muscle pain or muscle spasm, numbness, and weakness.[14] Some of the later symptoms include skin erosion, blistering, sloughing of the skin, and gangrene of the embolized area.[14]

Tests to diagnose arterial embolism include angiography, Doppler ultrasound examination of the extremity, MRI of the extremity, transesophageal echocardiography, Factor VII assay, platelet aggregation test, and tissue-type plasminogen activator levels.

The risk of arterial thromboembolism is increased in individuals who are smokers, inactive, overweight, and under increased emotional stress.

INFECTIVE ENDOCARDITIS

Infective endocarditis is an infection of the endocardial surface of the heart, which may include one or more heart valves, the mural endocardium, or a septal defect and is associated with several findings in the foot. Its intracardiac effects include severe valvular insufficiency, which may lead to congestive heart failure (CHF) and myocardial abscesses. If left untreated, infective endocarditis is often fatal.

Low-grade, often intermittent, fever is present in 90% of patients with infective endocarditis. Heart murmurs are also heard in approximately 85% of patients. Other systemic symptoms include joint pain, hypotension, and hematuria. A generalized, gradual flulike syndrome has also been reported in some cases of subacute bacterial endocarditis. In addition, there are several other classic signs of endocarditis, many seen in the lower extremity. These include petechiae, subungual (splinter) hemorrhages (Fig. 3-4), Osler nodes (Fig. 3-5), Janeway lesions (Fig. 3-6), and Roth spots.

Splinter hemorrhages are dark red, linear lesions in the nail beds. Osler nodes are tender, subcutaneous nodules usually found on the distal pads of the digits and are associated with subacute bacterial endocarditis (approximately 10% to 23%).[15] Osler nodules demonstrate a temporary course lasting hours to days. Janeway lesions are nontender, hemorrhagic macules on the palms and soles, typically associated with acute bacterial endocarditis. These lesions are a result of septic microemboli and represent microabscesses in the dermis with thrombosis of small vessel without vasculitis. Janeway lesions typically

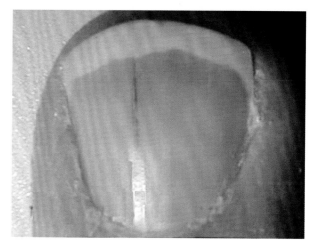

FIGURE 3-4. Splinter hemorrhage in a patient with endocarditis.

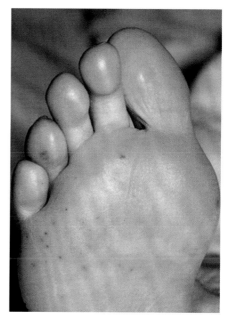

FIGURE 3-5. Osler nodes.

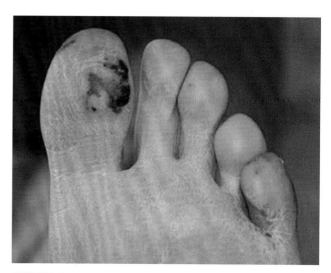

FIGURE 3-6. Janeway lesions.

last for several days to weeks.[16] Finally, Roth spots are retinal hemorrhages with a small clear center.

The etiologies of infective endocarditis are many, but include native valve endocarditis, prosthetic valve endocarditis, intravenous drug endocarditis, and nosocomial endocarditis.

The following are the main underlying causes of native valve endocarditis:

- Rheumatic valvular disease involving the mitral valve followed by the aortic valve
- Congenital heart disease etiologies including patent ductus arteriosus, ventricular septal defect, or tetralogy of Fallot
- Mitral valve prolapse
- Degenerative heart disease, including calcific aortic stenosis caused by a bicuspid valve, Marfan syndrome, or syphilitic disease

Approximately 70% of infections in native valve endocarditis are caused by *Streptococcus* species, including *Streptococcus viridans*, *Streptococcus bovis*, and enterococci. *Staphylococcus* species cause about a quarter of all cases and frequently are associated with a more aggressive course.

Infection associated with aortic valve prostheses is commonly associated with local abscess and fistula formation, often resulting in valvular dehiscence. Shock, heart failure, heart block, shunting of blood to the right atrium, pericardial tamponade, and peripheral emboli to the central nervous system and elsewhere may later ensue.

Diagnosis of infective endocarditis in intravenous drug users can be difficult. Two-thirds of patients have no previous history of heart disease or murmur. A murmur may be absent in those with tricuspid infective endocardial disease, as a result of the relatively small pressure gradient across this valve. Pulmonary manifestations may be prominent in patients with tricuspid infection: one-third have pleuritic chest pain, and three-quarters demonstrate chest radiographic abnormalities. *Staphylococcus aureus* is the most common (50% of cases) etiologic organism in patients with intravenous drug infective endocarditis. *Methicillin-resistant S. aureus* accounts for an increasing portion of *S. aureus* infections and has been associated with previous hospitalizations, long-term addiction, and prior antibiotic use. Fungal infective endocarditis is also found in intravenous drug users and intensive care unit patients who receive broad-spectrum antibiotics. Blood cultures are often negative, and diagnosis is frequently made after microscopic examination of subsequent emboli.

Nosocomial infective endocarditis may be associated with intravascular devices such as central or peripheral intravenous catheters, rhythm control devices such as pacemakers and defibrillators, hemodialysis shunts and catheters, and chemotherapeutic and hyperalimentation lines. These patients tend to have significant comorbidities, more advanced age, and predominant infection with *S. aureus*. The mortality rate is high in this group.

Of all cases of infective endocarditis, males are more than three times at risk compared with females. Infective endocarditis has no racial predilection.

LIVEDO RETICULARIS

Livedo reticularis is a condition caused by an interruption of blood flow in the dermal arteries, resulting from spasm, inflammation, or vascular obstruction, and is associated with diseases of varying etiology and severity. It appears as a mottled, blotchy, reddish-violet reticulated discoloration of the skin, often on the legs or soles of the feet. Vascular obstruction can, in turn, be caused by thrombosis, embolic events, or vessel wall abnormalities.

On occasion, livedo reticularis is simply the result of being exposed to a cold environment. It may be a symptom, however, of a serious underlying condition, such as vascular disease, an endocrine disorder, or a rheumatologic disease, such as systemic lupus erythematosus, polyarteritis nodosa, or rheumatoid arthritis. Livedo reticularis may also be related to a complication of kidney dialysis known as calciphylaxis. It may also result from certain medications, such as warfarin, and medications used to treat multiple sclerosis.

Livedo reticularis, without vasculitis or thrombosis, can also occur in systemic lupus erythematosus and rheumatoid arthritis. In such cases, the condition may be secondary to a slowing of the blood flow (caused by increased viscosity or thrombophilic states), to an intense vasoconstrictor reaction induced by cold, or to a combination of both these mechanisms.

Left atrial myxomas are benign tumors that originate in endothelial cells. Atrial myxomas are the most frequent cardiac neoplasm and typically present with fatigue, murmur, and arrhythmias.[17] Tumor fragments can break off, causing distal emboli and characteristic symptoms such as livedo reticularis, necrosis, distal cyanosis, and splinter hemorrhages.

Livedo reticularis may also result from cholesterol emboli secondary to rupture of atheromatous plaques in the aorta or other great arteries, either spontaneously or as the result of surgical procedures, catheterization, angioplasties, angiography, or following initiation of treatment with anticoagulants or thrombolytic agents. Skin lesions secondary to the presence of emboli in skin arteries and arterioles are very common and tend to be one of the first signs of cholesterol embolization (**Fig. 3-7**).

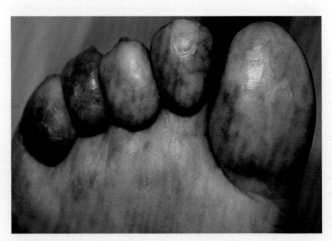

FIGURE 3-7. Livedo reticularis.

Vessel wall disorders can also result in livedo reticularis. Disorders of calcium and phosphorus metabolism in patients with advanced renal failure and secondary hyperparathyroidism can cause metastatic calcifications in the arteries, soft tissues, joints, and organs. Calciphylaxis refers to the calcification of the media of arteries and can result in the sudden appearance of livedo reticularis, hemorrhagic infarcts, necrosis, and ulceration. The plaques are well defined and are extremely painful; the condition is often fatal. There is a high risk of calciphylaxis when the calcium–phosphorus product is greater than 65 mg per mL.

CONGESTIVE HEART FAILURE

Symptoms of CHF consist of palpitations, orthopnea, cough with frothy sputum, jugular venous distension, systolic murmurs, and rales on auscultation of the base of both lungs. Left-sided heart failure results in pulmonary edema and eventually progresses to right-sided heart failure. In the lower extremity, a major sign of CHF is pitting edema. Pitting edema occurs when the hydrostatic pressure increases or the oncotic pressure decreases within the vasculature, forcing fluid into the interstitium. This form of edema can be identified by pressing a finger into the swollen lower extremity and an imprint can be observed.[18] Pitting edema is often painful with associated hemosiderin deposition and often results in ulceration. Another sign of CHF in the lower extremity is decreased walking velocity. Pepera et al.[19] showed that patients with CHF have a shorter step length and walk more slowly and that these altered gait mechanics may contribute to limited exercise capacity.

NAIL CHANGES

Nail findings may provide important clues to the diagnosis of systemic illness, limit the differential diagnosis, and focus on further workup.

Clubbing, spooning, pitting, depressions, pigmented bands, and color changes must always be evaluated.

A Quincke pulse is one example of cardiac issues, specifically aortic insufficiency, presenting as changes in the nail bed. This manifestation represents regurgitant blood flow during diastole in the cardiac cycle. This decrease in diastolic pressure causes an increase in stroke volume that can be seen in the nail bed as alternating blanching and flushing.

Clubbing of the distal fingers and toes is a condition in which Lovibond angle is increased and the nail seems to float instead of being firmly attached to the nail bed (Fig. 3-8). There is a thickening of the soft tissue beneath the proximal nail plate that results in sponginess of the proximal plate and thickening in that area of the digit. The distal portion of the finger or toenail may appear enlarged or bulging. The exact pathophysiology remains unknown, but theories of vasodilation (causing distended blood vessels) or oversecretion of growth factors from the lungs (such as platelet-derived growth factor and hepatocyte growth factor) have been proposed. It has also

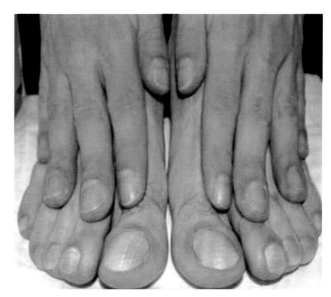

FIGURE 3-8. Clubbing of digits.

been hypothesized that the overproduction of prostaglandin E2 from other tissues is a causative factor for clubbing of the digits.[20] It can develop quickly, often within weeks. If the cause is treatable, clubbing may disappear quickly as well. Unfortunately, most clubbing occurs as a result of pulmonary neoplasms.[20] Clubbing may also be present in children with congenital heart disease such as tetralogy of Fallot. It is also seen in cystic fibrosis, chronic lung infections, asbestosis, pulmonary fibrosis, inflammatory bowel disease, and Hodgkin disease.

Koilonychia is noted by the presence of transverse and longitudinal concavity of the nail, resulting in a "spoon-shaped" nail. Although koilonychia may also result from trauma, constant occupational exposure of the hands to petroleum-based solvents, or nail–patella syndrome, koilonychia has been associated with iron deficiency. Occasionally, koilonychia has been seen in patients with hemochromatosis.

Pitting of the nails appears as punctate depressions in the nail plate. It is usually associated with psoriasis, affecting 10% to 50% of patients with that disorder. Individuals with psoriatic pitting have a high incidence of psoriatic bone disease.

Transverse linear depressions in the nail plate have been called Beau lines. Beau lines occur at the same spot of the nail plate in most or all of the person's nails and may be caused by any disease severe enough to disrupt normal nail growth. Knowing that nails grow about 1 mm every 6 to 10 days, the timing of the disease process may be estimated by measuring the distance from the line to the nail bed. The finding of Beau lines may indicate previous severe illness, trauma, or exposure to cold temperatures in patients with Raynaud disease.

Longitudinal pigmented bands are normal findings in the nails of dark-skinned persons, occurring in more than 77% of blacks older than 20 years. These findings present a diagnostic problem because they must be differentiated from subungual melanoma, which also occurs in older age groups and constitutes 50% of melanomas in dark-skinned populations.

Color and size changes in the lunula may be indicative of chronic disease. In patients with Wilson disease (hepatolenticular degeneration), the lunula takes on a blue coloration, a phenomenon called azure lunula. Patients with chronic renal failure and increased melanin production may cause the distal part of the nail bed to turn brown. Heart failure can turn the lunula red, and tetracycline therapy can turn it yellow. Silver poisoning will turn the nail itself a blue-gray color. Excessive fluoride ingestion can turn nails brown or black.

In patients with Terry nails, most of the nail plate turns white, and the lunula is obliterated. The condition may occur on only one digit, but more commonly all digits are affected. This condition was described originally in relation to hypoalbuminemia secondary to severe liver disease, usually cirrhosis, with 80% of these patients having Terry nails. In patients with severe renal disease, the proximal portion of the nail bed often turns white, obliterating the lunula and giving a half-brown, half-white appearance, also called half-and-half nails, and also known as Lindsey nails. Seventy percent of renal dialysis patients have Lindsay nails.

Differential cyanosis is a condition whereby the patient will have well-perfused pink upper extremities evident by the pink fingernails, whereas the lower extremities will have both cyanosis and clubbing of the toes. In adults, it is commonly seen in patients with patent ductus arteriosus when pulmonary hypertension has developed (right to left shunting of blood, or Eisenmenger syndrome). This occurs because venous blood shunts through the ductus and enters the aorta distal to the subclavian arteries.

In summary, many acute and chronic pathologies that manifest in the lower extremity can provide important information regarding the general health of the patient.

REFERENCES

1. Fowkes FG, Rudan D, Rudan I, et al. Comparison of global estimates of prevalence and risk factors for peripheral artery disease in 2000 and 2010: a systematic review and analysis. *Lancet.* 2013;382(9901):1329–1340.
2. Hirsch AT, Criqui MH, Treat-Jacobson D, et al. Peripheral arterial disease detection, awareness, and treatment in primary care. *JAMA.* 2001;286(11):1317–1324.
3. Bhatt DL, Steg PG, Ohman EM, et al. International prevalence, recognition, and treatment of cardiovascular risk factors in outpatients with atherothrombosis. *JAMA.* 2006;295(2):180–189.
4. Steg PG, Bhatt DL, Wilson PW, et al. One-year cardiovascular event rates in outpatients with atherothrombosis. *JAMA.* 2007;297(11):1197–1206.
5. Kownator S, Cambou JP, Cacoub P, et al. Prevalence of unknown peripheral arterial disease in patients with coronary artery disease: data in primary care from the IPSILON study. *Arch Cardiovasc Dis.* 2009;102(8-9):625–631.
6. Rutherford RB, Baker JD, Ernst C, et al. Recommended standards for reports dealing with lower extremity ischemia: revised version. *J Vasc Surg.* 1997;26(3):517–538.
7. Aboyans V, Criqui MH, Abraham P, et al. Measurement and interpretation of the ankle-brachial index: a scientific statement from the American Heart Association. *Circulation.* 2012;126(24):2890–2909.
8. Ankle Brachial Index Collaboration, Fowkes FG, Murray GD, et al. Ankle brachial index combined with Framingham risk score to predict cardiovascular events and mortality: a meta-analysis. *JAMA.* 2008;300(2):197–208.
9. Newman AB, Shemanski L, Manolio TA, et al. Ankle-arm index as a predictor of cardiovascular disease and mortality in the cardiovascular health study. The cardiovascular health study group. *Arterioscler Thromb Vasc Biol.* 1999;19(3):538–545.
10. Wild SH, Byrne CD, Smith FB, et al. Low ankle-brachial pressure index predicts increased risk of cardiovascular disease independent of the metabolic syndrome and conventional cardiovascular risk factors in the Edinburgh artery study. *Diabetes Care.* 2006;29(3):637–642.
11. Allison MA, Hiatt WR, Hirsch AT, et al. A high ankle-brachial index is associated with increased cardiovascular disease morbidity and lower quality of life. *J Am Coll Cardiol.* 2008;51(13):1292–1298.
12. Londahl M, Katzman P, Fredholm O, et al. Is chronic diabetic foot ulcer an indicator of cardiac disease? *J Wound Care.* 2008;17(1):12–16.
13. Crandall MA, Bradley DJ, Packer DL, et al. Contemporary management of atrial fibrillation: update on anticoagulation and invasive management strategies. *Mayo Clin Proc.* 2009;84(7):643–662.
14. Johnson JA, Everett BM, Katz JT, et al. Clinical problem-solving. Painful purple toes. *N Engl J Med.* 2010;362(1):67–73.
15. Yee J, McAllister CK. Osler's nodes and the recognition of infective endocarditis: a lesion of diagnostic importance. *South Med J.* 1987;80(6):753–757.
16. Gunson TH, Oliver GF. Osler's nodes and Janeway lesions. *Australas J Dermatol.* 2007;48(4):251–255.
17. Bursztejn AC, Bellut A, Weber-Muller F, et al. Erythematous macules on the feet in a case of cardiac myxoma. *Acta Derm Venereol.* 2009;89(3):321–322.
18. Navas JP, Martinez-Maldonado M. Pathophysiology of edema in congestive heart failure. *Heart Dis Stroke.* 1993;2(4):325–329.
19. Pepera GK, Sandercock GR, Sloan R, et al. Influence of step length on 6-minute walk test performance in patients with chronic heart failure. *Physiotherapy.* 2012;98(4):325–329.
20. Sarkar M, Mahesh DM, Madabhavi I. Digital clubbing. *Lung India.* 2012;29(4):354–362.

CHAPTER 4

Infectious Disease (Bone and Soft Tissue)

MARK KOSINSKI

THE HOST RESPONSE TO INFECTION

Infection can have a profound systemic effect on the human body. In the event of severe lower extremity infections, sepsis and even death can occur. In 1992, the American College of Chest Physicians (ACCP) and the Society of Critical Care Medicine (SCCM) introduced definitions for bacteremia, systemic inflammatory response syndrome (SIRS), sepsis, severe sepsis, septic shock, and multiple organ dysfunction syndrome. **Table 4-1** lists the definitions for sepsis and organ failure.[1]

Infection can be defined as an inflammatory response to the presence of microorganisms or the invasion of normally sterile host tissue by those organisms.[1] Bacteremia can be

Table 4-1. Definitions for Infection and Sepsis

Infection
The inflammatory response to the presence of microorganisms or the invasion of normally sterile host tissue by those organisms.
Bacteremia
The presence of viable bacteria in the blood.
Systemic Inflammatory Response Syndrome
The systemic response to inflammation, either infectious or noninfectious.   Two or more of the following conditions: 1. Temperature $>38°C$ or $<36°C$ 2. Heart rate >90 beats per minute   3. Respiratory rate >20 breaths per minute or $Paco_2 <32$ mm Hg   4. WBC count $>12,000$ per mm^3, $<4,000$ per mm^3, or $>10\%$ immature (band) forms
Sepsis
The systemic response to infection.   Two or more of the following conditions *as a result of infection:*   1. Temperature $>38°C$ or $<36°C$ 2. Heart rate >90 beats per minute   3. Respiratory rate >20 breaths per minute or $Paco_2 <32$ mm Hg   4. WBC count $>12,000$ per mm^3, $<4,000$ per mm^3, or $>10\%$ immature (band) forms.
Severe Sepsis
Sepsis is associated with organ dysfunction, hypoperfusion, or hypotension. Hypoperfusion and perfusion abnormalities may include, but are not limited to lactic acidosis, oliguria, or an acute alteration in mental status.
Septic Shock
Sepsis induced with hypotension despite adequate fluid resuscitation along with the presence of perfusion abnormalities that may include, but are not limited to, lactic acidosis, oliguria, or an acute alteration in mental status. Patients who are receiving inotropic or vasopressor agents may not be hypotensive at the time that perfusion abnormalities are measured.
Sepsis-Induced Hypotension
Systolic blood pressure <90 mm Hg or a reduction of >40 mm Hg from baseline in the absence of other causes of hypotension.
Multiple Organ Dysfunction Syndrome
Presence of altered organ function in an acutely ill patient such that homeostasis cannot be maintained without intervention.

Reprinted from Bone RC, Balk RA, Cerra FB, et al. American College of Chest Physicians/Society of Critical Care Medicine Consensus Conference: definitions for sepsis and organ failure and guidelines for the use of innovative therapies in sepsis. *Crit Care Med.* 1992;20:864–874, with permission.

defined as the presence of viable bacteria in the blood. Sepsis is defined as severe systemic inflammation in response to invading pathogens, or an uncontrolled hyperinflammatory response.[2] SIRS is the systemic response to an infectious or noninfectious insult and is characterized by two or more of the following: body temperature >38°C or <36°C, tachycardia (>90 beats per minute), respiratory rate >20 breaths per minute, $Paco_2 < 32$ mm Hg, and leukocytosis (>12,000 or <4,000 per mm³) or 10% immature (band) forms. It is non-specific as to etiology. Sepsis, on the other hand, is defined as the systemic response specifically to *infection*, its criteria being otherwise identical to SIRS.[3]

Purpura Fulminans as the Host Response to Sepsis

Sepsis is associated with multiple alterations in procoagulating and anticoagulating mechanisms,[4,5] which may lead to full-blown disseminated intravascular coagulation.

Sepsis-induced purpura fulminans (sometimes referred to as disseminated intravascular coagulation syndrome) is a relatively rare, multisystem disorder characterized by cutaneous hemorrhagic infarction, occlusion of dermal venules and capillaries by microthrombi. Skin necrosis may ultimately result in dry, gangrenous changes to the fingers and toes (**Fig. 4-1**).

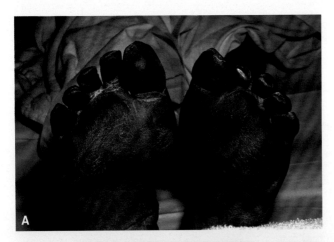

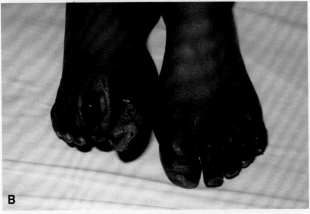

FIGURE 4-1. Patient with purpura fulminans. Note gangrenous changes to both feet and toes. (From Mark Kosinski, DPM, FIDSA, with permission).

It is caused by disseminated intravascular coagulation and dermal vascular thrombosis.

Acute infectious purpura fulminans presents concurrently with the signs and symptoms of sepsis. Clinically, the patient with purpura fulminans has concomitant disorders including septicemia, shock, and disseminated intravascular coagulation.[6]

Cutaneous necrosis begins with a region of skin discomfort that quickly progresses within hours to petechiae, which coalesce to form ecchymoses.[7] Purpuric skin lesions develop over the distal aspects of the feet and toes and tend to be symmetrical. These lesions can rapidly progress to hemorrhagic necrosis. Proximal extension of lower extremity lesions and diffuse patchy involvement of the abdomen and upper extremities can occur. Vascular changes are not limited to the skin; thrombosis and hemorrhagic necrosis are also common in other organ systems including the lungs, kidney, and adrenal glands, leading to multiorgan failure.

Once thought to be the result of septic embolization, purpura fulminans is caused by enhanced expression of the natural procoagulants and depletion of the natural anticoagulant proteins, particularly protein C.[6] Sepsis-related purpura fulminans is associated with severe, acute bacterial or viral infection, and has been most commonly associated with infections because of meningococci, *Neisseria meningitidis*, *Streptococcus pneumoniae* Gram-negative bacteria, *Haemophilus influenza*, group A and B streptococci, Staphylococci and rickettsia.[8–11] The cutaneous lesions of sepsis-induced purpura fulminans are similar, regardless of the causative organism. Cultures of skin lesions are usually negative, although bacterial colonization may occur with time. Amputation of the gangrenous portion of the extremity after demarcation may become necessary in severe cases.[12,13]

DIABETIC FOOT INFECTIONS

Diabetic foot infections (DFIs) are perhaps the most common and most limb-threatening infectious complications of systemic disease. It is estimated that approximately one in four people with diabetes will develop an ulcer during their lifetime and that as many as half of these ulcerations will develop an infection.[14] Approximately 15% to 20% of the estimated 16 million persons in the United States with diabetes mellitus will be hospitalized with a foot complication at some time during the course of their disease.[15] For those with diabetes, it has been estimated that the lifetime risk of developing a DFI is about 15% to 25%, although only about half of DFIs are clinically infected on presentation.[16,17]

Treatment of DFIs, whether bone or soft tissue, should be conducted as part of a multidisciplinary approach, with tight control of blood glucose and revascularization when necessary.

Most of the writings on DFI throughout the 1980s and into the early 1990s were based on studies from the 1970s that seemed to suggest that *all* DFIs were polymicrobial. We now know that mildly infected diabetic wounds harbor predominantly aerobic

Gram-positive cocci, not anaerobes. *Staphylococcus aureus* and Group B Streptococcus are by far the most common pathogens in the infected diabetic foot ulcerations. Unfortunately, there is a serious concern about increasing rates of multidrug-resistant organisms (MDROs) in general and methicillin resistance in *S. aureus* isolates in particular.

There have been many attempts to classify DFIs. Probably the most commonly used was introduced by Wagner,[18] which originally addressed only the dysvascular foot, but did not adequately address all diabetic foot ulcerations and infections.

The Infectious Diseases Society of America (IDSA) Practice Guidelines for the Diagnosis and Treatment of DFIs is perhaps the most widely used treatment-based classification system in current use and has been validated as a useful tool for grading foot infections.[19] This system can assist the clinician in deciding whether or not an antibiotic is indicated, which antibiotic to choose, when to use a parenteral versus an oral antibiotic agent, when to hospitalize a patient, and when to consider surgical intervention. Under these guidelines, DFIs are classified as being mild, moderate, or severe.

Noninfected Ulcerations

Noninfected wounds, by definition, do not require antibiotic therapy. Routine culturing of wounds that do not appear clinically infected (i.e., no cellulitis, purulence, erythema) should be avoided because even noninfected ulcerations are colonized with multiple organisms.[20]

The use of antibiotics to "prevent" infection is not supported by currently available medical evidence and may lead to the development of resistant organisms[21] that may make subsequent infections more difficult to treat. In at least one study, microbial load and diversity has been shown not to be predictive of weeks-to-closure or percent reduction in surface area per week.[22] Antibiotics should be used to treat infections, not heal wounds.

A common misconception is that patients with diabetes do not respond with cellulitis. Although there *may* be muted response to *some* of the signs of infection, it is extremely unlikely that there would be no evidence of cellulitis at all. Cellulitis is therefore a reliable indicator of infection in all but the most arterially compromised patients.

Mild Infection

The belief that all DFIs are polymicrobial has changed. Decades ago, it was thought that even mildly infected diabetic wounds harbored anaerobic bacteria such as *Bacteroides fragilis*, leading to treatment with broad spectrum antibiotics even in the face of negative anaerobic cultures.

We now know that mildly infected diabetic wounds harbor predominantly aerobic Gram-positive cocci. Whether the infection is mild, moderate, or severe, *S. aureus* and Group B Streptococcus are far and away the most common pathogens encountered.

Wounds with a mild infection show at least two of the signs and symptoms of a host response. There is usually localized cellulitis around the wound that extends <2 cm from the wound border. Purulent exudate may be present; however, the infection remains localized. There is no deep extension or proximal spread. There is no lymphangiitis or lymphadenopathy. There are no systemic signs or symptoms of infection, and the patient's white blood cell (WBC) count and blood glucose are not above the patient's usual range.

Mildly infected diabetic ulcers are treated no differently with respect to antibiotic choice and duration compared with similar wounds in nondiabetic patients and can usually be treated on an outpatient basis with oral antibiotic therapy. Antibiotic therapy should be directed against *S. aureus* and Streptococcus, with the caveat that there are increasing rates of methicillin-resistant *S. aureus* (MRSA) in these patients. Anaerobic coverage in these wounds is unnecessary. The use of broad spectrum agents such as amoxicillin/clavulanate or moxifloxacin, while not wrong, can be considered overkill.[23]

Some patients may require debridement or incision and drainage for a small abscess or offloading of pressure areas. It is recommended that the patient follow up in a few days to review the results of culture and sensitivity tests and to ensure there has been an adequate response to treatment.

Moderate and Severe Infections

Moderate and severe infections are often classified together. The choice of antibiotics to treat each group is often similar, owing to the similarity of the spectrum of infecting organisms. However, moderate infections are limb threatening, whereas severe infections are life threatening.

According to the 2012 IDSA guidelines,[19] moderate infections can be defined as those with cellulitis extending >2 cm from the wound margin or penetration of infection into the deeper tissues, such as fascia, tendon, muscle, or bone. Lymphadenopathy or lymphangiitis may be present. The patient is systemically well and metabolically stable, although there may be a mild elevation of the WBC count. Blood glucose levels may be higher than the patient's usual values.

Compared with a moderate infection, the hallmark of a severe infection is evidence of a septic state. The patient may be febrile, hypotensive, and confused or have significant metabolic imbalance (e.g., azotemia and acidosis). Distinct from mild infections, moderate and severe infections tend to be polymicrobial. *S. aureus*, including MRSA and Streptococci (Group B), are still the predominant pathogens, but Gram-negative organisms are commonly found.

There has been some debate as to the need to direct antibiotic therapy toward Gram-negative organisms in general and *Pseudomonas aeruginosa* in particular. Although an important pathogen in respiratory tract and urinary tract infections, there are data to suggest that *P. aeruginosa* when cultured from skin and soft tissue infections may exist as a commensal rather than a true pathogen, and therapy directed against this bacteria may not be necessary to effect a cure in diabetic lower extremity skin and skin structure infections.[23,24] Anaerobic bacteria such as *Bacteroides fragilis* are more frequently seen in these wounds, and whether suspected or cultured, it is often prudent to direct therapy toward them.[25,26] This is especially true in the case of infections in which gas is seen on X-ray.

THE ROLE OF ANAEROBES IN DFIS

The presence of anaerobic bacteria in DFIs is probably overestimated by most physicians. When present in lower extremity infections, anaerobes such as *Bacteroides* spp. are more commonly seen in moderate to severe infections, rarely if ever in mild infections, and almost never present as solitary organisms. Anaerobic bacteria require specialized culture media, rapid transport to the lab, and strict anaerobic conditions when cultured. Because of this, it may be more useful to employ 16s polymerase chain reaction (PCR) and pyrosequencing to detect their presence, rather than relying on traditional culture methods. Unfortunately, as of this writing, these tests are costly and not widely available.

There is a timeworn saying, "all that is gas is not clostridia." Although the presence of gas in soft tissue on X-ray can indeed indicate the presence of anaerobic bacteria, it is probably more often than not caused by gas-producing Gram-negative bacteria such as *Klebsiella*, *Proteus*, or *Escherichia coli* rather than obligate anaerobes. There are even nonbacterial causes of "gas in tissue," including the use of high-pressure irrigation in the operating room or the use of hydrogen peroxide flushes employed by the patient. In a recent literature review concerning the epidemiology, antibiotic susceptibility, and clinical significance of anaerobic isolates in patients with DFIs, 44 published studies were found, involving a total of 13,012 patients. Of these, the incidence of anaerobic pathogens was only 11%.[27] No epidemiologic survey to date has reported a worse outcome for wounds from which anaerobic bacteria were isolated compared with no-anaerobes, with the possible exception of *Clostridium* spp.[28]

Nonetheless, it has become standard practice by many to employ broad spectrum antibiotics with anaerobic activity in most if not all moderate to severe DFIs. Long-term coverage of anaerobic bacteria may not only be unnecessary, but may have the unwanted side effect of driving antibiotic resistance and increase health care costs. Antibiotics are not without their adverse events. In a recently published study from Istanbul, Turkey, almost 20% of patients receiving piperacillin/tazobactam for >10 days developed neutropenia (neutrophil count of <2,000 cells per mm^3).[29]

THE PROBLEM OF DRUG-RESISTANT ORGANISMS IN DFIS

In the past decade, one of the important changes in the microbiology of DFIs is the increasing isolation of MDROs. An MDRO can be defined as an organism with decreased susceptibility to multiple (usually two or three) *classes* of antimicrobial agents to which the organism would normally be susceptible.[30]

One of the most important Gram-positive MDROs is MRSA. In a survey of 97 US hospitals conducted between 2003 and 2007, the prevalence of MRSA in hospitalized patients with a DFI almost doubled, from 11.6% to 21.9%.[31]

Despite the prevalence of MRSA, treating every DFI for MRSA is unnecessary and likely to lead to a further increase in resistance as well as raise the cost of health care.[32] Although the isolation of MRSA would seem to be a factor associated with treatment failure in patients with DFIs,[33] it has not been demonstrated to be associated with longer hospitalization or a higher incidence of amputations.[32,34] In fact, studies by Hartemann-Huertier et al.[35] as well as Richard et al.[36] found that the presence of MDROs, most notably MRSA, had no significant impact on healing time of diabetic foot wounds when compared with methicillin-susceptible *S. aureus*.

Empiric coverage for MRSA should be started for patients with known risk factors, and for those patients with severe infections in whom failure to promptly treat would lead to loss of life or limb.

Risk factors associated with MRSA infection of foot ulcers include the presence of MDROs, history of an MRSA DFI, and a positive MRSA nasal culture.[32]

There are currently two newly approved antibiotics to treat MRSA infections. Ceftaroline is a parenteral-only extended spectrum cephalosporin that is active against MRSA and has the Gram-negative activity of a third-generation cephalosporin. Tedizolid is a newer oxazolidinone, similar to linezolid, except with once-daily dosing and without the serotonin syndrome risk.

The other MDRO seen with an increasing incidence is extended spectrum β-lactamase (ESBL)–producing Gram negatives (so named because they produce enzymes that hydrolyze *extended spectrum* cephalosporins). The increase in ESBL-producing strains jeopardizes the usefulness of β-lactam agents, leading to increases in costs and treatment failures. These organisms are being found with increasing frequency in DFIs.[37,38]

ESBLs are found in many commonly encountered Gram-negative organisms including *Klebsiella*, *E. coli*, *Acinetobacter*, *Citrobacter*, *Enterobacter*, *Morganella*, *Proteus*, *Pseudomonas*, *Salmonella*, and *Serratia*. ESBLs can hydrolyze oxyimino cephalosporins (ceftazidime, ceftriaxone, cefepime, cefotaxime) and monobactams (aztreonam) but cannot hydrolyze carbapenems (imipenem, meropenem, ertapenem).

Unfortunately, Gram-negative active agents such as aminoglycosides, trimethoprim–sulfamethoxazole (TMP/SMX), and quinolones may not be effective either. Plasmids w/genes encoding for ESBLs may also carry genes conferring resistance to aminoglycosides, TMP/SMX, and quinolones. Even when plasmid-encoded decrease in quinolone susceptibility is not present, there is a strong association between quinolone resistance and ESBL production.

The carbapenems have therefore emerged as the "go-to" class of antibiotics for treatment of ESBL Gram-negative infections, and for many years have held the top spot in this regard.

Unfortunately, some Gram-negative organisms have developed resistance to even the carbapenems. Collectively known as CRE (carbapenem-resistant Enterobacteriaceae), these organisms are resistant to not only carbapenems, but to penicillins, cephalosporins, and monobactams as well.[39] The most common type of carbapenemase (enzyme) currently seen in the United States is Klebsiella pneumonia carbapenemase. However, other enzymes capable of inactivating carbapenems have been discovered as well; among them are New Delhi metallo β-lactamase[40,41] and Verona integron-encoded metallo β-lactamase-1.[42]

Current treatment options for CRE infections are limited and include tigecycline and colistin. Newer drugs are under development. One such drug, avibactam, has been shown to inhibit extended spectrum β-lactamase and carbapenemase enzymes produced by Gram negatives in much the same way that tazobactam, sulbactam, and clavulanic acid inhibit β-lactamase produced by *S. aureus*. The addition of avibactam to existing antibiotics such as aztreonam and ceftaroline will result in a new compound with extended activity against a wide range of multidrug-resistant Gram-negative organisms.

DIABETIC FOOT OSTEOMYELITIS

It has been estimated that approximately 15% of diabetic foot ulcers are complicated by osteomyelitis, and in some centers approximately 20% of patients who present with a DFI have involvement of the underlying bone.[43] Most cases of diabetic foot osteomyelitis are chronic by the time they present. Infection of bone in the foot of a patient with diabetes usually occurs via contiguous spread from an overlying soft tissue ulceration. The presence of osteomyelitis increases the likelihood of lower extremity amputation. Thus, accurately diagnosing and treating diabetic foot osteomyelitis is of critical importance. Bone biopsy with culture and histopathology is still considered the criterion standard for diagnosing diabetic foot osteomyelitis, whereas magnetic resonance imaging (MRI) is currently considered the imaging modality of choice.

It has long been held that, with the possible exception of *S. aureus*, there exists little or no correlation between organisms cultured from a sinus tract and the infecting organism in bone. The question therefore arises as to the reliability of swab cultures in determining the bone pathogen.

In his seminal study, Mackowiak et al.[44] found only 44% of the sinus tract cultures contained the operative pathogen, with *S. aureus* having the highest correlation. Since then, however, there have been several studies that suggest that a carefully obtained culture of a sinus tract may indeed correlate well with bone cultures, depending on how they are performed.[45–47] Bernard et al.[46] demonstrated that

deep sinus tract cultures *in contact with bone* correlate well with bone biopsy specimens obtained through adjacent, noninfected skin. The reason for this may simply be that bacteria in the superficial portion of a sinus tract originate from skin, whereas bacteria in the deeper portion of a sinus tract originates from bone. Bernard found that performing two consecutive deep sinus tract cultures with bone contact accurately predicted the pathogen of diabetic foot osteomyelitis in 90% of cases.[46]

As mentioned, bone biopsy remains the criterion standard for diagnosis. Although rarely performed routinely, a bone biopsy can yield a wealth of information. A percutaneous 11ga or 13ga Jamshidi needle bone biopsy is simple to do, can be performed at the bedside or in an outpatient setting under local anesthesia, and is safe. The specimen should be obtained by going through adjacent, noninfected skin, if possible. In addition to confirming the presence of osteomyelitis, a bone biopsy can identify the causative organism and its antibiotic susceptibilities. In a retrospective cohort study of 50 consecutive patients with diabetic foot osteomyelitis treated nonsurgically, Senneville et al.[48] found that bone culture–based antibiotic therapy was the only variable significantly associated with remission of infection. There is, however, one important caveat to performing a percutaneous bone biopsy: chronic osteomyelitis can be a patchy disease, and there is no guarantee that a specimen of bone harvested "by feel" during a blind procedure will be "on the money." False negatives can result if infected bone is missed. It may therefore be advisable to perform the procedure under ultrasound guidance in order to increase the chances for a positive yield.

TREATING DIABETIC FOOT OSTEOMYELITIS

Osteomyelitis is still considered by many to be primarily a surgical disease.

The long-held standard (and, for some, dogmatic) approach to treating diabetic foot osteomyelitis has been to aggressively resect all infected and devitalized bone, and to follow up with 6 weeks of parenteral antibiotic therapy directed against a bone biopsy–recovered pathogen.

Surgical removal of all infected bone probably gives the best chance for a cure, as leaving infected bone behind increases the possibility for recurrence. Factors that favor surgical intervention include major bone destruction, acute infections requiring drainage, problems in limb perfusion, the presence of MDROs, and contraindication for or patient refusal of prolonged antibiotic therapy.

The surgeon, in an attempt to preserve gait and function, may opt for partial resection rather than aggressively pursuing amputation. However, patients with positive margins for residual osteomyelitis after surgical resection have been found to be at greater risk for treatment failure, including the need for more proximal amputation despite the longer duration of antibiotic therapy.[49]

Treating osteomyelitis can therefore be likened to treating certain forms of cancer. Wide excision and removal of *all* affected bone is optimal. Residual affected bone requires chemotherapy (antibiotics). As long as there remains infected bone, there remains the chance for recurrence. In the case of incomplete excision, remission may be the best that can be hoped for.

The notion that diabetic foot osteomyelitis is *always* a surgical disease is changing.

There are instances when surgery is not a viable option, such as when it is the patient's choice to avoid surgery or comorbidities confer an unacceptably high risk. In such situations, and when there are no contraindications to prolonged antibiotic therapy, medical-only (nonsurgical) management may be considered. A recent systematic review of patients treated for diabetic foot osteomyelitis found that there is currently no evidence that surgical debridement of the infected bone is routinely necessary, nor are there sufficient data to support the superiority of any particular antibiotic agent or route of delivery.[50] Zeun et al.[51] conducted a retrospective study of consecutive patients with diabetes presenting to a tertiary center between 2007 and 2011 with foot osteomyelitis initially treated with nonsurgical management. Almost two-thirds of patients presenting with osteomyelitis healed without undergoing surgical bone resection or the requirement for further antibiotic therapy.

The evidence for selecting an arbitrary 6-week duration of treatment is weak, largely resting on the results of experimental studies of acute staphylococcal osteomyelitis in rabbits[52,53]

and observations of the time it takes for bone healing to occur. Applying a standardized regimen to every patient may end up overtreating some, and undertreating others. Likewise, there are currently no data to indicate the superiority or inferiority of any particular route of administration (oral vs. parenteral) or any antibiotic over another for treating osteomyelitis. For some, this may seem counterintuitive.

Over the past few years, there have been a number of studies to support the use of oral (as opposed to parenteral) antibiotics as the sole therapy in the treatment of diabetic foot osteomyelitis, and to date there are no studies that appear to favor one particular antibiotic over another. The most important factors are that they have high bioavailability and are active against the infecting organism. Highly bioavailable antibiotics that are effective in the presence of biofilm[54] and can enter host cells[15] have changed the way we think about treating chronic osteomyelitis and may make nonsurgical management feasible in some cases. This is a somewhat iconoclastic view because parenteral antibiotics have remained for many (for better or worse) the perceived gold standard of treatment. Despite emerging evidence to the contrary, many clinicians still doggedly cling to the notion that parenteral is superior to oral for treating chronic bone infection. Adherence to such dogma leads to overutilization of parenteral antibiotics (which should be best reserved for treating acute infection), increases health care costs (increased length of hospital stay, placement of peripherally inserted central catheter lines, infusion nurses, materials associated with IV meds etc.), and presents the possibility of infection of the IV line itself.

Table 4-2. Suggested Route, Setting, and Duration of Antibiotic Therapy, by Clinical Syndrome

Site of Infection, by Severity or Extent	Route of Administration	Setting	Duration of Therapy
Soft-Tissue Only			
Mild	Topical or oral	Outpatient	1–2 wk; may extend up to 4 wk if slow to resolve
Moderate	Oral (or initial parenteral)	Outpatient/inpatient	1–3 wk
Severe	Initial parenteral, switch to oral when possible	Inpatient, then outpatient	2–4 wk
Bone or Joint			
No residual infected tissue (e.g., postamputation)	Parenteral or oral	—	2–5 d
Residual infected soft tissue (but not bone)	Parenteral or oral	—	1–3 wk
Residual infected (but viable) bone	Initial parenteral, then consider oral switch	—	4–6 wk
No surgery, or residual dead bone postoperatively	Initial parenteral, then consider oral switch	—	≥3 mo

Reprinted from Lipsky BA, Berendt AR, Cornia PB, et al. 2012 Infectious Diseases Society of America clinical practice guideline for the diagnosis and treatment of diabetic foot infections. *Clin Infect Dis.* 2012;54(12):e132–e173, with permission.

In a retrospective study by Embil et al.,[55] remission was achieved in over 80% of 93 episodes of diabetic foot osteomyelitis treated with oral antibiotic agents, 78% of whom had no bone debridement or resection. Game et al.[56] noted similar results, with a remission rate of over 82% noted in patients treated with antibiotics alone, compared with 78% in those treated with antibiotics and only minor amputation.

Recent studies also suggest the optimal length of treatment may even be significantly shorter than once thought. Tone et al.[57] compared 6- versus 12-week duration of antibiotic treatment at five French general hospitals. Remission was obtained in 26 (65%) patients, with no significant differences between patients treated for 6 versus 12 weeks. Patients received oral antibiotics for either all or as a major part of their treatment.

Regardless of the mode or duration of therapy, patients who achieve remission must be carefully monitored for at least 1 year because they may develop a recurrence of osteomyelitis despite "appropriate" treatment. Algorithms are needed that would reliably predict which patients would be most responsive to nonsurgical treatment, and which could receive exclusively oral antibiotic therapy. Currently, the IDSA Clinical Practice Guidelines for the Diagnosis and Treatment of DFIs are useful for estimating the length of therapy required based on the extent of resection and viability of affected bone (**Table 4-2**).[19] In light of new studies, it will be interesting to see how the IDSA recommendations will change in their next incarnation.

OTHER LOWER EXTREMITY INFECTIOUS COMPLICATIONS OF SYSTEMIC DISEASE

SEPTIC EMBOLIZATION TO THE FEET AND TOES FROM INFECTIVE ENDOCARDITIS

Peripheral embolization to the feet and toes from a proximal source of infection has been described in patients with infective endocarditis. Thromboembolic complications occur when the vegetations adherent to the endocardium or heart valves fragment and seed to distal sites—including the lower extremities.[58] This can result in focal necrotizing lesions or painful localized erythema and swelling.[59] Staphylococcus and Streptococcus are the most common organisms responsible for infective endocarditis, with Strep accounting for the majority of all cases.

The extracardiac, physical findings of infective endocarditis may be extensive[60] and include Osler nodes (painful) and Janeway lesions (painless).[61] Janeway lesions have been described on the palms and soles.[62] Osler nodes have also been described in the foot in patients with enterococcal endocarditis and S. aureus endocarditis.[63] Splinter hemorrhages of the toenails as well as the fingernails may be seen in subacute bacterial endocarditis and should be differentiated from splinter hemorrhages of microtrauma.

REACTIVE ARTHRITIS

Heel pain is one of the most common foot complaints that drives patients to seek medical care.

More often than not, it is of biomechanical origin and the result of the pull of tight plantar fascia (or Achilles tendon in the case of retrocalcaneal pain) from its attachment on the calcaneus. The diagnosis of reactive arthritis must be included in the differential for cases of heel pain when the symptoms are bilateral and refractory to treatment.

Reactive arthritis (once commonly referred to as Reiter syndrome) is considered a form of spondyloarthritis. It is an immune-mediated, sterile synovitis caused by a host response to an extra-articular slow bacterial infection, producing arthritis without infecting the joint itself. Causative organisms of reactive arthritis include *Chlamydia*, *Salmonella*, *Shigella*, *Campylobacter*, *Ureaplasma*, and *Yersinia* species.[64]

Genitourinary tract infection with *Chlamydia trachomatis* is the more commonly recognized cause of reactive arthritis in developed countries and has been identified in the United States as the preceding infection in 42% to 69% of patients with urogenic reactive arthritis.[65]

Reactive arthritis is distinguished by the classic triad of symptoms best characterized by medical students as the patient who "can't see" (conjunctivitis), "can't pee" (urethritis), and "can't climb a tree" (arthritis). It is important to note that only about one-third of patients present with all three components.[66]

Additional manifestations include dactylitis, keratoderma blennorrhagicum, and nail changes or may present with a recent onset of diarrhea or urinary tract infection. Constitutional symptoms may include fever, malaise, fatigue, and weight loss. Obtaining a thorough medical history is therefore essential.

Radiographic evidence of reactive arthritis is not present in every case. An unusual or bifurcate plantar calcaneal spur often suggests that the heel pain is not of biomechanical origin. The calcaneus may exhibit a fluffy periostitis (the so-called "lover's heel" implying a sexually transmitted etiology) with a poorly defined, frayed appearance at the insertion of the plantar aponeurosis and Achilles tendon. Radiographic evidence of Reiter syndrome is present in only about 25% to 50% of patients.[67]

The clinical course of reactive arthritis is unpredictable and variable. In some patients, the disease takes a more chronic course. In others, initial attacks may last from a few months to a year or more, with relapses occurring after long disease-free intervals.

Reactive arthritis is thought to be linked to the human leukocyte antigen (HLA)-B27.[68]

HLA-B27 has become an overused diagnostic test, however, as not every HLA-B27–positive patient will develop Reiter syndrome.[69] Synovial fluid analysis reveals inflammatory changes, including elevated WBC count, turbidity, poor viscosity, and poor mucin clot tests. Synovial glucose level is not significantly reduced as it is in septic arthritis. Gram stains of synovial fluid are negative, as are cultures.

Diagnosis of reactive arthritis is supported by isolation of an infectious entity from a nonarticular site. However, because this is rarely achieved, an increased antibody titer of a suspected organism often serves as a sufficient diagnostic criterion to specify the etiologic agent. Intra-articular bacteria, when present, are nonculturable; however, microbial DNA and RNA have been detected in the joints of patients with reactive arthritis.[65,70]

OSTEOARTICULAR TUBERCULOSIS

Tuberculosis (TB) is alive and well in our modern world. One-third of the world's population is infected with TB. In 2014, 9.6 million people around the world became sick with TB disease. There were 1.5 million TB-related deaths worldwide.[71] Osteoarticular TB is perhaps one of the most frequently misdiagnosed infectious diseases of bone.

TB is a chronic disease caused by *Mycobacterium tuberculosis*. Transmission commonly occurs by inhalation of aerosolized droplets of respiratory secretions from a patient with active pulmonary TB. TB has been named the second great imitator after syphilis by Sievers[72] because of its multiple and unusual presentations.

Clinical symptoms of active pulmonary TB include fever, weight loss, and productive cough often with bloody sputum. Patients with skeletal TB may have no active pulmonary disease and hence no systemic symptoms other than pain at the affected site. A negative chest X-ray does not exclude the diagnosis, nor does a nonreactive purified protein derivative (PPD) skin test. Peripheral skeletal TB, however, can exist without evidence of pulmonary involvement either clinically or radiographically.[73] Patients with abnormalities of the immune system (such as advanced human immunodeficiency virus [HIV] disease), advanced age, and even overwhelming tuberculous infection may have a false-negative PPD skin test.[73,74] Quantiferon-TB Gold (QFT-G; Cellestis, Ltd., Carnegie, Australia) is useful for detecting both active and latent infection.

Peripheral skeletal TB is caused by subsequent dissemination of *M. tuberculosis* by hematogenous spread or lymphatic drainage early in the course of the infection.

Skeletal involvement is rare. Foot involvement is even rarer[75,76] and is estimated to account for just 10% of osteoarticular TB and 0.1% to 0.3% of all patients with extrapulmonary disease.[77] The initial lesion is either in the bone or in the synovium, and one subsequently infects the other.[78] It can occur at any age. Bozkurt et al.[79] presented a case of TB osteomyelitis of the medial cuneiform in a 3-year-old child.

The evolution of skeletal TB is subtle: pain is often the presenting symptom. Early radiographic signs are nonspecific and mimic osteoarthritis. Lesions may remain silent for years without significant progression until reactivation occurs via trauma or a similar event.[80] It is this slow indolent progression coupled with its ability to mimic other disease states that allows an accurate diagnosis to be delayed.

Vertebral lesions (Pott disease) may cause symptoms of radiculopathy. Lumbosacral involvement may cause numbness, tingling, and weakness of the lower extremities.

When found in the foot, it most commonly occurs in the calcaneus and the tarsal bones.[77]

The typical radiographic presentation is or often nonspecific and characterized by juxta-articular osteoporosis, peripheral osseous erosions, and gradual joint space narrowing, known as the Phemister triad.[78,81,82] MRI is accepted as the imaging modality most useful in aiding diagnosis and revealing the extent of the disease.[73] Tuberculomas can be synovial (rare), osseous (frequent), or articular (indicative of a late stage)[78] and present with or without sinus tracts or ulceration.

The cornerstone of diagnosis of osteoarticular TB depends on demonstration of *M. tuberculosis* on either a histologic study or culture. Molecular diagnostics such as TB-PCR, line probe assays, or nucleic acid amplification tests have also been shown to be useful diagnostic tools.[83]

One of the most useful procedures for the diagnosis of TB arthritis is the synovial membrane biopsy. A definitive diagnosis is based on identification of *M. tuberculosis* in granulomas, synovial fluid, or synovial membrane. Biopsy should be taken from the granulomatous or cystic area or from immediately adjacent synovium.[77] Samples can be harvested by either open biopsy or CT-guided percutaneous needle aspiration.

It is prudent for the clinician to order acid-fast stains and cultures on bone and synovial membrane biopsies. Acid-fast organisms grow slowly. Culture reports may take several weeks to return. Acid-fast stains may be ordered to aid in the empiric diagnosis in the interim. Molecular diagnostics in TB has enabled rapid detection of *M. tuberculosis* complex in clinical specimens.[84]

Cultures are more sensitive than stains, and can reliably identify mycobacteria in a concentration of 103 organisms per mL of specimen. A specimen of at least 1 mL should be sent for culture. In cases of multiple bone lesions, it is important to obtain cultures from each focus of infection. Different strains of *M. tuberculosis*, each with different sensitivities, may reside in each focus of infection.

A negative PPD does not exclude the possibility of TB. The question arises as to whether a negative reaction is caused by lack of infection with *M. tuberculosis* or the patient's inability to mount a response to the skin test antigen. Indeed, patients with immune abnormalities (such as advanced HIV disease), advanced age, and even overwhelming TB infection may have a false-negative PPD.

It is important to remember that pyogenic bacteria such as *S. aureus* can coexist with *M. tuberculosis* in infected bone and soft tissue.[85] Mycobacterial osteomyelitis should be suspected when improvement does not occur with appropriate antibiotic therapy directed toward pyogenic bacteria. Unless acid-fast stains and cultures are specifically performed, a mycobacterial infection will be missed. A high index of suspicion is needed.

OSTEOMYELITIS IN SICKLE CELL DISEASE

Sickle cell disease is a congenital hemolytic anemia caused by inheritance of abnormal hemoglobin genes. It is one of the most common inherited blood diseases, and has worldwide distribution.[86] Sickle cell disease is characterized by acute episodes of painful vaso-occlusive crises.[87]

Osteomyelitis is a well-known complication of sickle cell disease. Bones are the second most affected organs after the spleen. During sickle cell crises, bone and muscle infarcts with necrosis occur, providing a nidus for infection. Recurrent vascular infarctions cause end-organ damage to the bone, lung, liver, kidney, skin, and spleen.[87] Autosplenectomy and surgical splenectomy render sickle cell disease patients susceptible to various types of infections, mainly from encapsulated bacteria.[88]

A French study of a cohort of 299 patients followed in four Parisian centers found a prevalence of osteomyelitis of 12%.[89] In another study, a relative rate of occurrence of almost 18% was found for osteomyelitis and 7% for septic arthritis.[90]

Osteomyelitis most commonly affects the long bones, but can involve other bones including those of the foot[87]; multifocal bone involvement has been recognized to occur in as many as a quarter of patients diagnosed with sickle cell osteomyelitis.[91]

The most common cause of osteomyelitis in sickle cell disease is Salmonella (especially the nontypical serotypes *Salmonella typhimurium*, *Salmonella enteritidis*, *Salmonella choleraesuis*, and Salmonella paratyphi B), followed by S. *aureus* and Gram-negative enteric bacilli, perhaps because intravascular sickling of the bowel leads to patchy ischemic infarction.[92]

Osteomyelitis caused by vancomycin-resistant *Enterococcus faecium* has also been reported.[91]

Dactylitis, also known as hand–foot syndrome, is an acute vaso-occlusive complication characterized by pain and edema in both hands and feet, frequently with increased local temperature and erythema.[93]

Sickling crisis are thought to be many times more common than bacterial osteomyelitis. Distinguishing between acute osteomyelitis and vaso-occlusive crisis bone infarction remains challenging, particularly in culture-negative cases.[94] Failure to correctly diagnose osteomyelitis in sickle cell disease may result in severe bone damage, whereas an erroneous diagnosis subjects the patient to unnecessary long-term antibiotic therapy.

Blood culture is positive in 50% of cases of acute osteomyelitis and is often required to diagnose infection accurately. If infection is not suspected and blood is sampled later in the course of management, cultures usually are unhelpful. Even the culture of biopsy specimens is not completely reliable.[95] Ultrasound and advanced imaging modalities such as MRI and single-photon emission computed tomography (SPECT)/CT[87] in combination with C-reactive protein and WBC count may assist in distinguishing bone infarct from osteomyelitis.[94]

HUMAN IMMUNODEFICIENCY VIRUS

In the early stages of the HIV epidemic, it was estimated that more than half of all patients infected with HIV would experience some bone or joint symptom during the course of their disease.[96] With recent advances in antiretroviral therapy, these numbers have undoubtedly declined.

Nonetheless, HIV infection has been associated with several types of arthritis, of which reactive arthritides are the most common. Although it is questionable that HIV infection is capable of initiating reactive arthritis, it undoubtedly increases the severity of reactive arthritis.[97] HIV-associated reactive arthritis frequently follows an accelerated course with a strong tendency to relapse, develop early erosions and joint deformity, and become chronic.[98–100]

Septic arthritis caused by fungal and mycobacterial organisms (e.g., *Candida* species, *Cryptococcus neoformans*, *Histoplasma capsulatum*, *Mycobacterium avium-intracellulare*, *Sporothrix schenckii*, and *M. tuberculosis*) also has been associated with HIV infection and may occur as a result of hematogenous dissemination of systemic infection.

It is therefore recommended that when dealing with any infectious process in a patient with HIV, aerobic, anaerobic, acid-fast, and fungal stains and cultures be included.

REFERENCES

1. Bone RC, Balk RA, Cerra FB, et al. American College of Chest Physicians/Society of Critical Care Medicine Consensus Conference: definitions for sepsis and organ failure and guidelines for the use of innovative therapies in sepsis. *Crit Care Med*. 1992;20:864–874.
2. Yao YM, Luan YY, Zhang QH, et al. Pathophysiological aspects of sepsis: an overview. *Methods Mol Biol*. 2015;1237:5–15.
3. Nierhaus A, Klatte S, Linssen J, et al. Revisiting the white blood cell count: immature granulocytes count as a diagnostic marker to discriminate between SIRS and sepsis—a prospective, observational study. *BMC Immunol*. 2013;14:8.
4. Levi M. The coagulant response in sepsis and inflammation. *Hamostaseologie*. 2010;30(10–12):14–16.
5. Levi M, van der Poll T. Inflammation and coagulation. *Crit Care Med*. 2010;38:S26–S34.
6. Betrosian AP, Berlet T, Agarwal B. Purpura fulminans in sepsis. *Am J Med Sci*. 2006;332(6):339–345.
7. Alexander G, Basheer HM, Ebrahim MK, et al. Idiopathic purpura fulminans and varicella gangrenosa of both hands, toes and integument in a child. *Br J Plast Surg*. 2003;56:194–195.
8. Deshmukh PM, Camp CJ, Rose FB, et al. Capnocytophaga canimorsus sepsis with purpura fulminans and symmetrical gangrene following a dog bite in a shelter employee. *Am J Med Sci*. 2004;327:369–372.

9. Kravitz GR, Dries DJ, Peterson ML, et al. Purpura fulminans due to *Staphylococcus aureus*. *Clin Infect Dis*. 2005;40:941–947.

10. Huemer GM, Bonatti H, Dunst KM. Purpura fulminans due to *E. coli* septicemia. *Wien Klin Wochenschr*. 2004;116:82.

11. Olowu WA. Klebsiella-induced purpura fulminans in a Nigerian child: case report and a review of literature. *West Afr J Med*. 2002;21:252–255.

12. Adcock DM, Hicks MJ. Dermatopathology of skin necrosis associated with purpura fulminans. *Semin Thromb Hemost*. 1990;16:283–292.

13. Childers BJ, Cobanov B. Acute infectious purpura fulminans: a 15-year retrospective review of 28 consecutive cases. *Am Surg*. 2003;69:86–90.

14. Lavery LA, Armstrong DG, Murdoch DP, et al. Validation of the Infectious Diseases Society of America's diabetic foot infection classification system. *Clin Infect Dis*. 2007;44:562–565.

15. Reiber GE, Boyko EJ, Smith DG. Lower extremity foot ulcers and amputations in diabetes. In: National Diabetes Data Group (U.S.), ed. *Diabetes in America*. 2nd ed. Bethesda, MD: National Institutes of Health, National Institute of Diabetes and Digestive and Kidney Diseases; 1995. NIH publication no. 95–1468.

16. Lavery LA, Armstrong DG, Wunderlich RP, et al. Risk factors for foot infections in individuals with diabetes. *Diabetes Care*. 2006;29:1288–1293.

17. Singh N, Armstrong DG, Lipsky BA. Preventing foot ulcers in patients with diabetes. *JAMA*. 2005;293:217–228.

18. Wagner FW. The diabetic foot. *Orthopedics*. 1987;10(1):163–172.

19. Lipsky BA, Berendt AR, Cornia PB, et al. 2012 Infectious Diseases Society of America clinical practice guideline for the diagnosis and treatment of diabetic foot infections. *Clin Infect Dis*. 2012;54(12):e132–e173.

20. Wolcott RD, Hanson JD, Rees EJ, et al. Analysis of the chronic wound microbiota of 2,963 patients by 16S rDNA pyrosequencing. *Wound Repair Regen*. 2016;24:163–174.

21. Abbas M, Uçkay I, Lipsky BA. In diabetic foot infections antibiotics are to treat infection, not to heal wounds. *Expert Opin Pharmacother*. 2015;16(6):821–832.

22. Gardner SE, Haleem A, Jao YL, et al. Cultures of diabetic foot ulcers without clinical signs of infection do not predict outcomes. *Diabetes Care*. 2014;37(10):2693–2701.

23. Kosinski MA, Lipsky BA. Current medical management of diabetic foot infections. *Expert Rev Anti Infect Ther*. 2010;8(11):1293–1305.

24. Lipsky BA, Armstrong DG, Citron DM, et al. Ertapenem versus piperacillin/tazobactam for diabetic foot infections (SIDESTEP): prospective, randomized, controlled, double-blinded, multicentre trial. *Lancet*. 2005;366(9498):1695–1703.

25. Brucato MP, Patel K, Mgbako O. Diagnosis of gas gangrene: does a discrepancy exist between the published data and practice. *J Foot Ankle Surg*. 2014;53(2):137–140.

26. Gardner SE, Hillis SL, Heilmann K, et al. The neuropathic diabetic foot ulcer microbiome is associated with clinical factors. *Diabetes*. 2013;62(3):923–930.

27. Charles PG, Uçkay I, Kressmann B, et al. The role of anaerobes in diabetic foot infections. *Anaerobe*. 2015;34:8–13.

28. Bahebeck J, Sobgui E, Loic F, et al. Limb-threatening and life-threatening diabetic extremities: clinical patterns and outcomes in 56 patients. *J Foot Ankle Surg*. 2010;49:43–46.

29. Uzun G, Mutluoğlu M, Ülçay A, et al. Incidence of piperacillin/tazobactam-induced neutropenia in patients with diabetic foot infection: a retrospective cohort study. *Gulhane Med J*. 2015;57(4):1.

30. Martin-Loeches I, Torres A, Rinaudo M, et al. Resistance patterns and outcomes in intensive care unit (ICU)-acquired pneumonia. Validation of European Centre for Disease Prevention and Control (ECDC) and the Centers for Disease Control and Prevention (CDC) classification of multidrug resistant organisms. *J Infect*. 2015;70(3):213–222.

31. Lipsky BA, Tabak YP, Johannes RS, et al. Skin and soft tissue infections in hospitalised patients with diabetes: culture isolates and risk factors associated with mortality, length of stay and cost. *Diabetologia*. 2010;53(5):914–923.

32. Lavery L, Fontaine JL, Bhavan K, et al. Risk factors for methicillin-resistant *Staphylococcus aureus* in diabetic foot infections. *Diabetic Foot Ankle*. 2014;5.

33. Vardakas KZ, Horianopoulou M, Falagas ME. Factors associated with treatment failure in patients with diabetic foot infections: an analysis of data from randomized controlled trials. *Diabetes Res Clin Pract*. 2008;80(3):344–351.

34. Aragon-Sanchez J, Lazaro-Martinez JL, Quintana-Marrero Y, et al. Are diabetic foot ulcers complicated by MRSA osteomyelitis associated with worse prognosis? Outcomes of a surgical series. *Diabet Med*. 2009;26:552–555.

35. Hartemann-Heurtier A, Robert J, Jacqueminet S, et al. Diabetic foot ulcer and multidrug-resistant organisms: risk factors and impact. *Diabet Med*. 2004;21(7):710–715.

36. Richard JL, Sotto A, Jourdan N, et al. Risk factors and healing impact of multidrug-resistant bacteria in diabetic foot ulcers. *Diabetes Metab*. 2008;34:363–369.

37. Shakil S1, Khan AU. Infected foot ulcers in male and female diabetic patients: a clinico-bioinformative study. *Ann Clin Microbiol Antimicrob*. 2010;9:2.

38. Varaiya AY, Dogra JD, Kulkarni MH, et al. Extended-spectrum beta-lactamase-producing *Escherichia coli* and *Klebsiella pneumoniae* in diabetic foot infections. *Indian J Pathol Microbiol*. 2008;51(3):370–372.

39. Candan ED, Aksöz N. *Klebsiella pneumoniae*: characteristics of carbapenem resistance and virulence factors. *Acta Biochim Pol*. 2015;62:867–874.

40. Ckakraborty A, Adhikari P, Shenoy S, et al. Molecular characterization and clinical significance of New Delhi metallo-beta-lactamases-1 producing *Escherichia coli* recovered from a South Indian tertiary care hospital. *Indian J Pathol Microbiol*. 2015;58(3):323–327.

41. Baliga S, Bhat G, Rao S, et al. Molecular characterization and clinical significance of New Delhi metallo-beta-lactamases-1 producing *Escherichia coli* recovered from a South Indian tertiary care hospital. *Indian J Pathol Microbiol*. 2015;58(3):323–327.

42. Cornaglia G, Mazzariol A, Lauretti L, et al. Hospital outbreak of carbapenem-resistant *Pseudomonas aeruginosa* producing VIM-1, a novel transferable metallo-beta-lactamase. *Clin Infect Dis*. 2000;31(5):1119–1125.

43. Yadlapalli N, Vaishnav A, Sheehan PD. Conservative management of diabetic foot ulcers complicated by osteomyelitis. *Wounds*. 2002;14(1):31–35.

44. Mackowiak PA, Jones SR, Smith JW. Diagnostic value of sinus-tract cultures in chronic osteomyelitis. *JAMA*. 1978;239(26):2772–2775.

45. Agarwal S, Zahid M, Sherwani MK, et al. Comparison of the results of sinus track culture and sequestrum culture in chronic osteomyelitis. *Acta Orthop Belg*. 2005;71:209–212.

46. Bernard L, Uçkay I, Vuagnat A, et al. Two consecutive deep sinus tract cultures predict the pathogen of osteomyelitis. *Int J Infect Dis*. 2010;14:e390–e393.

47. Ulug M, Avaz C, Celen MK, et al. Are sinus track cultures reliable for identifying the cuasative agent in chronic osteomyelitis? *Arch Orthop Trauma Surg*. 2009;129:1565–1570.

48. Senneville E, Lombart A, Beltrand E, et al. Outcome of diabetic foot osteomyelitis treated nonsurgically: a retrospective cohort study. *Diabetes Care*. 2008;31:637–642.

49. Kowalski TJ, Matsuda M, Sorenson MD, et al. The effect of residual osteomyelitis at the resection margin in patients with surgically treated diabetic foot infection. *J Foot Ankle Surg*. 2011;50(2):171–175.

50. Berendt AR, Peters EJ, Bakker K, et al. Diabetic foot osteomyelitis: a progress report on diagnosis and a systematic review of treatment. *Diabetes Metab Res Rev.* 2008;24:S145–S161.

51. Zeun P, Gooday C, Nunney I, et al. Predictors of outcomes in diabetic foot osteomyelitis treated initially with conservative (nonsurgical) medical management: a retrospective study. *Int J Low Extrem Wounds.* 2016;15:19–25.

52. Mader JT. Animal models of osteomyelitis. *Am J Med.* 1985;78:213–217.

53. Norden CW. Lessons learned from animal models of osteomyelitis. *Rev Infect Dis.* 1988;10:103–110.

54. Raad I, Hanna H, Jiang Y, et al. Comparative activities of daptomycin, linezolid, and tigecycline against catheter-related methicillin-resistant *Staphylococcus bacteremic* isolates embedded in biofilm. *Antimicrob Agents Chemother.* 2007;51:1656–1660.

55. Embil JM, Rose G, Trepman E, et al. Oral antimicrobial therapy for diabetic foot osteomyelitis. *Foot Ankle Int.* 2006;27:771–779.

56. Game FL, Jeffcoate WJ. Primarily non-surgical management of osteomyelitis of the foot in diabetes. *Diabetologia.* 2008;51: 962–967.

57. Tone A, Nguyen S, Devemy F, et al. Six-week versus twelve-week antibiotic therapy for nonsurgically treated diabetic foot osteomyelitis: a multicenter open-label controlled randomized study. *Diabetes Care.* 2015;38:302–307.

58. Novaro GM, Evans JM. 23-year-old woman with ankle pain and fever. *Mayo Clin Proc.* 1997;72(10):961–964.

59. Ho HH, Cheung CW, Yeung CK. Septic peripheral embolization from Haemophilus parainfluenzae endocarditis. *Eur Heart J.* 2006;27(9):1009.

60. Silverman ME, Upshaw CB Jr. Extracardiac manifestations of infective endocarditis and their historical descriptions. *Am J Cardiol.* 2007;100(12):1802–1807.

61. Khanna N, Roy A, Bahl VK. Janeway lesions: an old sign revisited. *Circulation.* 2013;127(7):861.

62. Hsu HS, Horne CC, Yang CC, et al. *Staphylococcus aureus* endocarditis with large vegetation and emboli: report of a case [in Chinese]. *Zhonghua Min Guo Xiao Er Ke Yi Xue Hui Za Zhi.* 1989;30(2):123–128.

63. Watanakunakorn C. Osler's nodes on the dorsum of the foot. *Chest.* 1988;94(5):1088–1090.

64. Canović P, Gajović O, Mijailović Z. Reiter's syndrome after Salmonella infection [in Serbian]. *Srp Arh Celok Lek.* 2004;132(3/4): 104–107.

65. Colmegna I, Cuchacovich R, Espinoza LR. HLA-B27-associated reactive arthritis: pathogenetic and clinical considerations. *Clin Microbiol Rev.* 2004;17(2):348–369.

66. Wu IB, Schwartz RA. Reiter's syndrome: the classic triad and more. *J Am Acad Dermatol.* 2008;59(1):113–121. doi: 10.1016/j.jaad.2008.02.047

67. Greenlaw SM, Alberta-Wszolek L, Garg A. Clinical images: beyond the classic triad: dermatologic manifestations of reactive arthritis. *Arthritis Rheum.* 2009;60(2):625.

68. Colbert R, Prahalad S. Predisposing factors in the spondyloarthropathies: new insights into the role of HLA-B27. *Curr Rheum Rep.* 2001;3:404–411.

69. Sonkar GK, Usha, Singh S. Is HLA-B27 a useful test in the diagnosis of juvenile spondyloarthropathies? *Singapore Med J.* 2008;49(10):795–799.

70. Gerard HC, Branigan PJ, Schumacher HR, et al. Synovial *Chlamydia trachomatis* in patients with reactive arthritis/Reiter's syndrome are viable but show aberrant gene expression. *J Rheumatol.* 1998;25:734–742.

71. Centers for Disease Control and Prevention Tuberculosis Data and Statistics. http://www.who.int/tb/publications/global_report/en/. Accessed December 22, 2015.

72. Sievers ML. The second "great imitator" tuberculosis. *JAMA.* 1961;176:809–810.

73. Chevannes W, Memarzadeh A, Pasapula C. Isolated tuberculous osteomyelitis of the talonavicular joint without pulmonary involvement-a rare case report. *Foot (Edinb).* 2015;25(1):66–68.

74. Gursu S, Yildirim T, Ucpinar H, et al. Long-term follow-up results of foot and ankle tuberculosis in Turkey. *J Foot Ankle Surg.* 2014;53(5):557–561.

75. Vijay V, Sud A, Mehtani A. Multifocal bilateral metatarsal tuberculosis: a rare presentation. *J Foot Ankle Surg.* 2015;54(1):112–115.

76. Muratori F, Pezzillo F, Nizegorodcew T, et al. Tubercular osteomyelitis of the second metatarsal: a case report. *J Foot Ankle Surg.* 2011;50(5):577–579.

77. Dhillon MS, Nagi ON. Tuberculosis of the foot and ankle. *Clin Orthop Relat Res.* 2002;(398):107–113.

78. Korim M, Patel R, Allen P, et al. Foot and ankle tuberculosis: case series and literature review. *Foot (Edinb).* 2014;24(4):176–179. doi:10.1016/j.foot.2014.07.006.

79. Bozkurt M, Doğan M, Sesen H, et al. Isolated medial cuneiform tuberculosis: a case report. *J Foot Ankle Surg.* 2005;44(1):60–63.

80. Vargaonkar G, Sathyamurthy P, Singh VK, et al. Posttraumatic tuberculous osteomyelitis of the foot. A rare case report. *Chin J Traumatol.* 2015;18(3):184–186.

81. Choi WJ, Han SH, Joo JH, et al. Diagnostic dilemma of tuberculosis in the foot and ankle. *Foot Ankle Int.* 2008;29:711–715.

82. De Backer AI, Mortelé KJ, Vanhoenacker FM, et al. Imaging of extraspinal musculoskeletal tuberculosis. *Eur J Radiol.* 2006;57:119–130.

83. Norbis L, Miotto P, Alagna R, et al. Tuberculosis: lights and shadows in the current diagnostic landscape. *New Microbiol.* 2013;36: 111–120.

84. Cheng VC, Yew WW, Yuen KY. Molecular diagnostics in tuberculosis. *Eur J Clin Microbiol Infect Dis.* 2005;24(11):711–720.

85. Chen SH, Wang T, Lee CH. Tuberculous ankle versus pyogenic septic ankle arthritis: a retrospective comparison. *Jpn J Infect Dis.* 2011;64(2):139–142.

86. Wang WC. Sickle cell anemia and other sickling syndromes. In: Greer JP, Foerster J, Rodgers GM, et al., eds. *Wintrobe's Clinical Hematology.* 12th ed. Philadelphia: Lippincott Williams & Wilkins; 2009:1038–1082.

87. Al-Jafar H, Al-Shemmeri E, Al-Shemmeri J, et al. Precision of SPECT/CT allows the diagnosis of a hidden Brodie's abscess of the talus in a patient with sickle cell disease. *Nucl Med Mol Imaging.* 2015;49(2):153–156.

88. Al-Salem AH. Splenic complications of sickle cell anemia and the role of splenectomy. *ISRN Hematol.* 2011;2011:864257.

89. Neonato MG, Guilloud-Bataille M, Beauvais P, et al. Acute clinical events in 299 homozygous sickle cell patients living in France. French Study Group on Sickle Cell Disease. *Eur J Haematol.* 2000;65(3):155–164.

90. Bahebeck J, Atangana R, Techa A, et al. Relative rates and features of musculoskeletal complications in adult sicklers. *Acta Orthop Belg.* 2004;70:107–111.

91. Bibbo C, Patel DV, Tyndall WA, et al. Treatment of multifocal vancomycin-resistant *Enterococcus faecium* osteomyelitis in sickle cell disease: a preliminary report. *Am J Orthop (Belle Mead NJ).* 2003;32(10):505–509.

92. Almeida A, Roberts I. Bone involvement in sickle cell disease. *Br J Haematol.* 2005;129(4):482–490.

93. da Silva GB Junior, Daher Ede F, da Rocha FA. Osteoarticular involvement in sickle cell disease. *Rev Bras Hematol Hemoter.* 2012;34(2):156–164.

94. Inusa BP, Oyewo A, Brokke F, et al. Dilemma in differentiating between acute osteomyelitis and bone infarction in children with sickle cell disease: the role of ultrasound. *PLoS One.* 2013;8(6):e65001. doi:10.1371/journal.pone.0065001.

95. Skaggs DL, Kim SK, Greene NW, et al. Differentiation between bone infarction and acute osteomyelitis in children with sickle-cell

disease with use of sequential radionuclide bone-marrow and bone scans. *J Bone Joint Surg Am*. 2001;83-A:1810–1813.

96. Biviji AA, Paiement GD, Steinbach LS. Musculoskeletal manifestations of human immunodeficiency virus infection. *J Am Acad Orthop Surg*. 2002;10:312–320.

97. Cuellar ML, Espinoza LR. Rheumatic manifestations of HIV-AIDS. *Baillieres Best Pract Res Clin Rheumatol*. 2000;14(3):579–593.

98. Lawson E, Walker-Bone K. The changing spectrum of rheumatic disease in HIV infection. *Br Med Bull*. 2012;103:203–221.

99. Maganti RM, Reveille JD, Williams FM.Therapy insight: the changing spectrum of rheumatic disease in HIV infection. *Nat Clin Pract Rheumatol*. 2008;4:428–438.

100. Njobvu P, McGill P. Human immunodeficiency virus related reactive arthritis in Zambia. *J Rheumatol*. 2005;32(7):1299–1304.

CHAPTER 5

Pedal and Lower Extremity Manifestations of Diabetes Mellitus

KHURRAM H. KHAN • TARA BLITZ-HERBEL

Management of diabetes in the past century has significantly changed diabetes from a primary cause to a secondary cause of mortality. With the introduction of insulin in the 1920s, not only could mortality from diabetes be prevented, but individuals were able to live a longer and more normal life. Although life span had increased with the advent of insulin, complications such as infections of lower extremity not previously seen began to emerge. These complications were even more apparent in patients with uncontrolled diabetes. The ramifications of uncontrolled diabetes include blindness, renal failure, stroke, and lower extremity amputations.[1]

The staggering growth of obesity in the United States directly influences the birth and growth of type 2 diabetes mellitus as an epidemic. Studying the past couple of decades confirms that 90% of individuals diagnosed with diabetes mellitus have type 2. Research has demonstrated that there is a 4.5% increased risk of developing type 2 diabetes for every kilogram of body mass gained.[2]

With regard to foot complication, foot ulcers and amputation is the main prevention goal. Over 85% of all diabetic-related lower extremity amputations were preceded by ulceration. It is well noted that quick resolution of a foot ulcer combined with appropriate intervention to reduce the rate of recurrence can lower the risk of developing a secondary infection and can decrease the probability of lower extremity amputation in the patient with diabetes.[3]

The multidisciplinary health care team approach for the treatment of the diabetic foot ulcer is efficacious and may improve the outcome and long-term prognosis of these patients. The foot specialist or primary care provider is often the first professional contacted for evaluation and management of the diabetic foot ulcer and therefore can serve as an effective "gatekeeper" for the purpose of integrating the other specialties in the treatment of this pathology.[4] This chapter incorporates the essential principles of diabetic wound care recommended by the American Diabetes Association (ADA), the Agency for Health Care Policy and Research, the Center for Disease Control (CDC), and the U.S. Department of Health and Human Services (HHS).

EPIDEMIOLOGY

Diabetes is the sixth leading cause of death in the United States. From 1990 to 2014, the prevalence of diabetes increased from 4.9% to 9.3%. According to the newest statistics from the 2014 CDC, 29.1 million Americans have diabetes, which is about 1 in every 11 people, and 1 out of 4 diabetics do not know they have the disease; 86 million Americans have prediabetes, which is 1 out of 3 adults in the United States, and of those 86 million 9 out of 10 do not realize they have prediabetes.[5]

The total medical costs and lost work and wages for people diagnosed with diabetes were estimated at 245 billion dollars. The risk of death for adults with diabetes is 50% higher than for adults without diabetes.[5]

In 2010, about 73,000 nontraumatic lower limb amputations were performed in adults aged 20 years or older with diagnosed diabetes.[5]

In 1991, the HHS, Public Health Service, published a report on "Diabetes and Chronic Disabling Conditions." Healthy People 2000 listed the national health promotion and disease prevention objectives. One goal of the Healthy People 2000 initiative was to reduce the incidence of diabetes to 2.5 cases per 1,000 people and reduce the prevalence to 25 cases per 1,000 people. These objectives were never met. Healthy People 2010 sought to continue on those goals and they too were never met. We are awaiting Healthy People 2020.[6,7]

NEUROPATHY

Many types of neuropathies can be associated with diabetes including polyneuropathy (many nerves affects both limbs), mononeuropathy (asymmetric and localized to one or several branches of a nerve trunk), and multifocal neuropathy (start in specific parts of the limb—usually the symptoms are more severe on one side of the body).[8] Peripheral neuropathy is the most common type of neuropathy affecting diabetic patients. It is a key factor in the development of diabetic foot ulcerations. Neuropathy is generally considered to be a multifactorial disorder.[9]

Over the past 20 years, there have been three main theories to explain diabetic neuropathy: the polyol pathway theory, the microvascular theory, and the glycosylation end product theory. It has become increasingly apparent that several pathophysiologic factors probably operate simultaneously, and it may be too simplistic to attempt to explain the many clinical presentations and pathologic findings of diabetic neuropathy by a single theory.[10]

The causes are probably different for different types of diabetic neuropathy. Nerve damage is likely caused by a combination of factors: metabolic factors, such as high blood glucose, long duration of diabetes, abnormal blood fat levels, and possibly low levels of insulin[11]; neurovascular factors leading to damage to the blood vessels that carry oxygen and nutrients to nerves; autoimmune factors that cause inflammation in nerves; mechanical injury to nerves, such as carpal tunnel syndrome; inherited traits that increase susceptibility to nerve disease; lifestyle factors such as smoking or alcohol use all may play a role in the cause of neuropathy.[12]

The effects of these mechanisms produce a combination of sensory, motor, and autonomic deficits.

Characteristics of diabetic neuropathy are symmetrical, stocking and glove distribution that starts distal and progresses proximally. Symptoms may not be present at diagnosis and are usually found on clinical exam. It is a length-dependent process, and its sensory manifestations are most pronounced in the lower limbs and, in more severe cases, in the fingers and hands.[13]

Sensory deficiency as a result of diabetic peripheral polyneuropathy is a commonly associated finding and has been identified as an important risk factor in the development of diabetic foot ulcers. The probability of developing wounds increases dramatically when sensation is lost in the presence of faulty biomechanics and resultant deformity.

Various diagnostic tests are employed when the clinician is assessing the level and degree of peripheral sensory neuropathy. Two of the more commonly used tests are the 5.07 Semmes-Weinstein Monofilament and the Vibration Perception Threshold exam. The Semmes-Weinstein device is a simple monofilament of nylon that delivers 10 g of force when applied to the skin and is an easily reproduced exam. A number of cross-sectional studies have assessed the sensitivity of the 10-g monofilament to identify feet at risk of ulceration. Sensitivities vary from 86% to 100%.[14]

The Vibration Perception Threshold exam is commonly performed with a graduated Rydel-Seiffer tuning fork.[15] This fork uses a visual optical illusion to allow the assessor to determine the intensity of residual vibration on a 0 to 8 scale at the point of threshold (disappearance of sensation),[16] but is more accurately performed with a calibrated electrical device known as the Biothesiometer. These tests should be repeated two to three times yearly for progressively developing neuropathic conditions and for those at identified high risk for developing loss of protective sensation in their feet.[17]

A small fiber neuropathy occurs when damage to the peripheral nerves predominantly or entirely affects the small myelinated (Aδ) fibers or unmyelinated C fibers. The specific fiber types involved in this process include both small somatic and autonomic fibers. The sensory functions of these fibers include thermal perception and nociception. These fibers also are involved in a number of autonomic and enteric functions.[18]

Diagnosis of small fiber neuropathy is determined primarily by the history and physical exam, specifically asking questions such as, Do your feet ever feel numb? Do they ever tingle? Do they ever burn? Do they ever feel as if insects are crawling on them?[17]

Functional neurophysiologic testing and skin biopsy evaluation of intraepidermal nerve fiber density can provide diagnostic confirmation.[19]

That is the absence of protective sensation with no significant vascular disease, no history of ulceration or Charcot arthropathy, and no foot deformity, a patient is 1.7 times more likely to ulcerate.[17]

Type 2 diabetic patients may have muscle weakness at the ankle and knee related to presence and severity of peripheral neuropathy. Motor deficit is exemplified by weakness of the anterior tibial compartment and pedal intrinsic muscular atrophy, leading to digital instability and associated increased peak pressures around the resultant deformities. High compressive and frictional forces occur around the areas of deformity. These deformities can include simple foot ailments such as bunions, hammer toes, and prominent metatarsals.[20] Long-term insulin-dependent diabetes mellitus patients have increased endurance but reduced strength and work performance of leg muscles. The combined effect of the motor abnormalities is suggested to give rise to functional impairment, including an increased risk of falls and injuries.[21] Patients with absent protective sensation, no significant vascular disease, no history of ulceration or Charcot arthropathy, and a foot deformity present (focus of stress) are 12.1 times more likely to ulcerate.[17]

Recognizing biomechanically altered gait patterns and prescribing the appropriate off-loading is imperative if one is to attain healing of an ulcer and decrease the probability of developing a new one.[22]

Hyperkeratosis often forms at the site of pressure or shear and repetitive injury. Calluses on the sole of the feet and corns on the top or sides of toes are important clues that an area may be at risk of ulceration. The presence of callus formation was associated with an 11-fold increased risk of developing an ulcer. Likewise, simple debridement of the callus tissue achieved a 26% reduction in peak pressure at the site of the callus.[23]

Clinical symptoms of autonomic neuropathy generally do not occur until long after the onset of diabetes. Subclinical autonomic dysfunction can, however, occur within a year of diagnosis in type 2 diabetic patients and within 2 years in type 1 diabetic patients. Autonomic neuropathy affects bodily functions including cardiovascular (resting tachycardia, exercise intolerance, orthostatic hypotension, silent myocardial ischemia), genitourinary (incontinence, frequent urination), gastrointestinal (difficulty swallowing, gastroparesis—stomach is slow to empty), and reproductive (erectile dysfunction).[24]

Sudomotor foot complications including dry, fissured skin are secondary to insufficient sweat gland activity. The fissured skin can lead to ulceration and infection if left untreated. Bounding pedal pulses and a pathologic increase in pedal perfusion can develop from decreased arteriolar tone and the resultant uncontrolled vasodilatation reactive to the autonomic dysfunction.[25]

VASCULAR DISEASE

The risk factors associated with development of peripheral atherosclerosis disease are similar to those associated with the development of coronary atherosclerosis.[26] These are:

- Genetics
- Obesity
- Diabetes
- Smoking
- Dyslipidemia
- Hypertension
- Hypercoagulability
- Hyperhomocysteinemia

Cardiovascular disease is the leading cause of morbidity and mortality in patients with diabetes mellitus. Patients with diabetes mellitus have two to four times higher risk of cardiovascular disease and up to three times increase in mortality than in the case of nondiabetics. The accelerated rate of atherosclerosis seen in diabetes mellitus predisposes patients to coronary artery disease and to higher rates of myocardial infarction (MI) and death.[27–30]

Peripheral arterial disease (PAD) is also a major risk factor for lower extremity amputation, especially in patients with diabetes. Moreover, even for the asymptomatic patient, PAD is a marker for systemic vascular disease involving coronary, cerebral, and renal vessels, leading to an elevated risk of events, such as MI, stroke, and death.[31]

The endothelial cell lining of the arterial vasculature is a biologically active organ. Most patients with diabetes, including those with PAD, demonstrate abnormalities of endothelial function and vascular regulation and abnormalities of endothelial function can render the arterial system susceptible to atherosclerosis and its associated adverse outcomes.[31]

The most common symptom of PAD is intermittent claudication, defined as pain, cramping, or aching in the calves, thighs, or buttocks that appears reproducibly with walking exercise and is relieved by rest. More extreme presentations of PAD include rest pain, tissue loss, or gangrene; these limb-threatening manifestations of PAD are collectively termed critical limb ischemia.[31]

PAD is often more subtle in its presentation in patients with diabetes than in those without diabetes. In contrast to the focal and proximal atherosclerotic lesions of PAD found typically in other high-risk patients, the lesions in diabetic patients are more likely to be more diffuse and distal. Persons with diabetes and lower extremity PAD have a very consistent pattern noted anatomically: multisegmental occlusion distal to the trifurcation of the popliteal artery at the level just distal to the knee.[31]

The initial assessment of PAD in patients with diabetes should always begin with a thorough history and physical. Ensure a complete walking history comparing function today with that in years past to assess functional status and claudication symptoms, which may or may not be the classical variation. In regard to physical exam, the absence of both pedal pulses is highly suggestive of vascular disease.[32]

Noninvasive vascular studies are a helpful screening tool for peripheral vascular disease in the patient with diabetes. The ankle-brachial index (ABI), is the ratio of the systolic blood pressure in the ankle divided by the systolic blood pressure at the arm and is a reproducible and reasonably accurate, noninvasive measurement for the detection of PAD and the determination of disease severity.[33]

The diagnostic criteria for PAD based on the ABI are interpreted as follows:

- Normal if 0.91 to 1.30
- Mild obstruction if 0.70 to 0.90
- Moderate obstruction if 0.40 to 0.69
- Severe obstruction if <0.40
- Poorly compressible if >1.30

It has been validated against angiographically confirmed disease and found to be 95% sensitive and almost 100% specific. There are some limitations, however, in using the ABI. Calcified, poorly compressible vessels in the elderly and some patients with diabetes may give you false values. The ABI may also be falsely negative in symptomatic patients with moderate aortoiliac stenoses. These issues complicate the evaluation of an individual patient, but are not prevalent enough to detract from the usefulness of the ABI as an effective test to screen for and to diagnose PAD in patients with diabetes. In diabetic patients, an ABI within normal range needs to be taken in context with history and physical to ensure proper diagnosis.[34]

Angiograms and other invasive vascular studies are more conclusive and are generally warranted in patients who are most likely going to benefit from a peripheral arterial bypass. Coordinated care with an interventional radiologist and a vascular specialist is an integral component of the team approach.[35,36] No angiographic factors were predictive of limb salvage.[37] Vascular reconstructive surgery of the impaired limb may be required prior to debridement and/or partial amputation foot surgery. Other options include endovascular surgery (i.e., stents/balloon angioplasty) for which long-term yields have not currently been reported. Vasodilator medications have not been found to promote wound healing in the ischemic foot. Treatment for such patients is individualized taking into account all the contributing factors.

Musculoskeletal Complications of Diabetes Mellitus

Diabetes leads to changes in connective tissue by glycosylation of proteins, microvascular abnormalities with damage to blood vessels and nerves, and collagen accumulation in skin and periarticular structures.[38] Musculoskeletal complications are most commonly seen in patients with a long-standing history of type 1 diabetes. Some have a known direct association with diabetes.[38]

Limited Joint Mobility

Limited joint mobility in the hands is also known as diabetic cheiroarthropathy, and is characterized by thick, tight, waxy skin mainly on the dorsal aspect of the hands, with flexion deformities of the metacarpophalangeal and interphalangeal joints (increased resistance to passive extension of the joints). In the early stages, paresthesias and slight pain develop from causes thought to be multifactorial, most likely increased glycosylation of collagen in the skin and periarticular tissue and decreased collagen degradation.[39]

Dupuytren Disease (Contracture)

Dupuytren disease is a fibroproliferative disorder of unknown origin causing palmar nodules and flexion contracture of the digits. About 5% of individuals with Dupuytren disease are diabetic, with an increased prevalence that is proportional to the duration of the diabetes. The association with diabetes mellitus is well recorded, with a reported prevalence of between 3% and 32%.[40]

Carpal Tunnel Syndrome

Carpal tunnel syndrome and diabetic polyneuropathy are common conditions in patients with type 1 and type 2 diabetes. The prevalence of carpal tunnel syndrome is thought to be higher in patients with diabetic polyneuropathy than in the general population, and the treatment less successful,[41] but recent studies seem to disparage the relationship. A retrospective, case-control study looked at all patients diagnosed with carpal tunnel syndrome between January 2011 and July 2012 and compared them with a control group of herniated nucleus pulposus patients. A total of 997 patients with carpal tunnel syndrome and 594 controls were included. Prevalence of type 2 diabetes was 11.5% in the carpal tunnel syndrome group versus 7.2% in the control group (odds ratio [OR] 1.67; 95% confidence interval [CI] 1.16 to 2.41). In multivariate analyses adjusting for gender, age, and body mass index, type 2 diabetes was not associated with carpal tunnel syndrome (OR 0.99; 95% CI 0.66 to 1.47). No differences in duration of diabetes mellitus, microvascular complications, or glycemic control between groups were detected.[42]

Frozen Shoulder

One of the most disabling musculoskeletal problems seen in diabetics is adhesive capsulitis, which is also known as frozen shoulder, shoulder periarthritis, or obliterative bursitis. It is characterized by progressive, painful restriction of shoulder movement, specifically external rotation and abduction. The thickened joint capsule is closely applied and adherent to the humeral head, resulting in considerable reduction in the volume of the glenohumeral joint.[43]

Recognizing biomechanically altered gait patterns and prescribing the appropriate off-loading is imperative if one is to attain healing of an ulcer and decrease the probability of developing a new one.

High compressive and frictional forces occur around areas of deformity. These deformities can include simple foot ailments such as bunions, hammer toes, and prominent metatarsals.[44] Multiple techniques are available to off-load areas of increased peak pressure. Use of simple felt or plastazote insoles for redistribution of weight-bearing forces is common in the treatment of the acute ulcer.[45] Recently, some removable walking casts have been shown to be very effective and statistically as efficacious as the total contact cast.[46] However, the total contact cast is still considered the gold standard for off-loading since it is a custom-molded device and applied on a weekly basis to allow for regular wound care to the site.[47,48] Once healed, long-term management of the patient may incorporate use of custom-molded orthoses and/or specialized supportive footwear to decrease the probability of redeveloping an ulcer.[49]

Dermatologic Manifestations of Diabetes Mellitus

The skin of all diabetic patients is affected in some form or another, and cutaneous disease can appear as the first sign of diabetes or may develop at any time in the course of the disease. The manifestations are secondary to long-term effects of diabetes on the microcirculation and skin collagen.[50] It has been suggested that increased cross-linking of collagen in diabetic patients is responsible for the fact that their skin is generally thicker than that of nondiabetics. Advanced glycosylation end products are probably responsible for yellowing of skin and nails, increased viscosity of blood resulting from stiff RBC membranes, and engorgement of the postcapillary venules in the papillary dermis. It is suggested that these skin changes may eventually be used as a reflection of the patient's current as well as past metabolic status.[51] Whereas type 2 diabetics more often have skin infection, type 1 diabetics have more autoimmune-related skin lesions. Skin manifestations of diabetes may also serve as ports of entry for secondary infection.[52]

Specific cutaneous markers for diabetes are as follows:

Necrobiosis lipoidica
Generalized granuloma annulare
Diabetic bullae
Scleredema diabeticorum
Acanthosis nigricans
Eruptive xanthomatosis
Diabetic dermopathy

Nonspecific condition associated with diabetes:

Acrochordons
Yellow skin/nails

Pruritus
Thick skin
Rubeosis faciei
Palmar erythema
Pigmented purpuric dermatosis

Conditions that are more common in diabetics:

Perforating dermatosis
Vitiligo
Lichen planus
Eruptive xanthomas
Kaposi sarcoma
Bullous pemphigoid
Psoriasis
Dermatitis herpetiformis[52,53]

One of the more devastating dermatologic complications from diabetes is a foot wound.[54] The lifetime risk for foot ulceration in a person with diabetes is estimated at 15%. Most foot ulcerations are plantar lesions that result from neuropathy in the face of increased pressure.[55,56]

The pivotal events that cause skin breakdown, and ultimately foot ulceration, can be identified in three main categories[57]:

1. Low pressure over prolonged periods of time, that is, pressure sores from bed rest. It takes ~2 lb per in^2 to cause blanching of the skin. This amount of pressure over 15 minutes affects microcirculation and tissue oxygenation. Common anatomic sites for these ulcers to present are the heel and the sacrum. These are also known as pressure ulcers, bed sores, or decubitus ulcerations.
2. High pressure over a short period of time, that is, puncture wounds from a foreign object. Pressure >100 lb per in^2 (70 N per cm^2) will puncture the skin. This is seen most commonly on the plantar surfaces of the foot from puncture wounds caused by a metallic or wooden object. These generally present as acute infections and can have a high risk for amputation because of the possible inoculation from a penetrating object.
3. Moderate pressure in a repetitive setting, that is, neuropathic ulcers from weight bearing. This is the primary causative factor in plantar foot ulcer development. Multiple studies have attempted to quantify this pressure, but no clear pressure threshold has been demonstrated. However, peak plantar pressures analyzed with computerized gait analysis systems have demonstrated 70 N per cm^2 (100 psi) as a focal point. Pressures in excess of this have a high risk for neuropathic ulceration (sensitivity of 70.0% and specificity of 65.1%).[58,59]

Wound Classifications

Wound assessment calls for the use of a common language that can be easily interpreted from one practitioner to the next. Wounds should be described by location, size (such as cross-sectional measurements), depth and/or level of tissue involved, color and type of wound surface (i.e., red granulation tissue, fibrous or necrotic), exudate, odor, sinus track, and/or tunneling. A description of the surrounding tissue should note such factors as cellulitis, edema, and/or callus tissue.[60] Classifications were developed to bring these descriptions together to help simplify and help standardize charting so as to be reproducible from clinician to clinician.

Basis for classification, including:

- Staging
- Predicting outcome
- Identifying management strategy

One of the first and most often used classification systems is the Meggitt/Wagner Classification 0 to 5, where[61]:

0—Skin intact
1—Superficial ulcer without penetrating to the deep layers
2—Deeper tissues involved and there is abscess
3—Deep involvement with osteomyelitis
4—Gangrene, localized
5—Gangrene, generalized

The basic structure of this classification is:

0 to 2: Graduation based on depth
3: Deep and infected
4 to 5: Gangrene (i.e., critical ischemia)

A problem with this type of wound classification system is that one cannot combine different categories of pathology in order to accurately identify and define the multiple processes occurring concurrently. For example, an infected wound is easily classified according to the Meggitt/Wagner system, but an infected/ischemic wound is difficult to properly assess and describe with this limited system.[62]

A wound classification system for diabetic foot wounds was developed at the University of Texas (UT) Health Science Center at San Antonio, Texas. The UT classification system is based on depth of wound and state of wound (i.e., ischemic, infected) (see **Table 5-1**).

The UT Wound Classification System takes into account only the known risk factors that ultimately influence the prognosis of a given wound site (depth, infection, ischemia). Many factors (i.e., wound size, drainage, quality) are not taken into direct account because these have not been demonstrated to directly determine the outcomes of the wound site (**Table 5-2**).

NATURAL HISTORY

Treatment Options

The essential therapeutic objectives for the management of any plantar ulcer include[36]:

- Establishing the level of arterial supply
- Eradicating/protecting against infection via appropriate debridement
- Maintaining a moist wound environment
- Off-loading the areas of greatest pressure

Table 5-1. University of Texas Classification System for Diabetic Foot Wounds

| | | Grade/depth: "How deep is the wound?" | | | |
		0	I	II	III
	A	Grade/depth: "How deep is the wound?"	Superficial wound not involving tendon, capsule, or bone	Wound penetrating to tendon or capsule	Wound penetrating to bone or joint
Stage/comorbidities	B	Pre- or postulcerative lesion completely epithelialized with infection	Superficial wound not involving tendon, capsule, or bone with infection	Wound penetrating to tendon or capsule with infection	Wound penetrating to bone or joint with infection
"Is the wound infected, ischemic, or both?"	C	Pre- or postulcerative lesion completely epithelialized with ischemia	Superficial wound not involving tendon, capsule, or bone with ischemia	Wound penetrating to tendon or capsule with ischemia	Wound penetrating to bone or joint with infection and ischemia
	D	Pre- or postulcerative lesion completely epithelialized with infection and ischemia	Superficial wound not involving tendon, capsule, or bone with infection and ischemia	Wound penetrating to tendon or capsule with infection and ischemia	Wound penetrating to bone or joint with infection and ischemia

From Armstrong DG, Lavery LA, Harkless LB. Validation of a diabetic wound classification system. The contribution of depth, infection, and ischemia to risk of amputation. *Diabetes Care.* 1998;21:855–859; Lavery LA, Armstrong DG, Harkless LB. Classification of diabetic foot wounds. *J Foot Ankle Surg.* 1996;35:528–531.

Table 5-2. University of Texas Risk Classification System for Diabetic Foot Wounds

Category 0: No Neuropathy	Category 1: Neuropathy, No Deformity	Category 2: Neuropathy, with Deformity	Category 3: History of Pathology
Patient diagnosed with DM Protective sensation intact ABI >0.80 and toe systolic pressure >45 mm Hg Foot deformity may be present No history of ulceration TREATMENT: Possible shoe accommodations Patient education Follow-up every 6–12 mo	Protective sensation absent ABI >0.80 and toe systolic pressure >45 mm Hg No history of ulceration No history of neuroarthropathy No foot deformity TREATMENT: Possible shoe accommodations Patient education Visits every 3–4 mo	Protective sensation absent ABI >0.80 toe systolic pressure >45 mm Hg history of ulceration No history of neuroarthropathy Foot deformity present TREATMENT: Custom-molded, extra depth shoes Possible prophylactic surgery Patient education Follow-up every 2–3 mo	Protective sensation absent ABI >0.80 and toe systolic pressure >45 mm Hg History of ulceration, amputation, or neuroarthropathy Foot deformity present TREATMENT: Custom-molded, extra depth shoes Possible prophylactic surgery Patient education Follow-up every 1–2 mo
Category 4A: Neuropathic Wound	**Category 4B: Acute Charcot Joint (Neuroarthropathy)**	**Category 5: Infected Diabetic Foot**	**Category 6: Ischemic Limb**
All UT stage A wounds protective sensation absent ABI >0.80 and toe systolic pressure >45 mm Hg Foot deformity present No acute neuroarthropathy TREATMENT: Wound care regimen Pressure reduction program Possible surgical intervention Patient education Frequent follow-up visits	Protective sensation absent ABI >0.80 and toe systolic pressure >45 mm Hg Noninfected neuropathic ulceration may be present Diabetic neuroarthropathy present TREATMENT: Wound care regimen if ulcer present Pressure reduction program Thermometric and radiographic monitoring Patient education Frequent follow-up visits	All UT stage B wounds Protective sensation may be present Infected wound Neuroarthropathy may be present TREATMENT: Debridement of infected, nonviable tissue and/or bone as indicated Possible hospitalization, antibiotic treatment regimen Medical management of diabetes	All UT stage C, D wounds Protective sensation may be present ABI <0.80 or toe systolic pressure <45 mm Hg or pedal transcutaneous oxygen tension <40 mm Hg Ulceration may be present TREATMENT: Vascular consultation, possible revascularization If infection present, treatment same as for category 5

From Armstrong DG, Lavery LA, Harkless LB. Treatment-based classification system for assessment and care of diabetic feet. *J Am Podiatr Med Assoc.* 1996;86:311–316; Armstrong DG, Lavery LA, Harkless LB. Who is at risk for diabetic foot ulceration? *Clin Podiatr Med Surg.* 1998;15(1):11–19; Lavery LA, Armstrong DG, Vela SA, et al. Practical criteria for screening patients at high risk for diabetic foot ulceration. *Arch Intern Med.* 1998;158(2):157–162.

- Maintaining metabolic control and nutritional status
- Frequently evaluating with response-directed treatment
- Patient education and compliance

Management of the diabetic foot ulcer should be initiated with an assessment of its etiology. This incorporates a careful medical history and physical examination with appropriate use of noninvasive studies. A complete examination involves assessing many factors, such as: serum glucose levels including glycosylated hemoglobin (HbA1c), complete blood count with differential, hepatic and renal profiles with electrolyte balance, nutritional status, the peripheral vascular status, neuropathy and sensory deficiency, limited joint mobility, and signs that may suggest the presence of soft tissue infection or osteomyelitis.[63]

Members of a team approach may include: podiatry, vascular surgery, internal medicine, infectious disease, endocrinology, cardiology, radiology, orthopedics, orthotist/prosthetist, nursing, and a certified diabetic educator.[64] Depending on the degree of severity and the contributing factors, additional specialists may need to be consulted. Patient compliance and knowledge of their disease has been identified as a significant factor in the expected prognosis and the prevalence of both ulceration and limb loss.[65]

DEBRIDEMENT

The removal of necrotic tissue is an integral component in the treatment of ulcerative wounds.[66] The types of debridement available include: surgical, mechanical, autolytic, and enzymatic. Autolytic debridement occurs naturally in a moist wound environment when arterial perfusion and venous drainage are maintained. The use of enzymatic debridement and its efficacy has been questioned in the literature and seems to have limited indications.[67] Mechanical debridement, however, has been demonstrated to be of direct benefit to the wound site by ridding the site of necrotic tissue, allowing cell activation through active bleeding and through stimulation of the healing pathways.[68] Wet-to-dry dressings were previously used as a common means of mechanically debriding the wound site, but debridement is now done primarily with surgical instrumentation in the form of sharp debridement and rapid tissue demarcation.[69] Irrigation is another form of mechanical debridement and is commonly utilized at the time of surgery as well as during dressing changes. Flush irrigation under pressure ($>$8 psi) appears to be more effective in reducing the bacterial count than low-pressure flush or scrubbing with a saline-soaked sponge. In addition, pulse lavage systems can be very efficacious in removing foreign debris. An 18-gauge needle or a 19-gauge angiocath is an alternative measure for providing pressure irrigation when pulse lavage is not available in the operating room or not practical for daily dressing changes.[70]

INFECTION

Surgical debridement is a key component in the management of necrotic wounds and includes the removal of all nonviable tissue from the surgical wound as well as the surrounding callus tissue. Necrotic tissue removed on a regular basis can expedite the rate at which a wound heals and has been shown in a recent study to increase the probability of attaining full secondary closure. Osteomyelitis may or may not require bone and possible joint resection or partial amputation of the foot.[71] With respect to the assessment of infection, it is indeed the overall clinical impression that is of primary importance; culture results are viewed as one aspect of the patient's total presentation.

Medical therapy should be guided, based on culture and sensitivity. For non–limb-threatening infections, treatment should be aimed at Staph and Strep. Most diabetic foot infections are polymicrobial and thus require broad spectrum and/or mixed antibiotic coverage initiated empirically. The medications utilized are modified primarily on the basis of clinical response; culture results; and, when needed, repeated cultures, which are also considered in the overall therapeutic management of the diabetic foot infection.[72]

WOUND CARE

Generally, a moist wound environment has been shown to facilitate the healing process. In addition, the bandage applied should provide protection from trauma and local contamination, allow gaseous exchange, thermally insulate the wound, absorb excess exudate, and provide for removal without traumatizing the wound surface. The type of dressing used varies according to the size and depth of the defect, its location on the foot, and the quality of the wound surface. Normal sterile saline method of wound management may require frequent reassessment and dressing changes up to several times daily to balance the wound between maceration and desiccation. Selection of the type of product to use varies between different degrees of absorbent dressings for exudative wounds versus those that encourage moisture for dry nonexudative defects.[73]

Categories of wound dressings include the following[74]:

1. Hydrocolloids, alginates, or foams: absorbent dressings for exudative wounds
2. Films or hydrocolloids: occlusive or semiocclusive dressings for dry nonexudative wounds
3. Hydrogels: add moisture to dry wounds
4. Impregnated dressings: decrease drying, prevent dressing adherence, and reduce bacterial content within the wound (i.e., Adaptic or Xeroform)
5. Topical medications such as antibiotics and antiseptics

Chronic wounds are those in which healing has terminated or is not occurring in a timely fashion. The length of time a wound must exist without signs of appreciable healing until it is considered chronic is not well defined. Regular reassessment of an ulcer's response to a given treatment program is necessary to avoid continuing ineffective interventions and to prevent overutilization of health care resources. Once it has been established that a particular treatment is ineffective, a systematic evaluation of the basic etiologic factors usually provides the information necessary to alter the plan of care and reestablish the healing process.[75]

The primary goal in treating the chronic ulcer is to convert it into an acute wound that will then contain the active matrix needed for healing. The basic principles of treatment discussed for the acute ulcer apply here and include: providing the required arterial perfusion, off-loading the involved area, resolving any infective processes, surgically debriding necrotic tissue, and assessing prior patient compliance.[76] Overall systemic management is imperative. Such factors as chronic hyperglycemia with serum levels of 180 to 200 or higher (HbA1c > 9) can interfere with wound healing.[77] Thus, reassessment requires analysis of all aspects of the patients' care and, as mentioned previously, a multidisciplinary approach is most efficacious toward achieving that end.

When all of the above have been addressed and active signs of healing have not developed, specifically 50% area reduction over 4 weeks, then engineered wound care products, such as endogenous or exogenous growth factors or cultured skin replacement, may be helpful to resolve the chronic wound.[78,79] These agents have been shown to provide an optimal wound environment and encourage chemotaxis and mitogenesis of platelets, neutrophils, fibroblasts, monocytes, as well as other components that form the cellular basis for good wound healing.

OFF-LOADING

Pedorthics is concerned with the design, manufacture, fit, and modification of shoes and related foot appliances as prescribed for the reduction of painful or disabling conditions of the foot or limb. Pedorthics help reduce shear, shock, and transfer from sensitive or painful areas. They can correct or support flexible deformities or accommodate fixed deformities. They also control or limit motion of joints.

Many modifications can be made to shoes to enable treatment of symptoms. Some of these modifications can be made to the flare of the shoe, whereas rocker soles can also be used to treat ulcers and Charcot.[80]

Extended steel shank modifications can be used for amputations of the forefoot and metatarsal ulcers. Cushion heel modifications can be used to absorb impact, reduce stress on heel and ankle. One can diminish the moment of force that bends the knee as well as reduce demand for ankle plantarflexion.[81]

Total contact orthoses are used to help relieve or eliminate pressure and support/control joint motion.[82] There are many materials that are available to help with the proper function of the orthoses including trilaminar material to make an orthotic accommodative. Rigid material can be used to make an orthotic functional. There are many moldable and nonmoldable coverings, and all these materials can be used in combination.[82]

Custom-molded shoes can be used for those with a severe deformity that will not be accommodated in over-the-counter shoes. People with amputations or unusual sizes may also benefit. Reducing pressure on the diabetic foot ulcer is an integral component of effective wound management.[82] Ill-fitting shoes should be replaced. A small or superficial ulcer can benefit from the use of a healing sandal made from a surgical shoe containing an insole of felt or plastazote, which can then be apertured to properly off-load ulcers. Plastazote can be custom molded to the foot or, depending on its density, dynamically molded around areas of increased pressure during ambulation using its thermoplastic properties, thus redistributing weight-bearing forces effectively.[82] Total avoidance of weight bearing with the use of bed rest, crutch-assisted ambulation, or utilizing a wheel chair is the most effective method to off-load the ulcerated foot.[75] The total contact cast has been accepted as the best overall method to reduce weight from a specific area of increased pressure and apply a more even distribution of weight-bearing forces across the entire forefoot.[83]

Following healing of ulcer, walking/running-style footwear and in-depth shoes can be accommodated with various orthoses for long-term management. In the presence of significant deformity, custom-molded shoes can be used to accommodate deformity and decrease pressure on areas of prominence and thus decrease the possibility of recurrence of a diabetic ulcer. Molded ankle foot orthoses and similar devices may support the otherwise unstable foot and ankle segments and thus decrease ulcerative risk.[82] Reducing the possibility (or the degree) of obesity may be helpful in decreasing plantar pressures in the ulcer-prone foot and should be part of the overall goals of a nutrition management program.[82]

SURGERY

The goal of surgery is to heal any existing ulcer and/or prevent the development of future ulcers. It is achieved by decreasing focal pressures through surgical reduction of associated bony prominence while preserving pedal functional stability. Surgery is performed either in response to an ulcer history (prior or current) or as prophylactic surgery to decrease the probability of developing future ulcers.[84] It is also indicated in cases of nonreversible ischemia resulting in amputation. Surgery includes incision and drainage of a deep abscess, debridement of necrotic tissue for the acute active infection, ablative with partial or total foot and possible leg amputation. Definitive surgery is applied with vascular analysis and intervention as needed.[85] The literature supports the conclusion that diabetes is not a contraindication for prophylactic foot surgery and is especially worth considering for those patients who cannot be accommodated by footwear modifications and related orthoses.[86]

Amputation is a common sequela, and the level of amputation is determined by the area in which viable bone and soft tissue are noted. In addition, the specific procedure selected takes into consideration the anticipated postoperative functional capacity of the patient. A variety of forefoot, midfoot, rearfoot, and leg amputations are available.

Closure can be achieved through secondary, primary, or delayed primary closure. Secondary wound healing is commonly utilized for patients when dealing with an infection that necessitates tissue resection to the extent that primary closure is not a viable option.[87] Keeping the wound open allows for daily flush, and wound packing may be required.[88] Delayed primary closure may be used when a wound infection has resolved. Plastic surgical techniques utilizing split- and full-thickness skin grafts and flaps are other options that may be used to avoid secondary wound healing and accelerate ulcer resolution. Primary closure can be considered for noninfected wounds or those where there is confidence that the infection has been fully eradicated during the definitive surgery. All patients must be assessed individually for the selection of the surgical procedure and closure technique that best meets their needs. Transmetatarsal amputation healing can be expected in a majority of diabetic patients after adequate revascularization, but cannot be predicted by angiographic findings. Efforts should be made to achieve primary wound closure.[37] Thirty-day readmission rates following primary lower extremity amputation in patients with diabetes were high at >10%. Both medical and surgical complications, many of which were unavoidable, contributed to readmission.[89]

CONCLUSION

The literature consistently demonstrates that the pedal complications of diabetes are significant, with the ultimate goal of prevention of foot ulcers. The treatment of diabetic foot ulcers is best accomplished by utilizing a multidisciplinary team. The primary care doctor is key in coordinating the integration of the necessary specialists in the management of the ulcerated patient. Members of the "team approach" may include physicians in any of the following specialties: family practice, internal medicine, endocrinology, infectious disease, neurology, radiology and imaging, vascular disease, podiatrists/orthopedics, orthotics and prosthetics, and others as necessary.

Treatment of diabetic foot ulcers requires a thorough understanding of the factors involved in the development of open wounds and their healing mechanisms. Necrotic tissue must be removed and excised. In addition, weight-bearing forces and shear must be removed from the wound surface through effective off-loading.

REFERENCES

1. American Diabetes Association. Foot care in patients with diabetes mellitus: position statement. *Diabetes Care*. 1998;21(suppl 1):S23–S31, S54–S55.
2. Wallach JB, Rey MJ. A socioeconomic analysis of obesity and diabetes in New York City. *Prev Chronic Dis*. 2009;6(3). http://www.cdc.gov/pcd/issues/2009/jul/08_0215.htm. Accessed January 3, 2017.
3. Caputo GM, Cavanagh PR, Ulbrecht JS, et al. Assessment and management of foot disease with diabetes. *N Engl J Med*. 1994;331:854–860.
4. Frykberg RG. The team approach in diabetic foot management. *Adv Wound Care*. 1998;11:71–77.
5. Centers for Disease Control and Prevention. *National Diabetes Statistics Report: Estimates of Diabetes and Its Burden in the United States*. Atlanta, GA: U.S. Department of Health and Human Services; 2014.
6. U.S. Department of Health and Human Services, Public Health Service: Diabetes and Chronic Disabling Conditions. *Healthy People 2000: Nation Health Promotion and Disease Prevention Objectives*. Washington, DC: Government Printing Office; 1991:442–474. DHHS publ. no. PHS 91-50212.
7. National Center for Health Statistics. *Healthy People 2010 Final Review*. Hyattsville, MD: NCHS; 2011.
8. Thomas PK. Classification, differential diagnosis, and staging of diabetic peripheral neuropathy. *Diabetes*. 1997;46(suppl 2):S54–S57.
9. Brand P, Yancey P. *Pain: The Gift Nobody Wants*. New York, NY: Harper Collins; 1993.
10. Kelkar P. Diabetic neuropathy. *Semin Neurol*. 2005;25(2):168–173.
11. American Diabetes Association. Diagnosis and classification of diabetes mellitus. *Diabetes Care*. 2008;31(suppl 1):S55–S60. doi:10.2337/dc08-S055.
12. http://www.niddk.nih.gov/health-information/health-topics/Diabetes/diabetic-neuropathies-nerve-damage-diabetes/Documents/Neuropathies_508.pdf. NIH Publication No. 09–3185; February 2009.
13. Boulton AJ, Malik RA, Arezzo JC, et al. Diabetic somatic neuropathies. *Diabetes Care*. 2004;27(6):1458–1486. doi:10.2337/diacare.27.6.1458.
14. Miranda-Palma B, Basu S, Mizel MD, et al. The monofilament as the gold standard for foot ulcer risk screening: a reappraisal [Abstract]. *Diabetes*. 2003;52(suppl 1):A63.
15. Young MJ, Breddy JL, Veves A, et al. The prediction of diabetic neuropathic foot ulceration using vibratory perception thresholds: a prospective study. *Diabetes Care*. 1994;17:557–560.
16. Hilz MJ, Axelrod FB, Hermann K, et al. Normative values of vibratory perception in 530 children, juveniles and adults aged 3–79 years. *J Neurol Sci*. 1998;159:219–225.
17. Lavery LA, Armstrong DG, Vela SA, et al. Practical criteria for screening patients at high risk for diabetic foot ulceration. *Arch Intern Med*. 1998;158(2):157–162. doi:10.1001/archinte.158.2.157.
18. Tavee J, Zhou L. Small fiber neuropathy: a burning problem. *Cleve Clin J Med*. 2009;76(5):297–305.
19. Myers MI, Peltier AC. Uses of skin biopsy for sensory and autonomic nerve assessment. *Curr Neurol Neurosci Rep*. 2013;13(1):323. doi:10.1007/s11910-012-0323-2.
20. Andersen H, Nielsen S, Mogensen CE, et al. Muscle strength in type 2 diabetes. *Diabetes*. 2004;53:1543–1548.
21. Andersen H. Muscular endurance in long-term IDDM patients. *Diabetes Care*. 1998;21(4):604–609.
22. Fernando DJS, Masson EA, Veves A, et al. Relationship of limited joint mobility to abnormal foot pressures and diabetic foot ulceration. *Diabetes Care*. 1991;14:8–11.
23. Young MJ, Cavanagh PR, Thomas G, et al. The effect of callus removal on dynamic plantar foot pressures in diabetic patients. *Diabet Med*. 1992;9:55–57. doi:10.1111/j.1464-5491.1992.tb01714.
24. Vinik AI, Maser RE, Mitchell BD, et al. Diabetic autonomic neuropathy. *Diabetes Care*. 2003;26(5):1553–1579. doi:157910.2337/diacare.26.5.1553.
25. McNeely MJ, Boyko E, Ahroni JH, et al. The independent contributions of diabetic neuropathy and vasculopathy in foot ulceration: how great are the risks? *Diabetes Care*. 1995;18:216–219.
26. Brevetti G, Giugliano G, Brevetti L, et al. Contemporary reviews in cardiovascular medicine. *Circulation*. 2010;122:1862–1875.
27. Li YW, Aronow J. Diabetes mellitus and cardiovascular disease. *J Clin Exp Cardiolog*. 2011;2:1.
28. Brand FN, Abbott RD, Kannel WB. Diabetes, intermittent claudication and risk of cardiovascular events. The Framingham study. *Diabetes*. 1989;38:504–509.
29. Haffner SM, Lehto S, Rönnemaa T, et al. Mortality from coronary artery disease in subjects with type 2 diabetes and in non-diabetic subjects with and without prior myocardial infarction. *N Eng J Med*. 1998;339:229–234.
30. Garg A, Grundy SM. Management of dyslipidemia in NIDDM. *Diabetes Care*. 1990;13:153–169.

31. American Diabetes Association. Peripheral arterial disease in people with diabetes. *Diabetes Care*. 2003;26(12):3333–3341.

32. Carman TL. A primary care approach to the patient with claudication. *Am Fam Physician*. 2000;61(4):1027–1034.

33. Rac-Albu M, Iliuta L, Guberna SM, et al. The role of ankle-brachial index for predicting peripheral arterial disease. *Maedica (Buchar)*. 2014;9(3):295–302.

34. American Diabetes Association. Peripheral arterial disease in people with diabetes. *Clinical Diabetes*. 2004;22(4):181–189.

35. Toursarkissian B, Shireman PK, Harrison A, et al. Major lower-extremity amputation: contemporary experience in a single Veterans Affairs institution. *Am Surg*. 2002;68(7):606–610.

36. Thomson FJ, Veves A, Ashe A, et al. A team approach to diabetic foot care—the Manchester experience. *The Foot*. 1991;2:75–82.

37. Toursarkissian B, Hagino RT, Khan K, et al. Healing of transmetatarsal amputation in the diabetic patient: is angiography predictive? *Ann Vasc Surg*. 2005;19(6):769–773.

38. Kim RP, Edelman SV, Kim DD. Musculoskeletal complications of diabetes mellitus. *Clin Diabetes*. 2001;19:132–135.

39. Cherqaoui R, McKenzie S, Nunlee-Bland G. Diabetic cheiroarthropathy: a case report and review of the literature. *Case Rep Endocrinol*. 2013;2013:257028. doi:10.1155/2013/257028.

40. Geraci A, Bianchi R, Sanfilippo A, et al. Dupuytren contracture in diabetic hand. *Endocrinol Stud*. 2011;1(1):e2.

41. Perkins BA, Olaleye D, Bril V. Carpal tunnel syndrome in patients with diabetic polyneuropathy. *Diabetes Care*. 2002;25(3):565–569.

42. Hendriks SH, van Dijk PR, Groenier KH, et al. Type 2 diabetes seems not to be a risk factor for the carpal tunnel syndrome: a case control study. *BMC Musculoskelet Disord*. 2014;15:346. doi:10.1186/1471-2474-15-346.

43. Smith L, Burnet SP, McNeil JD. Musculoskeletal manifestations of diabetes mellitus. *Br J Sports Med*. 2003;37:30–35. doi:10.1136/bjsm.37.1.30.

44. Veves A, Murray H, Young MJ, et al. The risk of ulceration in diabetic patients with high foot pressures: a prospective study. *Diabetologia*.1992;35:660–663.

45. Guzman B, Fisher G, Palladino SJ, et al. Pressure removing strategies in neuropathic ulcer therapy. *Clin Podiatr Med Surg*. 1994;11:339–353.

46. Gutekunst DJ, Hastings MK, Bohnert KL, et al. Removable cast walker boots yield greater forefoot off-loading than total contact casts. *Clin Biomech*. 2011;26:649–654.

47. Armstrong DG, Lavery LA, Bushman TR. Peak foot pressures influence the healing time of diabetic foot ulcers treated with total contact casts. *J Rehabil Res Dev*. 1998;35(1):1–5.

48. Lewis J, Lipp A. Pressure-relieving interventions for treating diabetic foot ulcers. *Cochrane Database Syst Rev*. 2013;1:CD002302. doi:10.1002/14651858.CD002302.pub2.

49. Armstrong DG, Peters EJ, Athanasiou KA, et al. Is there a critical level of plantar foot pressure to identify patients at risk for neuropathic foot ulceration? *J Foot Ankle Surg*. 1998;37(4):303–307.

50. Levy L, Zeichner JA. Dermatologic manifestations of diabetes. *J Diabetes*. 2012;4:68–76.

51. Huntley AC, Walter RM. Quantitative determination of skin thickness in diabetes mellitus: relationship to disease parameters. *J Med*. 1990;21(5):257–264.

52. Simone VH. Skin manifestations of diabetes. *Cleve Clin J Med*. 2008;75(11):772–787.

53. Pavlović MD. The prevalence of cutaneous manifestations in young patients with type 1 diabetes. *Diabetes Care*. 2007;30(8):1964–1967.

54. Frykberg RG. Diabetic foot ulcers: current concepts. *J Foot Ankle Surg*. 1998;37:440–446.

55. Anderson RN. *Leading Causes for Deaths, 1999 National Vital Statistics Report*. Hyattsville, MD: National Center for Health Statistics; 2001:49(11).

56. National Institute of Diabetes and Digestive and Kidney Diseases. *National Diabetes Statistics Fact Sheet. General Information and National Estimates on Diabetes in the US, 2000*. Bethesda, MD: US Dept. of Health & Human Services, National Institutes of Health; 2002.

57. Lazarus GS, Cooper DM, Knighton DR, et al. Definitions and guidelines for assessment of wounds and evaluation of healing. *Arch Dermatol*. 1994;130:489–493.

58. Levin ME. Preventing amputation in patients with diabetes. *Diabetes Care*. 1995;18:1383–1394.

59. Reiber GE, Vileikyte L, Boyko EJ, et al. Causal pathways for incident lower-extremity ulcers in patients with diabetes from two settings. *Diabetes Care*. 1999;22(1):157–162.

60. Frykberg RG, Armstrong DG, Giurini J, et al. Diabetic foot disorders: a clinical practice guideline. American College of Foot and Ankle Surgeons. *J Foot Ankle Surg*. 2000;39(5, suppl): S1–S60. Review.

61. Wagner FW. The dysvascular foot: a system for diagnosis and treatment. *Foot Ankle*. 1981;2:64–122.

62. Armstrong DG, Lavery LA, Harkless LB. Validation of a diabetic wound classification system. The contribution of depth, infection, and ischemia to risk of amputation. *Diabetes Care*. 1998;21(5):855–859.

63. American Diabetes Association. Consensus development conference on diabetic foot wound care. *Diabetes Care*. 1999;22(8):1354–1360.

64. Edmonds ME, Blundell MP, Morris ME, et al. Improved survival of the diabetic foot: Podiatr role of a specialized foot clinic. *Q J Med*. 1986;232:763–771.

65. Frykberg RG. Team approach toward lower extremity amputation prevention in diabetes. *J Am Podiatr Med Assoc*. 1997;87:305–312.

66. Steed DL, Donohue D, Webster MW, et al. Effect of extensive debridement and treatment on the healing of diabetic foot ulcers. *J Am Coll Surg*. 1996;183.61–64.

67. Alvarez OM, Fernandez-Obregon A, Rogers RS, et al. Chemical debridement of pressure ulcers: a prospective, randomized, comparative trial of collagenase and papain/urea formulations. *Wounds*. 2000;12:15–25.

68. Steed DL. Debridement. *Am J Surg*. 2004;187(5A):71S–74S.

69. Tomic-Canic M, Ayello E, Golinko M, et al. Bar Coding a wound: a molecular guide to surgical debridement. *Adv Skin Wound Care*. 2008;21(10):487–494.

70. Gross A, Cutright DE, Bhaskar SN. Effectiveness of pulsating water jet lavage in treatment of contaminated crushed wounds. *Am J Surg*. 1972;124:373–377.

71. Lipsky BA, Aragón-Sánchez J, Diggle M, et al; International Working Group on the Diabetic Foot (IWGDF). IWGDF guidance on the diagnosis and management of foot infections in persons with diabetes. *Diabetes Metab Res Rev*. 2015. doi:10.1002/dmrr.2699.

72. Lipsky BA, Peters EJ, Berendt AR, et al; International Working Group on Diabetic Foot. Specific guidelines for the treatment of diabetic foot infections 2011. *Diabetes Metab Res Rev*. 2012;28(suppl 1):234–235. doi:10.1002/dmrr.2251.

73. Snyder RJ, Kirsner RS, Warriner RA 3rd, et al. Consensus recommendations on advancing the standard of care for treating neuropathic foot ulcers in patients with diabetes. *Ostomy Wound Manage*. 2010;56(4 suppl):S1–S24.

74. Ovington LG. Advances in wound dressings. et al, *Dermatol*. 2007;25(1):33–38.

75. Kozak GP, Campbell DR, Frykberg RG, et al, eds. *Management of Diabetic Foot Problems*. Philadelphia, PA: WB Saunders; 1995.

76. Frykberg RG, Banks J. Challenges in the treatment of chronic wounds. *Adv Wound Care (New Rochelle)*. 2015;4(9):560–582.

77. Christman AL, Selvin E, Margolis DJ, et al. Hemoglobin A1c predicts healing rate in diabetic wounds. *J Invest Dermatol*. 2011;131(10):2121–2127. doi:10.1038/jid.2011.176.

78. Sheehan P, Jones P, Caselli A, et al. Percent change in wound area of diabetic foot ulcers over a 4-week period is a robust predictor of complete healing in a 12-week prospective trial. *Diabetes Care*. 2003;26(6):1879–1882.

79. Snyder RJ, Cardinal M, Dauphinée DM, et al. A post-hoc analysis of reduction in diabetic foot ulcer size at 4 weeks as a predictor of healing by 12 weeks. *Ostomy Wound Manage*. 2010;56(3):44–50.

80. Lavery LA, Vela SA, Lavery DC, et al. Reducing dynamic foot pressures in high-risk diabetic subjects with foot ulcerations. *Diabetes Care*. 1996;19:818–821.

81. Janisse DJ. A scientific approach to insole design for the diabetic foot. *The Foot*. 1993;3:105–108.

82. Bus SA, Armstrong DG, van Deursen RW; on behalf of the International Working Group on the Diabetic Foot (IWGDF). IWGDF Guidance on footwear and offloading interventions to prevent and heal foot ulcers in patients with diabetes. http://www.iwgdf.org/files/2015/website_footwearoffloading.pdf.

83. Shaw JE, His WL, Ulbrecht JS, et al. Mechanism of plantar unloading in total contact casts: implications, designs, and clinical use. *Foot Ankle Int*. 1997;18:809–817.

84. Catanzariti AR, Blitch EL, Karlock LG. Elective foot and ankle surgery in the diabetic patient. *J Foot Ankle Surg*. 1995;34:23–41.

85. Pearce BJ, Toursarkissian B. The current role of endovascular intervention in the management of diabetic peripheral arterial disease. *Diabet Foot Ankle*. 2012;3. doi:10.3402/dfa.v3i0.18977.

86. Armstrong DG, Lavery LA, Stern S, et al. Is prophylactic diabetic foot surgery dangerous? *J Foot Ankle Surg*. 1996;35:585–589.

87. Shaikh N, Vaughan P, Varty K, et al. Outcome of limited forefoot amputation with primary closure in patients with diabetes. *Bone Joint J*. 2013;95-B:1083–1087.

88. Hamer ML, Robson MC, Krizek TJ, et al. Quantitative bacterial analysis of comparative wound irrigations. *Ann Surg*. 1975;181:819–822.

89. Ries Z, Rungprai C, Harpole B, et al. Incidence, risk factors, and causes for thirty-day unplanned readmissions following primary lower-extremity amputation in patients with diabetes. *J Bone Joint Surg Am*. 2015;97(21):1774–1780. doi:10.2106/JBJS.O.00449.

CHAPTER 6

Neuromuscular Disease and Presentation Involving the Lower Extremity

PETER Z. YAN • ALYSSA G. REHM • CAROLINE MIRANDA • DEXTER Y. SUN

This chapter provides an overview of neuromuscular diseases in the lower extremities. As entire books have been written on the subject, the goal is to provide the reader with a pertinent rather than a comprehensive review of neuromuscular disease in the lower extremities. For completeness, the chapter begins with an anatomical description of the lumbar spine and cauda equina followed by selected common complications in this region, which while not part of the lower limbs per se, produce significant neurologic deficits affecting the lower extremities. The remainder of the chapter is organized anatomically, rostral to caudal, beginning with the lumbosacral plexus, followed by thigh, leg, ankle, and foot, and ending with peripheral neuropathies. Each section begins with an anatomic description, followed by an approach to diagnosis, and ends with a discussion of specific etiologies.

THE LUMBAR SPINE AND CAUDA EQUINA

Lumbar Spine Anatomy

Bone and Soft Tissue

The lumbar spine exhibits a normal lordosis starting at L1. As the patient bends forward, reducing the lordosis, the spinal canal straightens, giving more room to the cord, often alleviating symptoms in patients with lumbar spinal stenosis.

The vertebral body sits anterior to the spinal cord, supported by an intervertebral disc consisting of a soft nucleus pulposus and a thick annulus fibrosis. The disc slowly desiccates over time, leading to height loss, and in combination with trauma, obesity, and genetic predisposition can lead to lumbar disc herniation more frequently at L4–L5, L5–S1.[1]

There are five lumbar vertebrae. For each vertebra, the pedicle extends laterally and posteriorly on both sides, forming the margin of the intervertebral foramen (e.g., the L1 pedicle forms the superior margin of the L1–L2 foramen, and the L2 pedicle forms the inferior foramen margin). Superior and inferior articulating processes extend from the pedicles and form the articulating facet joints that lock the adjacent

vertebrae into place. As the pedicle extends more posteriorly, they turn medially, forming the lamina. The lamina then fuses at the midline and extends posteriorly and inferiorly as the spinous process (**Fig. 6-1**).

The supraspinous ligament covers the spinous processes and interspinous ligament posteriorly. The interspinous ligament fills the space between the spinous processes. The ligamentum flavum covers the spinous processes and interspinous ligament anteriorly. The anterior and posterior longitudinal ligaments cover the vertebral bodies and the intervertebral discs.

Spinal Cord and Cauda Equina

The spinal cord normally terminates in the lumbar spine at L1/2–L2/3 as the conus medullaris. The filum terminale, an extension of the pia, tethers the conus medullaris apex to the dorsal coccyx. Filum traction on the conus, most commonly from developmental abnormalities, can produce a tethered cord syndrome consisting of weakness and sensory loss in the legs as well as fecal and urinary incontinence.[2]

Spinal nerves of the lumbar and sacral region originate from the cauda equina, the bundle of nerves that originates from the start of the conus medullaris. The nerve roots have a very specific orientation within the cauda equina, with the most anterior nerves exiting as the L5 root and exiting in an anterior to posterior order as the S1–S5 roots (**Fig. 6-2**).[3] Compression of these nerves produces the cauda equina syndrome (CES).

Spinal Cord Vascular Supply

Arterial supply to L1 (starting from T1) is provided by the radicular arteries that branch from the intercostal arteries from the aorta. The artery of Adamkiewicz, which branches from the aorta, enters the spinal cord between T8 and L4, usually on the left, and supplies most of the lower spinal cord; emboli to this vessel usually lead to infarction of the anterior two-thirds of the spinal cord, causing weakness, pain, and loss of temperature sensation. The general orientation of arteries relative to the spinal column is shown in **Figure 6-3**.

Inside the spinal canal, from the radicular artery, the radiculopial artery branches and moves posteriorly to form

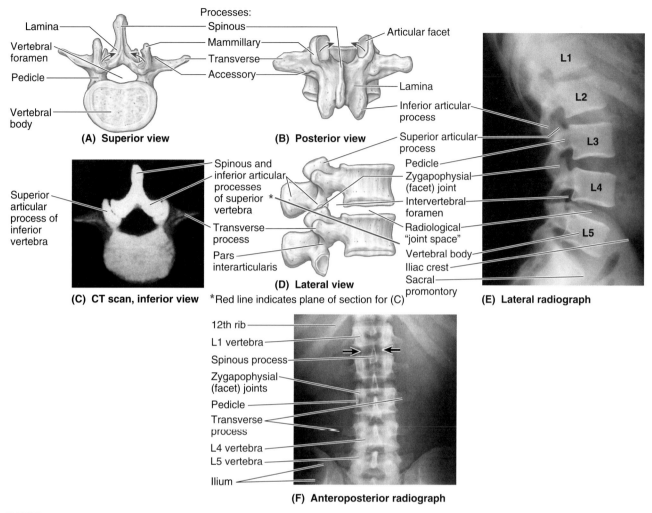

FIGURE 6-1. Illustrative and radiographic views of the lumbar spine (From Moore KL, Agur AM, Dalley AF. *Clinically Oriented Anatomy.* 7th ed. Philadelphia, PA: Wolters Kluwer; 2009, with permission).

the posterior spinal arteries and supply the posterior one-third of the spinal cord. In addition, the radiculomedullary branch of the radicular artery forms the anterior spinal artery. These arteries supply the anterior two-thirds of the spinal cord (**Fig. 6-4**).[4,5]

Venous drainage from the lower spinal cord is the same as from the rest of the cord. They drain into an irregular epidural venous plexus that communicates with the pedicular veins and ultimately drains into the vena cavae (**Fig. 6-5**). Lumbar needle procedures can puncture these veins and produce bleeding, and can lead to significant hematomas in patients with coagulopathies.

Common Lumbar Spine and Cauda Equina Complications

Epidural Steroid Injection

Low back pain is a common complaint, has its highest incidence in the third decade, with 1-year incidence of any back pain between 1% and 36% and recurrence between 24% and 80%.[6] Epidural steroid injections (ESIs) remain a popular nonsurgical intervention for low back pain. Although there is literature supporting its efficacy,[7,8] the Food and Drug Administration has not approved epidural corticosteroid injections for low back pain at this time because serious neurologic events, including paraplegia, quadriplegia, and brain and spinal cord infarction, have been reported with and without use of fluoroscopy.[9]

Complication rates for ESI remain low overall at 2.4%,[10] for intralaminar and interlaminar and transforaminal approaches, with conflicting reports comparing relative complication rates between the techniques.[10,11] Infectious complications, including epidural abscess, meningitis, discitis, and osteomyelitis, are about 1% to 2%.[12] The incidence of epidural hematoma is about 1 per 150,000 and increases to 2% in patients using anticoagulants.[13] Ideally, oral anticoagulation should be discontinued, and prothrombin time normalized. This usually takes 1 to 2 days. In patients taking coumadin, the International Normalized Ratio (INR) should be definitely less than 3, but there are no definitive guidelines for

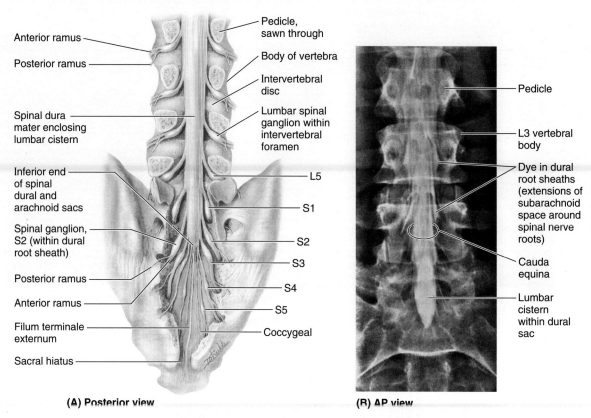

FIGURE 6-2. Illustrative and radiographic views of the lumbar spinal cord and cauda equina relative to their surrounding osseous structure (From Moore KL, Agur AM, Dalley AF. *Clinically Oriented Anatomy.* 7th ed. Philadelphia, PA: Wolters Kluwer; 2009, with permission).

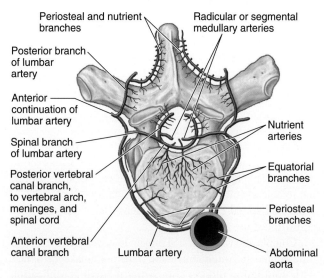

FIGURE 6-3. The spinal arteries relative to the lumbar spine (From Moore KL, Agur AM, Dalley AF. *Clinically Oriented Anatomy.* 7th ed. Philadelphia, PA: Wolters Kluwer; 2009, with permission).

INR between 1.5 and 3. Platelet function should also be normalized, which can mean holding the antiplatelet agent for 5 to 10 days.[14]

Surprisingly, intravascular injection can be frequent, as high as 21.3% in the transforaminal approach with fluoroscopic guidance.[15] Although this does not lead to an adverse outcome per se, instilling the local corticosteroid intravascularly subjects the patient to pain and anxiety associated with needle procedures without ensuing benefits. Dural puncture is another notable complication in ESI. Cerebrospinal fluid (CSF) flashback indicative of dural puncture may not necessarily be present, especially in the transforaminal approach.[16] Aside from a CSF leak that may require blood patching, injection of intrathecal anesthetic can lead to transient ascending weakness or sensory loss, which can spread as high as C2. Rarely, serious complications such as respiratory depression can also occur. Notably, the usual 6 to 8 mL of anesthetic used in ESI is not typically sufficient to produce significant adverse events.[12]

Epidural Anesthesia

Epidural anesthesia can lead to dural puncture in 0.4% to 6% of patients when used in a variety of abdominal and lower extremity surgeries.[17] A persistent CSF leak after dural puncture can lead to a postural headache alleviated with recumbence. There is no evidence correlating the length of postpuncture recumbence to incidence of postdural puncture headache. However, there is an association with needle gauge (11% to 28% with 20 gauge, 3% to 25% with 25 gauge, 3% to 8% with 26 gauge, and 0% to 2% with 29 gauge).[18] In cases of persistent headache, an epidural blood patch is usually applied, with a success rate of 36% to 57% for the first patch, increasing with subsequent patching. Interestingly, although theorized to spread, clot, and occlude the leak, the exact mechanism

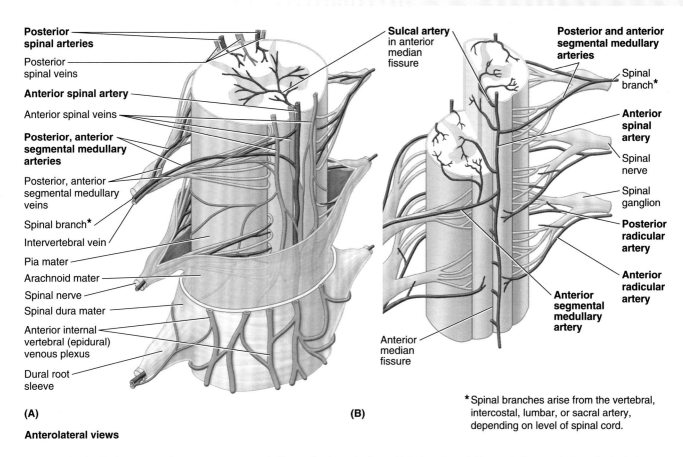

(A)

(B)

Anterolateral views

*Spinal branches arise from the vertebral, intercostal, lumbar, or sacral artery, depending on level of spinal cord.

Most proximal spinal nerves and roots are accompanied by **radicular arteries**, which do not reach the posterior or anterior spinal arteries. **Segmental medullary arteries** occur irregularly *in the place of* radicular arteries—they are really just larger vessels that make it all the way to the spinal arteries.

FIGURE 6-4. The major arteries supplying the spinal cord and the associated veins (From Moore KL, Agur AM, Dalley AF. *Clinically Oriented Anatomy.* 7th ed. Philadelphia, PA: Wolters Kluwer; 2009, with permission).

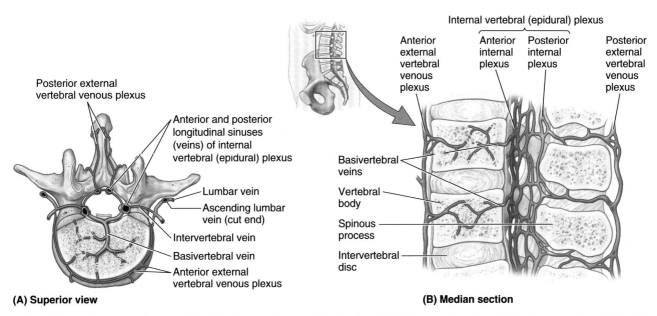

(A) Superior view

(B) Median section

FIGURE 6-5. The spinal venous plexuses relative to the lumbar spine (From Moore KL, Agur AM, Dalley AF. *Clinically Oriented Anatomy.* 7th ed. Philadelphia, PA: Wolters Kluwer; 2009, with permission).

for blood patching has not been determined.[19] Further, there is no consensus between blind patching and patching after a radiologic CSF study. Although targeted patching seems to provide higher symptom relief rate, in cases of indeterminate leak location, traditional blind patching in the lumbar spine is generally applied. In addition, the lumbar epidural space can accommodate a larger volume of blood without concern for compressive effects on the spinal cord.[20]

The process of epidural puncture can itself injure the vertebral venous plexus, around 6% incidence, leading to repeat procedure half the time,[21] and sometimes epidural hematomas. In these cases, the majority were associated with anticoagulant use or clotting disorder. Patients frequently present with motor weakness (46%) and back pain (38%). Notably, back pain can be masked in cases of continuous anesthesia.[22]

Lumbar Puncture

Headache after lumbar puncture is very common; roughly one-third of patients experience it.[23] These headaches are typically associated with rapid removal of roughly 15% (20 mL) of total CSF volume, provoked by sitting or standing, and relieved by recumbence.[24] The mechanism involves a combination of meningeal traction from intracranial hypotension as well as dilation of cerebral veins and venous sinuses.[25] Spontaneous intracranial hypotension has a similar presentation; however, its pathophysiology and diagnostic criteria differ (see **Table 6-1**). Conservative treatment with hydration and intravenous caffeine often offers symptomatic relief, but in refractory cases, blood patching is required.

The infection rate from lumbar puncture is low (1 to 2 per 10,000), the most common organism is *Streptococcus* two-thirds of the time.[26] Bleeding is a significant complication in coagulopathic and thrombocytopenic patients and can lead

to paraplegia. The diagnosis is often delayed, with about 50% of lumbar puncture–induced hematomas discovered after 12 hours of paraplegia.[27] Complication rates are significantly higher in anticoagulated patients who undergo lumbar puncture.[28] Guidelines for anticoagulation and lumbar puncture are the same as those of ESI and other epidural/dural puncture procedures. Notably, clear CSF does not preclude risk of hematoma formation, as up to half of patients who later develop hematomas have initially clear CSF.[27]

Degenerative Disc Disease and Spinal Stenosis

The cause of degenerative disc disease is multifactorial and includes lifestyle (smoking, occupation), mechanical loading, nutrition, and genetics (aggrecan gene polymorphism), which all lead to degenerative changes beginning in the 20s to early 30s.[29] Symptomatic lumbar disease contributes to an estimated 60% to 80% of low back pain cases and is most commonly caused by lumbar disc herniations.[30]

Sciatica is a common complication of degenerative disc disease. The hallmark presentation is radiating pain down the buttock, following the course of the sciatic nerve. Disc compression of the nerve roots at L4–S1 can produce unilateral sciatica symptoms. However, compression of the pelvic plexus or cauda equina and lumbar stenosis can produce bilateral symptoms. Clinically, worsening pain with coughing, sneezing, or Valsalva is indicative of disc disease rather than other etiologies such as spondylolisthesis or piriformis syndrome.[31] Fortunately, sciatica self-resolves in 75% of patients after 3 months.[32] The mainstay of treatment is with nonopiate analgesics to allow for physical therapy. Disc surgery is another option, but in terms of pain or disability, there seems to be limited benefit compared with conservative measures at 1 year.[33]

Table 6-1. Internal Headache Society Diagnostic Criteria for Headaches Related to Intracranial Hypotension

Diagnostic Criteria for Postdural (Postlumbar) Puncture Headache	Diagnostic Criteria for Headache Attributed to Spontaneous (or Idiopathic) Low CSF Pressure

A. Headache that worsens within 15 min after sitting or standing and improves within 15 min after lying, with at least one of the following and fulfilling criteria C and D:
  1. neck stiffness
  2. tinnitus
  3. hyperacusis
  4. photophobia
  5. nausea
B. Dural puncture has been performed
C. Headache develops within 5 d after dural puncture
D. Headache resolves either:
  1. spontaneously within 1 wk or
  2. within 48 h after effective treatment of the spinal fluid leak (usually by epidural blood patch)
	A. Diffuse and/or dull headache that worsens within 15 min after sitting or standing, with at least one of the following and fulfilling criterion D:
	  1. neck stiffness
	  2. tinnitus
	  3. hyperacusis
	  4. photophobia
	  5. nausea
	B. At least one of the following:
	  1. evidence of low CSF pressure on MRI (e.g., pachymeningeal enhancement)
	  2. evidence of CSF leakage on conventional myelography, CT myelography, or cisternography
	  3. CSF opening pressure <60 mm H_2O in sitting position
	C. No history of dural puncture or other cause of CSF fistula
	D. Headache resolves within 72 h after epidural blood patching

Spinal stenosis typically develops in the 50s to 60s. The stenosis can occur centrally or laterally. Aside from discogenic causes, central stenosis often develops from ligamentum flavum hypertrophy, which can be from aging or mechanical instability of the spine. Patients with central stenosis often present with neurogenic claudication: radiating pain down both legs while standing or walking, relieved with sitting down and bending forward, the kyphosis of which increases the spinal canal diameter. In contrast, lateral spinal stenosis produces radiculopathies, with weakness or sensory decrease along the corresponding myotome and dermatome and decreased reflexes corresponding to the levels of stenosis. Aside from direct disc compression, foraminal stenosis from articular hypertrophy, pedicular kinking, and uncinate spur can compress the nerve root as it enters, passes through, and exits the neural foramen.[34] Conservative treatment for lumbar spinal stenosis includes a combination of physical therapy, intermittent pelvic traction, oral analgesics, and epidural steroids. Depending on the degree of stenosis, 70% of patients can have symptom improvement.[35] For severe stenosis or refractory cases, decompressive surgeries such as laminectomies, foraminotomies, and spinal fusion in cases of instability can be tried, and when successful, patients can have complete resolution of symptoms.

Cauda Equina Syndrome

CES consists of low back pain, including radicular pain or numbness, tingling or electrical sensation traveling down the leg, as well as sensation change in the perineal region, or "saddle anesthesia," and bowel or bladder dysfunction. In practice, many patients present with a partial syndrome.[3,36]

Compression, whether by trauma, disc herniation, abscess, hematoma, or tumors, is the main etiology of CES. The degree and timing of compression affect clinical presentation, because patients with chronic mild compression are largely asymptomatic and show only changes in electrodiagnostic studies, whereas those with acute significant compression, such as from a hematoma, can manifest the entire CES syndrome.

When CES is suspected, imaging confirmation is required. Although magnetic resonance imaging (MRI) is the study of choice, CT with myelography can be useful for determining pathology that requires immediate surgical intervention. Intervention should be urgent, as patients have significant symptom improvement with decompression within 48 hours, though earlier is often preferred in practice.[37] More than half of patients who undergo decompression within 48 hours can have complete recovery of urinary incontinence versus only one third in patients outside of 48 hours.[38] Overall, surgery is very effective, with 43% of patients eventually gaining complete recovery and 87% gain functional recovery.[39]

THE LUMBOSACRAL PLEXUS

Lumbosacral Plexus Neuroanatomy

All spinal nerves exit the intervertebral foramen and divide into anterior (ventral) and posterior (dorsal) rami. The anterior rami of L1–S4 form the lumbosacral plexus, which has three components: (1) the lumbar plexus (L1–L4), (2) the sacral plexus (S1–S4), and (3) the lumbosacral trunk (L4–L5) that connects the lumbar and sacral plexus (**Fig. 6-6**).

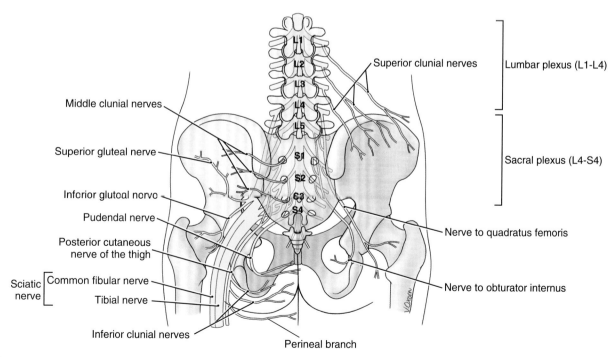

FIGURE 6-6. The lumbosacral plexus and their associated roots and nerves (From Agur AM, Dalley AF. *Grant's Atlas of Anatomy.* 13th ed. Philadelphia, PA: Wolters Kluwer; 2012, with permission).

The lumbar plexus forms on the psoas major muscle along the posterior abdominal wall, making it prone to compression from psoas muscle damage or retroperitoneal (RP) hematoma. It then branches into an anterior and posterior division. The anterior division forms the obturator nerve, which goes into the medial compartment of the thigh. The posterior division forms the femoral nerve, which innervates the leg extensors, and, owing to medial rotation during development, ends up in the *anterior compartment* of the thigh. The lumbar plexus nerve, roots, and functions are summarized in **Table 6-2**.

The roots of the sacral plexus lie on the piriformis muscle and form the sciatic nerve, which also divides into an anterior and posterior division. The anterior division forms the tibial branch of the sciatic nerve, which is more medial, while the posterior division forms the peroneal branch of the sciatic nerve, which is more lateral. The sacral plexus nerve, roots, and functions are summarized in **Table 6-3**.

Table 6-2. Lumbar Plexus, Nerves, Roots, and Their Functions

Nerve	Root	Motor	Sensory
Iliohypogastric	T12, L1	Internal oblique and transversus abdominis (supports abdominal wall)	Posterolateral gluteal skin
Ilioinguinal	L1	None	Medial thigh, pubis, and external genitalia
Genitofemoral	L1, L2	*Genital branch:* cremasteric reflex *Femoral branch:* none	*Genital branch:* external genitalia *Femoral branch:* upper anterior thigh-femoral triangle
Lateral cutaneous nerve of the thigh	L2, L3	None	Anterior and lateral thigh to the knee
Obturator (medial compartment of the thigh)	L2–L4	*Anterior division:* ■ Adductor longus and brevis (adducts) ■ Gracilis (adducts hip, internally rotates and flexes knee) *Posterior division:* ■ Adductor magnus (adducts) ■ Obturator externus (laterally rotates knee)	*Cutaneous branch of obturator nerve:* ■ Comes off the anterior division after it pierces the fascia lata. ■ It supplies the inferomedial thigh
Femoral (anterior compartment of the thigh)	L2–L4	■ Pectineus, psoas (hip flexors) ■ Iliacus (hip flexor, internal rotator thigh) ■ Quadriceps (rectus femoris, vastus lateralis, medialis and intermedius)—(knee extensor) ■ Sartorius (hip flexor, abductor, external rotator)	■ Anterior cutaneous: supplies anteromedial thigh ■ Saphenous (terminal branch): supplies anterior/medial leg and foot

Table 6-3. Sacral Plexus Nerves, Roots, and Their Functions[a]

Nerve	Root	Motor	Sensory
Superior gluteal	L4–S1	■ Gluteus minimus and medius (abduct thigh) ■ Tensor fascia latae (medial rotation thigh)	None
Inferior gluteal	L5–S2	■ Gluteus maximus (extend hip)	None
Sciatic (posterior compartment of thigh)	L4–S3	■ *Hamstring muscles:* semitendinosus, semimembranosus, short head of bicep femoris (extend the hip and flex the knee) *One muscle in medial compartment of thigh:* ■ Hamstring portion of adductor magnus (adducts the thigh) Terminates as tibial and fibular nerve	No direct innervations, but indirectly innervates via its terminal branches (tibial and fibular nerve)
Posterior femoral cutaneous	S1–S3	None	Posterior thigh, posterior leg, perineum
Pudendal	S2–S4	■ External anal sphincter ■ Internal urethral sphincter ■ Muscles of perineum	Clitoris, penis, skin of perineum

[a]Nerve to the piriformis, nerve to the obturator internus, nerve to the quadratus femoris also come off the sacral plexus and directly innervate the muscles that share the same name as the nerve.

Diagnosing Lumbosacral Plexopathy

Diagnosis

Clinical features of a lumbosacral plexopathy (LSP) depend on location and the underlying etiology. One should consider LSP if a patient's symptoms cannot be localized to a peripheral nerve or a single nerve root. If the lumbar plexus is damaged, there will be weakness of hip flexion, knee extension (femoral), and hip adduction (obturator). Sensory loss and paresthesia tend to occur over the lateral, anterior, and medial thigh, but may extend down to the medial calf. If pain is present, it is most often located in the pelvis, with radiation to the anterior thigh. Lesions of the sacral plexus tend to present with weakness of hip extensors (gluteus maximus), adductors, and internal rotators (gluteus medius and tensor fasciae latae), and hamstring muscles or distal foot muscles. Sensory symptoms are seen over the posterior thigh, and posterior lateral calf and foot.[40] Pain may be present in the pelvis.

The first step in diagnosing an LSP is the exam. The physician should assess for weakness and sensory loss in the distributions discussed above. Loss of reflexes, or diminished reflexes, may indicate specific nerve root involvement (adductor [L3], patellar [L4], Achilles [S1]). One should also palpate the inguinal region to feel for hematoma or mass, and palpate the greater trochanter of the hip for bursitis. Straight leg raise (L5, S1) can also help distinguish an LSP from a radiculopathy (a common mimic). Maneuvering the hip can also help determine whether the pain is related instead to sacroiliitis.

The imaging of choice is an MRI. If abscess, neoplasm, or inflammatory changes are suspected, the MRI should be ordered with contrast. More recently, MR neurography can more closely examine at the plexus nerve roots.[40] Electrodiagnostic studies help localize a lesion to the lumbosacral plexus, and exclude radiculopathies or neuropathies that may clinically mimic an LSP. Nerve conduction studies (NCS) should be performed to look for specific nerve abnormalities, and electromyogram (EMG) of lower extremities and paraspinal muscles can aid in localizing weakness or muscle denervation. Specifically on NCS, decreased sensory nerve action potentials imply that the lesion is at or distal to the dorsal root ganglion, but *not* at the level of the nerve roots. Important muscles to test on EMG include gluteal, thigh adductor muscles, and paraspinal muscles. Testing the gluteal muscles can distinguish a sciatic neuropathy from a lower LSP. Abnormalities in the adductor muscles (obturator nerve) in addition to femoral innervated muscles indicate an upper LSP, rather than an isolated femoral neuropathy. Abnormalities in the paraspinal muscles localize the lesion to the nerve root, rather than the plexus. An upper limb EMG should be used if there is bilateral involvement, to help exclude polyneuropathy.

The clinician should consider hemoglobin A1c, erythrocyte sedimentation rate (ESR), C-reactive protein, infectious studies (Epstein–Barr virus [EBV], varicella-zoster virus, syphilis, Lyme), and rheumatologic studies (anti-nuclear antibody [ANA], anti-neutrophilic cytoplasmic antibody [ANCA], angiotensin converting enzyme [ACE], serum protein electrophoresis [SPEP], Anti Ro/La) because these tests help rule out the common causes of neuropathy. A lumbar puncture can also be used to look for occult infection or malignancy.

COMMON ETIOLOGIES OF LUMBOSACRAL PLEXOPATHY

Systemic Etiologies

Diabetes

Diabetic LSP (or diabetic amyotrophy) typically occurs in long-term type 2 diabetics. Persistently high blood sugar produces an ischemic microvasculopathy. Although only 1% of diabetics develop an LSP, those who do have significant morbidity. Patients present with acute onset of unilateral neuropathic pain (stabbing, burning, aching) and allodynia in the thigh or leg, usually lasting weeks. As the pain subsides, patients experience proximal more than distal weakness out of proportion to the pain. Over months, the symptoms become bilateral and diffuse. Autonomic involvement is common. NCS reveal multifocal primary axonal degeneration.[41] Unfortunately, many patients have long-term disability requiring wheelchairs or walkers. Because proximal segments of the plexus reinnervate earlier, foot drop is the most notable chronic symptom.

Idiopathic Plexitis

For most idiopathic plexitis, the underlying pathology remains unclear; inflammation is thought to be the primary culprit. Presentation is acute-onset severe pain in the proximal pelvis or upper leg that subsides over several weeks, followed by weakness that subsides over months. Sometimes, patients report a preceding illness or vaccination. In cases of progressive LSP, ESR may be elevated, indicating a systemic inflammatory response, and steroids or immunosuppressive therapy can be used.

Infectious, Inflammatory, and Infiltrative

Infectious, inflammatory, and infiltrative causes of LSP are very rare. They should be considered in patients with HIV; who have concomitant infections with echovirus, EBV, cytomegalovirus, Lyme; or who are undergoing HIV seroconversion. Although patients most often experience radicular symptoms, LSP can also occur. Other considerations include compression from an abscess, sarcoidosis, and amyloidosis.[42,43]

Compressive Etiologies

Postpartum

Postpartum LSP occurs in about 1/2,600 births, and tends to affect the lumbosacral trunk (L4/L5). Risk factors include large infant size, prolonged or arrested labor, and maternal short stature. The mechanism is compression of the plexus by the fetal head as it passes through the pelvic brim, where the plexus is no longer cushioned by the psoas muscle. Because the peroneal fibers of the sciatic nerve are located posteriorly, nearest to bone, they are most vulnerable to compression. For this reason, "foot drop" is the most common presenting feature, and women are often misdiagnosed as having a compressive peroneal neuropathy (from positioning during labor). Subtle weakness of knee flexion, hip flexion, abduction, and internal rotation may help localize the lesion to the lumbosacral plexus, rather than a peripheral nerve.[44] NCS may show signs of demyelination. However, if there is prolonged compression, leading to severe ischemic damage, axonal loss may occur. Prognosis is usually excellent, and recovery is expected within 2 to 3 months; if longer, axonal loss should be suspected.

Neoplastic

Neoplasms typically injure the lumbosacral plexus via direct invasion, or infiltration. Colorectal carcinoma is the most common tumor leading to an LSP, but other common culprits include pelvic tumors and peripheral nerve sheath tumors.[45,46] Distant tumors can cause LSP via bone metastases or meningeal carcinomatosis, which is seen more commonly in leukemia, lymphoma, melanoma, and lung and breast cancer.[47]

In neoplasm-induced LSP, the primary symptom is severe pain (91%), characterized as aching or lancinating, which is worse with movement or standing. Weakness (typically in the distribution of the sacral plexus), sensory loss, and areflexia follow the pain. Fifty percent of patients have radicular signs with positive straight leg raise. Urinary incontinence is most commonly associated with epidural extension of tumor, but only 12% of patients have loss of sphincter tone.[48]

Gadolinium-enhanced MRI of the pelvis can show compression or direct invasion of the pelvis. If leptomeningeal spread of tumor is considered, MRI of the lumbar spine should be ordered, and if this is negative, a lumbar puncture can help with the diagnosis. Therapy response and prognosis depend on the tumor type. Earlier diagnosis, with less neurologic involvement, predicts a better treatment response. Unfortunately, patients are often resistant to traditional pain management methods. Radiation can give pain relief in up to 50% of patients.[47] Dorsal rhizotomy can be considered for refractory pain, because it can significantly reduce pain rating and daily narcotic use, but additional research is needed in this area.[49]

Vascular Etiologies

Vascular causes of LSP include RP hematoma, aneurysms or pseudoaneurysms, and ischemia. Because of its rich vascular supply, ischemia is a rare etiology, but when it does occur, it is thought to be at the microvascular level. Arterial pseudoaneurysms can occur postoperatively in the setting of infection or defective vascular anastomoses.[50–52] Common locations include the abdominal aorta; internal, external, and common iliac arteries; superior and inferior gluteal arteries; and hypogastric arteries. Because the roots of the sacral plexus lie in close proximity to the internal iliac vessels, they are more prone to vascular compression.

LSP from RP hematoma occurs most commonly in the setting of anticoagulation, but can also occur in patients with clotting disorders, after femoral artery catheterization, or after lumbar plexus nerve block. RP hematomas most often occur in the psoas muscle, and thus cause compression of the lumbar plexus. Smaller RP hematomas often affect the femoral nerve alone, whereas larger ones involve more of the lumbar plexus.

Common symptoms include tenderness or fullness in the inguinal or suprainguinal region, severe back pain, lower quadrant pain, and weakness of hip flexion and knee extension, with reduced or absent patellar reflex. Neurologic recovery is generally complete, or near complete.[53] For anticoagulated patients, coagulopathy should be immediately reversed, and physicians should be vigilant-in treating hypovolemic shock. In stable patients, conservative management with blood transfusions and bed rest is appropriate.

Iatrogenic Etiologies

Radiation Plexopathy

Radiation-induced LSP rarely occurs with conventional radiation methods and dosing. It occurs more frequently with higher dosing used in intracavitary radiation, and some reports show increased risk with radiation doses exceeding 60 Gy. Doses above 10 Gy have been shown to cause changes in Schwann cells, endoneural fibroblasts, perineural cells, and cells of small vessel walls.[54]

Symptoms of radiation plexopathy injury typically occur 1 year after treatment, with a peak onset at 5 years. Unlike malignant LSP, radiation-induced LSP is typically painless, and presents with bilateral leg weakness, sometimes accompanied by sensory loss. EMG can be very useful in diagnostically challenging patients, as about half of patients with radiation plexopathy demonstrate myokymia.

There are no effective therapies for radiation plexopathy. Although some physicians assert benefit from hyperbaric oxygen, at least one randomized, double-blinded trial has shown otherwise.[55] Dysesthesias can be treated with neuropathic pain medications such as amitriptyline, venlafaxine, or gabapentin. Physical therapy is sometimes helpful in patients with weakness.

Traumatic Etiologies

Indirect Trauma

Since the lumbosacral plexus is protected by bone and multiple muscle layers, direct trauma is uncommon. However, sacral, pelvic, or acetabular fractures, or sacroiliac dislocation, can cause indirect trauma to the lumbosacral plexus. The sacral plexus is more commonly damaged than the lumbar plexus, and it is more prone to injury with sacral fractures or sacroiliac joint dislocation, when compared with pelvic or acetabular fractures.[56] In most cases, diagnosis is explained by the mechanism of injury, and a suggestive exam. However, EMG can be used to help confirm the diagnosis.

Postoperative

The lumbosacral plexus can be damaged mechanically during operations of the neighboring kidneys and internal genital organs. Ischemia to the LSP has been shown to occur in renal transplant patients if the internal iliac artery is used for allograft revascularization. Postoperative abscess or hematoma formation in the psoas muscle, or elsewhere in the retroperitoneum, can cause LSP through mass effect. Some investigators propose that postoperative LSP may be related to inflammatory mechanisms, based on nerve biopsy findings that indicate ischemic injury and microvasculitis. When this is the case, treatment with immunomodulatory therapy may help improve outcomes.[57]

THE THIGH

Obturator Nerve

Anatomy

The obturator nerve originates from the anterior division of the lumbosacral plexus medial to the femoral nerve. It then passes along the medial side of the psoas muscle, along the lateral pelvic wall, and enters the obturator foramen, where it divides into two. The anterior division emerges from the obturator canal, runs over the obturator externus, deep to the pectineus, and then passes between the adductor longus and brevis, where it innervates these muscles. The pectineus is typically innervated by the femoral nerve, but sometimes can be innervated by the obturator nerve. The obturator nerve also innervates the gracilis muscle and a small cutaneous area in the medial thigh. The posterior division of the obturator nerve passes through the obturator externus and then runs between the adductor brevis and the adductor magnus, where it innervates the obturator externus, and the adductor portion of the adductor magnus. It also gives off cutaneous supply to the inferomedial portion of the thigh, just above the knee.

Modes of Injury, Diagnosis, Treatment

Neuropathies of the obturator nerve are uncommon, but can occur from pelvic trauma, surgery, or compression from pelvic tumors, most commonly bladder cancer. There is no evidence that entrapment in the obturator foramen occurs. The most common symptoms are pain, leg adduction weakness, and sensory loss over a small area of the medial thigh. Diagnosis is clinical, but can be confirmed with electrodiagnostic testing.

Sciatic Nerve

Anatomy

The sciatic nerve arises from the lumbosacral trunk and upper part of the lumbosacral plexus (L4–S3 nerve roots). It then travels down the wall of the pelvis and enters the thigh through the greater sciatic foramen in the hip. In the thigh, it passes under the piriformis muscle, where it is prone to compression, and between the ischial tuberosity and greater trochanter of the femur, where it can be prone to injury from trauma. It terminates at the superior border of the popliteal fossa as the tibial nerve (medial) and common peroneal nerve (lateral). It innervates the hamstring muscles (long and short head of biceps femoris, semitendinosus, semimembranosus), which are all extensors of the hip except the biceps femoris long head, which is a flexor of the knee (**Fig. 6-7A**). It also innervates the adductor magnus, which aids with hip extension. It has no direct sensory innervations in the thigh, but its distal branches (tibial and common peroneal nerves) provide sensation to most of the limb below the knee.

Modes of Injury, Diagnosis, Treatment

The primary cause of sciatic neuropathy can occur after mechanical trauma to the hip. Sciatic nerve injury most often occurs in the gluteal region or area of sciatic notch, from hip trauma, fracture, dislocation, and occasionally after hip replacement. Other less common reasons for sciatic nerve injury in the gluteal region include incorrect injections to the buttock (lateral side is safe, medial side is unsafe, **Fig. 6-7B**), compression from prolonged bed rest, and mass or hematoma in the pelvic area.

Piriformis syndrome can also injure the sciatic nerve in the region of the sciatic notch, as it comes in contact with a hypertrophied piriformis muscle. Common causes of piriformis syndrome are repetitive movements of the muscles in the gluteal region, which occur with skating, cycling, or climbing. This diagnosis, however, is one of exclusion and often controversial.[58] Cardiac surgery and intra-aortic balloon pumps can also be associated with sciatic nerve injury. More rarely, lesions of the sciatic nerve can occur at the mid-thigh from a femur mass or fracture, or nerve infarction.

Patients typically present with pain shooting down the posterior aspect of the leg to the foot. If the lesion is in the gluteal region, weakness occurs in the distribution of the hamstrings (knee flexion), in addition to the muscles below the knee. If the damage is in the mid-thigh, knee flexion is spared, and weakness only occurs below the knee. No matter where the nerve is injured, there is always sparing of hip flexion, extension, abduction and adduction, and knee extension. Interestingly, the peroneal distribution of the sciatic nerve is often more affected than the tibial distribution, despite the entire nerve being affected. Sensory loss involves the entire peroneal, tibial, and sural territories. Sensation is spared above the knee and below the knee in the distribution of the saphenous nerve (the medial calf and arch of the foot). The knee reflex is spared, whereas the ankle reflex is often missing.

Sciatic neuropathy is mainly a clinical diagnosis, but if the damage is severe enough, findings may be seen on EMG and NCS. Some typical findings include reduced peroneal and sural sensory responses, normal saphenous sensory response, reduced tibial and peroneal motor response amplitudes, and denervation/reinnervation muscle patterns.

Prognosis in sciatic injury is favorable, with one study reporting good recovery in 75% of patients over a 3-year period without treatment. Lack of plantarflexion and dorsiflexion involvement at initial evaluation is a favorable prognostic sign.

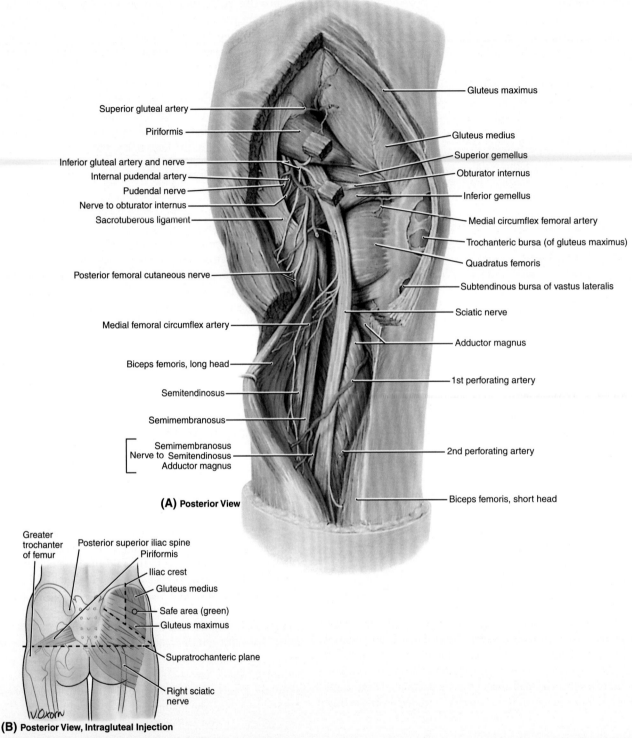

Superior gluteal artery

Piriformis

Inferior gluteal artery and nerve

Internal pudendal artery

Pudendal nerve

Nerve to obturator internus

Sacrotuberous ligament

Posterior femoral cutaneous nerve

Medial femoral circumflex artery

Biceps femoris, long head

Semitendinosus

Semimembranosus

Semimembranosus
Nerve to Semitendinosus
Adductor magnus

(A) Posterior View

Gluteus maximus

Gluteus medius

Superior gemellus

Obturator internus

Inferior gemellus

Medial circumflex femoral artery

Trochanteric bursa (of gluteus maximus)

Quadratus femoris

Subtendinous bursa of vastus lateralis

Sciatic nerve

Adductor magnus

1st perforating artery

2nd perforating artery

Biceps femoris, short head

Greater
trochanter
of femur

Posterior superior iliac spine

Piriformis

Iliac crest

Gluteus medius

Safe area (green)

Gluteus maximus

Supratrochanteric plane

Right sciatic
nerve

(B) Posterior View, Intragluteal Injection

FIGURE 6-7. A: Nerves of the thigh as they course posteriorly. **B:** Illustration of the safe area for gluteal injections (From Agur AM, Dalley AF. *Grant's Atlas of Anatomy.* 13th ed. Philadelphia, PA: Wolters Kluwer; 2012, with permission).

Femoral Nerve

Anatomy

The femoral nerve is the largest nerve that emerges from the lumbar plexus (roots L2, L3, and L4). It forms in the psoas muscle, descends between the psoas and iliacus muscle, and then tucks beneath the inguinal ligament, lateral to the femoral artery and vein, to enter the thigh. Here it innervates several muscles, including the iliacus muscle (hip flexion and internal rotation), and the quadriceps, which are knee extensors (rectus femoris, vastus lateralis, vastus intermedius, vastus medialis). It also innervates the sartorius muscle, which flexes, abducts, and externally rotates the hip. It provides sensation to the anterior medial thigh via the anterior cutaneous branches. It ends as the saphenous nerve, which provides sensation from the medial aspect of the knee, to the medial malleolus and arch of the foot.

Modes of Injury, Diagnosis, Treatment

Similar to sciatic neuropathy, femoral neuropathy can occur for a variety of reasons. Because the femoral nerve is protected within the pelvis, direct compression here is uncommon, but can occur from hip or pelvic fractures, pelvic masses, or iliacus hematoma. Damage can also occur after hip replacements, abdominal or pelvic surgeries, inguinal lymph node biopsy, or childbirth, most likely from compression of the nerve along the inguinal ligament from prolonged lithotomy position.[59,60] Other mechanisms of injury include ischemia, toxic injury, and direct transection.

On examination, patients have weakness of the quadriceps muscle group with sparing of adduction (obturator nerve). If innervation to the iliopsoas muscle is lost, weakness may be present in hip flexion. Sensory loss occurs along the anterior thigh, medial thigh, and extends down along the medial leg to the arch of the foot. The knee jerk (L4) is generally decreased or absent.

Femoral neuropathy is usually a clinical diagnosis. Nevertheless, needle EMG can help confirm the diagnosis. Findings include weakness of muscles innervated by the femoral nerve, absence of weakness in muscles innervated by the obturator nerve, and compromised saphenous sensory nerve function.

Prognosis for incomplete femoral neuropathy is generally good, with about two-thirds of patients achieving satisfactory to excellent recoveries. The smaller the degree of axonal loss on EMG/NCS, the better the prognosis. In general, treatment is supportive, including physical therapy and appropriate analgesia. If the mechanism of injury is hematoma compression, drainage may be indicated. If the nerve is damaged directly, as in transection or ligation, surgical exploration and nerve repair or grafting may be considered.

Lateral Femoral Cutaneous Nerve

Anatomy

The lateral femoral cutaneous nerve branches directly off the lumbosacral plexus (L2, L3). It emerges lateral to the psoas muscle, crosses the iliacus, and then passes underneath the lateral part of the inguinal ligament to enter the thigh. It runs on top of the sartorius muscle and terminates as cutaneous sensory branches that innervate the lateral thigh. It innervates no muscles.

Modes of Injury, Diagnosis, Treatment

This nerve is most commonly injured as it passes beneath the inguinal ligament, where it can become compressed, causing a syndrome known as meralgia paresthetica. Common risk factors include obesity, old age, diabetes, pregnancy, and tight-fitting clothing.[61] Patients generally complain of paresthesias and pain, which radiate down the lateral thigh toward the knee. In severe cases, fixed sensory loss of the lateral thigh can occur.

Diagnosis is mainly clinical, based on the unique location of paresthesias. Also, there should not be weakness, and there should be no sensory loss below the knee. Electrodiagnostic studies have a limited role, but may show reduced response amplitude if damage is severe enough to produce axonal loss.[62] Electrodiagnostic studies can also be useful to help exclude plexopathy or radiculopathy.

Meralgia paresthetica is usually self-limited. Most patients respond to conservative measures such as avoiding tight-fitting clothing or weight loss. However, if symptoms recur, or are refractory, medications such as gabapentin or carbamazepine may be helpful for reducing symptoms of neuropathic pain. More rarely, a local nerve block or surgical decompression can be considered.

THE LEG, ANKLE, AND FOOT

Neuroanatomy of the Leg and Foot

Common Peroneal Nerve

The common peroneal nerve exits the popliteal fossa between the biceps femoris tendon and the lateral head of gastrocnemius, coursing anterolaterally across the fibular neck. It then gives off communicating branches to the sural nerve and the lateral cutaneous nerve of the calf. The nerve then pierces the peroneus longus muscle and divides into deep and superficial branches. The deep peroneal nerve runs between the extensor digitorum longus and the extensor hallucis longus 5 cm above the ankle mortise. At approximately 1 cm above the ankle joint, beneath the extensor retinaculum, the nerve divides into medial and lateral branches. The medial branch travels parallel to the dorsalis pedis artery. The lateral branch supplies proprioceptive fibers to the ankle joint and sensory fibers to the roof of the sinus tarsi, traveling in a fibrous tunnel beneath the extensor digitorum brevis. The deep peroneal nerve innervates the muscles of the anterior compartment, including tibialis anterior, extensor hallucis longus, extensor digitorum longus, peroneus tertius, and extensor digitorum brevis.[63] The superficial peroneal nerve innervates peroneus longus, peroneus brevis, and peroneus tertius. It exits the deep fascia of the leg 10 to 13 cm proximal to the tip of the lateral malleolus and remains subcutaneous. It then divides into the intermediate and medial dorsal cutaneous nerves. These divisions carry sensation from the anterior lower leg and dorsum of the foot.

The Tibial Nerve

The tibial nerve passes through the popliteal fossa below the arch of the soleus muscle. Within the popliteal fossa, it gives off branches to the gastrocnemius, popliteus, soleus, and plantaris muscles, as well as to the sural nerve. Distal to soleus, the tibial nerve innervates the tibialis posterior, flexor digitorum longus, and flexor hallucis longus muscles. It passes beneath the medial malleolus, where it is bound by the flexor retinaculum in the "tarsal tunnel." Here it divides into medial and lateral plantar branches. The medial plantar nerve passes beneath the insertion of the abductor hallucis and then travels within connective tissue attaching the flexor hallucis brevis to the tarsal bones. It innervates the abductor hallucis, flexor digitorum brevis, flexor hallucis brevis muscles, as well as the first lumbrical. Sensation is carried from the medial aspect of the sole, the medial three and one-half digits, and the nail beds. The lateral plantar nerve courses deep to the insertion of the abductor hallucis, passing between flexor digitorum brevis and quadratus plantae. It innervates quadratus plantae,

flexor digiti minimi, adductor hallucis, all interossei, the three remaining lumbricals, and the abductor digiti minimi muscles, and carries cutaneous sensation from the lateral sole and lateral one and one-half digits. Both the medial and lateral plantar nerves divide into interdigital nerves located beneath the transverse metatarsal ligament, terminating at the distal phalanges, and carry sensation from the plantar surfaces and web spaces between the toes. The medial plantar proper digital nerve supplies the skin on the medial aspect of the first digit.

Figures 6-8 and **6-9** provide both an anterior and posterior view of the peroneal and tibial nerves as well as the corresponding soft tissue and bones of the leg.

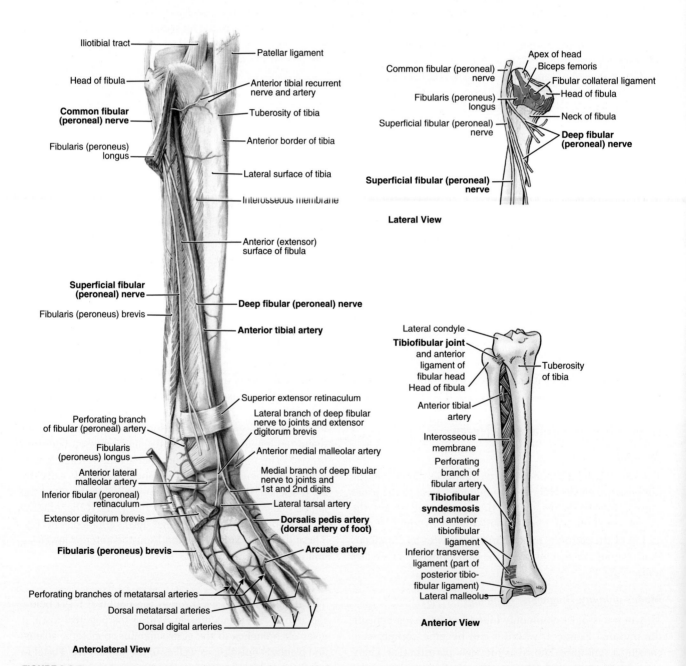

FIGURE 6-8. The peroneal and tibial nerves viewed anteriorly in the leg relative to associated bone and soft tissue (From Agur AM, Dalley AF. *Grant's Atlas of Anatomy.* 13th ed. Philadelphia, PA: Wolters Kluwer; 2012, with permission).

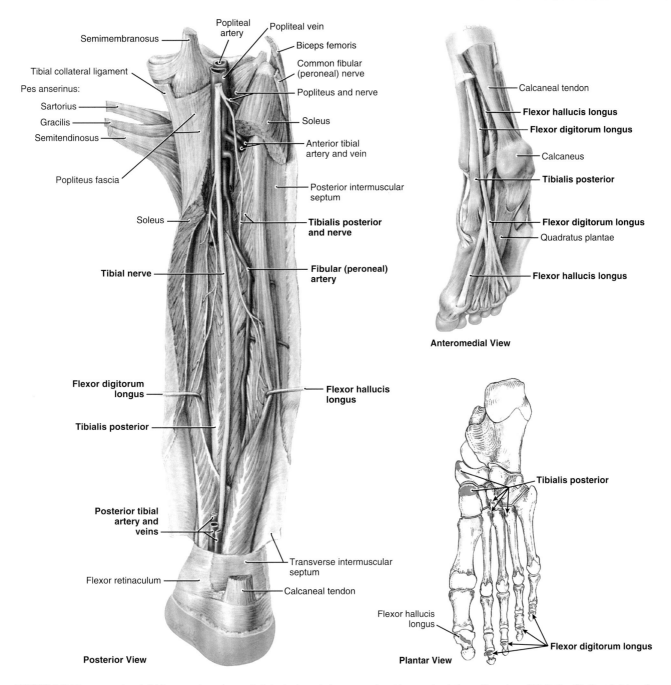

FIGURE 6-9. The peroneal and tibial nerves viewed posteriorly in the leg relative to associated bone and soft tissue (From Agur AM, Dalley AF. *Grant's Atlas of Anatomy.* 13th ed. Philadelphia, PA: Wolters Kluwer; 2012, with permission).

The Sural Nerve

The sural nerve originates from the tibial and common peroneal nerves, carrying cutaneous sensation from the lateral aspect of the ankle, heel, and fourth and fifth digits. It also mediates foot proprioception, measures stretch in the Achilles tendon, and provides sensation from deeper tissues. Traditionally, the sural nerve is considered a purely sensory nerve, although electrophysiologic studies have demonstrated motor fibers. **Figure 6-10** shows the position of the sural nerve relative to the peroneal and tibial nerves.

Diagnosing Nerve Injury in the Leg and Foot

The history should include questions about the nature of the injury and any sensory change or muscle weakness. Complaints of burning pain, paresthesias, and numbness suggest injury to small diameter sensory fibers. Allodynia may be present. Dysfunction of large diameter sensory fibers can cause proprioceptive loss and lead to ataxia, tremor, or disequilibrium. Involvement of motor fibers is suggested by weakness. Complaints of difficulty walking or a change in appearance of gait not explained by pain or limited range of

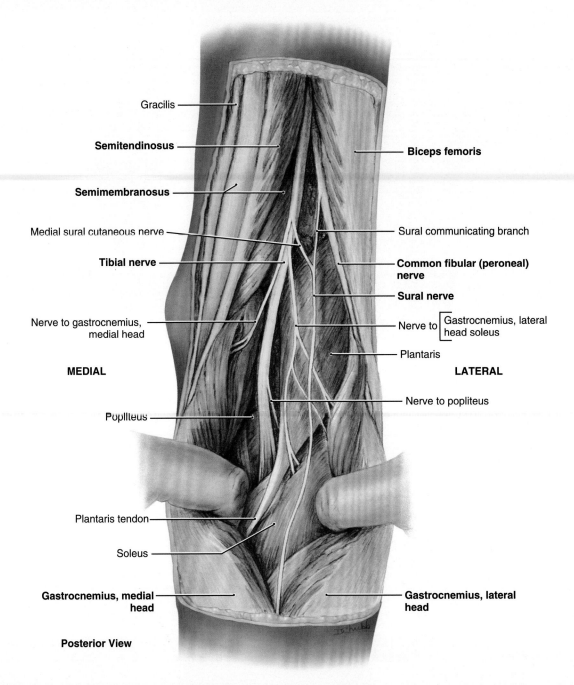

FIGURE 6-10. The sural nerve and its relative position to the tibial and peroneal nerves as it forms them (From Agur AM, Dalley AF. *Grant's Atlas of Anatomy.* 13th ed. Philadelphia, PA: Wolters Kluwer; 2012, with permission).

motion should raise suspicion for motor injury. The neurologic examination should include evaluation of sensation, motor function, reflexes, and gait. Abnormalities are more easily identified by comparison with the unaffected limb. The sensory examination should include assessment of pain, temperature, light touch, vibratory sensation, and proprioception. Appropriate mapping of the affected areas localizes to the corresponding nerve. Nerves can also be palpated and percussed to ascertain the site of compression or entrapment. Eliciting muscle weakness is a special

challenge when examining patients with acute injuries, because many suffer from severe pain. Analgesics may facilitate the examination. In addition to strength, muscle bulk and tone are assessed. Chronic motor nerve injury leads to atrophy. Weak joints may assume an abnormal position. The muscles should be closely inspected for signs of denervation, such as fasciculations or myokymia. The gait is often revealing. Patients with ankle dorsiflexion weakness excessively flex the hip and knee when ambulating in order to raise the leg. This compensation allows passage of the paretic foot through the swing phase. Lack of a controlled descent of the foot causes a characteristic slapping noise. The resulting appearance of the patient attempting to step over an object has led to the term "steppage gait."

Electrodiagnostics

NCS and needle EMG add certainty to the location of nerve injury and elucidate the nature and severity of impairment. The collective data from both NCS and EMG may help determine the temporal course of injury, differentiate neuropathy from myopathy, assess the severity of the axonal damage, and reveal signs of axonal regeneration. In addition, electrodiagnostic studies provide quantitative measurements, which can be followed over time.

Imaging Studies

Standard radiographs and computed tomography have little role in the characterization of neuropathies because of the inability to directly visualize nerves. The typical modalities to image peripheral nerve injury are mainly ultrasound (US) and MRI.

US has gained wide acceptance as a useful tool in the evaluation of the musculoskeletal system. High-resolution transducers can depict individual nerve fascicles. The advantages of this technique include dynamic, real-time examination, and quick assessment of entire nerve segments; US is also noninvasive, well tolerated, and affordable and can be performed in the office; however, image quality is operator dependent.[64] Inflamed nerves can be identified by increased caliber or internal signal changes, and focal thinning with proximal fusiform swelling occurs with nerve compression.[65] Analogous to EMG testing, US can yield important information about muscle by differentiating phases of muscle contraction.

MR provides resolution up to the level of the nerve fascicle. The signal characteristics of peripheral nerves using traditional MR pulse sequences are well described. Relative to adjacent muscle tissue, T1-weighted images of normal nerve fascicles are hypointense, with hyperintense perineurial and epineurial fat surrounding them. Roughly the reverse is seen in T2-weighted images.[66–69] Deviation from the normal signal characteristics of a nerve indicates pathology. T2 hyperintensity within the nerve is thought to reflect disruption of the blood–nerve barrier, leading to endoneurial or perineurial edema. However, the underlying pathogenesis remains uncertain.[66,67] Changes in nerve diameter should raise suspicion for pathology. The fascicles in nerves distal to the common peroneal nerve are poorly visualized with MRI. Neuropathy in distal nerves is suggested by changes consistent with denervation myopathy.[70,71] Denervated muscles are edematous in the subacute phase and atrophic in the chronic phase. T1-weighted images are useful for visualizing fatty deposits in chronically denervated muscle. Denervation myopathy is apparent on MRI up to 4 days after a traumatic nerve injury. The abnormal signal changes are reversible if there is reinnervation.

Individual Nerve Injuries

Common Peroneal Nerve

Table 6-4 lists common activities associated with injury of the peroneal nerve. Although frequently asymptomatic, peroneal neuropathy is a common complication of ankle injuries. Using electrodiagnostic studies, Nitz et al. found that 17% of patients with grade II ankle sprains and 86% with grade III sprains had evidence of subclinical motor impairment in the peroneal nerve.[72] Symptomatic ankle dorsiflexion and eversion weakness results from plantarflexion and inversion injuries as seen in severe sprains or fractures of the distal tibia and fibula. The common peroneal nerve can be torn by sudden, extreme ankle inversion, leading to internal hemorrhage and ischemia. After such injury, paralysis is usually immediate, but can be delayed for several days. Baccari et al. reported six cases of delayed paralysis because of peroneal nerve injury following ankle sprain by up to 3 days.[73] Patients with sensory injury to the common peroneal nerve may complain of numbness or burning pain from the knee to the top of the foot.

Deep Peroneal Nerve

Deep peroneal nerve compression may result from anterior compartment syndrome, which is associated with a painful, tight, and swollen lower leg. Intramuscular pressure measurements facilitate diagnosis, and electrodiagnostic studies may document the extent of involvement. Chronic compartment syndrome can occur in runners or other athletes experiencing repetitive lower extremity impact. Pain that increases on passive stretching and active contraction may be present. Generally, symptoms disappear once the offending activity is stopped. The deep peroneal nerve can also be compressed against the talonavicular joint in crush injuries, in postsurgical inflammation, and by tightly tied shoes. Compression occurs over the head of the talus when the ankle is plantarflexed and inverted.[74] Chronic compression beneath the extensor retinaculum has been referred to as the "anterior tarsal tunnel

Table 6-4. Activities Associated with Injury to the Peroneal Nerve	
Activity	**Associated Nerve Injury**
Running	Entrapment at the fibular neck; anterior tibial compartment syndrome; compression at the capitulum peronei by a mucous cyst
Dancing	Footwear compression
Martial arts	Impact nerve contusion
Football	Knee dislocation and/or ligamentous injury with subsequent nerve trauma (incidence of 24%)
Soccer	Entrapment at the fibular neck
Auto racing	Compression within small cockpit
Surfing	Chronic nerve trauma
Roller skating	Entrapment secondary to footwear

syndrome."[63] Patients with lateral branch compression typically complain of pain radiating to the lateral tarsometatarsal joints, whereas medial nerve compression causes symptoms within the first web space. The precise site of compression can be confirmed with a focal nerve block.

Superficial Peroneal Nerve

The superficial peroneal nerve can sustain traction injury during inversion ankle sprain or become entrapped as it exits the deep fascia. Entrapment can be seen in dancers with a technique flaw referred to as "sickling" in which the foot is either inverted or everted during dancing. Hypertrophied peroneal muscles may also lead to entrapment by causing increased compartment pressure. In dancers with lateral ligament deficiency or ankle instability, the superficial peroneal nerve may be tethered and stretched. Pain at the distal third of the lateral leg is precipitated by dancing and relieved by rest. The examiner may reproduce sensory symptoms over the dorsum and lateral aspect of the foot by dorsiflexing and everting the ankle. Nerve percussion can also reproduce symptoms.

Tibial Nerve

Table 6-5 lists common activities associated with injury of the tibial nerve. Entrapment of the tibial nerve within the tarsal tunnel has been frequently described in athletes. Any swelling of structures in or adjacent to the tunnel can lead to the so-called tarsal tunnel syndrome. Inflammatory tenosynovitis, edema related to trauma, and ganglia of adjacent joints or tendon sheaths are potential causes. The classic symptoms are pain in the heel and sole of the foot with accompanying sensory changes.

Morton's neuroma is a well-known cause of impingement of the interdigital nerves. Although the name implies a nerve tumor, histologic analysis reveals fibrosis and demyelination instead. It is suspected that repetitive dorsiflexion of the toes against the transverse metatarsal ligament causes nerve trauma and subsequent fibrosis. Inflammation of the intermetatarsal bursa is another potential cause. Morton's neuroma can be found between any of the metatarsals, but most commonly occurs in the third followed by the second interdigital space.[75,76] Although the exact incidence is unknown, it is considered to be a common cause of forefoot pain. Symptoms are exacerbated by running and tight-fitting footwear. Female predominance may be due to footwear differences. MRI is 90% sensitive and 100% specific for detecting Morton's neuroma. The diameter of the mass is usually 5 mm or larger with T1 and T2 hypointensity and occasional enhancement. A fluid collection may be seen within the intermetatarsal bursa. Greater than 3 mm of fluid is considered abnormal.[77] US is also commonly used to image neuromas, with reported sensitivity >90%.[78]

Treatment

Once the diagnosis is established, intervention should focus on minimizing further injury, treating symptoms, and accelerating recovery. Acute ankle and foot trauma may require surgery. Anti-inflammatory drugs can be used acutely as adjuvant or primary therapy to decrease edema and inflammation.

The approach to chronic injuries is different, and likewise depends on the mechanism of injury. Interventions for compressive neuropathy may be as simple as apparel adjustment, as in deep peroneal nerve compression from tight footwear. In other cases, decompression may require surgery. Pain can be a disabling result of peripheral nerve injury. It is important to identify and treat neuropathic pain to prevent morbidity, given the high prevalence of comorbid depression in chronic pain patients.[79] Gabapentin, carbamazepine, and pregabalin are anticonvulsants used to treat neuropathic pain. Gabapentin is used most frequently, and has proven efficacy.[80] Carbamazepine is an older drug. It was the initial anticonvulsant investigated in the treatment of trigeminal neuralgia and is still considered first-line therapy. Tricyclic antidepressants such as amitriptyline or nortriptyline are also very effective. N-methyl D-aspartate receptor antagonists, opioid analgesics, and topical agents are also useful treatment options. Combination therapy may be necessary to achieve adequate pain control.

Recovery from peripheral nerve injury is variable. Currently, physical medicine and rehabilitation offer the best options. Rigorous rehabilitation programs produced improved outcomes with improved strength, agility, and balance.

Surgical treatment continues to be investigated. Neurotization is a technique by which an autologous nerve of little functional significance is transplanted to the site of disabling nerve injury. This technique has been used extensively in patients with brachial plexus injuries. In patients with tibialis anterior denervation, Schwann cell transplant has been shown to enhance reinnervation after neurotization.[81] These approaches are currently experimental and should be considered only on a case-to-case basis.

PERIPHERAL NEUROPATHIES

Peripheral Nerve Anatomy

Peripheral sensory nerves originate at the dorsal root ganglia and exit dorsally from the spinal cord. The peripheral motor nerves emerge from the anterolateral horn cells in the spinal cord and brain stem motor nuclei. They exit the spinal cord

Table 6-5.	Activities Associated with Injury to the Tibial Nerve
Activity	**Associated Nerve Injury**
Running	Chronic trauma within the tarsal tunnel caused by repetitive ankle dorsiflexion; Morton neuroma; entrapment at the calcaneal nerve; injury of lateral and medial branches
Dancing	Morton neuroma
Martial arts	Morton neuroma
Hiking	Chronic trauma within the tarsal tunnel caused by repetitive ankle dorsiflexion
Hockey	Footwear compression at the tarsal tunnel

Table 6-6. Nerve Fiber Types and Their Function

Type	Fiber Type	Function
A	Large myelinated	Motor, proprioception, vibratory, touch, pressure sensation
B	Small myelinated	Autonomic (preganglionic fibers)
C	Small unmyelinated	Pain/temperature sensation, autonomic (postganglionic fibers)

via the ventral roots. Finally, the peripheral preganglionic autonomic nerve fibers exit the spinal interomedial column, also via the ventral roots. All these fibers exit through the intervertebral foramina. Peripheral nerves are categorized into three types (A, B, C) by size and myelin thickness (Table 6-6).

Myelinated axons are individually enveloped by a myelin sheath and Schwann cell membrane, whereas unmyelinated nerve fibers are bundled together and are covered by a single Schwann cell membrane. In general, nerve fibers are additionally enveloped by multiple connective tissue sheaths rich in vascular supply: endoneurium, which covers individual nerve fibers; perineurium, which surrounds each fascicle or bundle of nerve fibers; and epineurium, which envelopes all the fascicles of a nerve.

Diagnosing Peripheral Neuropathy

Symptoms

Peripheral neuropathy or polyneuropathy refers to a disease process involving the cell body, axon, and/or myelin of sensory, motor, or autonomic peripheral nerves. It is distinct from mononeuropathy (injury to a single nerve) and mononeuropathy multiplex (disease of two or more noncontiguous nerve trunks). As a result, its clinical presentation is largely symmetric in the limbs or trunk. The main categories of peripheral neuropathy involve damage to either the axon or myelin, and their clinical presentations differ (Table 6-7). Many times, both the axon and myelin are affected, although usually one more so than the other. Electrodiagnostic testing

can indicate whether the pathologic process is predominately axonal or demyelinating, or reveal a subclinical process.

Electrodiagnostics

NCS can indicate whether a peripheral neuropathy is predominately axonal or demyelinating and can rule out radiculopathy and myopathy. Demyelination implies decreased conduction that manifests as temporal dispersion of compound action potentials, conduction block, partial conduction block at noncompressible nerve sites, prolonged distal latencies, prolonged or absent F waves, and prolonged or absent H waves. In contrast, axonal injury decreases the total amount of charge carried via the nerve and results in decreased area under the curve of the action potential. Specifically for motor neuropathies, the muscle itself can be affected. The EMG can demonstrate fibrillations, fasciculations, decreased recruitment of motor units, and motor unit recruitment that is long in duration and polyphasic.

Biopsy

A nerve biopsy can be helpful in cases of inconclusive EMG/NCS. Nerve biopsy is also informative when certain conditions are suspected, for example, infiltrative diseases such as amyloid or sarcoidosis.[82] Biopsy can also aid in diagnosing suspected cases of autonomic or small fiber neuropathy where EMG/NCS testing will be normal or impractical.[83] The sural nerve is most commonly biopsied.

Laboratory Studies

High-yield serology tests prior to EMG/CNS include B12, fasting glucose, methylmalonic acid, and serum electrophoresis.[82] The clinician should otherwise refrain from sending most tests until after EMG/NCS is done. If axonal neuropathy, screening for systemic diseases is indicated. If demyelinating, screening for an inflammatory process using lumbar puncture is often necessary (Table 6-8).

Common Etiologies of Peripheral Neuropathy

Many etiologies of peripheral neuropathy have been identified over the years (see Table 6-9 for a comprehensive list by etiology). Despite this, up to 25% of peripheral neuropathies, mostly axonal neuropathies, remain idiopathic.

Table 6-7. General Symptoms of Peripheral Neuropathies

Symptoms	Axonal	Demyelinating
Motor	Symmetric weakness	Symmetric weakness is the typical presenting complaint
Sensory	Symmetric sensory loss/numbness, burning/pain, mild gait disturbances prior to weakness	Distal dysesthesias, impaired proprioception and vibratory sensation, hand clumsiness and gait disturbance
Duration	Both chronic over years but can have acute fulminant symptoms	Weeks to years
Exam findings	Intrinsic hand and foot muscle wasting; distal sensation loss to all sensation modalities; hypoactive or absent reflexes, usually ankle reflexes affected first	Generalized weakness (distal more than proximal), sensory loss (vibratory and proprioceptive loss more than pain and temperature), globally decreased reflexes, autonomic instability

Table 6-8. Screening Tests for Peripheral Neuropathies

Screening Tests if EMG/NCS Show Predominately Axonal Neuropathy

TSH, HbA1c	Cell count and complete metabolic panel
B12, folate, B1, methylmalonic acid +/– homocysteine	Lyme, HIV, RPR, hepatitis screen
Serum and urine electrophoresis	ANA, ESR, RF, Anti-Ro/La
Heavy metals	Porphyrins

Screening Tests if EMG/NCS Show Predominately Demyelinating Neuropathy

Serum and urine electrophoresis	Hepatitis screen, HIV
Lumbar puncture for elevated CSF protein	Anti-myelin-associated glycoprotein (MAG) (if predominately sensory symptoms)
Genetic testing for Charcot–Marie–Tooth disease (if "inverted champagne bottle" phenotype observed in legs)	Anti-GM1 (if predominately motor symptoms, indicative of AIDP)

Table 6-9. Etiologies of Peripheral Neuropathies

Systemic Disease

Diabetes mellitus	Critical illness/sepsis	Carcinoma	Uremia
Vitamin deficiency	B12 deficiency	Chronic liver disease	Malabsorption (sprue, celiac)
HIV	Lyme	Lymphoma	Multiple myeloma
Benign monoclonal gammopathy (IgA, IgG, IgM)	Porphyria	Hypoglycemia	Primary biliary cholangitis
Primary systemic amyloidosis	Hypothyroidism	Chronic obstructive lung disease	Acromegaly
Polycythemia vera	Cryoglobulinemia	Sjögren syndrome	Rheumatoid arthritis
Systemic lupus erythematosus	Systemic sclerosis	Mixed connective tissue disease	Sarcoidosis
Hypereosinophilic syndrome	Celiac disease	Inflammatory bowel disease	Leprosy
Herpes varicella-zoster virus	Hepatitis	Paraneoplastic	

Drugs/Medications

Amiodarone	Aurothioglucose	Cisplatin	Dapsone
Disulfiram	Hydralazine	Isoniazid	Leflunomide
Linezolid	Metronidazole	Misonidazole	Nitrofurantoin
Nucleoside analogues	Oxaliplatin	Phenytoin	Pyridoxine
Suramin	Taxol	Vincristine	Cytarabine
Etoposide	Bortezomib	Hydroxychloroquine	Colchicine
Podophyllin	Thalidomide	Ethambutol	Lithium

Toxins

Acrylamide	Arsenic	Diphtheria toxin	Gamma-diketone hexacarbons
Lead	Organophosphates	Thallium	Carbon disulfide
Ethylene oxide	Mercury	Gold	

Genetic

CMT type 1	CMT type 2	CMT 1, X-linked	CMT type 4a
Porphyric neuropathy	Hereditary liability to pressure palsy	Fabry disease	Adrenomyeloneuropathy
Hereditary sensory and autonomic neuropathy type I	Hereditary sensory and autonomic neuropathy type II	Dejerine–Sottas syndrome	Hereditary amyloid polyneuropathies
Refsum disease	Ataxia-telangiectasia	Abetalipoproteinemia	Giant axonal neuropathy
Metachromatic leukodystrophy	Friedrich ataxia	Hereditary neuralgic amyotrophy	Tangier

Axonal Predominant Neuropathies

Axonal polyneuropathies are predominately manifestations of systemic disease. The most common is diabetes mellitus, characterized by distal symmetric sensory loss, paresthesias, and autonomic dysfunction (commonly postural hypotension or gastroparesis). Critical illness polyneuropathy is common in critically ill patients, frequently presenting as weakness and inability to wean from the ventilator. Autoimmune and inflammatory conditions can also produce axonal neuropathies. Examples include Sjögren disease, scleroderma, various mixed connective tissue disorders, sarcoidosis, and inflammatory bowel disease (IBD). Infectious causes include leprosy, Lyme disease, diphtheria, and HIV.[84] Other systemic conditions that lead to axonal peripheral neuropathy include lymphoproliferative disorders (multiple myeloma, Waldenström macroglobulinemia, lymphoma, other plasmacytomas) and endocrinopathies such as hypothyroidism, which presents as carpal tunnel syndrome or sensory neuropathy with painful paresthesias.

Toxin exposure can also lead to axonal neuropathy. The most common example is alcohol. Others include mercury, lead, arsenic, thallium, and hexa-carbons. Taxane, platinum, or vinca alkaloid–based chemotherapy has antimicrotubule effects that are particularly toxic to axons.[85] Onset and time course vary depending on intensity and duration of exposure. Most patients present with sensory and motor symptoms, but some toxins lead to primarily sensory neuropathies (pyridoxine, oxaliplatin, cisplatin), whereas others are primarily motor neuropathies (dapsone). Some toxins affect both the axon and myelin, including aurothioglucose, suramin, paclitaxel, amiodarone, and vincristine.

Other causes of axonal neuropathy include vitamin or nutritional deficiencies (B12, B6, B1, E, niacin, copper), environmental exposures (cold and hypoxemia), and rare mitochondrial disorders (Charcot–Marie–Tooth [CMT] type 2A and syndrome of neuropathy, ataxia, and retinitis pigmentosa).[86]

Axonal peripheral neuropathies have predominantly sensorimotor involvement, though primary sensory axonal peripheral neuropathies can be seen in B12 deficiency, primary biliary cholangitis, hypothyroidism, acromegaly, and polycythemia vera. Hypoglycemia has been linked to motor-only neuropathy, and systemic diseases such as diabetes and primary systemic amyloidosis often injure the peripheral autonomic nervous system as well.

Demyelinating Predominant Neuropathies

Demyelinating polyneuropathies are broadly classified into two categories, acute and chronic inflammatory demyelinating polyneuropathies (AIDP and CIDP, respectively), depending on whether symptoms persist >2 months. AIDP is otherwise known as Guillain–Barré syndrome (GBS). There is usually, though not always, a preceding infection weeks prior (*Campylobacter jejuni* is a well-known offender), followed by symmetric ascending numbness and weakness affecting the legs and then arms as well as loss of distal reflexes. The Miller Fisher variant of GBS preferentially affects cranial nerves first.

Diagnosis is made based on history and supportive diagnostic studies including lumbar puncture (albuminocytologic dissociation—normal CSF cell count with elevated protein) and NCS/EMG (absent F waves are an early sign). Note that during the first week, these studies may be normal. For the Miller Fisher variant of GBS, a positive ganglioside antibody panel is diagnostic. Gangliosides specific to cranial nerve myelin are thought to be the antigen mistakenly targeted by the immune system.

Treatment for GBS is primarily supportive, including intubation if the disease ascends to the diaphragm. Intravenous immunoglobulin (IVIG) and plasma exchange (PLEX) temporize symptoms. Steroids are not helpful. With physical therapy, most patients have full recovery after 2 months.

CIDP is characterized by progressive weakness (symmetric proximal and distal, although there are atypical forms) with or without sensory loss over more than a 2-month period. CSF typically demonstrates albuminocytologic dissociation. NCS and nerve biopsy can additionally be helpful in the diagnosis of CIDP. When CIDP is suspected, paraproteinemia and other alternative etiologies should be excluded.

Chronic demyelinating neuropathies are commonly a manifestation of systemic disease. These diseases include monoclonal gammopathies, paraneoplastic syndromes (anti-CV2), celiac disease, and IBD.[87] Notably, an additional demyelinating component can be seen in diabetes. Certain toxin exposures can cause demyelinating neuropathy, including n-hexane, thalidomide, and arsenic.[85]

Multiple genetic diseases produce demyelinating polyneuropathies. CMT disease is a more common example. CMT type 1 presents during childhood or early adulthood, with progressive distal sensory loss and weakness. It is an autosomal dominant duplication of the PMP-22 gene on chromosome 17. CMT type 3 is also autosomal dominant, but presents in infancy, and is characterized by severe motor weakness. Common metabolic diseases of childhood can present with a demyelinating neuropathy, including Krabbe disease, metachromatic leukodystrophy, and adrenoleukodystrophy.

Treatments

For axonal polyneuropathies, treatment is focused on the underlying disease, that is, tight glucose control in diabetes or avoiding toxins in exposure cases. For demyelinating polyneuropathy, in autoimmune cases, IVIG or PLEX is usually helpful, but it is also crucial to treat the underlying disease if possible. In CIDP, steroids can also be of help. For refractory CIDP, alternative immunomodulatory agents can be used such as azathioprine, cyclosporine, mycophenolate mofetil, methotrexate, and rituximab.

There are many ways to treat neuropathic pain. Gamma aminobutyric acid (GABA)ergic agents such as gabapentin or pregabalin (note that they do not act directly on GABA receptors but rather on voltage-gated calcium channels) and tricyclic antidepressants are first line. Second-line agents include certain antiepileptics (carbamazepine, lamotrigine) and serotonin norepinephrine reuptake inhibitors. Third-line agents are a mix of nonsteroidal anti-inflammatories, capsaicin, baclofen, and low-dose narcotics. Many patients require multiple agents of various drug classes. In these cases, referral to a pain management specialist is recommended.

REFERENCES

1. Battié MC, Videman T. Lumbar disc degeneration: epidemiology and genetics. *J Bone Joint Surg Am.* 2006;88(Suppl 2):3–9.
2. Lew SM, Kothbauer KF. Tethered cord syndrome: an updated review. *Pediatr Neurosurg.* 2007;43(3):236–248.
3. Gitelman A, Hishmeh S, Morelli BN, et al. Cauda equina syndrome: a comprehensive review. *Am J Orthop (Belle Mead NJ).* 2008;37(11):556–562.
4. Melissano G, Bertoglio L, Rinaldi E, et al. An anatomical review of spinal cord blood supply. *J Cardiovasc Surg (Torino).* 2015;56(5):699–706.
5. Saliou G, Theaudin M, Join-Lambert Vincent C, et al. *Practical Guide to Neurovascular Emergencies.* Paris: Springer Paris; 2014.
6. Hoy D, Brooks P, Blyth F, et al. The epidemiology of low back pain. *Best Pract Res Clin Rheumatol.* 2010;24(6):769–781.
7. Benyamin RM, Manchikanti L, Parr AT, et al. The effectiveness of lumbar interlaminar epidural injections in managing chronic low back and lower extremity pain. *Pain Physician.* 2012;15(4):E363–E404.
8. Buenaventura RM, Datta S, Abdi S, et al. Systematic review of therapeutic lumbar transforaminal epidural steroid injections. *Pain Physician.* 2009;12(1):233–251.
9. Epidural Steroid Injections (ESI) and the Risk of Serious Neurologic Adverse Reactions. *FDA Brief Doc—Anesth Analg Drug Prod Advis Comm Meet.* 2014;(24–25):1–63.
10. McGrath JM, Schaefer MP, Malkamaki DM. Incidence and characteristics of complications from epidural steroid injections. *Pain Med.* 2011;12:726–731.
11. Manchikanti L, Malla Y, Wargo BW, et al. A prospective evaluation of complications of 10,000 fluoroscopically directed epidural injections. *Pain Physician.* 2012;15:131–140.
12. Goodman BS, Posecion LWF, Mallempati S, et al. Complications and pitfalls of lumbar interlaminar and transforaminal epidural injections. *Curr Rev Musculoskelet Med.* 2008;1(3–4):212–222.
13. Epstein NE. The risks of epidural and transforaminal steroid injections in the Spine: Commentary and a comprehensive review of the literature. *Surg Neurol Int.* 2013;4(Suppl 2):S74–S93.
14. Horlocker TT. Regional anaesthesia in the patient receiving antithrombotic and antiplatelet therapy. *Br J Anaesth.* 2011;107:96–106.
15. Furman MB, Giovanniello MT, O'Brien EM. Incidence of intravascular penetration in transforaminal cervical epidural steroid injections. *Spine (Phila Pa 1976).* 2003;28(20):21–25.
16. Goodman BS, Bayazitoglu M, Mallempati S, et al. Dural puncture and subdural injection: a complication of lumbar transforaminal epidural injections. *Pain Physician.* 2007;10(5):697–705.
17. Berger CW, Crosby ET, Grodecki W. North American survey of the management of dural puncture occurring during labour epidural analgesia. *Can J Anaesth.* 1998;45(2):110–114.
18. Morewood GH. A rational approach to the cause, prevention and treatment of postdural puncture headache. *CMAJ.* 1993;149(8):1087–1093.
19. Turnbull DK. Post-dural puncture headache: pathogenesis, prevention and treatment. *Br J Anaesth.* 2003;91(5):718–729.
20. Cho KI, Moon HS, Jeon HJ, et al. Spontaneous intracranial hypotension: efficacy of radiologic targeting vs blind blood patch. *Neurology.* 2011;76(13):1139–1144.
21. Pan PH, Bogard TD, Owen MD. Incidence and characteristics of failures in obstetric neuraxial analgesia and anesthesia: a retrospective analysis of 19,259 deliveries. *Int J Obstet Anesth.* 2004;13(4):227–233.
22. Vandermeulen EP, Van Aken H, Vermylen J. Anticoagulants and spinal-epidural anesthesia. *Anesth Analg.* 1994;79:1165–1177.
23. Evans R, Armon C, Frohman E, et al. Assessment: prevention of post–lumbar puncture headaches: Report of the Therapeutics and Technology Assessment Subcommittee of the American Academy of Neurology Randolph W. Evans, Carmel Armon, Elliot M. Frohman and Douglas S. Goodin This informa. *Neurology.* 2000;55:909–914.
24. Grant R, Condon B, Hart I, et al. Changes in intracranial CSF volume after lumbar puncture and their relationship to post-LP headache. *J Neurol Neurosurg Psychiatry.* 1991;54(5):440–442.
25. Mokri B. Headaches caused by decreased intracranial pressure: diagnosis and management. *Curr Opin Neurol.* 2003;16(3):319–326.
26. Baer ET. Post-dural puncture bacterial meningitis. *Anesthesiology.* 2006;105(2):381–393.
27. Sinclair AJ, Carroll C, Davies B. Cauda equina syndrome following a lumbar puncture. *J Clin Neurosci.* 2009;16(5):714–716.
28. Ruff RL, Dougherty JH. Complications of lumbar puncture followed by anticoagulation. *Stroke.* 1981;12(6):879–881.
29. Choi Y-S. Pathophysiology of degenerative disc disease. *Asian Spine J.* 2009;3(1):39–44.
30. Baldwin NG. Lumbar disc disease: the natural history. *Neurosurg Focus.* 2002;13(2):1–4.
31. Longo DL, Ropper AH, Zafonte RD. Sciatica. *N Engl J Med.* 2015;372(13):1240–1248.
32. Vroomen PC, de Krom MC, Knottnerus JA. Predicting the outcome of sciatica at short-term follow-up. *Br J Gen Pract.* 2002;52(475):119–123.
33. Peul WC, van Houwelingen HC, van den Hout WB, et al. Surgery versus prolonged conservative treatment for sciatica. *N Engl J Med.* 2007;356(22):2245–2256.
34. Botwin KP, Gruber RD. Lumbar spinal stenosis: anatomy and pathogenesis. *Phys Med Rehabil Clin N Am.* 2003;14(1):1–15.
35. Simotas AC. Nonoperative treatment for lumbar spinal stenosis. *Clin Orthop Relat Res.* 2001;(384):153–161.
36. Gardner A, Gardner E, Morley T. Cauda equina syndrome: a review of the current clinical and medico-legal position. *Eur Spine J.* 2011;20(5):690–697.
37. Ahn UM, Ahn NU, Buchowski JM, et al. Cauda equina syndrome secondary to lumbar disc herniation: a meta-analysis of surgical outcomes. *Spine (Phila Pa 1976).* 2000;25(12):1515–1522.
38. Shapiro S. Cauda equina syndrome secondary to lumbar disc herniation. *Neurosurgery.* 1993;32(5):743–746; discussion 746–747.
39. Lawton MT, Porter RW, Heiserman JE, et al. Surgical management of spinal epidural hematoma: relationship between surgical timing and neurological outcome. *J Neurosurg.* 1995;83(1):1–7.
40. Soldatos T, Andreisek G, Thawait GK, et al. High-resolution 3-T MR neurography of the lumbosacral plexus. *Radiographics.* 2013;33(4):967–987.
41. Tracy J, Dyck J. The spectrum of diabetic neuropathies. *Phys Med Rehabil Clin N Am.* 2013;18(9):1199–1216.
42. Gainsborough N, Hall SM, Hughes RA, et al. Sarcoid neuropathy. *J Neurol.* 1991;238(3):177–180.
43. Ladha SS, Dyck PJB, Spinner RJ, et al. Isolated amyloidosis presenting with lumbosacral radiculoplexopathy: description of two cases and pathogenic review. *J Peripher Nerv Syst.* 2006;11(4):346–352.
44. Katirji B, Wilbourn AJ, Scarberry SL, et al. Intrapartum maternal lumbosacral plexopathy. *Muscle Nerve.* 2002;26(3):340–347.
45. Ladha SS, Spinner RJ, Suarez GA, et al. Neoplastic lumbosacral radiculoplexopathy in prostate cancer by direct perineural spread: an unusual entity. *Muscle Nerve.* 2006;34(5):659–665.
46. Planner AC, Donaghy M, Moore NR. Causes of lumbosacral plexopathy. *Clin Radiol.* 2006;61(12):987–995.

47. Brejt N, Berry J, Nisbet A, et al. Pelvic radiculopathies, lumbosacral plexopathies, and neuropathies in oncologic disease: a multidisciplinary approach to a diagnostic challenge. *Cancer Imaging*. 2013;13(4):591–601.

48. Jaeckle KA, Young DF, Foley KM. The natural history of lumbosacral plexopathy in cancer. *Neurology*. 1985;35(1):8–15.

49. Son B, Yoon J, Kim D, et al. Dorsal rhizotomy for pain from neoplastic lumbosacral plexopathy in advanced pelvic cancer. *Stereotact Funct Neurosurg*. 2014;92(2):109–116.

50. Yurtseven T, Zileli M, Goker ENT, et al. Gluteal artery pseudoaneurysm, a rare cause of sciatic pain—case report and literature review. *J Spinal Disord Tech*. 2002;15:330–333.

51. Gardiner MD, Mangwani J, Williams WW. Aneurysm of the common iliac artery presenting as a lumbosacral plexopathy. *J Bone Joint Surg Br*. 2006;88(11):1524–1526.

52. Ozkavukcu E, Cayli E, Yagci C, et al. Ruptured iliac aneurysm presenting as lumbosacral plexopathy. *Diagn Interv Radiol*. 2008;14(1):26–28.

53. Aveline C. Delayed retroperitoneal haematoma after failed lumbar plexus block. *Br J Anaesth*. 2004;93(4):589–591.

54. Klimek M, Kosobucki R, Łuczyńska E, et al. Radiotherapy-induced lumbosacral plexopathy in a patient with cervical cancer: a case report and literature review. *Współczesna Onkol*. 2012;2(2):194–196.

55. Pritchard J, Anand P, Broome J, et al. Double-blind randomized phase II study of hyperbaric oxygen in patients with radiation-induced brachial plexopathy. *Radiother Oncol*. 2001;58(3):279–286.

56. Kutsy RL, Robinson LR, Routt ML. Lumbosacral plexopathy in pelvic trauma. *Muscle Nerve*. 2000;23(11):1757–1760.

57. Staff NP, Engelstad J, Klein CJ, et al. Post-surgical inflammatory neuropathy. *Brain*. 2010;133(10):2866–2880.

58. Kirschner JS, Foye PM, Cole JL. Piriformis syndrome, diagnosis and treatment. *Muscle Nerve*. 2009;40(1):10–18.

59. Wong CA, Scavone BM, Dugan S, et al. Incidence of postpartum lumbosacral spine and lower extremity nerve injuries. *Obstet Gynecol*. 2003;101(2):279–288.

60. Moore AE, Stringer MD. Iatrogenic femoral nerve injury: a systematic review. *Surg Radiol Anat*. 2011;33(8):649–658.

61. Parisi TJ, Mandrekar J, Dyck PJB, et al. Meralgia paresthetica: relation to obesity, advanced age, and diabetes mellitus. *Neurology*. 2011;77(16):1538–1542.

62. Seror P, Seror R. Meralgia paresthetica: clinical and electrophysiological diagnosis in 120 cases. *Muscle Nerve*. 2006;33(5):650–654.

63. Akyüz G, Us O, Türan B, et al. Anterior tarsal tunnel syndrome. *Electromyogr Clin Neurophysiol*. 2000;40(2):123–128.

64. Martinoli C, Bianchi S, Gandolfo N, et al. US of nerve entrapments in osteofibrous tunnels of the upper and lower limbs. *Radiographics*. 2000;20 Spec No:S199–S213; discussion S213–S217.

65. Bianchi S. Ultrasound of the peripheral nerves. *Joint Bone Spine*. 2008;75(6):643–649.

66. Spratt J, Stanley A, Grainger A, et al. The role of diagnostic radiology in compressive and entrapment neuropathies. *Eur Radiol*. 2002;12:2352–2364.

67. Grant G, Britz G, Goodkin R. The utility of magnetic resonance imaging in evaluating peripheral nerve disorders. *Muscle Nerve*. 2002;25:314–331.

68. Hörmann M, Traxler H. Correlative high-resolution MR-anatomic study of sciatic, ulnar, and proper palmar digital nerve. *Magn Reson Imaging*. 2003;21:879–885.

69. Jarvik J, Kliot M, Maravilla K. MR nerve imaging of the wrist and hand. *Hand Clin*. 2000;16:13–24.

70. Bendszus M, Wessig C. MR imaging in the differential diagnosis of neurogenic foot drop. *Am J Neuroradiol*. 2003;24:1283–1289.

71. Bendszus M. Sequential MR imaging of denervated muscle: experimental study. *Am J Neuroradiol*. 2002;23:1427–1431.

72. Nitz A, Dobner J, Kersey D. Nerve injury and grades II and III ankle sprains. *Am J Sport*. 1985;13:177–182.

73. Baccari S, Turki M. Une étiologie rare de paralysie du nerf sciatique poplité externe: L'entorse de la cheville: A propos de 6 cas. *Journal de Traumatologie du Sport*. 2000;17:208.

74. Kennedy J, Brunner J. Clinical importance of the lateral branch of the deep peroneal nerve. *Clin Orthop Relat Res*. 2007;459:222–228.

75. Bencardino J, Rosenberg Z. Morton's neuroma: is it always symptomatic? *Am J Roentgenol*. 2000;175:649–653.

76. Perini L, Del Borrello M, Cipriano R. Dynamic sonography of the forefoot in Morton's syndrome: correlation with magnetic resonance and surgery. *Radiol Med*. 2006;111:897–905.

77. Arnow B, Hunkeler E, Blasey C. Comorbid depression, chronic pain, and disability in primary care. *Psychosom Med*. 2006;68:262–268.

78. Quinn TJ, Jacobson JA, Craig JG, et al. Sonography of Morton's neuromas. *AJR Am J Roentgenol*. 2000;174(6):1723–1728.

79. Mossey J, Gallagher R. The longitudinal occurrence and impact of comorbid chronic pain and chronic depression over two years in continuing care retirement community residents. *Pain Med*. 2004;5:334–348.

80. Gilron I, Bailey J, Tu D. Morphine, gabapentin, or their combination for neuropathic pain. *N Engl J Med*. 2005;352:1324–1334.

81. Fukuda A, Hirata H, Akeda K, et al. Enhanced reinnervation after neurotization with Schwann cell transplantation. *Muscle Nerve*. 2005;31(2):229–234.

82. England JD, Gronseth GS, Franklin G, et al. Evaluation of distal symmetric polyneuropathy: the role of laboratory and genetic testing (an evidence-based review). *Muscle Nerve*. 2009;39(1):116–125.

83. Sommer C, Lauria G. Skin biopsy in the management of peripheral neuropathy. *Lancet Neurol*. 2007;6(7):632–642.

84. Hehir MK, Logigian EL. Infectious neuropathies. *Continuum (Minneap Minn)*. 2014;20(5 Peripheral Nervous System Disorders):1274–1292.

85. Staff NP, Windebank AJ. Peripheral neuropathy due to vitamin deficiency, toxins, and medications. *Continuum (Minneap Minn)*. 2014;20(5 Peripheral Nervous System Disorders):1293–1306.

86. Pareyson D, Piscosquito G, Moroni I, et al. Peripheral neuropathy in mitochondrial disorders. *Lancet Neurol*. 2013;12(10):1011–1024.

87. Muppidi S, Vernino S. Paraneoplastic neuropathies. *Continuum (Minneap Minn)*. 2014;20(5 Peripheral Nervous System Disorders):1359–1372.

CHAPTER 7

Edema in the Lower Extremity: Pathophysiology and Differential Diagnosis

JEFFREY S. BORER • BRIAN SHAFFER • ROCK C.J. POSITANO • LORETTA CACACE

*I*njuries of the foot are commonly associated with edema, a concomitant of local inflammation and mechanical obstruction to local venous blood flow. Edema also can result from a variety of systemic conditions, some of which are potentially life threatening. However, "swelling, like fever, is not a disease itself but a sign of an underlying disorder."[1] Therapy, both in its form and urgency, must be targeted to the causative process, not to the physical sign. The objective of this chapter is to review the pathophysiology of edema, differentiate the pathophysiologic characteristics associated with local injury from those associated with other diseases, and present the differential diagnosis of peripheral edema, with particular reference to the clinical signs and symptoms by which the edema of localized injury might be differentiated from that resulting from other causes.

This chapter represents an update of a chapter we published earlier (Shaffer B, Borer JS. Edema and foot injuries: pathophysiology and differential diagnosis. In: Ranawat CS, Positano RG, eds. *Disorders of the Heel, Rearfoot, and Ankle*. New York, NY: Churchill Livingstone; 1999:116–124). Much of that material is integrated and incorporated herein by direct quotation or paraphrasing (with permission of the publisher), with addition of new material as appropriate.

PATHOPHYSIOLOGY OF PERIPHERAL EDEMA

Ultimately, edema results from transudation of fluid across the capillary or proximal venular wall. Such fluid movement results from an imbalance between capillary permeability and the flow of fluid through the capillaries. Fluid flow is determined by capillary hydrostatic and oncotic pressures[2–4]; capillary permeability is a function of the performance of the endothelial cells (through which solute and fluid can move) and size of the spaces between these cells (which also serve as pathways for fluid and solute egress).[3,5]

Interstitial and Capillary Hydrostatic Pressure

The usual cause of abnormal capillary hydrostatic pressure is increased total intravascular volume. Concomitant with the increased intraluminal pressure, the pressure gradient between the capillary lumen and the interstitium must rise, at least transiently, precipitating fluid transudation through interendothelial interstices. Most commonly, intravascular volume expansion results from abnormal sodium retention, as is found in the setting of chronic heart failure (CHF). In CHF, cardiac output is subnormal (low-output CHF) or relatively inadequate (high-output CHF). In either case, renal perfusion is compromised by a combination of neural and humoral responses triggered by signals emanating from a series of baroreceptors and chemoreceptors; these signals are influenced by cardiac output.[3,4,6–8] Subnormal renal perfusion (plasma volume deficiency) increases the release of renin through stimulation of the β-adrenoceptors in the juxtaglomerular cells of the renal cortex, which enhances the production of angiotensin I. In the bloodstream, angiotensin I is rapidly converted to angiotensin II. Angiotensin II causes increased secretion of the salt-retaining hormone aldosterone from the adrenal cortex, renal vasoconstriction (specifically, constriction of efferent renal glomerular arterioles), and sodium reabsorption from the proximal convoluted tubule. Angiotensin-mediated vasoconstriction increases blood pressure and decreases renal perfusion, thus increasing filtration fraction and proximal tubular reabsorption of water and sodium in the kidney. Aldosterone acts on the distal convoluted tubule and collecting duct to reabsorb sodium. Thus, the result of activating the renin–angiotensin–aldosterone system is increased plasma volume potentiating the development of edema.[6–10]

Intravascular volume also can be expanded iatrogenically by intake of large fluid volumes at a rate that exceeds renal excretory potential.[11] Effective capillary volume can be increased even without an increase in total vascular volume by relaxation of precapillary arteriolar muscular sphincters, as occurs iatrogenically by administration of certain vasodilators, like nifedipine.[12] Similarly, capillary volume, and concomitant intracapillary hydrostatic pressure, can be increased by obstruction to venous flow, as by venous thrombosis. Such obstruction can prevent egress of fluid from the capillary lumen into the venular lumen while forward flow continues from the precapillary arterioles, resulting in abnormal filling of the capillary lumen. Similarly, in CHF, increased central venous pressure is reflected backward throughout the venous system, and the effects of relative obstruction to outflow potentiate those resulting from the increase in total vascular volume.[6,11,13]

Interstitial and Capillary Colloid Oncotic (Osmotic) Pressure

Capillary osmotic pressure primarily is a function of plasma protein concentration and, most specifically, the concentration of the relatively small protein, albumin. Thus, capillary osmotic pressure is reasonably approximated as capillary oncotic pressure. Generally, plasma proteins do not pass through the capillary endothelial cells or the intercellular capillary pores. Therefore, the osmotic effects of the intraluminal plasma albumin counteract the effects of abnormal hydrostatic pressure and even tend to promote resorption of interstitial fluid. Plasma oncotic pressure is diminished by various systemic, renal, and hepatic diseases (e.g., nephrotic syndrome, malnutrition, cirrhosis, loss of protein in the gastrointestinal tract, severe catabolic state).[6,11]

The effects of intravascular proteins are opposed by the interstitial colloid concentration. Tissue colloid osmotic pressure can be altered by extravascular protein accumulation as a result of abnormal capillary permeability or obstruction of flow within the lymphatic system.[3,6,13] Physiologically, the lymphatics remove the fluid, which is filtered by normal capillaries. Thus, normally, there is a slight flow gradient from the arterial to the venous side of the capillaries; the fluid and protein, which enter the capillaries from the arterioles, exceed the capacity of the capillaries, which filter the excess into the interstitial space. Some of this excess is resorbed into the capillary as this vessel communicates with the more compliant venule. However, the amount filtered generally exceeds the efficiency of the resorption process. The excess is removed directly by the lymphatic vessels, which drain the interstitial space, thus enabling tissue homeostasis to be maintained for water and solute.[3–6,13] The lymph is returned to the venous system via anastomoses between lymphatic vessels and the larger central veins.

If the lymphatic system is obstructed (as may occur with certain malignancies and central venous obstruction), excess fluid and protein can accumulate in the extravascular space, increasing interstitial osmotic pressure and potentiating edema formation.[3,5,6,13]

Capillary Permeability

Generally, only noncolloid solutes permeate the capillary wall freely. Injury to the capillary wall from chemical, bacterial, immunologic, thermal, or mechanical sources (as is characteristic of inflammation) can increase capillary transmural permeability to larger molecules, like albumin and other plasma proteins. Thus, for example, in extreme cases of capillary endothelial cell hypoxia (as might be seen with the ischemia of arteriolar or arterial obstruction or in the context of poison gas, burns, or allergic reactions), increases in permeability of capillaries and small venules can allow fluid, high in protein content, to enter the extravascular space within the injured tissue. Such abnormalities in microvascular permeability generally are not important factors in the pathophysiology of the common generalized edematous states, but can be important in the genesis of localized edema.[3,6,11]

Several mechanisms may underlie pathologic alterations in capillary permeability. During acute and non-necrotizing injury to the skin, release of endogenous autacoids (e.g., histamine, serotonin), presumably most often from mast cells, can cause arterial constriction, possibly associated with capillary injury (itself potentially affecting capillary endothelial function and integrity). A period of constriction generally is followed by arterial dilation, which increases flow into the capillaries. Release of autacoids appears to be triggered by local release of calcium ions from injured cells. The effects of the autacoids are highly selective, resulting in separation of the lateral borders only of the endothelial cells lining the postcapillary venules of 10 to 30 μm in diameter and not, strictly speaking, of the capillaries themselves. Indeed, the effect can be quite marked: the width of the intercellular clefts can be greatly enlarged, sufficiently even to accommodate 7 to 10 μm of formed blood elements.[14] Although the microvascular basement membrane, which limits movement of colloidal particles (e.g., lipoproteins), is not affected by autacoid release, this barrier can be traversed by plasma proteins and smaller solutes, allowing edema formation.[14]

Alteration in the function of the endothelial cells themselves also can be important in the pathophysiology of edema formation. Endothelium lining the microvasculature forms the critical barrier controlling the exchange of molecules between blood and interstitial fluid. Interaction of blood with the endothelial cell surface (the glycocalyx) can restrict or increase transendothelial transport of specific ligands. Excessive movement of osmotically active molecules into the interstitium can promote edema formation, whereas their transport out of the interstitial space can have the opposite effect. Because these endothelial transport mechanisms depend on endothelial expression of cell surface glycoproteins, regional variations in endothelial transport can be expected and may be useful in developing tissue-directed drug therapies, which might limit edema formation in certain settings.[15]

The composition of the serum also can affect capillary permeability. This influence depends on the capacity of serum components to affect the configuration of the electrical charge of the glycocalyx. Normally, the net negative charge configuration at the cell surface tends to restrict transcapillary transport of polyanionic molecules to a greater degree than neutral or polycationic molecules. Endothelial cell surface binding of certain plasma anionic macromolecules, such as albumin and orosomucoids, increases the charge negativity at the glycocalyx, resulting in greater polyanion exclusion.[15] In addition to its effects via surface charge alteration, serum albumin acts as a steric molecular "filter" that can resist the transport of water, small solutes, and macromolecules across the microvascular wall.[15] Thus, reduction in serum proteins can promote edema formation both by reducing serum oncotic pressure and minimizing the electrostatic and physical effects that retard movement of osmotically active molecules into the extravascular space.

DIFFERENTIAL ETIOLOGIC DIAGNOSIS OF PERIPHERAL EDEMA

The pathophysiologic processes described previously can occur in various combinations among the many disease processes characterized by peripheral edema. Clues to the underlying cause can be inferred from associated clinical symptoms and physical signs. In approaching the differential diagnosis of edema, a useful framework for separating localized processes from systemic or diffuse diseases can be based on consideration of the following characteristics:

1. **History**
   a. Known potential causes or contributing factors (recent trauma, surgery, concurrent illness, drug therapy)
   b. Temporal factors
      1. Rapidity of onset (gradual, more commonly associated with systemic diseases, versus sudden, more commonly associated with localized processes)
      2. Temporal pattern (short duration/first episode, chronic, recurrent, cyclic; note that variations in edema during 24-hour periods have limited diagnostic value because, irrespective of cause, peripheral edema is greatest in dependent regions and, therefore, typically is greater in feet and ankles during the daytime, when upright posture is most common)
   c. Symptoms (painless, more common in systemic diseases, versus painful, very uncommon in most systemic diseases)[1,2,4,6,11]
2. **Physical signs**
   a. Laterality (unilateral, more common in localized processes, versus bilateral, more common in systemic diseases)
   b. Condition of overlying skin (taut, thick, fibrotic skin generally is associated with a chronic process, more likely a result of systemic disease or venous insufficiency than musculoskeletal condition)
   c. Density of edema (edema that is relatively low in protein commonly is soft and "pitting," typical of CHF or hypoproteinemia; edema that is relatively high in protein content or involves extensive subcutaneous fibrosis generally is nonpitting, as in pretibial myxedema)
   d. Location (anasarca, edema plus ascites, simultaneous upper and lower extremity edema, and other generalized patterns suggest systemic diseases; localized edema, even if bilateral, may be more closely associated with a localized process)[1,2,4,6,11]

Laterality of edema is perhaps the most efficient initial discriminator of systemic versus localized processes. Therefore, the etiologic differential diagnosis of peripheral edema, presented next, is keyed to this characteristic, as modified from the classification schemes of Ruschhaupt and Graor[2] and Young.[1]

Bilateral Edema

Bilateral edema commonly begins simultaneously in both legs at feet and ankles and proceeds symmetrically up the legs.[2] Possible causes include the following:

Chronic Heart Failure

History of potential causes/contributing factors: hypertension, angina, or myocardial infarction; valvular diseases; cardiomyopathy; etc. Symptoms: dyspnea on exertion, orthopnea, paroxysmal nocturnal dyspnea; associated signs: tachypnea, rales, rhonchi, distended neck veins, tachycardia, hepatomegaly, ventricular gallop, heart murmur, etc.[1,2,11] Edema of CHF typically is soft and easily pitting, occurs predominantly in dependent parts of body, and, therefore, diminishes in legs after a period of recumbency.[1,2,11] CHF edema can be distinguished from other forms of dependent edema by the presence of engorged cervical veins, particularly if evidence of diffusely elevated systemic venous pressure (e.g., hepatomegaly) also is present.[6]

Pulmonary Hypertension

Causes of pulmonary hypertension are left-sided heart failure, chronic obstructive pulmonary disease (COPD), and sleep apnea.[16] Sleep apnea is an underrecognized cause of edema and can cause hypertension due to sympathetic nervous system overactivity secondary to intermittent hypoxia.[17] Pulmonary hypertension has been reported to be common in those with obstructive sleep apnea, and pretibial edema is a common sign of pulmonary hypertension in those with sleep apnea.[18] Studies suggest that patients who are at risk for pulmonary hypertension and over the age of 45 with nonspecific leg edema should undergo echocardiogram in order to rule out obstructive sleep apnea.[16]

Nephrotic Syndrome

History of causative/contributing factors: renal disease/uremia, proteinuria, hypoalbuminemia, hypercholesterolemia; symptoms: polyuria/polydipsia, nocturia. Renal biopsy can confirm the diagnosis.[1,2,6]

Acute Glomerulonephritis

History of causative/contributing factors: history consistent with recent group A β-hemolytic streptococcal infection; proteinuria, hematuria, markedly subnormal creatinine clearance, recent-onset hypertension.[2]

Hepatic Cirrhosis

History of causative/contributing factors: history of continuing jaundice or abdominal swelling, hepatosplenomegaly, gynecomastia, ascites, spider angiomas, palmar erythema[2]; abnormal fecal loss of albumin,[6] diagnostic liver biopsy or scan, abnormal serum liver enzymes, etc.[1]

Hypoproteinemia

History of causative/contributing factors: malnutrition, diarrhea, known malabsorption syndrome of any cause.[1,2]

Idiopathic Cyclic Edema

History of temporal factors: onset is quick and marked and disappearance is complete, with recurrences of a similar pattern; edema affects hands, face, legs, abdomen, and lower extremities. It often is related to the menstrual cycle and is limited almost entirely to obese women aged 20 to 40 years; may cause a 3- to 4-lb weight gain from morning to evening, reversed by bed rest; syndrome may be self-limited, sometimes disappearing after a few cycles (months). More commonly, it recurs during 1 to 20 years after initial episode. Associated symptoms: headache, irritability, anxiety, and depression.[1,2,19]

Position-Related Edema

History of causative/contributing factors: any condition that severely limits ambulation (e.g., various arthritides[2]). History of temporal factors: temporal association with sitting and standing for long periods without use of calf and leg muscles (increasing capillary hydrostatic pressure by relative obstruction to capillary outflow because of gravity-mediated venous pressure elevation in lower extremities). Symptoms: generally painless, but if pain exists for other reasons (e.g., musculoskeletal injury), hanging affected foot over bed at night to relieve pain may result in unilateral edema[2]; sitting (to relieve ischemic pain) can result in bilateral edema.[2] Physical signs: skin generally increasingly compliant with age, resulting in diminishing interstitial fluid pressure and enabling considerable fluid accumulation[2]; edema can be unilateral if arterial insufficiency coexists with dependency or if dependency is systematically unilateral.

Lipedema

History of causative/contributing factors: bilateral symmetric distribution of fat confined to or predominantly present in the lower extremities, characteristically sparing the feet (and thus distinguishable from lymphedema[1,2]), occurring only in women, often familial. Symptoms: generally painless,[1] although if complicated by exogenous obesity can be painful. Physical signs: this is not true edema and is not associated with pitting unless a comorbid condition causes water retention.[1] Support hose, often useful in other forms of edema, does not provide benefit and can potentiate pain; avoidance of abnormal weight gain may be useful, but intensive weight loss generally is not effective therapy because site of abnormal fat accumulation (buttocks and legs) generally does not respond to dietary alteration.[1]

Drug Effects

History of causative/contributing factors: temporally related use of nonsteroidal anti-inflammatory medications (e.g., phenylbutazone, oxyphenbutazone, ibuprofen[2]), certain vasodilating and antihypertensive drugs (e.g., dihydropyridine calcium channel blockers like nifedipine, α-methyldopa,

guanethidine sulfate, hydrazaline, diazoxide, rauwolfia alkaloids),[1] hormone therapy (e.g., progesterone, estrogen, testosterone, corticosteroids, adrenocorticotropins), monoamine oxidase inhibitor antidepressant drugs, etc. Physical signs: edema is soft and pitting, similar to that observed with cyclic edema or hypoproteinemia.[1]

In rare instances, the antibiotic class of fluoroquinolones has been associated with causing peripheral leg edema. Levofloxacin, which is commonly prescribed for treatments of the respiratory tract, urinary tract, and skin/soft tissue infections, has been associated with acute leg edema and stasis dermatitis.[20] Furthermore, antibiotics that are excreted through the kidneys need to be monitored, as leg edema could be a sign of kidney pathology secondary to antibiotic regimen. Antibiotics that have been associated with acute renal failure are aminoglycosides, amphotericin B, vancomycin, and β-lactam antibiotics.[21]

Primary Lymphedema

History of temporal factors: onset gradual, over days, weeks, or months[2] (and thus distinguishable from idiopathic cyclic edema) and is chronic. Symptoms: generally painless unless a concurrent painful process is extant. Physical signs: often accompanied by abnormal epidermal proliferation and dermal subcutaneous fibrosis[22] but rarely by skin ulceration; often not bilateral and, in any event, generally less uniformly distributed and extensive than edema caused by lymphatic or venous obstruction.[1] A positive Kaposi-Stemmer's sign is pathognomonic lymphedema and an accepted way to differentiate from lipedema. A positive outcome of this clinical evaluation is when there is failure of the skin overlying the dorsum of the second toe to tent when a "pincer grasp" is applied.[23]

Extreme High-Temperature Exposure

History of causative/contributing factors: temporally related exposure to high temperatures (which cause peripheral vasodilation, increasing flow through, and hydrostatic pressure in affected capillary beds), typically occurring in healthy individuals.[2] History of temporal factors: moderately rapid onset (many minutes to hours depending on temperatures, dependency of limbs, etc.), moderately rapid resolution (again depending on temperature change, as well as intercurrent ambulation).

Unilateral Edema

The causes of unilateral edema are more numerous than bilateral edema and, most commonly, are because of local rather than systemic conditions.[2]

Chronic Venous Insufficiency

This is the most common cause of unilateral edema,[1,2] occasionally resulting from congenitally absent or abnormal valves of the deep veins but more commonly caused by acquired deep venous valvular dysfunction; in either case, valvular insufficiency results in abnormal venous pressure when affected body parts are dependent, with associated relative obstruction to capillary outflow. History of causative/contributing factors: remote deep venous thrombosis (veins subjected to engorgement distal to thrombi often are permanently dilated because of damage and remodeling vascular wall, commonly rendering valves incompetent; additionally, venous valves often are damaged or destroyed during the healing process[1]). Deep venous thrombophlebitis can be symptomatic, but often is asymptomatic and must be detected by objective testing. A specific "subacute" form of this syndrome regularly is observed after coronary artery bypass grafting in which a venous bypass conduit is used; removal of the saphenous vein leads to transient volume overload of the remaining veins in the ipsilateral leg, with resulting soft, pitting edema that resolves over several months as the deep veins remodel to handle their new load. Chronic stasis changes (see later) seldom occur unless additional, preexisting venous disease is present. Physical signs: in early stages, edema typically is soft and pitting, consisting mainly of fluid transudation resulting from excessive microvascular hydrostatic pressure[1,2]; with time, inefficient capillary inflow and abnormal interstitial pressure lead to chronic skin changes, including pigmentation (iron deposition can occur as a result of extravasation of red blood cells), dermatitis, and fibrosis, occasionally accompanied by indurated cellulitis and ulceration.[1] The result is so-called brawny edema, which can be contrasted with the soft, easily pitting edema of hypoproteinemia. These changes commonly are associated with venous stasis. Prominent superficial veins may appear shortly after an attack of phlebitis and may become varicose in the chronic stage of venous insufficiency. In the very late stages, chronic venous insufficiency can result in secondary hemodynamic stresses in the superficial veins, which are sufficient to cause soft, pitting edema in addition to the chronic, brawny edema.[1] Edema secondary to chronic venous stasis causes blood to pool in the venous system, which activates inflammatory process and causes capillary damage. Furthermore, venous stasis ulcers tend to demonstrate impaired wound healing due to intracellular edema, platelet aggregation, and leukocyte activation. Venous stasis ulcers are the most common form of ulceration present on the lower extremity. These ulcers tend to be superficial, be painful, and have irregular borders and are located over bony prominences. Ulcerations are an important sequela of edema secondary to chronic venous insufficiency, accounting for approximately 80% of lower extremity ulcerations.[23]

Superficial Thrombophlebitis

History of causative/contributing factors: temporally related development of tender, indurated superficial "cord" extending a variable distance along the path of superficial vein, associated with erythema, warmth, and tenderness during the acute stage; thrombus usually remains palpable for days or weeks after diminution of the acute inflammation. Although systemic symptoms usually are absent, a low-grade fever may be present.[1,24] Physical signs: although pitting, edema is not soft, because inflammatory process can be expected to alter

microvascular permeability; importantly, edema usually is uniform in consistency in the area drained by the obstructed vein.[24]

Deep Vein Thrombosis and/or Thrombophlebitis

History of causative/contributing factors: temporally related conditions associated with enforced bed rest or physical inactivity, particularly if extremities are immobilized (e.g., orthopedic or abdominal surgery, prolonged airplane flight, childbirth, traumatic injury, or any particularly debilitating illness). Diagnosis generally requires support from objective testing (e.g., contrast venography, Doppler ultrasonography, radionuclide-based thrombus imaging) and leads to chronic venous hypertension of the affected lower extremity when the leg is dependent.[2] History of temporal factors: edema may develop gradually, over a few days, or more rapidly over hours, depending on the location and extent of the underlying process.[1,2,24] When thrombosis is unusually extensive, edema can occur relatively abruptly, with massive sudden swelling and intense cyanosis of extremity. The latter presumably results from particularly complete oxygen extraction from blood flowing very slowly through the capillaries, combined with compromise of arterial and arteriolar flow resulting from the external mechanical pressure of the rapidly accumulating edema and engorged veins. Indeed, in this setting, pulses in the limb are subnormal or absent; gangrene can result if the obstruction to the arterial flow is particularly severe,[1] as in the condition known as phlegmasia cerulean dolens, which can cause shock by trapping a large quantity of blood in the swollen extremity. Phlegmasia cerulean dolens primarily is associated with advanced or metastatic malignancies.[1] Even in somewhat less severe deep venous obstruction, fluid can accumulate beneath the deep fascia. Symptoms: deep venous thrombosis or thrombophlebitis can cause localized dull, aching pain, which can be quite severe, particularly when limb is dependent,[4] but lack of pain does not rule out this cause. Low-grade fever may be common, but rigors are uncommon and lymphadenopathy and lymphangitic streaking are absent.[1] Physical signs: soft, pitting edema often develops within 24 to 48 hours of the thrombosis and can be extensive. Associated inflammation can cause local warmth, tenderness, erythema, and even cyanosis; it can occur as in chronic venous insufficiency.[1,2] Superficial veins can be prominent[1] (a single "sentinel" vein may be observed), and tenderness on deep palpation can be present.[1,2]

Lymphedema

History of causative/contributing factors: any condition associated with obstruction of lymphatics or incompetence of lymphatic valves, resulting in lymph stasis, increased intralymphatic pressure, and inefficient drainage of the interstitium (e.g., femoral artery bypass surgery, which appears to damage and interfere with surrounding lymphatics, or local infection).[1] Lymphedema can be subclassified according to the cause: (1) primary lymphedema (idiopathic) can be congenital or acquired, commonly affects drainage of cutaneous or subcutaneous lymphatics in the legs[1,2]; primary lymphedema can be further subclassified into (a) lymphedema tarda, which becomes apparent only after age 40, raising concern of other common causes (e.g., malignancy)[1]; (b) primary congenital lymphedema (either nonfamilial ["simple"] or familial [Milroy disease]), present at birth, and usually involving only one lower extremity that manifests aplasia, hypoplasia, or varicose dilation of the lymphatic vessels[1,2]; (c) primary acquired lymphedema (lymphedema praecox), idiopathic but apparently involving a subnormally developed lymphatic system, not seen before adolescence but usually presenting before age 30 and predominately affecting women.[2] Characteristically, this form is associated with a "hump" on the dorsum of the foot, although upper extremities can be involved, and edema development is slow, typically involving an entire limb over the course of months to years; although commonly unilateral, both limbs may be affected. In early stages, edema is soft and painless and disappears overnight. Lymphangitis and/or cellulitis occurs within weeks to months of edema in a minority of cases[1,2]; (2) secondary (obstructive) lymphedema may be inflammatory or noninflammatory[1] and most commonly is secondary to malignancy. The noninflammatory form almost always is unilateral and typically results from metastatic carcinoma involving regional lymph nodes or after irradiation or surgical lymph node resection,[2] but can occur with retroperitoneal fibrosis and other conditions[1]; the inflammatory form results from lymphangitis (sometimes recurrent) or cellulitis, commonly caused by infection, local traumatic injury, filariasis, etc.,[1] and is often associated with fever. History of temporal factors: all forms usually develop slowly over months or years. Symptoms: usually painless.[1] Physical signs: soon after onset, edema is soft and pitting; in chronic stages, as subcutaneous fibrosis develops, the skin thickens, and edema may resist pitting and is firmer than that associated with chronic venous obstruction; superficial veins are not dilated, another point of differentiation from chronic venous obstruction.[1] Clinically, differentiation from deep venous thrombosis may be difficult unless pain is present (generally not present with lymphatic obstruction); venograms can rule out venous obstruction, but lymphangiograms then may be necessary to confirm lymphangitic abnormality.[1]

Lymphangitis

Like lymphedema, lymphangitis features lymphatic obstruction, in this case by thrombosis and fibrosis, which occurs secondary to local parasitic (dermatophytoses) and bacterial infections, typically introduced in the foot and ankle. The lymph stasis that is produced predisposes to recurrent cellulitis, in turn causing recurrent lymphangitis. Physical signs: although typically restricted to the foot and ankle, inflammation and edema may spread up the leg.[1,2]

Infection

Although infection can cause lymphangitis and lymphedema, occasionally a particularly virulent infection presents acutely with characteristics that justify a separate classification. History of causative/contributing factors: trauma breaking the skin

(wound, cut, abrasion, ulcer, contusion, scratch, hangnail, pinprick, or vesicle) allows for invasion of microorganisms; the area between the toes is the most common site, because it is often softened from chronic tinea pedis infection.[1,2] History of temporal factors: dramatic development of edema, with subsequent complete disappearance, occasionally featuring similarly characterized recurrences.[2] Infections that commonly cause sudden, unilateral edema include filariasis, particularly in tropical climates, clostridia infections causing gas gangrene, and agents associated with chronic osteomyelitis.[1] Symptoms and physical signs: pronounced fever, rigors, malaise, other nonspecific systemic symptoms, and localized pain[2] associated with rapid and even explosive development of local warmth, tenderness, erythema, "lymphangitic" streaks following the course of affected lymphatics from the infection site, and regional lymphadenopathy. Dermatophytosis of the toes may enable recurrent attacks, probably caused by secondary bacterial invaders; inflammation and edema are restricted to the foot and ankle but can spread up the leg.[2]

Trauma

Mechanical injury can affect characteristics of microvasculature directly resulting in edema.[1,2] In addition, traumatic injury to veins can result in venous thrombosis and provide a skin portal for entry of infectious agents.

Position-Related Edema

See Bilateral Edema.[2]

Vascular Anomalies

Arteriovenous fistulas must be considered in the differential diagnosis of edema because they can cause edema (e.g., by mechanical pressure or microvasculature) and can result in limb enlargement, which can mimic edema. History of causative/contributing factors: traumatic penetrating injury. Physical signs: thrill and bruit overlying the lesion, abnormal limb circumference; hemangiomas or other vascular anomalies and severe, unilateral, varicose, or dilated veins in unusual places may indicate a congenital fistula.[1] Angiography and venous oxygen saturation determinations can confirm the diagnosis.[2]

Klippel–Trenaunay–Weber Syndrome

Presentation of muscular, bony, and soft tissue hypertrophy, persistent nevus flammeus, and varicose veins usually involving a single lower limb may be associated with arteriovenous fistulas.[1]

Tumors

Lipomas, hemangiomas, hemangiolymphangiomas, sarcomas, neuroepitheliomas, and osteosarcomas can cause unilateral limb edema, usually relatively localized to the proximity of the tumor,[1,2] unlike the more extensive and diffuse edema of several other common processes. Tumors also can cause more extensive edema by extrinsic mechanical compression of vascular structures.

Factitious Edema

Edema cause by self-inflicted constriction of veins, as with a tourniquet. When reported, such edema generally follows no pattern suggestive of a known cause; on examination, there may be a sharply defined region of edema consistent with the application of the constricting apparatus.[2]

Gastrocnemius Rupture

Typically the result of athletic effort, gastrocnemius rupture is sudden, acutely painful (usually mid-calf), commonly associated with a large ecchymosis in dependent areas (foot, ankle) from internal hemorrhage. The increased limb circumference must be differentiated from edema and also causes edema as vascular structures are compressed by the internal hemorrhage and hematoma.[1,2]

Popliteal Cyst, Popliteal Syndrome

Mechanical compression of venous structures by cyst or aneurysm can cause edema like that of venous thrombosis; differential clue is the palpation of the cystic structure on examination.[2]

Compartment Syndrome

Increased tissue pressure in the region of the anterior tibial artery as a result of trauma, thrombosis, or embolism can cause severe ischemia, edema, and pain over the anterior tibial compartment.[2] Edema within the confined space may compress arterial structures sufficiently to compromise viability of muscle and nerve structures within the compartment, requiring fasciotomy to prevent gangrene.[1] Compartment syndrome within the foot and lower leg can be identified by four main symptoms: pain, paresthesia, paresis, and pain with stretch. Pulse examination and pink skin color can also aid in diagnosis. Within the foot, intracompartmental pressure should be correlated with the diastolic pressure. Today, indication for surgical intervention (fasciotomy) depends on a differential pressure between compartment pressure and diastolic pressure of less than 30 mmHg.[25] Certain injuries have a higher risk in developing compartment syndrome; for example, within the foot, Chopart and Lisfranc joint dislocations are frequently associated with compartment syndrome whereas in isolated midfoot fractures, compartment syndrome is rarely observed.[25]

Retroperitoneal Fibrosis

As noted previously, this entity can cause secondary lymphedema. In addition, retroperitoneal fibrosis can compromise arterial flow to the affected limb.[1,2]

Angioneurotic Edema (Hereditary Angioedema)

This is a noninflammatory and hereditary disease characterized by localized swelling of the skin, internal organs, and mucous membranes and caused by lack of C1 esterase inhibitor of the first component of complement C1 esterase, resulting in increased capillary permeability and precapillary arteriolar dilation.[2] History of temporal factors: attacks are episodic, usually begin in adolescence, and are often preceded by anxiety and triggered by trauma or infection, although an identifiable trigger may not exist. Initial site of edema may be one of minor trauma (e.g., athletic contact).[26] Frequency of attacks varies, from weekly to yearly or longer. Symptoms: abdominal pain, tightness, or tingling of skin, followed by a nonpruritic and painless rash. Symptoms are usually short lived.[27] Attacks commonly are preceded by bloating, anorexia, vomiting, constipation, and nausea.[26] Signs: stridor (resulting from potentially lethal edematous airway obstruction), edema in upper extremities and oropharynx (upper face, trunk, extremities; lower trunk and lower extremities are rarely swollen); lesions are nonpitting and erythematous.[26]

Pretibial Myxedema

Unlike the myxedema associated with hypothyroidism, which may result from alterations in capillary permeability and in the synthesis and degradation rates of plasma proteins, pretibial myxedema is an unusual manifestation of hyperthyroidism.[1,2,28] The pathogenesis may be related to an increase in osmotically active mucopolysaccharide production in the interstitium, producing a brawny, nonpitting edema, often with plaque formation of the overlying skin, affecting the pretibial region and dorsum of the foot. The basis for the rarity of this finding in the hyperthyroid population is unclear. Pretibial myxedema is seen in combination with exophthalmos and may not resolve with treatment of the underlying disease.[29]

Thermal Injury and Exposure to Extreme High Temperatures

See Bilateral Edema.[2]

Baker Cyst

This synovial structure can rupture behind the knee into the calf muscle, producing severe pain,[2] swelling, and tenderness, which can mimic the presentation of thrombophlebitis.[1] Baker cysts have been associated with rheumatoid arthritis, osteoarthritis, and internal knee malfunction[1]; may be bilateral; and can be confirmed by arthrography.[2]

CONCLUSION

Peripheral edema results from well-defined pathophysiologic processes that can be variously combined in many disease entities. The clinical presentation, specifically, the character and distribution of edema, depends on the pathophysiologic mechanisms involved in each case. The operative pathophysiology is at least partially inferable from the clinical evaluation. Although beyond the scope of this chapter, such recognition is important in selection among therapeutic modalities for the conditions of which edema is a feature.

REFERENCES

1. Young JR. The swollen leg. *Am Fam Physician*. 1977;15(1):163–173.
2. Ruschhaupt WF, Graor RA. Evaluation of the patient with leg edema. *Postgrad Med*. 1985;78:132–139.

3. Tobian L. The influence of hydrostatic pressure and colloid osmotic pressure and fluid transfer across the capillary membrane. In: Moyer JH, Fuchs M, eds. *Edema: Mechanisms and Management: A Hahnemann Symposium on Salt and Water Retention.* Philadelphia, PA: WB Sanders; 1960:3–6.

4. Johnson HD, Pflug J. *The Swollen Leg: Causes and Treatment.* Philadelphia, PA: J. B. Lippincott; 1975:70–86, 134–146.

5. Witte CL, Witte MH, Dumont AE. Pathophysiology of chronic edema, lymphedema, and fibrosis. In: Staub NC, Taylor AE, eds. *Edema.* New York, NY: Raven Press; 1984:521–542.

6. Friedberg CK. Edema and pulmonary edema: pathologic physiology and differential diagnosis. *Prog Cardiovasc Dis.* 1971;13(6):546–579.

7. Harris P. Role of arterial pressure in the oedema of heart disease. *Lancet.* 1988;1:1036–1038.

8. Braunwald E. Pathophysiology of heart failure. In: *Heart Disease: A Textbook of Cardiovascular Medicine.* 4th ed. Philadelphia, PA: WB Saunders; 1992:411–412.

9. Firth JD, Raine AE, Ledingham JG. Raised venous pressure: a direct cause of renal sodium retention in oedema? *Lancet.* 1988;1:1033–1036.

10. Pastan SO, Braunwald E. Renal disorders and heart disease. In: Braunwald E, ed. *Heart Disease: A Textbook of Cardiovascular Medicine.* 4th ed. Philadelphia, PA: WB Saunders; 1992:1856–1858.

11. Braunwald E. Edema and heart failure. In: Wilson JD, Braunwald E, Isselbacher KJ, et al, eds. *Harrison's Principles of Internal Medicine.* 12th ed. New York, NY: McGraw-Hill; 1991:228–232, 890–900.

12. Rutherford JD, Braunwald E. Chronic ischemic heart disease. In: Braunwald E, ed. *Heart Disease: A Textbook of Cardiovascular Medicine.* 4th ed. Philadelphia, PA: WB Saunders; 1992:1311–1313.

13. Streeten DHP. *Othostatic Disorders of the Circulation: Mechanisms, Manifestations, and Treatment.* New York, NY: Plenum Medical; 1987:13–57.

14. Wissig SL, Charonis AS. Capillary ultrastructure. In: Staub NC, Taylor AE, eds. *Edema.* New York, NY: Raven Press; 1984:117–142.

15. Schnitzer JE. Update on the cellular and molecular basis of capillary permeability. *Trends Cariovasc Med.* 1993;3:124–130.

16. Ely JW, Osheroff JA, Chambliss ML, Ebell MH. Approach to leg edema of unclear etiology. *J Am Board Fam Med.* 2006;19(2):148–160.

17. Gharibeh T, Mehra R. Obstructive sleep apnea syndrome: Natural history, diagnosis, and emerging treatment options. *Nat Sci Sleep.* 2010;2:233–255.

18. O'Hearn DJ, Gold AR, Gold MS, Diggs P, Scharf SM. Lower extremity edema and pulmonary hypertension in morbidly obese patients with obstructive sleep apnea. *Sleep Breath.* 2009;13(1):25–34.

19. Streeten DH. Idiopathic edema: pathogenesis, clinical features, and treatment. *Metabolism.* 1978;27:353–383.

20. Hyman DA, Cohen PR. Stasis dermatitis as a complication of recurrent levofloxacin-associated bilateral leg edema. *Dermatol Online J.* 2013;19(11):20399.

21. Khalili H, Bairami S, Kargar M. Antibiotics induced acute kidney injury: Incidence, risk factors, onset time and outcome. *Acta Med Iran.* 2013;51(12):871–878.

22. Gniadecka M. Localization of dermal edema in lipodermatosclerosis, lymphedema, and cardiac insufficiency. High-frequency ultrasound examination of intradermal echogenicity. *J Am Acad Dermatol.* 1996;35:37–41.

23. Collins L, Seraj S. Diagnosis and treatment of venous ulcers. *Am Fam Physician.* 2010;81(8):989–996.

24. Young JR. Evaluation of the patient with spontaneous thrombophlebitis. *Postgrad Med.* 1985;78:149–156.

25. Frink M, Hildebrand F, Krettek C, Brand J, Hankemeier S. Compartment syndrome of the lower leg and foot. *Clin Orthop Relat Res.* 2010;468(4):940–950.

26. Elnicki ME, Mansmann PT. Hereditary angioedema. In: Conn RB, Borer WZ, Snyder JW, eds. *Current Diagnosis.* Philadelphia, PA: WB Saunders; 1997:1172–1180.

27. Granger DN, Barrowman JA. Gastrointestinal and liver edema. In: Staub NC, Taylor AE, eds. *Edema.* New York, NY: Raven Press; 1984:645.

28. Kleeman CR, Mackovic-Basic M. The kidneys and electrolyte metabolism in hypothyroidism. In: Braverman LE, Uitger RD, eds. *Werner and Ingbar's The Thyroid: A Fundamental and Clinical Text.* Philadelphia, PA: J. B. Lippincott; 1991:1009–1016.

29. Smith TJ. Localized myxedema. In: Braverman LE, Uitger RD, eds. *Werner and Ingbar's The Thyroid: A Fundamental and Clinical Text.* Philadelphia, PA: J. B. Lippincott; 1991:676–681.

CHAPTER 8

Deep Venous Thrombosis, Thromboembolism, Thrombophlebitis in the Lower Extremity

ISHAAN SWARUP • JOHN BOLES • GEOFFREY H. WESTRICH

Significant morbidity and mortality are associated with the development of thromboembolic disease after orthopedic surgery.[1] Thromboembolic disease encompasses the development of deep venous thrombosis (DVT) and pulmonary embolism (PE). Both of these complications are considered to be life threatening, and they are both associated with significant patient morbidity and influence management after foot and ankle trauma and surgery.[2] As a result, knowledge about the etiology, risk factors, diagnosis, and management of thromboembolic disease is essential to any surgeon who treats patients with foot and ankle disorders.

Although the rates of thromboembolic disease have been thoroughly studied after total joint replacement, hip fracture surgery, and orthopedic trauma, only recently have authors begun to study the rates of thromboembolism after foot and ankle trauma and surgery.[3,4] The rates of thromboembolic disease after foot and ankle surgery are considered to be lower than those of thromboembolism after hip and knee surgery.[5] The current incidence of DVT after foot and ankle surgery ranges from 0.12% to 5.7%,[4–12] with highest rates reported after surgery for acute Achilles tendon rupture and hallux valgus.[8,11] The current incidence of PE after foot and ankle surgery ranges from 0.15% to 1.1%.[4–10,12] Generally, the rate of thromboembolic disease after foot and ankle surgery is considered to be less than 1%, but it may be higher in patients with certain risk factors. The reported incidence rates from the most recent studies in foot and ankle surgery are listed in **Table 8-1**.[5]

In this chapter, we describe the etiology of thromboembolic disease and also its risk factors, clinical presentation, diagnosis, and management. Since disease prevention is an essential component of patient care and an important institutional measure, we also discuss prophylactic strategies for preventing thromboembolic disease after foot and ankle trauma and surgery.

Table 8-1. Reported Incidences of Venous Thromboembolism (VTE) Including Deep Venous Thromboembolism (DVT) and Pulmonary Embolism (PE) Following Foot and Ankle Surgery

Study	Incidence of VTE	
	DVT	PE
Griffiths et al.[6]	0.27	0.15
Shibuya et al.[7]	0.28	0.21
Saragas and Ferrao[8]	5.7	1.1
Wukich and Waters[5]	0.4	0.3
Hanslow et al.[4]	4	1.3
Mizel et al.[9]	0.22	0.15
Solis and Saxby[13]	3.5	0
Barg et al.[10]	3.9	0
Radl et al.[11]	4	0
Jameson et al.[12]	0.1	0.1

THROMBOEMBOLIC DISEASE OVERVIEW

Although Rudolf Virchow, a German pathologist and biologist, initially described the phenomenon of venous thromboembolism (VTE) in 1856, its true morbidity and mortality was not appreciated until many years later. Approximately 90% of clinically significant PEs arise from proximal DVT of the lower extremities, and it is estimated that PEs are associated with 5% to 10% of all hospital deaths in the United States annually.[3]

VTE is the third most common vascular disease, following acute ischemic attacks and cerebrovascular accidents.[3] A DVT occurs when one or more of the calf veins become obstructed to venous blood flow. The formation of DVT is multifactorial and best described by Virchow.[14] In fact, Virchow's triad of hypercoagulability, endothelial injury, and venous stasis provides the foundation for understanding the pathogenesis of DVT formation after foot and ankle surgery and trauma.[15] For example, orthopedic surgery causes the release of thromboplastins that can activate the coagulation cascade and result in a hypercoagulable state. Similarly, endothelial injury is common in surgery, and venous stasis occurs with the use of a tourniquet or postoperative immobilization after foot and ankle surgery. Postoperative swelling and limited ambulation further contribute to venous stasis, and provide an ideal environment for clot formation.[3]

The majority of these thrombi occur in the deep veins of the calf; however, clot propagation to more proximal veins is known to occur as well. More specifically, the rate of propagation after total knee replacement surgery has been documented at 23%,[16] which underscores the importance of longitudinal follow-up. A PE occurs when a DVT in the pelvis or lower extremity embolizes through the right heart and gets lodged in the pulmonary vasculature. This event results in an obstruction of pulmonary perfusion and subsequent oxygenation of blood. Although the majority of PEs are asymptomatic, these events may be fatal. The size and location of the PE determine the associated morbidity and mortality, with large saddle-type PEs being the most fatal type.[3]

RISK FACTORS FOR THROMBOEMBOLIC DISEASE

Multiple risk factors have been identified as increasing a patient's predisposition to thromboembolic disease. Given the multifactorial nature of thromboembolic disease, it is important to recognize the presence of multiple risk factors in each patient and to stratify the risk of thromboembolic disease in each patient accordingly. A few studies have looked at the most important risk factors for thromboembolic disease in patients undergoing lower extremity surgery, some of which are listed in **Table 8-2**. For example, Barg et al.[10] concluded that obesity, history of previous thromboembolic disease, and absence of full weight-bearing status postoperatively are independent risk factors for developing symptomatic DVT after total ankle replacement. Similarly, Jameson et al.[12] found increasing age and multiple comorbidities as being risk factors for thromboembolic events after foot and ankle trauma surgery in a British National Health Service registry. More recently, Shibuya et al.[7] found that older age, obesity, and higher injury severity score are significantly associated with the development of DVT and PE after foot and ankle trauma. Other known risk factors for thromboembolic disease include rheumatoid arthritis, recent air travel, malignancy, hypercoagulable states, pregnancy, and oral contraceptive use.[3,4]

Table 8-2. Reported Relative Risk (RR) or Odds Ratio (OR) of VTE Risk Factors

Study	VTE Risk Factors	RR or OR
Shibuya et al.[7]	Older age	1.02 (OR for DVT); 1.02 (OR for PE)
	Obesity	2.35 (OR for DVT); 3.06 (OR for PE)
	Higher injury severity score	1.22 (OR for DVT); 1.21 (OR for PE)
Wukich and Waters[5]	Many listed	No RR or OR provided
Mayle et al.[17]	Many listed	No RR or OR provided
Hanslow et al.[4]	History of rheumatoid arthritis	No RR or OR provided
	Recent history of air travel	No RR or OR provided
	Previous DVT or PE	No RR or OR provided
	Limb immobilization	No RR or OR provided
Wang et al.[2]	Anticoagulant prophylaxis not prescribed	No RR or OR provided
	Immobilization with a cast or splint	No RR or OR provided
	Age over 40 y	No RR or OR provided
	Obesity	No RR or OR provided
Mizel et al.[9]	Postoperative nonweight bearing and immobilization	0.4% increase in RR for VTE
Solis and Saxby[13]	Hind foot surgery	5.64 (Wald Chi-Square test)
	Increasing age	4.39 (Wald Chi-Square test)
	Tourniquet time	4.80 (Wald Chi-Square test)
	Obesity	3.37 (Wald Chi-Square test)

(continued)

Table 8-2. Reported Relative Risk (RR) or Odds Ratio (OR) of VTE Risk Factors (*continued*)

Study	VTE Risk Factors	RR or OR
Cirlincione et al.[18]	Many listed	No RR or OR provided
Barg et al.[10]	Age	1.06
	Women	1.20
	Obesity	6.54 or 6.94
	ASA classification	1.69
	Tobacco use	2.98
	Previous DVT	5.43 or 7.07
	Surgery duration >120 min	1.77
	Spinal anesthesia	0.99
	Additional surgical procedures	1.36
	Bilateral simultaneous TAR	1.07
	Postoperative mobilization with cast	1.37
	No full weight bearing postoperatively	3.57 or 4.53
Jameson et al.[12]	Age 50–60	2.32 (OR for ankle ORIF); 1.14 (OR for hind foot arthrodesis)
	Age 60–70	3.20 (OR for ankle ORIF); 7.52 (OR for first MTO); 0.88 (OR for hind foot arthrodesis)
	Age >70	4.37 (OR for ankle ORIF); 5.69 (OR for first MTO); 2.24 (OR for hind foot arthrodesis)
	Charlson score 1	1.53 (OR for ankle ORIF); 2.65 (OR for first MTO); 0.84 (OR for hind foot arthrodesis)
	Charlson score ≥2	5.37 (OR for ankle ORIF)
	Past medical Hx: IHD	2.54 (OR for ankle ORIF)
	Past medical Hx: COPD	5.47 (OR for ankle ORIF)
	Past medical Hx: NIDDM	14.6 (OR for ankle ORIF); 1.70 (OR for hind foot arthrodesis)

History of Thromboembolism

Patients with a history of thromboembolic disease are at a significant risk for a repeat thromboembolic event. A hospitalized patient with a history of thromboembolic disease has an almost eightfold increased risk in acute thromboembolism compared to patients without such a history. As a result, patients with a history of thromboembolic disease who undergo major surgery or immobilization should be considered as being at a very high risk for repeat thromboembolic disease.

Lower Extremity Surgery

Orthopedic surgery of the lower extremity should be considered an important risk factor in the development of thromboembolic disease. Without prophylaxis, DVT can develop in more than 50% of patients undergoing elective total joint replacement surgery.[19] Similarly, more than 90% of proximal thrombi occur on the ipsilateral side after total hip replacement, which may be because of twisting and kinking of local veins as well as endothelial damage.[3] As previously discussed, lower extremity surgery affects all components of Virchow's triad, and subsequently could increase the incidence of thromboembolic disease.

Lower Extremity Fractures

Fractures of the hip, pelvis, and long bones of the lower extremity are associated with the development of thromboembolic disease. Patients with pelvic or lower extremity fractures were shown by venography to have an overall DVT incidence of 69%, with the incidence of DVT after tibial fractures being as high as 77%.[20] Postoperative immobilization or cast immobilization may contribute to the development of thromboembolic disease in patients with lower extremity fractures.[3]

Multiple Trauma and General Surgery

It has been shown that polytrauma patients are at a significantly increased risk for the development of thromboembolic disease. This risk is particularly high when the primary site of injury includes the face, chest, or abdomen. In fact, the risk is as high as 40% in this group of patients,[21] and without prophylaxis, the risk of DVT exceeds 50%.[20] In patients with foot and ankle trauma, a higher injury severity score is associated with a higher risk of DVT (odds ratio [OR] 1.22) and PE (OR 1.21).[7] Abdominal surgeries that require general anesthesia greater than 30 minutes also increases the risk of thromboembolic disease, which is often necessary in polytrauma patients.[21]

Patient Age

The risk of thromboembolic disease increases exponentially between the ages of 20 and 80 years.[22] Even though 40 years is traditionally used as the transition point for an age-related increase in the risk of thromboembolic disease, the risk continues to increase as a patient ages and nearly doubles with each successive decade. Older age has been shown to be significantly associated with the development of DVT and PE in patients with foot and ankle trauma.[7,12] The risk of thromboembolism is low for children, but the risk increases in certain situations, such as multiple trauma and lower extremity fracture.[3]

Malignancy

Patients with malignancy are at an increased risk for thromboembolic disease because of the hypercoagulable state that results from malignancy. The hypercoagulable state occurs because of an increase in procoagulant activity and a reduction in fibrinolysis. Advanced pancreatic cancer, gynecologic cancer, lung cancer, breast cancer, gastrointestinal cancer, and brain tumors are specifically associated with an increased risk.[23] Chemotherapy also has a toxic effect on the endothelium and may increase the risk of thrombus formation. Surgery for malignant disease results in a two- to threefold increase in the risk for thromboembolism compared to surgery for nonmalignant conditions.[3]

Immobilization

It is well known that immobility increases the risk for the development of thromboembolic disease. An autopsy study showed a 15% incidence of thrombosis in patients at bed rest for less than 1 week compared to 80% in patients at bed rest for greater than 1 week.[24] As a result, early mobilization should be an important goal after foot and ankle trauma and surgery in order to prevent thromboembolic disease. Immobilization after spinal cord injury and paralysis of lower extremities has an associated risk of thromboembolic disease that approaches 40%.[3]

Obesity

In foot and ankle trauma and surgery, obesity has been shown to be an important risk factor for the development of thromboembolic disease.[7,10] In fact, obesity has been shown to significantly increase the risk of symptomatic DVT (OR 2.35) and PE (OR 3.06) in a national trauma database.[7] The etiology of this increased risk is unclear, but it may be related to general health states, hyperestrogenic states, or immobility.

Oral Contraceptive and Estrogen Therapy

Historically, oral contraceptives were associated with an increased risk for thromboembolic disease. Although estrogen therapy may increase the incidence of thromboembolism in patients with prostate cancer, estrogen therapy in women does not appear to increase the risk of thromboembolic disease.[25,26]

Hypercoagulable States

Systemic hematologic abnormalities may predispose patients to the development of thromboembolic disease. For example, the presence of lupus anticoagulant; deficiencies in protein S, C, and antithrombin III; and factor V Leiden are all shown to increase the risk of thromboembolism.[3] These abnormalities should be considered in all patients undergoing foot and ankle surgery and the thromboembolic prophylaxis should be adjusted accordingly.

CLINICAL PRESENTATION AND DIAGNOSIS

The signs and symptoms of DVT and PE are nonspecific. However, the signs and symptoms of DVT include swelling, pain, redness, superficial venous dilatation, and Homan's sign (pain in the calf or behind the knee with ankle dorsiflexion). Similarly, the signs and symptoms of PE include dyspnea, pleuritic chest pain, cough, hemoptysis, and tachycardia.[27] Since these signs are unreliable and nonspecific, screening tests such as venography, ultrasound, and computed tomography (CT) have become increasingly popular.

Historically, contrast venography is considered to be the gold standard for detecting the presence of DVTs.[28] Venography of the lower extremity is performed by cannulation of a dorsal vein in the foot.[28–41] This test has several limitations since it is expensive, technically demanding, invasive, and exposes patients to radiation.[42] As a result, Doppler ultrasound has become the most commonly used modality to detect DVT formation and has essentially replaced venography in the clinical setting. This technique utilizes ultrasound to depict flow in the venous system, and the advantages of this modality include lower cost and lack of radiation. In the hands of an experienced technician or radiologist, the overall sensitivity of ultrasound in detecting DVT is 85% and the specificity is 97%,[42] and this method has an even higher sensitivity in symptomatic patients for proximal DVT.[27]

Historically, the gold standard for the detection of PE was pulmonary angiography. This method is invasive, requires expertise, and had significant morbidity. This technique was then replaced by ventilation-perfusion scintigraphy scanning, but this was difficult to administer and the results were equivocal in many instances. In fact, this test is nondiagnostic in approximately 50% of cases and requires additional testing.[27] Similar to the detection of DVT, alternative technologies have been developed and have become increasingly popular in determining the presence of a PE. The most commonly used contemporary method is multislice spiral CT of the chest, which can help to detect the presence of PE as well as other pathology in symptomatic patients.

THROMBOEMBOLISM PROPHYLAXIS

The goal of a prophylactic regimen is to prevent the formation of a DVT, as well as the occurrence of a PE. Since the incidence of symptomatic PE is low, comparative studies of prophylactic regimens would have to include thousands of patients. As a result, the majority of studies have focused on the prevention of DVT. Several prophylactic regimens have been studied in orthopedic surgery, the majority of which include intraoperative and postoperative modalities. Intraoperatively, the type of anesthesia (general, epidural, or hypotensive epidural anesthesia) and the duration of surgery have been shown to affect the incidence of thromboembolic disease. Postoperative prophylaxis includes mechanical devices such as compression stockings and foot pumps, as well as pharmacologic prophylaxis such as warfarin, aspirin, and low-molecular-weight heparin (LMWH).[43] Newer pharmacologic regimens such as rivaroxaban and dabigatran are starting to be used in orthopedic surgery, and are increasing in popularity as they are administered orally and do not require any monitoring.[3]

In foot and ankle surgery, DVT prophylaxis is not consistently used by all surgeons. In a recent study from the United Kingdom, only a fifth of surgeons used thromboprophylaxis after elective or trauma foot and ankle surgery.[44] Similarly, Wolf and DiGiovanni found that approximately 44% of surgeons used DVT prophylaxis after foot and ankle trauma surgery.[45] Although practice patterns vary throughout the world, it is imperative that foot and ankle surgeons understand the various modalities that are available to prevent the formation of DVTs and life-threatening PEs.

Mechanical Prophylaxis

Mechanical devices and physical agents have been used for DVT prophylaxis after a variety of surgical procedures and trauma. These devices increase fibrinolysis and decrease stasis by accelerating venous emptying.[3] Early mobilization, continuous passive motion machines, and graded compression stockings have all been proposed and studied. A compression boot or stocking can be applied to the nonoperative leg preoperatively, and applied to the operative side postoperatively. These devices are usually continued until the patient is ambulating, and in fact, sequential compression devices (SCDs) are the most commonly used prophylactic modality used by foot and ankle surgeons.[45]

Several studies have demonstrated the efficacy of mechanical devices in reducing the rate of DVT following total joint arthroplasty.[16,20,23,28,33,34,36,37,41,46–63] The incidence of DVT with the use of calf and thigh length devices has been reported to be between 7.5% and 33% after unilateral total knee arthroplasty.[54,64–69] In a randomized prospective study comparing compression stockings to aspirin, the incidence of DVT was reduced to 22% with pneumatic compression stockings compared to 47% with aspirin.[54] Foot pump devices have been shown to be effective in total knee arthroplasty as DVT prophylaxis.[70] These devices increase venous circulation by applying a rapid increase in pressure to the plantar plexus.[52] However, proximity to the operative site as well as the use of a postoperative splint or cast may limit the use of a foot pump device in foot and ankle surgery.

Overall, mechanical prophylaxis modalities offer several advantages over pharmacologic prophylaxis such as high patient tolerance, no known risk of bleeding, and low monitoring requirements.[3] These devices have been shown to be efficacious after orthopedic surgery, and continue to be a popular method of prophylaxis after foot and ankle surgery.[45] In general, newer impulse compression high-flow devices appear to be more efficacious than older, traditional slow-flow SCD-type devices.

Pharmacologic Prophylaxis

Several pharmacologic prophylaxis regimens have been studied in orthopedics. Traditionally, aspirin, heparin, and LMWH have been used and studied, but more recently, factor X inhibitors and thrombin inhibitors have been studied as well. LMWH continues to be a popular agent for DVT prophylaxis, and it has been specifically studied in the setting of foot and ankle surgery.[18,45]

Aspirin (acetylsalicylic acid) is a nonsteroidal anti-inflammatory agent that irreversibly inhibits the cyclooxygenase enzyme in platelets, thereby inhibiting the synthesis of thromboxane A2,[71] which causes platelet aggregation and vasoconstriction. The use of aspirin in orthopedic surgery has received mixed reviews. Its advantages include ease of use, low cost, and low monitoring requirements. However, its limitations include several medical complications such as gastritis, gastric ulcers, and upper gastrointestinal bleeding, as well as limited efficacy after total joint replacement surgery and trauma.[3] A recent study by Griffiths et al.[6] showed that there was no protective effect of aspirin against VTE after elective foot and ankle surgery. As a result, aspirin alone is not commonly used as a prophylactic regimen after foot and ankle surgery.

Warfarin (Coumadin) is another form of pharmacologic prophylaxis that has become increasingly popular in orthopedic surgery. Warfarin works by inhibiting the synthesis of vitamin K–dependent coagulation factors (factors II, VII, IX, X, protein C). Since warfarin affects the synthesis of coagulation factors and does not affect activated factors, it takes approximately 24 to 72 hours to become therapeutic.[3] The dose of warfarin is titrated daily to maintain an international normalized ratio (INR) of 2.0 to 2.5. The disadvantages of warfarin include frequent prothrombin time monitoring, bleeding, and, less frequently, warfarin-induced skin necrosis. More specifically, bleeding complications have been reported in 0% to 4% of patients receiving warfarin prophylaxis.[72–74] The advantages of warfarin prophylaxis include its oral form of administration, and the fact that it can be continued as treatment if a DVT is detected. Although warfarin is an effective agent in reducing the incidence of DVT after total joint arthroplasty, its efficacy has not been specifically studied in foot and ankle surgery. It may by an effective strategy in high-risk patients, since it has been shown to be effective after orthopedic trauma. However, the risks and benefits must be carefully assessed since not all polytrauma patients may be candidates for anticoagulation due to head or major organ involvement.[3]

LMWHs have become a popular form of DVT prophylaxis in orthopedic surgery. These agents were developed in the 1970s and have been shown to have good antithrombotic activity. When compared to heparin, LMWH have less bleeding per unit of equivalent antithrombotic effect. LMWHs are the fractionated form of heparin and contain a tetrasaccharide that binds antithrombin III. As a result, this complex can inactivate coagulation factors (factor Xa greater than factor IIa) and inhibit coagulation. The advantages of LMWHs include fixed daily dose and lack of need for daily monitoring of partial thromboplastin time. Its disadvantages include its invasive mode of administration, since it is available as a subcutaneous injection. The risks of LMWH include bleeding and heparin-induced thrombocytopenia. Major bleeding has been reported in 0% to 2.8% of patients, and the frequency of bleeding complications with LMWH is greater than that associated with warfarin.[75] In a recent study by Barg et al.,[10] 3.9% of patients undergoing total ankle replacement and treated with LMWH developed a symptomatic DVT. This rate is comparable to the rates of DVT after total knee or hip arthroplasty.

Newer pharmacologic prophylaxis regimens include factor X inhibitors such as rivaroxaban and direct thrombin inhibitors such as dabigatran. Rivaroxaban has been studied in total hip and knee arthroplasty, and compared to LMWH, rivaroxaban demonstrated superiority with regards to primary efficacy outcome, the prevention of VTE, and secondary efficacy outcome, the prevention of major VTE. There were no significant differences seen in bleeding risk between rivaroxaban and LMWH, with major bleeding seen in 0.3% to 1.3% of patients receiving daily doses of 10 mg or

less.[28,29,47,72,76] On the other hand, dabigatran is a prodrug with a half-life of approximately 12 to 17 hours that also does not require daily monitoring. In a multicenter double-blinded randomized study comparing dabigatran to LMWH after total hip and knee arthroplasty, VTE was significantly lower in patients receiving higher doses of dabigatran compared to LMWH. However, major bleeding complications were significantly lower in the low-dose groups and elevated with higher doses.[77] As a whole, further study is needed to clearly define the role of these agents in the prevention of DVT and PE after foot and ankle trauma and surgery.

Recommended Prophylaxis

It is clear that patients undergoing major orthopedic procedures are at a high risk for the development of thromboembolic disease. However, the majority of authors still consider foot and ankle surgery to be a lower-risk procedure compared to total hip or knee arthroplasty. Regardless, an individual patient's risk factors as well as the type and extent of the surgical intervention must be taken into consideration in order to determine the optimal prophylactic regimen. A combination of mechanical and pharmacologic prophylaxis has been shown to reduce the incidence of DVT in a synergistic manner,[70] and it is the optimal strategy to prevent thromboembolism after foot and ankle trauma and surgery. Aspirin alone may be inadequate, while LMWH is associated with greater complications. Warfarin requires frequent patient monitoring, but may be the optimal strategy in a high-risk patient. The advent of newer anticoagulants may change the landscape of thromboprophylaxis after orthopedic surgery, and they can be considered for DVT prophylaxis after foot and ankle trauma and surgery.

The American Academy of Orthopaedic Surgeons (AAOS) has no specific recommendations for DVT prophylaxis after foot and ankle surgery, and the American Orthopaedic Foot and Ankle Society (AOFAS) does not support or discourage the use of DVT prophylaxis after surgery.[78] Similarly, the American College of Chest Physicians (ACCP) does not recommend the routine use of thromboprophylaxis in patients with isolated lower extremity injuries distal to the knee.[79] However, clinical judgment is recommended in determining patients that may require thromboprophylaxis. More specifically, patients with certain risk factors, undergoing higher risk procedures, exposed to general anesthesia, and subject to postoperative immobilization should be managed accordingly.

TREATMENT OF THROMBOEMBOLISM

Treatment of DVT and PE in the postoperative patient is not without complication and requires a clear discussion of treatment goals. Prevention of clot embolization or life-threatening PE is the primary goal, but postphlebitic syndrome and pulmonary hypertension are also potential causes of morbidity. Unfortunately, PE is difficult to diagnose and has the potential to be rapidly fatal. In fact, among patients who will eventually die of a PE, two-thirds of patients will survive less than 30 minutes after the event, which is insufficient for most forms of treatments to be effective.[46] This fact underscores the importance of treating DVT. Treatment regimens for DVT include anticoagulants, vena caval interruption devices, thrombolytics, or surgery.

Anticoagulants

The most widely used anticoagulants are heparin and warfarin. LMWH and newer anticoagulants such as factor X inhibitors, however, are becoming increasingly popular for the treatment of DVT. Patients without contraindications to anticoagulation are generally treated with initial administration of heparin along with the initiation of warfarin therapy. Heparin is administered intravenously or by subcutaneous injection, with the goal of activated partial thromboplastin time set to 1.5 to 2.5 times the control.[80] When the warfarin dosage is therapeutic with an INR between 2.0 and 2.5, the heparin may be discontinued. This overlap is necessary to allow warfarin to inactivate vitamin K–dependent factors and reduce the likelihood of warfarin-induced skin necrosis. Treatment is typically continued for 3 months for isolated DVT and 6 months for PE.[81] Complications associated with heparin include bleeding at the operative site, gastrointestinal bleeding, and thrombocytopenia.[3]

LMWH has been advocated for the management of DVT as well, and it has become increasingly popular in clinical medicine today. These medications are administered by subcutaneous injection, and several studies have showed equal effectiveness as intravenous heparin. Furthermore, factor X inhibitors such as rivaroxaban were recently approved by the Food and Drug Administration for the treatment of DVT.[82] However, few studies have specifically investigated the use of anticoagulants in the treatment of DVT after foot and ankle surgery.

Vena Caval Filter Devices

Indications for an inferior vena cava (IVC) filter include recurrent embolism despite anticoagulation (anticoagulation failure) and DVT with a contraindication to or a complication of anticoagulation therapy. These devices, typically placed by interventional radiologists or vascular surgeons, can be permanently or temporarily inserted. These devices halt the proximal migration of emboli from the distal venous system to the lungs. IVC filters have been shown to be effective in reducing PE, and long-term follow-up revealed a recurrent embolism rate of 4% and patency rate of 98%.[83] Complications associated with IVC filters are unusual but include filter misplacement (2.6%) and risk of bleeding at the insertion site. Rarely, an IVC filter can migrate or can cause bleeding secondary to perforation of the vena cava.[3]

Thrombolytics

Thrombolytics such as streptokinase and tissue plasminogen activator dissolve thrombi. They are used in patients with PE and significant hemodynamic changes (systolic blood pressure less than 90 to 100 mm Hg).[27] Complete clot lysis occurs in 30% to 40% of patients medicated with these agents; however, there is a very high risk of bleeding.[84] In fact, cerebral hemorrhage has been reported in as high as 1% of cases.[80]

Surgical Intervention

Surgical intervention such as venous thrombectomy or pulmonary embolectomy is only performed when thrombolysis has failed or is contraindicated. Surgery is also performed when venous obstruction exists, which can lead to cerulea dolens (massive clotting of the leg) and further limit the viability of the leg.[3]

Recommended Treatment

It is clear that large proximal thrombi and symptomatic PE should be treated aggressively. In addition to medical treatment with intravenous hydration and supplemental oxygen, these patients require treatment with anticoagulants or vena caval filter devices. The choice to use medications or vena caval filter devices should be individualized for each patient. The use of thrombolytics is restricted to patients with significant hemodynamic disturbances in the setting of a PE. Clinical judgment takes precedence over any guidelines in the treatment of thromboembolic disease. There are no specific guidelines for the treatment of thromboembolic disease after foot and ankle trauma or surgery. An open discussion is important with patients in determining the optimal treatment strategy for DVT in the setting of foot and ankle trauma and surgery.

CONCLUSION

Thromboembolic disease is associated with significant morbidity and mortality. It is an important complication that can occur after foot and ankle trauma and surgery. Several factors contribute to the development of thromboembolic disease after foot and ankle trauma and surgery, including stasis and endothelial injury. Patient risk factors further increase this risk, and as a result, patients should be screened in order to determine the risk of thromboembolic disease. The diagnosis of DVT and PE is made by physical exam and imaging, and the treatment is dictated by a patient's condition as well as risks and benefits of treatment. Even though there are no specific DVT prophylaxis guidelines issued by any of the major advisory associations including AAOS, AOFAS, and ACCP, DVT prophylaxis is recommended for all patients with risk factors for thromboembolic disease. In general, although thromboembolic disease is rare in the setting of foot and ankle trauma and surgery, clinical judgment is paramount in preventing the development of thromboembolic disease in this setting and a patient's risk factor profile must be ascertained.

In the future, randomized controlled trials with solid methodology are needed to further determine the efficacy and risks of anticoagulants in the treatment and prevention of thromboembolic disease after foot and ankle surgery. Studies focusing on newer anticoagulants such as factor X inhibitors and direct thrombin inhibitors will be particularly interesting. Studies specifically defining risk after foot and ankle trauma and specific types of foot and ankle surgery will further help to stratify risk and prevent the development of thromboembolic disease. With an increasing emphasis being placed on disease prevention at an institutional and national level, we are hopeful that future research will improve outcomes for patients after foot and ankle trauma and surgery.

REFERENCES

1. Hentges MJ, Peterson KS, Catanzariti AR, et al. Venous thromboembolism and foot and ankle surgery: current updates 2012. *Foot Ankle Spec.* 2012;5(6):401–407.
2. Wang F, Wera G, Knoblich GO, et al. Pulmonary embolism following operative treatment of ankle fractures: a report of three cases and review of the literature. *Foot Ankle Int.* 2002;23(5):406–410.
3. Westrich GH, Dlott JS, Cushner FD, et al. Thromboembolic disease: state of the art diagnosis, prophylaxis and treatment. *Instructional Course Lecture, The American Academy of Orthopedic Surgeons.* 2013.
4. Hanslow SS, Grujic L, Slater HK, et al. Thromboembolic disease after foot and ankle surgery. *Foot Ankle Int.* 2006;27(9):693–695.
5. Wukich DK, Waters DH. Thromboembolism following foot and ankle surgery: a case series and literature review. *J Foot Ankle Surg.* 2008;47(3):243–249.
6. Griffiths JT, Matthews L, Pearce CJ, et al. Incidence of venous thromboembolism in elective foot and ankle surgery with and without aspirin prophylaxis. *J Bone Joint Surg Br.* 2012;94(2):210–214.
7. Shibuya N, Frost CH, Campbell JD, et al. Incidence of acute deep vein thrombosis and pulmonary embolism in foot and ankle trauma: analysis of the National Trauma Data Bank. *J Foot Ankle Surg.* 2012;51(1):63–68.
8. Saragas NP, Ferrao PN. The incidence of venous thromboembolism in patients undergoing surgery for acute Achilles tendon ruptures. *Foot Ankle Surg.* 2011;17(4):263–265.
9. Mizel MS, Temple HT, Michelson JD, et al. Thromboembolism after foot and ankle surgery. A multicenter study. *Clin Orthop Relat Res.* 1998;348:180–185.
10. Barg A, Henninger HB, Hintermann B. Risk factors for symptomatic deep-vein thrombosis in patients after total ankle replacement who received routine chemical thromboprophylaxis. *J Bone Joint Surg Br.* 2011;93-B(7):921–927.
11. Radl R, Kastner N, Aigner C, et al. Venous thrombosis after hallux valgus surgery. *J Bone Joint Surg Am.* 2003;85(7):1204–1208.
12. Jameson SS, Augustine A, James P, et al. Venous thromboembolic events following foot and ankle surgery in the English National Health Service. *J Bone Joint Surg Br.* 2011;93-B(4):490–497.
13. Solis G, Saxby T. Incidence of DVT following surgery of the foot and ankle. *Foot Ankle Int.* 2002;23(5):411–414.
14. Kraritz E, KarinoT. Pathophysiology of deep venous thrombosis. In: Leclerc JR, ed. *Venous Thromboembolic Disorders.* Philadelphia, PA: Lea and Febiger; 1998·54–64.
15. Virchow R. Neuer fall von todlicher emboli der kungerarteries. *Arch Path Anat.* 1856;10:225.
16. Grady-Benson JC, Oishi CS, Hannson PB, et al. Postoperative surveillance for deep venous thrombosis with duplex ultrasound after total knee arthroplasty. *J Bone Joint Surg Am.* 1994;76-A:1649–1657.
17. Mayle RE, DiGiovanni CW, Lin SS, et al. Current concepts review: venous thromboembolic disease in foot and ankle surgery. *Foot Ankle Int.* 2007;28(11):1207–1216.
18. Cirlincione AS, Mendicino R, Catanzariti AR, et al. Low-molecular-weight heparin for deep vein thrombosis prophylaxis in foot and ankle surgery: a review. *J Foot Ankle Surg.* 2001;40(2):96–100.
19. Paiement GD, Bell D, Wessinger SJ, et al. New advances in prevention, diagnosis, and cost effectiveness of venous thromboembolic disease in patients with total hip replacement. In: *The Hip,* Proceedings of the fourteenth open scientific meeting of the Hip Society. St. Louis, MO: C.V. Mosby; 1987:94–119.
20. Geerts WH, Jay RM, Code KI, et al. A comparison of low-dose heparin with low-molecular-weight heparin as prophylaxis against venous thromboembolism after major trauma. *N Engl J Med.* 1996;335:701–707.
21. Clagett GP, Reisch JS. Prevention of venous thrombosis in general surgical patients. Results of meta-analysis. *Ann Surg.* 1988;208(2):227–240.
22. Anderson FA, Wheeler HB. Venous thromboembolism: risk factors and prophylaxis. *Clin Chest Med.* 1995;16(2):235–251.
23. Rahr HB, Sorenson IV. Venous thromboembolism and cancer. *Blood Coagul Fibrinolysis.*1992;3:451–460.
24. Gibbs N. Venous thrombosis of the lower limbs with particular reference to bed-rest. *Br J Surg.* 1957;45:209–236.
25. Devor M, Barrett-Connor E, Renvall M, et al. Estrogen replacement therapy and the risk of venous thrombosis. *Am J Med.* 1992;92:275–282.
26. Lundgren R, Sundin T, Colleen S, et al. Cardiovascular complications of estrogen therapy for nondisseminated prostatic carcinoma. A preliminary report from a randomized multicenter study. *Scand J Urol Nephrol.* 1986;20:101–105.
27. Rosendaal FR, Biller HR. Venous thrombosis. In: Kasper DL, Fauci AS, Longo DL, et al, eds. *Harrison's Principles of Internal Medicine.* 17th ed. New York, NY: McGraw-Hill; 2008:733–735.
28. Bergqvist D, Benoni G, Björgell O, et al. Low-molecular-weight heparin (enoxaparin) as prophylaxis against venous thromboembolism after total hip replacement. *N Engl J Med.* 1996;334:696–700.
29. Britt LD, Zolfaghari D, Kennedy E, et al. Incidence and prophylaxis of deep venous thrombosis in a high risk trauma population. *Am J Surg.* 1996;172:13–14.
30. Caprini JA, Arcelus JI, Hoffman K, et al. Prevention of venous thromboembolism in North America: results of a survey among general surgeons. *J Vasc Surg.* 1994;20:751–758.
31. Fauno P, Suomalainen O, Rehnberg V, et al. Prophylaxis for the prevention of venous thromboembolism after total knee arthroplasty. A comparison between unfractionated and low-molecular-weight heparin. *J Bone Joint Surg Am.* 1994;76:1814–1818.
32. Frim DM, Barker FG, Poletti CE, et al. Postoperative low-dose heparin decreases thromboembolic complications in neurosurgical patients. *Neurosurgery.* 1992;30:830–832.
33. Green D, Lee MY, Lim AC, et al. Prevention of thromboembolism in spinal cord injury: role of low-molecular weight heparin. *Arch Phys Med Rehabil.* 1995;75:290–292.
34. Hamilton MD, Hull RD, Pineo GF. Prophylaxis of venous thromboembolism in brain tumor patients. *J Neurooncol.* 1994;22:111–1289.
35. Imperiale TF, Speroff T. A meta-analysis of methods to prevent venous thromboembolism following total hip replacement [see comments] [published erratum appears in JAMA 1995 Jan 25;273(4):288]. *JAMA.* 1994;271:1780–1785.
36. Janku GV, Paiement GD, Green HD. Prevention of venous thromboembolism in orthopaedics in the United States. *Clin Orthop Relat Res.* 1996;325:313–321.
37. Kakkar VV, Cohen AT, Edmonson RA, et al. Low molecular weight versus standard heparin for prevention of venous thromboembolism after major abdominal surgery. The Thromboprophylaxis Collaborative Group. *Lancet.* 1993;341:259–265.

38. Leclec J, Geerts W, Desjardins L, et al. Prevention of deep venous thrombosis after major knee surgery—a randomized, double blind trial comparing a low molecular weight heparin fragment (enoxaparin) to placebo. *Thromb Haemost.* 1992;67:417–423.

39. Nurmohamed MT, Verhaeghe R, Haas S, et al. A comparative trial of a low molecular weight heparin (enoxaparin) versus standard heparin for the prophylaxis of postoperative deep venous thrombosis in general surgery. *Am J Surg.* 1995;169:567–571.

40. Pellegrini VD, Langhans MJ, Totterman S, et al. Embolic complications of calf thrombosis following total hip arthroplasty. *J Arthroplasty.* 1993;8:449–457.

41. Warwick D, Williams MH, Bannister GC. Death and thromboembolic disease after total hip replacement. *J Bone Joint Surg Br.* 1995;77-B:6–10.

42. Westrich GH, Allen ML, Tarantino SJ, et al. Ultrasound screening for deep venous thrombosis after total knee arthroplasty. 2-year reassessment. *Clin Orthop Relat Res.* 1998;356:125–133.

43. Westrich GH, Farrell C, Bono JV, et al. The incidence of venous thromboembolism after total hip arthroplasty: a specific hypotensive epidural anesthesia protocol. *J Arthroplasty.* 1999;14:456–463.

44. Gadgil A, Thomas RH. Current trends in thromboprophylaxis in surgery of the foot and ankle. *Foot Ankle Int.* 2007;28(10):1069–1073.

45. Wolf JM, DiGiovanni CW. A survey of orthopedic surgeons regarding DVT prophylaxis in foot and ankle trauma surgery. *Orthopedics.* 2004;27(5):504–508.

46. Agnelli G. Anticoagulation in the prevention and treatment of pulmonary embolism. *Chest.* 1995;107:39S–44S.

47. Cade JF. High risk of the critically ill for venous thromboembolism. *Crit Care Med.* 1982;10:448–450.

48. Carter C, Gent M. The epidemiology of venous thrombosis. In: Coleman RW, Hirsh J, Marder VJ, et al, eds. *Hemostasis and Thrombosis: Basic Principles and Clinical Practice.* Philadelphia, PA: JB Lippincott; 1987:805–819.

49. Collignon F, Frydman A, Caplain H, et al. Comparison of the pharmacokinetic profiles of three low molecular mass heparins: dalteparin, enoxaparin, and nadroparin administered subcutaneously in healthy volunteers (doses for prevention of thromboembolism). *Thromb Haemost.* 1995;73:630–640.

50. Flinn WR, Sandaraer GP, Silva MB, et al. Prospective for surveillance for perioperative venous thrombosis. *Arch Surg.* 1996;131:472–480.

51. Frampton JE, Faulds D. Pamaparin: a review of its pharmacology, and clinical application in the prevention and treatment of thromboembolic and other vascular disorders. *Drugs.* 1994;47:652–676.

52. Friedel HA, Balfour JA. Tinzaparin: a review of its pharmacology and clinical potential in the prevention and treatment of thromboembolic disorders. *Drugs.* 1994;48:638–660.

53. Garlund, B. Randomised, controlled trial of low-dose heparin for prevention of fatal pulmonary embolism in patients with infectious diseases. *Lancet.* 1996;347:1357–1361.

54. Geerts WH, Code KI, Jay RM, et al. A prospective study of venous thromboembolism after major trauma. *N Engl J Med.* 1994;331:1601–1606.

55. Halkin H, Goldberg J, Modan M, et al. Reduction of mortality in general medical inpatients by low-dose heparin prophylaxis. *Ann Intern Med.* 1982;96:561–565.

56. Howell R, Fidler J, Letsky E, et al. The risks of antenatal subcutaneous heparin prophylaxis: a controlled trial. *Br J Obstet Gynaecol.* 1983;90:1124–1128.

57. Jorgensen LN, Willie-Jörgensen P, Hauch O. Prophylaxis of postoperative thromboembolism with low molecular weight heparins. *Br J Surg.* 1993;80:689–704.

58. Keane MG, Ingenito FP, Goldhaber SZ. Utilization of venous prophylaxis in the medical intensive care unit. *Chest.* 1994;106:13–14.

59. Keith SL, McLaughlin DJ, Anderson FA, et al. Do graduated compression stocking and pneumatic boots have additive effect on the peak velocity of venous blood flow? *Arch Surg.* 1992;127:727–730.

60. Knudson MM, Collins JA, Goodman SB, et al. Thromboembolism following multiple trauma. *J Trauma.* 1992;32:2–11.

61. Nicolaides AN, Fernandes JF, Pollack AV. Intermittent sequential pneumatic compression of the legs in the prevention of venous stasis and postoperative deep venous thrombosis. *J Surg.* 1980;87:69–73.

62. Noble S, Peters DH, Goa KL. Enoxaparin: a reappraisal of its pharmacology and clinical applications in the prevention and treatment of thromboembolic disease. *Drugs.* 1995;49:388–410.

63. Ziomek S, Read RC, Tobler HG, et al. Thromboembolism in patients undergoing thoracotomy. *Ann Thorac Surg.* 1993;56:223–227.

64. Graor RA, Davis AW, Borden LS, et al. Comparative evaluation of deep venous thrombosis prophylaxis in total joint replacement patients. Presented at AAOS; February 1989; Las Vegas.

65. Hodge WA. Warfarin and sequential calf compression in the prevention of deep venous thrombi following total knee replacement. Presented at the Knee Society; 1989; Las Vegas.

66. Hood RW, Flawn LB, Insall JN. The use of pulsatile compression stockings in total knee replacement for prevention of venous thromboembolism: a prospective study. Presented at the ORS; 1982; New Orleans.

67. Hull RD, Raskob GE, Gent M, et al. Effectiveness of intermittent pneumatic leg compression for preventing deep venous thrombosis after total hip replacement. *J Am Med Assoc.* 1990;263:2313–2317.

68. Kaempffem FA, Lifeso RM, Meinding C. Intermittent pneumatic compression versus coumadin: prevention of deep venous thrombosis in lower-extremity total joint arthroplasty. *Clin Orthop Relat Res.* 1991;269:79–89.

69. Lynch JA, Baker PL, Polly RE, et al. Mechanical measures in the prophylaxis of post-operative thromboembolism in total knee arthroplasty. *Clin Orthop Relat Res.* 1990;260:24–29.

70. Westrich GH, Sculco TP. Prophylaxis against deep venous thrombosis after total knee arthroplasty. Pneumatic plantar compression and aspirin compared to aspirin alone. *J Bone Joint Surg Am.* 1996;78-A:826.

71. Hirsh J, Salzman EW, Harker L, et al. Aspirin and other platelet active drugs: relationship among dose, effectiveness and side effects. *Chest.* 1989;95:12s–16s.

72. Bern MM, Lokich JJ, Wallach SR, et al. Very low doses of warfarin can prevent thrombosis in central venous catheters. A randomized prospective trial. *Ann Intern Med.* 1990;112:423–428.

73. Knight MTN, Dawson R. Effect of intermittent compression of the arms on deep venous thrombosis in the legs. *Lancet.* 1976;2:1265–1267.

74. Wells PS, Lensing AWA, Hirsch J. Graduated compression stockings in the prevention of postoperative venous thromboembolism. *Arch Intern Med.* 1994;154:67–71.

75. Salvati EA, Pellegrini VD, Sharrock NE, et al. Recent advances in venous thromboembolic prophylaxis during and after total hip replacement. *J Bone Joint Surg Am.* 2000;82:252–270.

76. Barritt DW, Jordan SC, Brist MB. Anticoagulant drugs in the treatment of pulmonary embolism: a controlled trial. *Lancet.* 1960;18:1309–1312.

77. Eriksson BI, Dahl OE, Büller HR, et al. A new oral direct thrombin inhibitor, dabigatran etexilate, compared with enoxaparin for prevention of thromboembolic events following total hip or knee replacement: the BISTRO II randomized trial. *J Thromb Haemost.* 2005;3(1):103–111.

78. American Orthopaedic Foot and Ankle Society. Position Statement: The Use of VTED Prophylaxis in Foot and Ankle Surgery. July 9, 2013. http://www.aofas.org/medical-community/health-policy/Documents/VTED%20Position%20Statement%20approv%207-9-13%20FINAL.pdf.

79. Stanton T. Routine DVT, PE prophylaxis questionable in foot, ankle surgery. June, 2011. http://www.aaos.org/news/aaosnow/jun11/clinical10.asp.

80. Wood MK, Spiro SG. Pulmonary embolism: clinical features and management. *Hosp Med.* 2000;61:46–50.
81. Della Valle CJ, Steiger DJ, Di Cesare PE. Thromboembolism after hip and knee arthroplasty: diagnosis and treatment. *J Am Acad Orthop Surg.* 1998;6:327–336.
82. United States Food and Drug Administration. FDA expands use of Xarelto to treat, reduce recurrence of blood clot. November 2, 2012. http://www.fda.gov/NewsEvents/Newsroom/PressAnnouncements/ucm326654.htm.
83. Greenfield LJ, Michna BA. Twelve year clinical experience with the Greenfield vena cava filter. *Surgery.* 1998;104:706–712.
84. Emerson RH, Cross R, Head WC. Prophylactic and early therapeutic use of the Greenfield filter in hip and knee joint arthroplasty. *J Arthroplasty.* 1991;6:129–135.

CHAPTER 9

Peripheral Arterial Disease

SACHIN KUMAR AMRUTHLAL JAIN • ARTHUR TARRICONE •
BHASKAR PURUSHOTTAM • PRAKASH KRISHNAN

Peripheral artery disease (PAD) most commonly results from atherosclerosis (plaque) of the arteries that carries blood to the upper and lower extremities, kidneys, and the splanchnic circulation. However, in this chapter, we focus on lower extremity arterial disease. Atherosclerotic plaque is primarily made up of cholesterol, inflammatory tissue, calcium, and fibrous tissue. Over time, they harden and narrow the arteries, thereby limiting the flow of blood. Impaired blood flow to your legs can cause pain and numbness. This can increase the risk of infection, especially in diabetic patients, and also prevent healing after foot surgeries. In addition, prolonged, persistent ischemia of the lower extremity can lead to gangrene (tissue death), nonhealing ulcers, and eventually amputation.

PAD is a very common condition affecting 12% to 20% of Americans who are 65 years and older. It is a leading cause of disability among patients who are 50 years and older and those who have diabetes. PAD affects men and women equally and is more prevalent in African Americans.[1] The Framingham Heart Study and the National Health and Nutrition Examination Survey (NHANES) have revealed that traditional coronary and cerebrovascular risk factors such as age, diabetes, hypertension, hypercholesterolemia, metabolic syndrome, and smoking increase the risk of PAD.[2] Importantly, patients with PAD have high cardiac and cerebrovascular event rates. Interestingly, though, only 10% to 35% of patients with PAD present with typical features. Most of the patients are either asymptomatic or present with atypical symptoms, which is associated with functional limitation. One to two percent of PAD patients present with critical limb ischemia (CLI) without any warning signs or symptoms. Given the fact that CLI has been associated with a high rate of morbidity and mortality, it makes it the most concerning category among PAD. Hence, it becomes of utmost importance to recognize CLI at the earliest.

The appropriate treatment may slow disease progression to some extent and reduce the burden of morbidity associated with PAD. Treatment can be broadly categorized into lifestyle changes, medical management, endovascular therapy, and surgery. The significant morbidity and mortality associated with PAD along with its adverse impact on economics makes it an important public health problem. The overlap of PAD with coronary artery disease (CAD) has led interventional cardiologists to be more involved in the care of these patients.

Finally, in the last few years, there has been a tremendous growth in endovascular techniques and devices, which has led to the preference of endovascular therapy over surgery when it comes to revascularization.

RISK FACTORS

Several risk factors as mentioned earlier have been associated with PAD. Smoking and diabetes remain the most important ones. Smoking is the main risk factor for PAD, which can increase the risk up to fourfold. Smokers with PAD become symptomatic 10 years earlier than their nonsmoking counterparts. Abstinence of smoking halts the progression of the disease. Diabetic patients who are also smokers are at the highest risk for developing PAD and its associated complications, such as gangrene. About one in three people older than 50 who have diabetes have PAD. PAD is twice as common in diabetics.[1] Diabetic PAD patients often have extensive involvement of infrapopliteal arteries. PAD increases the risk of CAD, myocardial infarction (MI), stroke, and transient ischemic attack. Of the people who have CAD, there is a one in three chance of having PAD. The prevalence of foot ulcers ranges from 4% to 10% among diabetic patients.[3] Annual incidence of ulcers in diabetics ranges from 1% to 4.1%, with a lifetime incidence being as high as 25%. Diabetic foot ulcers frequently become infected and are a major cause of hospital admissions. In a recent two-center study, PAD partially contributed to 30% of all foot ulcers.[4]

HISTORY AND PHYSICAL

A thorough history and physical examination is absolutely critical in the diagnosis of PAD and also for planning further management. PAD patients may present with typical claudication or with atypical symptoms on most occasions. Intermittent claudication is defined as a reproducible discomfort of a group of lower extremity muscles, which is brought on with exertion and typically relieved with rest. Claudication is derived from the Latin word, "Claudicato," which means limp. Atypical symptoms may vary from nonspecific pain, numbness, aching, or heaviness in the lower extremities. When the arteries of lower extremities start to develop obstruction and result in reduced blood flow, the respective muscle group accumulates lactic acid with exertion. This accumulation of lactic acid and other metabolites causes pain. With rest, lactic acid and other metabolites are washed away and the patient becomes free of pain. The longer the time needed for the pain to be relieved with rest, the worse is the obstruction. The presence of lower extremity resting pain, which improves when the lower extremities are dependent, herald CLI. The presence of gangrene and ulcers signifies CLI and needs urgent attention. Patients with a history of amputation or foot surgeries should undergo comprehensive evaluation with regard to the details of the amputation/foot surgery, such as the cause for it and the recovery or healing phase of the stump (Table 9-1).

Careful and meticulous examination should be performed in these patients. Blood pressure (BP) should be recorded from both the upper extremities as a difference (in systolic blood pressure [SBP]) exceeding 20 mm Hg indicates potential innominate, subclavian, or axillary occlusive arterial disease. Auscultation over the carotid, subclavian, and renal arteries is important, as the presence of bruit can be a clue to underlying stenosis and is also associated with higher cardiovascular mortality (especially with carotid bruit).[5] The presence of a pulsatile abdominal mass should raise the suspicion for an abdominal aortic aneurysm. It is absolutely imperative to make every effort possible to palpate all the peripheral pulses (radial, brachial, femoral, popliteal, dorsalis pedis, and posterior tibial). If the pulses are not palpable, the use of a handheld Doppler should be strongly considered. The dorsalis pedis pulse can be absent in 8% to 12% of healthy individuals, but the posterior tibial pulse is absent in only 2%. The lack of palpable pedal pulses strongly suggests the presence of PAD. However, the presence of a palpable pulse does not exclude PAD as collateral blood flow can give rise to a palpable distal pulse.[6] If pedal pulses are nonpalpable, there would be a need for further workup with noninvasive or invasive assessment based on the clinical presentation. Expansile and palpable masses in the femoral and popliteal arterial regions should raise the suspicion for aneurysms. Capillary filling time is assessed by squeezing the great toe to cause the skin to blanch and then letting go to see how long it takes for the skin to regain its original color. A capillary filling time of greater than 5 seconds is considered prolonged. Feet and nails should be examined thoroughly for

any calluses, discoloration, gangrenous changes, ulceration, and infections. The presence of the above should warrant an immediate assessment of the arterial circulation to the lower extremity. Consultation with a vascular specialist is recommended. It is important to understand that a large proportion of PAD patients are asymptomatic. Strict foot care is very important, especially so in diabetics, as they are prone to develop gangrene and eventually amputation.

Screening recommended per American Heart Association (AHA) as a screening initiative[7] recommends ankle-brachial index (ABI) in asymptomatic individuals who are:

- Older than 50 years of age with a history of diabetes mellitus or smoking
- Anyone older than 65 years of age

CLASSIFICATION OF PAD PATIENTS

There are two types of classification that are accepted internationally to clinically categorize the PAD patients.

The Fontaine classification, introduced by René Fontaine in 1954 for chronic limb ischemia,[8] is based on symptoms and walking distance:

Stage I: Asymptomatic
Stage II: Mild claudication
Stage IIA: Claudication distance of greater than 200 meters
Stage IIB: Claudication distance of less than 200 meters
Stage III: Rest pain, mostly in the feet
Stage IV: Necrosis and/or gangrene of the limb

The more recent classification by Rutherford consists of four grades and seven categories[9] based on symptom alone:

Grade 0, Category 0: Asymptomatic
Grade I,
Category 1: Mild claudication
Category 2: Moderate claudication
Category 3: Severe claudication

Grade II, Category 4: Rest pain
Grade III, Category 5: Minor tissue loss, ischemic ulceration not exceeding ulcer of the digits of the foot
Grade IV, Category 6: Major tissue loss, severe ischemic ulcers or frank gangrene

OTHER PAD DISORDERS

Two diseases need special mention because of their unique presentation and characteristics. Leriche syndrome is an atherosclerotic occlusive disease involving the abdominal aortic bifurcation and may extend into both the common iliacs. It is recognized with intermittent thigh claudication and impotence from hypogastric artery occlusion with decreased flow to the pudendal artery. Distal pulses are usually diminished. Any tissue loss implies distal disease, except in case of

Table 9-1. Site of Pain to Presumed Level of Obstruction

Site of pain	Presumed level of obstruction
Buttock and hip	Aortoiliac artery disease
Impotence	Bilateral aortoiliac artery disease (Leriche)
Thigh	Common femoral or aortoiliac artery disease
Upper two-thirds of calf	Superficial femoral artery
Lower one-third of calf	Popliteal artery disease
Foot claudication	Tibial or Peroneal artery disease

"blue toe" syndrome where multiple toes are involved from embolization of the iliac plaque. Blue toe is also associated with aortic aneurysms. Angioplasty is the treatment of choice.

The other one is Berger syndrome, which is also known as thromboangiitis obliterans. This inflammatory disease involves the small and medium arteries as well as the veins. The histopathology is characterized by inflammatory tissue, thrombus, and microabscess. It is distinctively seen in male smokers. Typically, the pedal pulses are not palpable.

As mentioned earlier, most of the PAD population do not have any signs or symptoms. Thus, screening and having a low threshold to perform noninvasive testing are of critical importance.

VASCULITIS OF THE LOWER EXTREMITIES

Vasculitis is inflammatory systemic or local syndromes, which is the result of autoimmune-mediated inflammation of the blood vessels. There are several types, and a significant proportion of the syndromes involve the lower extremity arteries. They are known to present with systemic symptoms such as fever, weight loss, fatigue, malaise, and constellation of symptoms, depending on which organs are involved. On physical examination, rash, nodules, ulcers, and gangrenous changes of upper and lower extremities can be identified. When there is a concern for vasculitis, an immediate consultation to a vascular specialist is warranted.

DIAGNOSTIC TOOLS

In this current era, there are multiple noninvasive tools and techniques available to diagnose PAD. They can be as simple as the ABI to a sophisticated magnetic resonance arteriography. It is important to understand the pros and cons of these tests, as a combination of these investigations may be used in the PAD population. Essentially, the testing is individualized to the patients. Nevertheless, ABI remains the first choice of investigation in screening as well as in diagnosing PAD.

Ankle-brachial Index

ABI = Highest SBP in ankle (dorsalis pedis and posterior tibial arteries)/highest SBP in upper arm (brachial artery)

This test has 95% sensitivity and 99% specificity to detect PAD. An ABI ≤ 0.90 is diagnostic of PAD. Depending on the ABI values, we can assess the severity of PAD. It is also used to follow patients subsequent to their endovascular or surgical intervention. Finally, ABI is an independent multivariate predictor of cardiovascular and cerebrovascular mortality (**Table 9-2**).

Alternate ABI is a variant of the standard ABI, which is derived by dividing the lowest SBP of the ankle (either dorsalis pedis or posterior tibial) by the highest SBP of the upper arm. An abnormal ABI by this method implies that

Table 9-2. Interpretation of ABIs	
≥0.9–1.4	Normal
>1.4	Calcified vessels, which prompts further studies
≤0.9	Diagnostic for occlusive arterial disease
0.4–0.9	Suggests arterial obstruction associated with claudication (mild to moderate)
<0.4	Multilevel disease (any combination of iliac, femoral, or tibial vessel disease), associated with nonhealing ulcers, ischemic rest pain, pedal gangrene

there is an isolated tibial artery disease, which is not identified by the standard ABI as it uses the higher SBP of the two tibial vessels. It is important to acknowledge that both these forms of ABIs can impact on your cardiovascular morbidity and mortality.[10] Segmental BP and pulse volume recordings (PVRs) may be useful for localizing the vascular lesions in the lower extremities, and are most useful in patients who have abnormal ABI scores at rest. Thus, they help in determining the level and extent of disease. The patient is placed in a supine position and standard size BP cuffs are placed at several segments of the lower extremity. The reference BP cuff is placed at the arm level. In the three-cuff technique, there is one cuff above and below the knee and at the ankle level. In the four-cuff technique, two narrower BP cuffs are placed at the thigh level (this helps in the differentiation between aortoiliac and superficial femoral artery [SFA] disease). A 20 mm Hg or greater reduction in SBP between two segments is indicative of a flow-limiting lesion. It is important to note that well-developed collaterals can diminish the gradients. In hypertensive patients, the gradients may falsely increase, and in low cardiac output states, the gradients may falsely decrease.

PVR may be especially useful in diabetic patients with noncompressible arteries as it is less affected by medial calcinosis than segmental BP recording. PVR detects changes in blood volume in the lower extremities and not the pressures. A normal PVR waveform is composed of a systolic upstroke with a sharp systolic peak followed by a downstroke that contains a prominent dicrotic notch. In calcified arteries, BPs are falsely elevated (as they are not compressible by the BP cuff) and thus can have normal ABIs and segmental pressures. Thus, the PVR becomes a valuable tool in detecting obstructive PAD in such calcified arteries. Mild to moderate disease is characterized by loss of the dicrotic notch and an outward "bowing" of the downstroke of the waveform. In severe disease, the amplitude of waveform is blunted (**Fig. 9-1**). As previously mentioned, calcification of the arteries can result in a falsely normal ankle-brachial pressure index. In addition to PVR, toe-brachial index (TBI) can be used to assess significant obstructive PAD as the smaller pedal arteries are relatively free from calcinosis. This is done by placing a pneumatic cuff on one toe (usually the great toe) and a photoelectrode on the tip of the toe to obtain a photoplethysmographic (PPG)

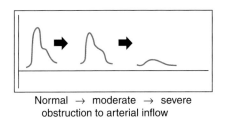

Normal → moderate → severe
obstruction to arterial inflow

FIGURE 9-1. Pulse volume recording.

signal using infrared light (an arterial waveform is created from these signals). The signal is proportional to the quantity of red blood cells in the cutaneous circulation. The toe cuff is inflated until the PPG waveform flattens and then the cuff is deflated. The systolic pressure is recorded when the waveform reestablishes. Pressure gradient of 20 to 30 mm Hg normally exists between the ankle and toe. Normal TBI values are 0.7 to 0.8. A toe pressure of >30 mm Hg is required for general wound healing. In diabetics, toe pressures >50 mm Hg are needed for better wound healing (as they have capillary dysfunction and thus need greater perfusion pressures to overcome this dysfunction). Patients with aortoiliac disease can have normal resting ABIs, but with exercise their ABIs fall to abnormal levels. Hence, exercise stress testing can increase the sensitivity of detecting obstructive PAD. In fact, every ambulatory patient should undergo rest and exercise ABIs. Normally, with exercise the perfusion pressures increase to the lower extremities. The two most commonly used exercise protocols are as follows: one involves walking on a treadmill at a constant speed with no change in incline and the other protocol involves walking on a treadmill at 2 mph at 12% incline for at least 5 minutes or until the symptoms are reproduced. The walking distance and time of onset of pain or symptoms are recorded. The ABIs are done at rest, 1 minute after exercise, and every minute thereafter (up to 5 minutes). The normal response is a slight increase or no change in ABI. The fall in ankle systolic pressure by more than 20% from baseline or below absolute 60 mm Hg that requires more than 3 minutes to recover is abnormal. Those patients whose postexercise systolic ankle pressure drops below 50 mm Hg have severe claudication and potentially multivessel or inflow disease. Also, with exercise, the gradients across stenotic lesions worsen. Patients with occlusive internal iliac disease present with typical buttock claudication and can have normal resting and exercise ABIs. Such patients should undergo computed tomography angiography (CTA) or invasive angiography to delineate the disease and undergo treatment if warranted. Transcutaneous oxygen tension measurement (TcPO$_2$) is a noninvasive diagnostic study, which measures the partial pressure of oxygen at the skin surface. The electrode element has a heating element that raises the temperature of the underlying tissue and results in an increase in capillary flow and partial pressure of oxygen. This then results in diffusion of oxygen through the skin, which can be measured by the electrode. It is important to remember that this device measures the underlying oxygen

tension in the tissue and not the arterial oxygen tension. As long as hemodynamic conditions are stable, transcutaneous measurements can be used as a surrogate of arterial oxygen tension. In simple words, this test quantifies the oxygen delivered to the microvascular tissue. Importantly, they have a prognostic value in predicting wound healing.[11]

Ultrasonography

Ultrasonography comprises B-mode imaging, pulse wave Doppler, continuous wave Doppler, and color Doppler. They are helpful in understanding the underlying anatomy, hemodynamics, and lesion morphology. It is cost-effective and can be done in an office setting. They are extremely useful in diagnosing obstructive PAD, localizing the stenosis, quantifying the severity of the disease, and assessing the patency of stents, grafts, and other interventions.[12] Hence, they are recommended in the surveillance period postendovascular and surgical interventions. B-mode ultrasonography with the help of color Doppler provides information on the anatomy of the lesion and also the morphology of the atherosclerotic plaque. Duplex ultrasonography helps in the accurate assessment of the severity of stenosis using pulsed and continuous Doppler techniques. Therefore, Duplex ultrasonography is a very important tool in following up patients who have undergone endovascular and surgical interventions. They help in the early recognition of restenosis.[13]

Computed Tomography Angiography and Magnetic Resonance Angiography

In recent years, the use of CT and magnetic resonance angiography (MRA) in the evaluation of PAD has increased. However, this varies from institution to institution, as it is highly dependent on the resources and the expertise available to perform these tests and interpret them. CTA has a sensitivity and specificity greater than 95% for identifying significant stenotic lesions.[14,15] MRA acquired with contrast (gadolinium) produces high-resolution images of the infrapopliteal vessels. MRA has a sensitivity of 90% and a specificity of 97% for identifying significant stenotic lesions.[16] CTA is associated with the risks seen with contrast and radiation exposure. The MRA test done with gadolinium contrast carries the risk of nephrogenic systemic fibrosis (especially so in patients with chronic kidney disease). It is important to note that the presence of metallic implants, calcified lesions, and total occlusions results in distorted images and artifacts with CT and MRI.

Peripheral Invasive Arteriography

Peripheral invasive angiography is considered the gold standard for the diagnosis of obstructive PAD. Invasive arteriography involves the use of radiation and contrast. Angiograms performed with digital subtraction angiography (DSA) are the preferred method. It enables to visualize the lumen better.

The DSA highlights only the blood vessel and it does so by eliminating the background bony structures using a complex computerized algorithm. During invasive angiography, in addition to diagnostic angiograms, hemodynamic assessments, intravascular ultrasonography (to visualize the vessel wall and define lesion morphology), and various revascularization therapies can be performed.

Acute Limb Ischemia

Acute limb ischemia (ALI) is the sudden cessation of blood flow to the limbs, which threatens the viability of the limb and the patient presents within 14 days. The incidence of ALI is rare and is approximately 1 to 2 per 10,000 persons per year. It is characterized by the six Ps, which are pain, pallor, pulselessness, paresthesia, paralysis, and poikilothermia (coolness). The most common cause is arterial thrombosis, which comprises about 80% to 85% of the total cases. Usually, these patients would have undergone some sort of endovascular or surgical procedures in the recent past. The second most common cause is embolic in origin, which constitutes the rest 10% to 15%. The most common source of embolism is cardiac in origin (atrial fibrillation with a left atrial or left atrial appendage clot, thrombosed prosthetic mechanical valve, infective endocarditis with septic emboli, severe cardiomyopathy with left ventricular thrombus, atrial myxoma, and other neoplasia which give rise to tumor emboli). The second most common cause of embolism is artery to artery in origin (from an atherosclerotic aorta or popliteal artery). There are several other causes, which make a minuscule piece of the whole pie. It is important to remember that a significant proportion of these patients do not present with the classic six Ps. Therefore, there needs to be a strong sense of suspicion in patients with a prior history of endovascular/surgical procedures who present with acute severe extremity pain. Such patients warrant a detailed examination of the circulation with handheld Dopplers and also an assessment of the neurologic function. When suspected, it should be treated as an emergency because rapid revascularization is the cornerstone for success. Treatment consists of medical, endovascular, and surgical arms. Every patient is started on antiplatelet therapy and heparin infusion. If the limb is viable or marginally threatened, then endovascular intervention is the treatment of choice. Multiple endovascular techniques are available (catheter-directed thrombolysis, rheolytic thrombectomy, mechanical aspiration thrombectomy). In patients with suprainguinal or purely embolic occlusions with significant neurologic impairment, surgery is preferred if the patient is a low surgical risk.

Critical Limb Ischemia

CLI is recognized by the presence of ischemic rest pain and lesions or gangrene attributable to arterial occlusive disease for more than 2 weeks. It is also recognized with ankle pressure less than 50 mm Hg or toe pressure <30 mm Hg in medial calcinosis or ischemic lesions with an ankle pressure <70 mm Hg

and toe pressure <50 mm Hg. A transcutaneous partial pressure of oxygen of less than 30 to 50 mm Hg also aids in the CLI diagnosis. CLI patients present with resting lower extremity pain, which is relieved temporarily by narcotics, and the patient prefers to dangle their legs down. The more frank presentations are gangrene and ulcers. The usual findings of CLI include weak or absent pulses in the feet, cooler feet, dependent pallor, poor growth of toe nails, decreased hair growth on the legs, dark discoloration of the toes, gangrene of toes, sores or wounds or ulcers on the toes, feet, or the legs that heal slowly or do not heal.[17] The ABI is usually ≤0.4, ankle systolic pressure ≤50 mm Hg, and toe systolic pressure ≤30 mm Hg. Microcirculation studies from the skin reveal a capillary density of less than 20 mm^2, absent reactive hyperemia on capillary microscopy, and transcutaneous oxygen tension of less than 10 mm Hg. One year after the diagnosis of CLI, 25% would have died and 30% would have undergone a major amputation. Patients with chronic CLI have a 3-year limb loss rate of approximately 40%. CLI patients have a quality-of-life index similar to that of patients with terminal cancer. There is an unacceptably high rate of amputation if aggressive revascularization strategies are not sought. Goodney et al.[18] studied 20,464 patients with CLI and found that 54% of the patients had no diagnostic or therapeutic vascular procedures performed in the year before the amputation. In another study, which used the Medicare registry, the authors found that among the 417 patients who underwent at least one infrainguinal amputation, only 35% had an ABI and 16% underwent angiography before primary amputation. Sixty-seven percent of these patients underwent primary amputation and only 33% underwent some form of revascularization procedure (23% underwent bypass surgery and 10% underwent balloon angioplasty) before undergoing an amputation. Majority of the wound complications (80%), MI (77.7%), stroke (81.2%), and death (100%) occurred in the primary amputation group.[19]

TREATMENT

The goals of therapy in PAD involve the following: (1) improve the patient's symptoms and quality of life; (2) prevention and management of gangrene, wounds, and ulcers related to PAD; (3) aggressive primary and secondary prevention of coronary and cerebrovascular disease. A multidisciplinary team approach is strongly advised in PAD management.

GLOBAL RISK FACTOR MODIFICATION AND LIFESTYLE CHANGES

SMOKING CESSATION

Cigarette smoking along with diabetes is most strongly correlated with PAD. Smoking cessation improves the outcomes associated with PAD and systemic atherosclerotic disease. Smoking cessation improved symptoms with claudicant by 40% at 10 months compared with patients who failed to quit smoking. Smoking cessation or a reduction improved the 3-year survival (from 40% to 65%) in patients undergoing vascular surgery for PAD.[20]

DIABETES MANAGEMENT

The American College of Cardiology (ACC)/AHA/American Diabetic Association (ADA) guidelines recommend that diabetics achieve a hemoglobin A_{1C} goal of <7.0% to reduce the frequency of cardiovascular complications and also to help in retarding the progression of PAD.[21] Podiatrists play a key role in these diabetic patients in the prevention of diabetic foot ulcers and early treatment if it occurs. Meticulous foot care with regular foot examination and appropriate footwear as a prevention strategy is of utmost importance. Thus, podiatrists play an indispensable role in achieving this foot care, and also the timely referral of these patients to vascular specialists improves limb salvage rates. The LEAP (Lower Extremity Amputation Prevention) study was done to determine the cost-effectiveness of lower extremity amputation prevention strategy compared to standard clinical practice in diabetic patients with CLI. The main aim of the LEAP strategy was to enhance salvage via aggressive revascularization. The study enrolled 388 patients in the LEAP arm and they were followed for 4 years. The LEAP arm had a cost savings of approximately 2,000 dollars per patient. Also, the LEAP strategy had lower amputation rates (29% vs. 76%), lower death rates (1% vs. 19%), and fewer in-hospital days (18 vs. 23 days) when compared to standard practice.[22]

HYPERTENSION MANAGEMENT

Aggressive control of hypertension to achieve a target BP of <140/90 mm Hg and a more strict goal of <130/80 mm Hg in diabetics and patients with renal insufficiency is highly recommended. In the HOPE (The Heart Outcomes Prevention Evaluation Study) trial, ramipril reduced the risk of MI by 22% in patients with PAD. Beta-blockers were once thought to worsen claudication, but this has not borne true in large studies. Therefore, patients with heart disease who are already on β-blockers should continue to be on it unless advised against it by the patient's cardiologists.

CHOLESTEROL MANAGEMENT

Lipid-lowering therapy with a statin to achieve a target low-density lipoprotein (LDL) of <70 mg per dL is strongly advocated by the ACC/AHA professional societies in patients with PAD and those who have had an MI. In fact, even if the LDL is <70 mg per dL, patients with PAD or any form of atherosclerotic disease should be started on a statin. Among 6,748 individuals with PAD in the Heart Protection Study, the use of simvastatin reduced the overall mortality by 12%, vascular mortality by 17%, adverse coronary events by 24%, and stroke by 27% (at a mean follow-up of 5 years). Also, lipid lowering improves claudication symptoms and extends walking times.

ANTIPLATELET THERAPY

Antiplatelet therapy receives a class I recommendation in the ACC/AHA guidelines for the prevention of adverse cardiovascular events in PAD. The Antithrombotic Trialists' Collaboration studied 42 clinical trials comprising 9,214 patients with PAD and found that patients who were on antiplatelet therapy had a 25% reduction in the rate of stroke, MI, or cardiovascular death when compared with patients who had received placebo. The ACC/AHA guidelines give the use of aspirin in PAD a class IA recommendation. The CAPRIE (clopidogrel vs. aspirin in patients at risk of ischemic events) trial, which studied 19,000 patients, found that, individuals taking clopidogrel had an 8.7% relative reduction in the composite endpoint of MI, stroke, or vascular death when compared to those taking aspirin alone. This effect was more pronounced in the subgroup analysis of patients with PAD, where the composite endpoint was reduced by 23.8% among individuals taking clopidogrel. In light of these findings, the ACC/AHA and TASC-II (Trans-Atlantic Society-II) guidelines[23] support the use of clopidogrel monotherapy as an alternative to aspirin in patients with PAD (class IB recommendation). The role of dual antiplatelet is not validated in any large trials. Dual antiplatelet therapy is recommended in PAD patients who undergo an intervention. Usually, for a month, and in patients who receive a drug-eluting stent (Zilver PTX stent), the dual antiplatelet therapy needs to be continued for at least 3 months. It is important to be mindful that patients with CAD who have stents in them need the dual antiplatelet therapy for at least 1 year (especially if they have drug-eluting stents).

EXERCISE THERAPY

Supervised exercise therapy along with cilostazol is the mainstay therapy for patients with intermittent claudication. Various mechanisms have been proposed on how exercise improves claudication, including collateral vessel angiogenesis, decreased inflammation, decreased free radical and lactic acid accumulation, better exercise pain tolerance, improved cellular metabolism, efficient muscle energy metabolism, reduced blood viscosity and red blood cell aggregation, and improved endothelial function. The recommendations are for three to five supervised exercise sessions per week with 35 to 50 minutes of exercise per session on a treadmill (to achieve near-maximal claudication pain) for more than 6 months. In a meta-analysis of 21 studies involving supervised walking programs, the mean walking distance to onset of claudication was increased by 180%. They also showed that the absolute walking distance was improved by 130% when compared with baseline.[24,25] It is important to note that the exercise program has to be supervised. Studies have shown that unsupervised exercise programs do not help the patients. Currently, supervised exercise program has a class IA recommendation for the management of intermittent claudication.

DRUG THERAPY FOR CLAUDICANTS

Two medications that are approved by the Food and Drug Administration (FDA) for claudication management are cilostazol and pentoxifylline. Cilostazol is a phosphodiesterase inhibitor (PDE-3) that promotes vasodilatation and inhibits platelet aggregation. In clinical trials, cilostazol statistically improved the walking distance after 12 weeks of therapy. The ACC/AHA and TASC-II guidelines recommend the use of cilostazol for the management of intermittent claudication in combination with supervised exercise therapy (class IA recommendation). It is important to bear in our minds that the use of cilostazol therapy has a black box warning from the FDA in patients with congestive heart failure.[26] In a meta-analysis of 11 clinical studies, pentoxifylline showed only modest improvement in walking distance. This agent exerts its beneficial effects by lowering blood viscosity and improving red blood cell flexibility. Pentoxifylline receives a class IIb recommendation for the management of intermittent claudication as per ACC/AHA and TASC-II guidelines.[27]

REVASCULARIZATION THERAPY

Revascularization therapy can be performed by either the endovascular or surgical route. Recently, there has been tremendous improvement and introduction of several new endovascular techniques. Revascularization remains the cornerstone of treatment for CLI. It is also indicated in claudication for symptom relief for those who fail medical therapy and the exercise program, and performed to reduce the level of amputation. The choice between endovascular and surgical revascularization should be individualized. Each of the therapies has its own merits and demerits.

Based on the TASC-II classification, the vascular society has come up with guidelines regarding the choice of revascularization therapies. The choice of revascularization therapy is dependent on the complexity and extent of PAD. TASC-II classification is purely based on the anatomy of the disease. There are two TASC classifications. One classification is for iliac disease and the other classification is for femoropopliteal disease. The classification is based on the location and severity of the stenosis, the length of the stenosis, number of stenosis, calcification, chronic total occlusions, level of reconstitution, prior endovascular interventions, etc. Type A is the simplest lesion and type D is the most complex lesion. The society recommends endovascular therapy as the treatment of choice for type A and B lesions and surgical therapy as the treatment of choice for type D lesions. Surgical therapy is preferred for type C lesions. In addition to the complexity and extent of PAD, the patient's comorbidities, patient preference, available resources and expertise, along with the operator's long-term success rate must be considered as well when making the treatment decisions for type C and D lesions. With surgical approach, the risk of MI is 1.9% to 3.4%, mortality is 1.3% to 6%, wound infection is 10% to 30%, and scar-related

neuropathic pain is 23%. About 30% of grafts will require revision during their lifetime. Endovascular treatment is associated with groin complications, contrast-related adverse reactions, risks associated with radiation exposure, restenosis, and repeat procedures. The field of endovascular therapy is so rapidly evolving that guidelines and consensus statements are yet to incorporate these new advances. It is suffice to say that the choice of revascularization therapy is dependent on the disease, patient, and the expertise available.

ENDOVASCULAR THERAPY

In the BASIL (bypass vs. angioplasty in severe ischemia of the leg) trial, 452 patients with severe chronic limb ischemia were randomized on an intention-to-treat basis to an initial strategy of bypass surgery or endovascular treatment with angioplasty (not stenting) for infrainguinal disease. This study showed no significant differences in the outcomes between the angioplasty and surgery groups at 3 years. However, this study has been criticized for bias and the lack of uniformity in the study population. Also, this study was done in an era where endovascular techniques were still quite primitive in its evolution. Recently, studies have demonstrated that stenting of SFA lesions yielded a better restenosis and clinical improvement when compared to angioplasty only. In fact, one study demonstrated that SFA stenting had a 24% restenosis rate at 6 months when compared to a 43% rate in those who underwent angioplasty alone. Thus, these findings suggest that endovascular therapy for SFA using nitinol stents may provide greater durability than angioplasty alone.[28] In addition, with the introduction of atherectomy debulking devices and drug-coated balloons (DCBs), the endovascular specialist is able to achieve results similar to that of stenting and thus has the tremendous advantage of not leaving a metal behind.

PERCUTANEOUS TECHNIQUES AND TOOLS

Various tools are available in the current era to treat PAD by the endovascular route. These include short and long angioplasty balloons, special cutting balloons, more recently FDA-approved DCBs, balloon-delivered and self-expanding stents, drug-eluting stents, debulking atherectomy devices, reentry devices, and special crossing devices to cross chronic total occlusions.

Angioplasty Balloons and Special Balloons

There are several balloons available to treat PAD. The standard balloons come in various lengths, different profiles on the same balloon and can be complaint, semi-compliant, and noncompliant (hence tailor-made for different kinds of lesions). Then we have the cutting balloons, which can have metal spikes, metal wires, or metal rings wound round the balloon. These cutting balloons give an excellent result in resistant calcified lesions causing minimal plaque shift, hence preserving side branches. The Chocolate percutaneous transluminal angioplasty (PTA) balloon catheter (Cordis, Fremont, CA) is a novel balloon catheter with a mounted nitinol-constraining structure specifically designed for uniform dilatation in resistant lesions. The Chocolate balloon angioplasty registry contains both 174 patients with above-the-knee (ATK) and 180 patients with below-the-knee (BTK) lesions. In the ATK cohorts, at 6 months postintervention, only 11% of patients required target lesion revascularization (TLR), 96% of patients had an amputation-free survival, and 89% of patients were free of any major adverse events. The success rate for BTK interventions was also similar at 3 months, only 7% required TLR, the amputation-free survival rate was 97%, and freedom from major adverse events was 90%. The other cutting balloons are the AngioScore (AngioScore Inc, Fremont, CA) and the Flextome cutting balloon (Boston Scientific, Marlborough, MA). DCBs will be discussed in the section below.

Stents

There are several stents such as the Supera (Abbott vascular, Abbott Park, IL), EverFlex (Covidien, Mansfield, MA), and Complete SE (Medtronics, Minneapolis, MN) that are available in the market to treat PAD. The only drug-eluting stent that is available in the USA is Zilver PTX stent (Cook, Bloomington, IN) to be used in SFA lesions. The Zilver PTX paclitaxel-eluting nitinol stent (Zilver PTX stent) trial enrolled 60 patients and showed 90% primary patency rates in Zilver PTX group when compared to 52% primary patency rates in the PTA control group (follow-up period of 9 months). Only 8% of all the patients who were treated with the Zilver PTX stent needed a reintervention in the first 12 months.[29,30]

Drug-Coated Balloons

Recently, DCBs were approved for its use in femoropopliteal lesions by the FDA. DCBs act by delivering the antiproliferative agent to the vessel wall without leaving any stent behind. Some of the advantages of the DCB are as follows: ability to treat bypass landing zones; preserves the original anatomy of the vessel; does not leave a metal or polymer behind, therefore removing any source for physical, chemical, or immunologic trigger; ability to treat segments where stents are not advised (common femoral and popliteal arteries), and a recent study showed that DCBs could potentially lower the projected budget impact over 2 years when compared to standard balloon angioplasty and bare-metal stents as they improve primary patency and reduce target vessel revascularization (thus reducing the need for further procedures). The THUNDER, FEMPAC, LEVANT, and PACIFIER trials showed a significant reduction in late lumen loss (an objective means of assessing restenosis) and TLR when compared to standard balloon angioplasty. These trials and few more recent trials led to its approval in the management of femoropopliteal

lesions by the FDA. DCBs have definitely started a new era in the endovascular management of PAD.

ATHERECTOMY DEVICES

The major disadvantage of angioplasty is restenosis, which may be overcome to some extent by debulking the plaque. Multiple studies have shown advantages of these debulking devices in specific conditions. There are four different kinds of atherectomy.

Directional Atherectomy

Directional atherectomy involves the resection of the atherosclerotic plaque with a cutting device in the longitudinal plane. It is preferred in diabetic patients. Two FDA-approved devices are SilverHawk and TurboHawk (Covidien, Mansfield, MA). The DEFINITIVE-LE (Determination of Effectiveness of the SilverHawk Peripheral Plaque Excision System [SilverHawk Device] for the Treatment of Infrainguinal Vessels/Lower Extremities) trial enrolled 799 patients (53% were diabetics) and found that with atherectomy, they were able to achieve a primary patency rate of 78% in the claudicant and 71% in the CLI group at 1 year follow-up.[31] There were no major differences in the results between diabetics and nondiabetics. Additionally, the use of DCBs after directional atherectomy in calcified resistant lesions yielded excellent results.

Orbital Atherectomy

This system employs a 360° rotational device with a diamond-coated crown that orbits eccentrically within the vessel contour. The only FDA-approved orbital atherectomy device is the CSI Diamondback Orbital atherectomy system (Cardiovascular Systems, Inc., Saint Paul, MN). The CALCIUM 360° (Comparison of Orbital Atherectomy plus Balloon Angioplasty vs. Balloon Angioplasty Alone in Patients with Critical Limb Ischemia) trial enrolled 50 patients with heavily calcified popliteal or infrapopliteal arteries, and they achieved a primary patency rate of 93% in the orbital atherectomy arm when compared to 82% in the PTA-only group.[32] The COMPLIANCE 360° (Comparing Balloon Angioplasty to Diamondback 360° Orbital Atherectomy System in Calcified Femoropopliteal Disease) study enrolled 50 patients with heavily calcified femoropopliteal vessels and showed a 72.7% freedom from TLR at 6 months in the group that received orbital atherectomy and PTA when compared to 8.3% in the PTA-only group.[33] Hence, orbital atherectomy is an excellent tool in calcified infrainguinal femoropopliteal and infrapopliteal lesions.

Rotational Atherectomy

Rotational atherectomy employs a high-speed rotating cutting blade (or "burr") coated with abrasive material such as microscopic diamond particles and at the same time aspirates the denuded particles.[34] The FDA-approved device is Pathway PV system (currently Jetstream; Pathway Medical Technologies, Kirkland, WA). The single-arm Pathway PVD trial that enrolled 172 patients (42% were diabetics) showed that 38.2% of the patients had evidence of vessel restenosis, and 26% of the patients underwent repeat TLR, which is better than PTA alone.[35] The other devices are the Rotablator (Boston Scientific, Marlborough, Fremont, CA) and the Phoenix atherectomy device (AtheroMed, Menlo Park, CA), which is still under investigation. Thus, it is very useful in the treatment of calcified lesions.[34]

Laser Atherectomy

This technique utilizes laser to remove atherosclerotic plaque by "photoablation." The Turbo-Booster/Turbo-Elite laser catheter (Spectranetics, Colorado Springs, CO) is the only FDA-approved device for the treatment of femoropopliteal in-stent restenosis. The CELLO (CliRpath Excimer Laser System to Enlarge Lumen Openings) study enrolled 65 patients and showed a primary patency of 54%.[35] The EXCITE ISR (EXCImer Laser Randomized Controlled Study for Treatment of FemoropopliTEal In-Stent Restenosis) was a prospective randomized multicenter study that compared excimer laser atherectomy (169 patients) with standard balloon angioplasty (81 patients) for femoropopliteal in-stent restenosis. The laser arm had significantly higher procedural success rate and safety rate and lower TLR than the standard balloon angioplasty arm. It was this study that led to its approval by the FDA.

CHRONIC TOTAL OCCLUSION DEVICES AND REENTRY DEVICES

There are many tools available to cross chronic total occlusions. The most commonly used are the Viance crossing catheter (Covidien, Mansfield, MA), Crosser (Bard, Tempe, AZ), Laser (Spectranetics, Colorado Springs, CO), and TruePath (Boston Scientific, Marlborough, MA). Reentry into the true lumen distally where it reconstitutes can be achieved by devices like the Pioneer (ultrasound guided, Volcano, San Diego, CA), Outback (fluoroscopy guided, Cordis, Fremont, CA), Ocelot (optimal computed tomography [OCT] guided), and Enteer reentry system (Covidien, Mansfield, MA).

SURGICAL THERAPY

Surgical therapy is dependent on the lesion complexity; patient's comorbidities; availability of venous conduits, adequate target distal vessels, resources, expertise; and finally the surgeon's track record. As per Medicare claims data from 1996 to 2006, there has been a >3-fold increase in endovascular intervention and bypass surgery decreased by 42%. Despite the decreasing rate of bypass, surgery remains an important treatment strategy in advanced multilevel vascular disease. Typically, surgical mode of revascularization is indicated in patients with acceptable surgical risk (and life expectancy of >2 years) who need a more durable long-lasting repair, those patients whose vascular disease cannot be managed by endovascular strategies, and finally those who have failed endovascular treatment. There has to be an adequate venous conduit available for bypass, otherwise the patency rates are the same as those for endovascular strategies. Mortality rates from surgery range from 3% to 8% depending on the comorbidities. On the other hand, the rates of major complications associated with endovascular interventions range from 1.9% to 2.9%. With the rising elderly population and its concomitant cardiovascular comorbidities, endovascular intervention is usually the preferred choice of revascularization. In this current era, several patients may benefit from a hybrid approach, where the inflow is taken care by one approach and the outflow via the other approach, depending on the arterial anatomy.

USING THE ANGIOSOME PRINCIPLE IN PLANNING THE OPTIMAL REVASCULARIZATION

Successful limb salvage is dependent on detailed knowledge of the vascular anatomy of the foot and ankle. The concept of angiosomes was first introduced in 1987 by Taylor and Palmer.[36] They divided the body into three-dimensional vascular territories supplied by specific source arteries and drained by specific veins. The foot and ankle are composed of six distinct angiosomes[37]; the six angiosomes of the foot and ankle originate from the three main source arteries. The posterior tibial artery supplies the medial ankle and the plantar foot which includes the calcaneal branch (heel), the medial plantar artery (instep), and the lateral plantar artery (lateral midfoot and forefoot). The anterior tibial artery supplies the anterior ankle and then becomes the dorsalis pedis artery, which supplies the dorsum of the foot. The peroneal artery supplies the anterolateral portion of the ankle and rear foot with two branches, the anterior perforating branch (lateral anterior upper ankle) and the calcaneal branch (lateral and plantar heel). Arterial–arterial connections allow for uninterrupted blood flow to the entire foot despite the occlusion of one or more arteries. The primary goal for CLI patients is to reestablish pulsatile straight-line flow to the distal extremity, especially to the respective angiosome where the ulcer or gangrene is present.[38] Unfortunately, 15% of surgical bypasses fail to improve ulcer healing because they do not provide blood supply to the affected angiosome.[39] Gooden and colleagues found that up to 25% of patients with heel ulcers ultimately succumbed to a proximal leg amputation despite a palpable pedal pulse.[40] The major reason is inadequate revascularization, because the supplying artery or the collaterals supplying the ischemic area are occluded or absent.[41] The failure rates of wound healing can be decreased if the bypassed vessel directly feeds the vessel that supplies the angiosome which is affected (straight-line flow), rather than revascularizing one of the other two vessels that may supply blood via collateral or arterial to arterial connections.[42] Clemens and Attinger retrospectively examined the results of direct versus indirect revascularization of 52 limbs. The direct revascularization group had fewer failures (9.1% vs. 38.1%) than the indirect revascularization group. Those who failed to heal underwent major amputation. The amputation rates were four times higher in the indirect revascularization group. There is increasing evidence to support the use of angioplasty in CLI patients with infrapopliteal disease. One study, with a 5-year follow-up, showed tibioperoneal angioplasty was effective with a clinical success rate of 95%. Among those patients who had a clinically successful angioplasty, 91% of those limbs were salvaged, only 8% underwent bypass surgery and only 9% needed significant amputations. Meta-analysis of infrapopliteal angioplasty by Romiti et al.[43] reported 12-month and 36-month results as follows: primary patency rates at 77.4% and 48.6%, secondary patency rates at 83.3% and 62.9%, limb salvage rates at 93.4% and 82.4%, and patient survival rates at 98.3% and 68.4%, respectively. Despite the marginal patency rates at 36 months, the wound healing is better and is definitely a better option than amputation.

ANGIOSOME TERRITORIES

Tables 9-3 and 9-4 show the area supplied by infrapopliteal arteries and its branches (Fig. 9-2).

SURVEILLANCE

As mentioned earlier, ABIs and duplex ultrasonography are the preferred surveillance tests to follow patients postendovascular

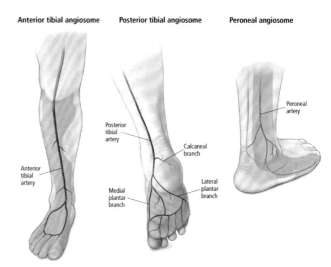

FIGURE 9-2. Angiosomes of the lower extremity. The foot and ankle can be divided into six territories called angiosomes, based on the artery supplying them. The concept can help in locating the obstruction in the specific artery in patients with lower extremity ischemic ulcers and in planning revascularization. (Reproduced from Shishehbor MH. Acute and critical limb ischemia: when time is limb. *Cleve Clin J Med.* 2014;81:209–216, with permission from The Cleveland Clinic Foundation© 2014. The Cleveland Clinic Foundation. All rights reserved.)

or surgical interventions. The benefit of surveillance is to improve the primary assisted patency rates. The recommended surveillance options from our experience are as follows. For iliac and BTK revascularization therapies, duplex ultrasonography should be performed at 6 months and yearly thereafter. For femoropopliteal and graft interventions, it should be performed every 3 months for a year and then 6 months thereafter.

CONCLUSION

PAD is a pandemic disease with multiple facets. It confers a high risk for significant cardiovascular and cerebrovascular morbidity and mortality. A multidisciplinary approach, involving an interventional cardiologist, vascular surgeon, radiologist, infectious disease specialist, and podiatrist is absolutely crucial. Podiatrists play a critical role as they are in the forefront of this battle against PAD and can be considered the "foot soldiers." Podiatrists see and manage the entire spectrum of

Table 9-3. Site of Pain to Culprit Arterial Obstruction

Heel	Peroneal or posterior tibial artery
Plantar foot	Posterior tibial artery
Lateral ankle wound	Peroneal artery
Dorsal foot	Anterior tibial artery

Table 9-4. Angiosome to Culprit Arterial Obstruction

Tibial Arteries	Areas Supplied (angiosomes)	Branch Distribution
Anterior tibial and dorsalis pedis	Anterior leg and the dorsum of the foot	
Posterior tibial	Inside of the heel, sole of the foot, plantar surface, and web spaces of toes	Heel—calcaneal branch Instep—medial plantar branch Lateral midfoot and the forefoot—lateral plantar branch
Peroneal	Lateral ankle and heel	Plantar aspect of heel—calcaneal branch Anterolateral part of upper ankle—anterior perforating branch

the disease and thus are in a critical position, wherein they can create a significant positive impact on this disease. The goals of the treatment should be symptom relief, improvement in the quality of life, prevention of cardiovascular events, and limb salvage.

REFERENCES

1. Gregg EW, Sorlie P, Paulose-Ram R, et al. Prevalence of lower-extremity disease in the US adult population >=40 years of age with and without diabetes: 1999–2000 national health and nutrition examination survey. *Diabetes Care*. 2004;27:1591–1597.

2. Hirsch AT, Haskal ZJ, Hertzer NR, et al. ACC/AHA 2005 Practice Guidelines for the management of patients with peripheral arterial disease (lower extremity, renal, mesenteric, and abdominal aortic): a collaborative report from the American Association for Vascular Surgery/Society for Vascular Surgery, Society for Cardiovascular Angiography and Interventions, Society for Vascular Medicine and Biology, Society of Interventional Radiology, and the ACC/AHA Task Force on Practice Guidelines (Writing Committee to Develop Guidelines for the Management of Patients With Peripheral Arterial Disease): endorsed by the American Association of Cardiovascular and Pulmonary Rehabilitation; National Heart, Lung, and Blood Institute; Society for Vascular Nursing; TransAtlantic Inter-Society Consensus; and Vascular Disease Foundation. *Circulation*. 2006;113(11):e463–e654.

3. Singh N, Armstrong DG, Lipsky BA. Preventing foot ulcers in patients with diabetes. *JAMA*. 2005;293(2):217–228.

4. Reiber GE, Vileikyte L, Boyko EJ, et al. Causal pathways for incident lower-extremity ulcers in patients with diabetes from two settings. *Diabetes Care*. 1999;22(1):157–162.

5. Pickett CA, Jackson JL, Hemann BA, et al. Carotid bruits as a prognostic indicator of cardiovascular death and myocardial infarction: a meta-analysis. *Lancet*. 2008;371(9624):1587–1594.

6. Olin JW, Sealove BA. Peripheral artery disease: current insight into the disease and its diagnosis and management. *Mayo Clin Proc*. 2010;85(7):678–692.

7. Mohler ER. Screening for peripheral artery disease. *Circulation*. 2012;126(8):e111–e112.

8. Fontaine R, Kim M, Kieny R. Die chirugische Behandlung der peripheren Durchblutungsstörungen. [Surgical treatment of peripheral circulation disorders.] *Helvetica Chirurgica Acta*. 1954;21(5/6):499–533.

9. Norgren L, Hiatt WR, Dormandy JA. Inter-society consensus for the management of peripheral arterial disease (TASC II). *Eur J Vasc Endovasc Surg*. 2007;33(suppl 1):S1–S75.

10. Nead KT, Cooke JP, Olin JW, et al. Alternative ankle-brachial index method identifies additional at-risk individuals. *J Am Coll Cardiol*. 2013;62(6):553–559.

11. Kruse I, Edelman S. Evaluation and treatment of diabetic foot ulcers. *Clinical Diabetes*. 2006;24(2):91–93.

12. Jager KA, Ricketts HJ, Strandness DE Jr. Duplex scanning for the evaluation of lower limb arterial disease. In: Bernstein EF, ed. *Noninvasive Diagnostic Techniques in Vascular Disease*. St Louis, MO: CV Mosby; 1985:619–631.

13. Olin JW, Kaufman JA, Bluemke DA, et al. Atherosclerotic Vascular Disease Conference. American heart association, imaging, writing group IV. *Circulation*. 2004;109(21):2626–2633.

14. Sun Z. Diagnostic accuracy of multislice CT angiography in peripheral arterial disease. *J Vasc Interv Radiol*. 2006;17(12):1915–1921.

15. Rubin GD, Schmidt AJ, Logan LJ, et al. Multi-detector row CT angiography of lower extremity arterial inflow and runoff: initial experience. *Radiology*. 2001;221(1):146–158.

16. Prince MR, Meaney JF. Expanding role of MR angiography in clinical practice. *Eur Radiol*. 2006;16(suppl 2):B3–B8.

17. Hiatt WR. Medical treatment of peripheral arterial disease and claudication. *N Engl J Med*. 2001;344:1608–1621.

18. Goodney PP, Travis LL, Nallamothu BK, et al. Variation in the use of lower extremity vascular procedures for critical limb ischemia. *Circ Cardiovasc Qual Outcomes*. 2012;5:94–102.

19. Allie DE, Hebert CJ, Lirtzman MD, et al. Critical limb ischemia: a global epidemic. A critical analysis of current treatment unmasks the clinical and economic costs of CLI. *EuroIntervention*. 2005;1(1):75–84.

20. Hobbs SD, Wilmink AB, Adam DJ, et al. Assessment of smoking status in patients with peripheral arterial disease. *J Vasc Surg*. 2005;41(3):451–456.

21. Goff DC, Lloyd-Jones DM, Sean Coady GB, et al. 2013 ACC/AHA Guideline on the Assessment of Cardiovascular Risk: A Report of the American College of Cardiology/American Heart Association Task Force on Practice Guidelines. *Circulation*. 2014;129:S49–S73.

22. Tan MLM, Feng J, Gordois A, et al. Lower extremity amputation prevention in Singapore: economic analysis of results. *Singapore Med J*. 2011;52(9):662–668.

23. Norgren L, Hiatt WR, Dormandy JA, et al. *Eur J Vasc Endovasc Surg*. 2007;33:S1–S70.

24. Gardner AW, Poehlman ET. Exercise rehabilitation programs for the treatment of claudication pain. A meta-analysis. *JAMA*. 1995;274:975–980.

25. Murphy TP, Cutlip DE, Regensteiner JG, et al. Supervised exercise versus primary stenting for claudication resulting from aortoiliac peripheral artery disease: six-month outcomes from the claudication: exercise versus endoluminal revascularization (CLEVER) study. *Circulation*. 2012;125(1):130–139. doi: 10.1161/CIRCULATIONAHA.111.075770.

26. Beebe HG, Dawson DL, Cutler BS, et al. A new pharmacological treatment for intermittent claudication: results of a randomized, multicenter trial. *Arch Intern Med*. 1999;159:2041–2050.

27. Dawson DL, Cutler BS, Meissner MH, et al. Cilostazol has beneficial effects in treatment of intermittent claudication: results from a multicenter, randomized, prospective, double-blind trial. *Circulation*. 1998;98(7):678–686.

28. Schillinger M, Sabeti S, Loewe C, et al. Balloon angioplasty versus implantation of nitinol stents in the superficial femoral artery. *N Engl J Med*. 2006;354:1879–1888.

29. Dake M. Interim Report on the Zilver PTX Trial. Presented at: 2009 Charing Cross Symposium; London, UK. http://www.aimsymposium.org/pdf/aim/2480.pdf. Accessed April, 2009.

30. Dake M. Interim Analysis of Two-year Results for the Zilver PTX Drug-eluting Peripheral Stent. Presented at: 2009 Vascular Annual Meeting; June 11–14, 2009; Denver, CO.

31. Regine R, Catalano O, De Siero M, et al. Endovascular treatment of femoropopliteal stenoses/occlusions with a SilverHawk directional atherectomy device: immediate results and 12-month follow-up. *Radiol Med*. 2010;115(8):1208–1218.

32. Shammas NW, Lam R, Mustapha J, et al. Comparison of orbital atherectomy plus balloon angioplasty vs. balloon angioplasty alone in patients with critical limb ischemia: results of the CALCIUM 360 randomized pilot trial. *J Endovasc Ther*. 2012;19(4):480–488.

33. Datilo R. 12 months results of compliance 360: a prospective, multicenter, randomized trial comparing orbital atherectomy to balloon angioplasty for calcified femoropopliteal lesions. *J Am Coll Cardiol*. 2012;59(13, suppl 1):E2085–E2085.

34. Zeller T, Krankenberg H, Steinkamp H, et al. One-year outcome of percutaneous rotational atherectomy with aspiration in infrainguinal peripheral arterial occlusive disease: the multicenter pathway PVD trial. *J Endovasc Ther*. 2009;16(6):653–662.

35. Dave RM, Patlola R, Kollmeyer K, et al. Excimer laser recanalization of femoropopliteal lesions and 1-year patency: results of the CELLO registry. *J Endovasc Ther*. 2009;16(6):665–675.

36. Taylor GI, Palmer JH. The vascular territories (angiosomes) of the body: experimental study and clinical applications. *Br J Plast Surg*. 1987;40:113–141.

37. Clemens MW, Attinger CE. Angiosomes and wound care in the diabetic foot. *Foot Ankle Clin N Am.* 2010;15:439–464. doi: 10.1016/j.fcl.2010.04.003.
38. Arain SA, White CJ. Endovascular therapy for critical limb ischemia. *Vasc Med.* 2008;13:267.
39. Berceli SA, Chan AK, Pomposelli FB, et al. Efficacy of dorsal pedal artery bypass in limb salvage for ischemic heel ulcers. *J Vasc Surg.* 1999;30:499.
40. Gooden MA, Gentile AT, Mills JL, et al. Free tissue transfer to extend the limits of limb salvage for lower extremity tissue loss. *Am J Surg.* 1997;174:644.
41. Attinger CE, Ducic I, Neville RF, et al. The relative roles of aggressive wound care versus revascularization in salvage of the threatened lower extremity in the renal failure diabetic patient. *Plast Reconstr Surg.* 2002;109:1281.
42. Neville RF, Attinger CE, Bulan EJ, et al. Revascularization of a specific angiosome for limb salvage: does the target artery matter? *Ann Vasc Surg.* 2009;23(3):367–373.
43. Romiti, M, Albers M, Brochado-Neto FC, et al. Meta-analysis of infrapopliteal angioplasty for chronic critical limb ischemia. *J Vasc Surg.* 2008;47:975–981.

CHAPTER 10

Gait Disorders

JOSEPH C. D'AMICO

Gait is the momentary loss and regaining of balance that takes place with each step. Of course most people never think about this complex, rhythmic process that takes place thousands of times each day which is dependent upon a myriad of three systems working interdependently to allow for a smooth-in-form bipedal gait. The visual, vestibular, and proprioceptive senses comprise the afferent sensory system. Nerves, muscles, bones, joints, and tendons comprise the locomotor efferent system, and all are monitored and under the control of the central nervous system (CNS).[1] It is only when one of these systems begins to falter either as a result of systemic disease or as a result of the inevitable aging process that the individual and those closest to them begin to notice these changes.

Most children take their first steps at approximately 1 year of age; however, complete adultlike coordination is not achieved until 6 years of age. It is at this time that the lower extremity nervous system receives its full myelin coating making it easier for the neuromotor system to orchestrate a mature gait pattern.[2] The act of adult walking begins with a confidence inherent in the human organism that instills in the individual the belief that if he or she thinks they can walk from point A to point B they automatically will be able to do so. They think they can because they have done it before and therefore should be able to do it again until one day that process is interrupted and their feet do not respond in the same coordinated manner as they once did. They begin to notice their gait is not as graceful, smooth, or spry as it once was. There may be an irregularity in arm–leg coordination and symmetry, increased sway, shorter steps, slower speed, trips, slips and falls, rigidity with motion, and an overall loss of confidence in being able to accomplish basic locomotor tasks. Compensatory adjustments made by the individual in an attempt to improve stability may result in further disassociation from a normal-appearing gait pattern. It is at this point that professional consultation is usually sought to determine whether or not this alteration in function is due to systemic disease, the manifestation of idiopathic gait changes associated with the aging process or as simple as an improperly fitting shoe.

Locomotion is the act of getting from one place to another and involves not only the lower extremity but the arm/hand complex as well. Gait is the means of achieving this action. Balance and gait are intimately connected. Walking is a form of gait with a particular pattern of footfalls and specific requirements (Table 10-1). It is a complex process involving the musculoskeletal and nervous systems, which represents the sum total of all the functional and structural capabilities of the individual. Walking is the response of the individual who is actively solving a specific motor problem. It is dictated by individual constraints and task environment, that is, walking on a wet, sloped cobblestone street is a much more difficult task than walking on a dry, flat, level sidewalk. Gait solutions to locomotor challenges emerge, which are task and individual neuromotor capability appropriate.

Speed is a key indicator of the functional status of the locomotor system. In fact, observation of the unprompted speed at which an individual walks is a cost effective determinant used to predict the overall health of the individual—the speedier live longer.[3,4] Walking speed inversely correlates with the ability of the individual to live independently, perform various activities of daily living such as being able to cross an intersection before the light changes, and the risk of falling.[5] An inevitable result of living a longer life is that at some point, usually somewhere in the sixth decade, people start slowing down.[6] This process can to some extent be delayed through exercise and proper nutrition; however, no one in their later years walks as spritely, runs as fast, or balances as well as they did in their youth.

Central pattern generators (CPGs) are groupings of neurons or neural circuits that can generate and control co-ordinated movements. It is an innate neuromotor and spinal reflexive neural network.[7] CPGs are modified by sensory input. Changes in neural output are dependent upon joint angle, interjoint relationships, center of gravity (COG), and the weightbearing status of the limb and are recognized by multisensorial afferent input or by peripheral receptors.[7] Activation patterns for the leg musculature and stance to swing phase transitions during ambulation are determined by local information received through mechanical receptors in the plantar aspect of the feet and from proprioceptive inputs in the extensor foot musculature.[8] Locomotor control is distributed across neural networks organized at higher and lower levels with parallel ascending and descending pathways for integration among different subsystems. Age-resistant neurospinal circuits control limb movements and modulate antigravity muscle tone and active propulsion. However, active propulsive power deteriorates with advancing age. The challenge for the aging individual is the precise regulation of their musculoskeletal system function while maintaining balance and propelling the body forward. The maintenance of dynamic neuromuscular equilibrium providing external stability essential for safe locomotion is adversely affected by age and systemic disease.

It has been stated that gait and balance are intimately connected, and when stepping is impaired there is an increased risk for falls. This may be due to the displaced COG, impaired CNS regions, an inability to correct perturbations or due to the manifestation of a gait disorder affecting postural stability.[1]

There are a number of factors that influence gait (**Table 10-1**). Most individuals experience an increasing difficulty in ambulation with increasing age.[9] Gait abnormalities increase with age even in otherwise healthy individuals. In 75% of the cases the etiology is multifactorial, but if solitary it is probably musculoskeletal in nature.[9]

Spielberg in his landmark study investigating the walking patterns of older people classified gait changes with advancing age into three stages (**Table 10-2**).[10] The challenge for health practitioners is to be able to ascertain whether or not alterations in gait can be ascribed to the expected changes accompanying the aging process, resulting in an idiopathic geriatric gait due to or aggravated by an underlying systemic disorder. Systemic disorders affecting gait may be divided into the following etiologic categories: neurosensory, metabolic, cardiovascular, musculoskeletal, and idiopathic.

Table 10-1. Walking Requisites

Upright posture
Ability to alternately swing from double limb support to single limb support
Single limb support
Lateral stability
Alternately generate and resist self-produced forward momentum
Intact central pattern generators

Table 10-2. Geriatric Gait Stage (by Age)

Stage 1: 60–72 y
Decreased velocity (>63 y = 1.6%/y)
Decrease cadence
Decrease vertical excursion (COG)
Decreased step length
Disturbed coordination of upper and lower extremities
Stage 2: 72–86 y
Arm–leg synergy is lost
Increased unwanted movements
Stage 3: 86–104 y
Rapid disintegration of gait patterns
Arrhythmic stepping patterns

OBSERVATIONAL GAIT ANALYSIS

Human gait should be effortless and efficient with minimal energy expenditure and minimal shift in the COG from its protected, balanced position anterior to the second sacral vertebrae as it moves forward to its intended destination.[11] The greater the number of contact points in the locomotor apparatus the simpler the effort. In the case of a wheel the number of contact points is infinite; however, in humans there are only two.[11]

Gait is virtually impossible to measure through observational gait analysis (OGA), and although it is an unreliable indicator of the body in motion, significant deviations from the norm should be relatively easy to discern even to the untrained clinician. The correlation of the biomechanical examination findings as well as knowledge of musculoskeletal constraints is critical in the evaluation of gait observations. When observing gait begin by obtaining a gross review of the organism in motion, that will provide a sense of flow to the action taking place. Begin from the foot upward and compare each segment with normal and with the contralateral side, paying particular attention to lower extremity articulations.[12] Note head tilt; shoulder, spinal, or pelvic deviations; arm swing; or limp. The eyes should be level to the horizon and the mouth parallel to the eyes. Shoulders should be level. The knee should be straight ahead at heel contact without excessive adduction or abduction of the femur. There should be neutral to inverted calcaneus at heel contact without undue impact and normal sequencing of the gait cycle. The heel should not be seen to "bounce" up prematurely during propulsion, and all observations should be symmetrical and expected. The gait angle and base of gait should be within normal ranges and symmetrical. During swing phase, the foot should clear the ground efficiently without excessive activity of the extensor group (**Table 10-3**).

Table 10-3. Gait Influences

Advancing age
Vision disorders
Inactivity
Chronic disease
Frailty
Medications
Alcohol
Balance disturbances
Musculoskeletal disease
Foot discomfort
Foot dysfunction
Foot deformity
Footwear
Idiopathic gait disturbances

PATHOLOGIC GAIT OBSERVATIONS

During heel contact phase of the gait cycle, the heel should contact the ground before any other part of the foot. A toe–heel gait would be an indicator of anterior leg musculature weakness and/or posterior group contracture with or without spasm. This may be observed in any disorder resulting in an imbalance between dorsiflexors and plantarflexors with secondary paralysis or weakness of the common peroneal nerve with triceps surae contracture resulting in a drop-foot (pes equinus) deformity such as post cerebrovascular accident. There may or may not be an accompanying or prodromal forefoot slap or forefoot scuff early in the disease evolution. A steppage gait, where the entire foot contacts the ground at heel strike, is seen in lower motor neuron disease such as common peroneal or popliteal nerve disease. In common peroneal nerve pathology gait, there is an accompanying foot slap with the steppage gait, and in popliteal involvement it is a more flaccid, exaggerated steppage gait that is observed. Steppage gait is a prominent distinguishing feature seen in Charcot-Marie-Tooth disease (CMT). During the midstance phase of gait, an early heel lift off may be observed and may be due to equinus influences on the lower extremity especially affecting the triceps surae. This may be seen in congenital spasticity as observed in cerebral palsy (CP), congenital contracture of the gastrocnemius-soleus musculature or bony block at the ankle. A scissor, ataxic, or Trendelenburg gait is seen in upper motor neuron (UMN) disease disorders such as CP. Propulsive phase of gait disorders may be due to cerebellar pathology, lower motor neuron lesion such as diabetic neuropathy, or an antalgic gait due to increased forefoot pressure due to hallux valgus or hammertoe deformities. A calcaneus gait due to gastroc/soleus paralysis may be seen in lower motor neuron lesion diseases such as diabetes mellitus, Guillain-Barré, porphyria, and others. Patients with diabetic neuropathy exhibit reduced active propulsion due to a deficit of gastroc/soleus function.

Antalgic gait is a compensatory gait in which the gait alteration is an alteration in gait designed to relieve pain. It ceases when the pain is absent. This is frequently seen in musculoskeletal disorders affecting the lower extremity such as inflammatory of degenerative disease disorders affecting the spine, hip, knee, ankle, or foot. Disorders affecting posture or balance may result in either a cautious or reckless gait. Cautious gait is caused by an overresponsiveness to gait instability and features slower shorter steps with increased double support. Patients walk with arms outstretched as if on ice and is linked to "fear of falling" syndrome or "fall phobia."[1] Reckless or careless gait is seen in individuals with poor assessment of their own falling risk. Ataxic gait from the Greek for "without order" is an example of reckless gait with wide base of support to neutralize medial to lateral instability commonly seen in CNS disorders.

NEUROSENSORY DISORDERS AFFECTING GAIT

Normal function of the foot and its ability to support a normal locomotor pattern is dependent on intact neural pathways. Neurosensory gait disorders include myopathy, neuromuscular junction disease, and upper or lower motor neuron lesions. Myopathic gait disorders are caused by impairment of the conduction of muscle impulses such as seen in Duchenne muscular dystrophy or alcoholic myopathy. The gait is described as dystrophic or atrophic with exaggerated lateral trunk movements resulting in a penguin- or duck-like gait. Commonly observed gait deviations include Trendelenburg, toe-walking, hyperlumbar lordosis, knee instability, recurvatum, and balance disorders.[13] Gowers sign, named by the renowned British neurologist Sir William Richard Gowers in the late 19th century, is an inability to stand from a kneeling position due to lower limb muscular weakness. The patient is forced to "walk" over his own body to achieve the upright position. Although classically a classic sign of Duchenne muscular dystrophy, it is also seen in centronuclear myopathy and myotonic dystrophy. Individuals with myopathic disease require arm assistance to rise from a chair.

Myasthenia gravis is an example of a neuromuscular junction disease in which the gait is labored as a result of their ability to easily fatigue. There is difficulty maintaining the upright posture as well as in climbing stairs. The accompanying double vision disorder magnifies these deficits.

UMN GAIT DISTURBANCES

UMN lesion pathology is associated with muscle paresis, overactivity-spasticity, and stiffness. CPGs may be intact in these individuals; however, due to dysfunctional spinal reflexes and supraspinal inputs motor control and gait patterns are pathologically affected.[7] UMN-induced gait disturbances are seen in cerebellar dysfunction secondary to tumor, abscess, cardiovascular accident, CP, multiple sclerosis (MS), or Parkinson disease (PD). There is axial instability with few focal neurologic signs. A wide base, slow and small steps, shuffling, unsteadiness, and lurching toward the affected side (vestibular ataxia) characterize the typical ataxic gait seen in these conditions. The patient has difficulty turning with severe truncal instability. At times, the individual may appear "frozen" with an inability to initiate a step. Sensory ataxia is due to proprioceptive sensory deficits and is exemplified by a staggering gait, which may include stomping, slapping, or heavy heel strike to increase sensory feedback as an aide to ambulation.[7] Patients with sensory ataxia exhibit a positive Romberg sign. UMN lesion patients may be unable to accomplish unsupported stance.

Cerebellar ataxia is caused by cerebellar dysfunction involved in limb movement and dynamic balance control. Cerebellar gait has been described as a "drunken" gait that is unstable, veering, and irregular. Studies have demonstrated that the main feature of ataxic gait is increased intrasubject performance variability.[14,15] Tandem walking, the act of placing one foot directly in front of the other while walking, is a sensitive clinical test for cerebellar dysfunction.[16]

Cerebrovascular Accident

In an average year, 0.2% of the population will suffer a stroke.[13] It is the most common neurologic deficit and leading cause of gait impairment in rehabilitation facilities.[13] Stroke results in a hemiparetic gait with marked asymmetry and increased stance time on the unaffected limb, decreased stance and decreased swing on the affected side, and increased double support time,[7] all in essence increasing stability by decreasing demands placed on the affected limb. Speed of ambulation in stroke patients is also negatively affected.[17] This has been shown to be due to weak ankle plantarflexors, hip flexors, and knee extensors.[18] Arm swing may be absent or diminished on the affected side. Initially, the arm may be flaccid or held in adduction and flexion.[7] The affected limb is held stiff-legged in extension, internal rotation, and equinovarus of the foot and ankle. This creates difficulty in achieving forefoot clearance during swing phase with compensatory adjustments including hip elevation, increased trunk sway, circumduction, and occasionally contralateral vaulting.[7] Swing phase initiation is difficult, delayed, and prolonged. Electromyogram (EMG) studies have revealed prolonged tibialis anterior function in an attempt to dorsiflex the forefoot to clear the ground.[19]

In patients with transient brain ischemia (TBI), the zone of neurologic insult is not as well circumscribed. Therefore, the range of neurologic deficits is wider. TBI patients generate increased step length and normal stance time on affected limb compared with stroke patients in spite of increased stance time on the unaffected extremity.[7]

Parkinson Disease

PD is a progressive asymmetrical disorder caused by a basal ganglia dopamine deficiency and is responsible for 10% of gait disturbances in adults.[20] Due to neurotransmitter imbalances, PD patients progressively lose flexibility and adaptability in locomotor responses and walk with a stereotypical shortened-step, narrow-base, shuffling gait. The ability to respond to gait challenges including cognitive demands made during ambulation and gait perturbations are significantly compromised in the PD patient.[21]

Although initially asymmetrical, the contralateral limb eventually becomes affected in 80% of cases though not as severely as the side of inception.[20] Approximately 1% of those over 50 years of age have PD.[13] In a community dwelling, 15% of those 65 to 74 years of age exhibit gait abnormality and one or more signs of PD. This number rises to 30% for the 75-to-84-year group and 50% in those over 85 years of age.[22] There has been reported a 35% incidence in gait disorders in community dwellers over 70 years of age.[23]

Like other UMN disease disorders, parkinsonian gait is ataxic in nature with distinctly different and distinguishing "hallmark of the disease" characteristics. These include pill rolling, tremor, festination, rigidity, postural instability, and an overall slowness of gait known as hypo- or bradykinesia (Table 10-4). In some severe cases, there may be akinesia or complete loss of mobility. Unlike pyramidal disorders, strength is preserved with the lower extremity that is rigid in nature. Festination is the inability of the parkinsonian patient to slow down once gait has been initiated. This is due to muscular hypertonicity manifested by ankle and knee stiffness along with pelvis and trunk flexion.[24]

Asymmetric arm swing and accompanying tremor as well as staggering and en-bloc turning are suggestive of early PD.[25] As the disease progresses, there is pronounced tendency to drag the ipsilateral leg and decreased foot clearance and reduced step length may be more clearly evident.[25] Patients with PD typically increase cadence in an attempt to compensate for the shorter step length and reduced velocity.[1] In addition to the above-mentioned deficits, it is significant to note that balance control is asymmetrical in about 75% of patients with PD.[20]

Parkinsonian gait is characterized by a foot flat strike placing the entire foot on the ground at the same time.[26] In advanced stages, a toe–heel gait may be observed. Patients have reduced foot lift during swing phase of gait with resultant reduced toe clearance between the foot and the ground.[27] There is reduced impact at heel strike in parkinsonian patients with additional decreases as the disease progresses.[28] The load on the forefoot is increased with a tendency toward medial displacement. The interpatient gait variability in foot strike pattern is less than in the normal population.[28] The vertical ground reaction force (GRF) has two peaks in the normal individual: one at heel contact and one at propulsion. In

Table 10-4. Parkinsonian Gait Characteristics

Increase muscle tone and tremor
Stiff arms held closely to body
Absent arm swing
Impaired postural reflexes
Stiffly stooped
Arms close to sides
Reduced stride length
Increased double limb support
Increased cadence
Slow, shuffling steps
Difficult to initiate steps or turns ("freezing")
Cog wheel rigidity
Pill rolling
Festination

early stages of PD, there are reduced forces in the heel and forefoot resembling those seen in the geriatric population.[29,30] As the disease progresses with a shuffling type gait, only one narrow peak in the vertical GRF is shown.

Freezing of gait is a disabling, episodic affectation in which the feet appear to be "glued to the floor." Falls and freezing of gait have been linked together since freezing in many instances may lead to falls. Both are more common in the latter stages of the disease process.[31] Freezing of gait is a common and disabling feature of PD and is most commonly experienced during gait initiation, turning, and negotiating obstacles of other tasks.[32] The pathophysiology of freezing of gait has been linked to asymmetries in leg coordination.[33,34] Falls may result from attempting sudden movements or changes in postural positions. The risk of falls is increased in the PD patient who attempts to perform more than one activity at a time such as carrying a shopping bag while ambulating. Most of these falls are forward (45%) and 20% laterally.[31]

Postural sway is the ability to maintain balance during upright stance and locomotion. Postural sway characteristically increases in most UMN lesion disorders, creating balance disorders. However, in PD it is diminished. This fact, coupled with an inability to maintain the center of mass over the base of support, increases the risk of falls in the parkinsonian patient.[21] EMG studies have demonstrated a significant reduction in tibialis anticus muscle activation in early stance and early and late swing phases of gait and a reduction in triceps surae action at propulsion.[35] The hamstrings and quadriceps show prolonged activation during stance.[35] The passive stiffness of ankle joints and co-contraction of leg muscles in stance result in abnormal postural sway in PD patients.[36]

Subcortical arteriosclerotic encephalopathy (SAE) also referred to as lower-body parkinsonism and cerebral ataxia are gait disorders that resemble that of PD but have common underlying mechanisms different from that of parkinsonism.[37]

Cerebral Palsy

CP is an idiopathic perinatal disorder with an incidence of 2 per 1,000 live births.[13] The underlying neurologic pathology is nonprogressive; however, the secondary effects including muscular contractures and abnormal bone growth continue and cause deterioration in function. Spasticity occurs in 80% of CP patients. Only 20% are quadriplegic, 30% hemiplegic, and 50% diplegic.[38] Seventy percent of those with CP are able to walk. The fundamental problems in this disorder include weakness, spasticity, and loss of selective motor control with retention of primitive reflexes and postural reactions. These neurologic deficiencies result in equinus function with knee and hip contractures, premature heel off, foot drop, and excessive limb flexion during swing. Foot deformities include hammer, claw, and mallet toe deformities; hallux flexus; equinus; varus; valgus; planovalgus; and the most commonly occurring equinovarus.[38] In weaker patients, excessive pronation, crouch gait with knee and hip flexion, and toe drag are observed. The crouch gait position deleteriously affects

loading patterns of the knee and surrounding structures, leading to a load that is two and one half times greater than that of the normal pain-free individual.[39]

Multiple Sclerosis

MS is a bilateral UMN autoimmune disease seen in young adults from 20 to 40 years of age that causes progressive neurodegeneration with subsequent ataxic, paraparetic, spastic, stiff-legged gait, which may or may not be symmetrical.[7] Gait changes seen in MS is dependent on areas of injury involved and neurologic function. Gait changes seen in spinal cord injury are similar to those seen in MS depending on the injury level, residual neurologic function, muscle weakness, spasticity, and secondary instability due to impaired coordination and sensory deficits.[7] A scissoring gait may be observed due to increased activity of the hip adductors.[7] Excessive hip adduction interferes with swing phase limb advancement, decreased base of support, decreased postural stability, and resultant increased risk for falls. MS patients have decreased muscle strength, proprioception and balance all of which further negatively impact gait. Symptoms vary with the disease severity and include sensory disturbances, limb weakness, awkward gait, and cognitive deficits.[40,41]

Patients with MS walk more slowly, take shorter steps, and exhibit a broader base of gait.[41] Gait abnormalities include decreased stride length, increased double support, and reduced joint torque and power. Variability of step length and step time is directly correlated with disease severity.[41] Individuals who use gait assistive devices had significantly greater step length variability than did MS patients who were able to walk independently.[41]

Peak ankle plantarflexory torque is significantly reduced in late stance as revealed by lowered ankle power generation for propulsion. This results in an inability to support forward progression of the trunk and to initiate the swing phase of gait.[42] MS patients that are able to walk faster are able to overcome this deficit by increasing the angular velocity of the segment resulting in increased ankle power during late stance.[40] MS patients are unable to adapt other compensatory strategies to overcome reduced power at one joint by increasing power at another.[40] As a result of the numerous gait disturbances associated with the disease, MS patients exhibit a significant degree of fatigue over the course of the day.[43]

LOWER MOTOR NEURON GAIT DISTURBANCES

Lower motor lesion gait disturbances may be linked to systemic disorders such as diabetes, amyotrophic lateral sclerosis (ALS), CMT, or Guillain-Barré syndrome or may be due to spinal disc or peripheral nerve compression (Table 10-5). Gait abnormalities are dependent on the level of involvement. For example, with common peroneal nerve compression or disease, there is a steppage gait with foot slap and difficulty climbing stairs. With sciatic nerve pathology, the limb may

Table 10-5. Etiology of Lower Motor Lesion Gait Disorders

Diabetes mellitus
Alcoholism
Vitamin B$_{12}$ deficiency
Malignancy
Medications
Collagen vascular disease
Guillain-Barré syndrome
Porphyria

be functionless with guarding and dragging of the extremity forward. Popliteal nerve involvement produces a more flaccid, exaggerated steppage gait and gastroc/soleus paralysis produces a calcaneus gait. A Trendelenburg gait is seen with gluteal paralysis.

Diabetic Neuropathy

Diabetic peripheral neuropathy is one of the most severe complications of diabetes, occurring in 30% to as high as 70% of all diabetic patients.[44–48] Diabetic neuropathy impairs the somatosensory and motor systems thereby affecting the quality and quantity of sensory information that is essential for the complexities involved in gait generation and control. Patients with diabetes frequently exhibit a conservative gait strategy, which includes slower speeds, decreased ankle range of motion, wider base of gait, decreased step and stride length, increased double limb support, differences in kinetic patterns with modified ground reactive forces and joint moments of force, as well as delayed activation.[49,50] Changes in gait parameters that appear to be specific to diabetes include shorter stride length, reduced speed, and altered lower limb and trunk mobility.[51] Diabetic neuropathy patients exhibit a significantly longer stance phase of gait and stride time.[47,51] There is an increase in cadence and swing phase with increased susceptibility to joint kinematic changes.[49]

Patients with diabetic neuropathy walk slower and more cautiously than healthy individuals and employ different knee and ankle adjustments with increasing speeds. Increasing cadence leads to loss of gait cycle stability due to a diminution of motor skills adaptive responsive mechanisms. Diabetes reduces the ability to accomplish shock absorption during gait.[51] At heel contact in the diabetic patient, the lack of sensory afferent input leads to delayed activation of ankle and knee musculature.[52] Muscle atrophy and weakness combined with fat pad degeneration and increased stiffness affect shock absorption.[53] The premature plantarflexion at heel contact observed in diabetic neuropathy patients results in increased foot flat phase and increased forefoot loading predisposing to ulcer production. Studies have demonstrated moderately higher plantar pressures in diabetic peripheral

neuropathy patients at the rearfoot, midfoot, and forefoot compared with controls.[47] This is probably due to increased time spent in the stance phase of gait and not solely due to increased ground reactive forces.[47]

Increased dermal thickness and inelasticity coupled with fat pad atrophy affect braking force at heel contact.[54–56] These changes affect the ability of the first rocker mechanism in the foot from functioning properly.[50] Lack of sensory afferent input with muscle weakness and limited joint mobility affect single limb support and gait instability.[50,57] There is a delayed peak activation of the gastroc/soleus group during stance phase of gait thereby extending midstance and delaying active propulsion. The tibialis anticus is also delayed in stance, affecting forthcoming swing and toe clearance and thereby compromising the entire gait cycle.[49] Limited joint mobility affects the second rocker mechanism necessary for normal gait. The third rocker mechanism is negatively affected because of an inability to generate adequate ankle plantarflexory torque necessary for propulsion. As a result, hip flexors may be used instead of ankle plantarflexors to assist in propulsion. Abnormal ankle mechanics further add to abnormal hip mechanics. A wider base of gait combined with skin and fat pad degeneration affect medial–lateral shear and pushing force.[57]

Looser extremity stiffness associated with diabetes negatively affects the swing phase of gait. Lack of afferent sensory input, muscle weakness and diminished joint mobility increases gait instability and impacts single limb support.[50,57]

Diabetes produces physiologic changes in the organism that in turn result in decreased lower extremity function. Additional comorbidities associated with elevated blood glucose levels, such as cardiovascular disease, may also contribute to, and magnify, disturbed lower extremity function.[45] The existence of a preexisting pathologic foot type in the diabetic patient determines the biomechanical behavior and functionality of the foot and has been shown to be clinically relevant.[51,58] It is this intrinsic deficiency in structure or alignment that is the primary underlying cause of hyperkeratoses and subsequent plantar ulceration in the diabetic especially one with neuropathy, which negatively alters the individual's response to effectively manage elevated plantar pressure.[58–61]

Charcot-Marie-Tooth Disease

CMT, also known as peroneal muscle atrophy, refers to a group of inherited autosomal dominant, and in some cases recessive, disorders resulting in symmetrical, progressive peripheral neuropathy, which typically begins in the feet. There is progressive loss of motor function with resultant weakness, muscle atrophy, and limb deformities secondary to muscle imbalance. These include a "hallmark of the disease" cavovarus foot type and claw toes with plantarflexed first ray and compensatory forefoot valgus. This is caused by peroneal weakness especially in the brevis segment along with weak tibialis anterior and sparing of the tibialis posterior.[39] The peroneal muscle atrophy evidenced in the lower segments of the legs gives rise to the "stork leg" or "inverted champagne bottle" appearance. The cavovarus foot type predisposes the patient to increased plantar pressures on the calcaneus, first, and fifth metatarsal heads. There is a sequential progression of weakness and atrophy beginning with the peroneus brevis, toe extensors, and tibialis anticus and ending with the intrinsic musculature.[39] As a result, there is clawing of the digits throughout swing phase due to extensor musculature substitution for a weakened tibialis anticus. This may result in foot slap or if more severe foot drop. During stance phase due to gastroc/soleus weakness, the ankle may buckle forward with anterior tibial migration on the talus. In more severe cases, a "crouch" gait may be observed.[39] As the disease progresses, there may be a progressive inability to ambulate from weakness, balance, and/or associated deformities.

Amyotrophic Lateral Sclerosis

ALS also referred to as Lou Gehrig disease named after the famed Yankee first baseman whose career was ended due to this debilitating progressive neurodegenerative disorder. ALS affects CNS motor neurons that directly or indirectly control muscular contractions during ambulation.[62–64] Neurologic dysfunction is caused by deterioration of motor neurons or their myelin sheath disrupting normal pathways of transmission to target muscle fibers.[62,63] The motor neurons are replaced by fibrous astrocytes causing muscle tissue atrophy, weakness, and ultimately paralysis.[62] Due to this interruption of cerebellum-to-muscle pathway, the lower limbs cannot properly perform voluntary movements thereby pathologically impacting gait. This results in slower walking speeds in ALS patients with an increased variability in gait rhythm time series compared with healthy individuals.[65] In fact gait variability patterns in ALS is more pronounced than in PD and Huntington disease.[66]

Onset of ALS is subtle so that early detection of the disease is uncommon. The patient may experience awkwardness in gait caused by difficulty in symmetrical use of the limbs thereby altering stride and swing phase intervals.[67] Stride time is longer and the magnitude of stride-to-stride variability is increased.[66,68] Stride time is defined as the time between initial contact of one foot to the successive contact of that same foot.[69] Gait asymmetry is a prominent feature in all ALS patients.

METABOLIC DISORDERS AFFECTING GAIT

Endocrine disorders affecting gait include hypothyroidosis and vitamin B_{12} deficiency. Medications, notably CNS depressant, antianxiety, antihypertensive, hypnotics, and so forth, will unfavorably affect gait, decreasing ability to balance and to resist gait perturbations. Psychological issues affecting gait include psychogenic gait, fear of falling, and gait associated with senile dementia.

Senile Dementia

Deterioration in spatial cognitive abilities with advancing age is compounded by disorders such as senile dementia present in at least 9% of older persons. Even mild forms may restrict travel in familiar environments in spite of an otherwise healthy locomotor system. In the older individual, lower extremity function involves intention and integration of higher cortical sensory information. Impairment in cognition impairs gait and these same gait impairments may be able to predict future decline and dementia.[70] Therefore, identification of the underlying disease process accompanying the gait abnormality may allow earlier treatment to be instituted. Alzheimer disease is the most common type of dementia with concomitant loss of independent and safe mobility due to balance and gait dysfunction. Even those in the early stages of the disease have been shown to have gait and balance deficits including decreased speed, shorten step length, and increased time in double support.[71] Recovery from a gait perturbation or the ability to complete simple cognitive tasks while walking is difficult for the early Alzheimer disease patient thereby negatively affecting gait.[72] This is accomplished by slower speeds, decreased step and stride lengths, decreased cadence, and increased double support.[73] In fact, Eggermont et al.[70] in their study suggest that walking speed could be evaluated as a predictor of gait impairment and falls in older individuals. Gait instability increases the risk of falls in the Alzheimer disease patient.[71,72] Advancing age further magnifies the effects of Alzheimer disease on gait by adversely affecting spatial knowledge required for traveling to goals not visible from the start.

Cardiovascular Disorders Affecting Gait

An intact cardiovascular system provides the hemodynamic requisites necessary to maintain an upright posture without collapsing. Peripheral arterial disease (PAD) especially when accompanied by intermittent claudication may severely restrict at individual's ability to walk longer distances. In addition, calf pain secondary to the diminished blood supply associated with PAD may result in an antalgic gait with diminished propulsive activity due to increased demands placed on this muscle. The individual walks more slowly and less propulsively to reduce muscle oxygen requirements, thereby lessening the likelihood of cramping and the ability to walk longer distances. Orthostatic hypotension, a precipitous drop in pressure upon standing, disrupts gait stability by affecting one's ability to balance well. Vertebrobasilar insufficiency may result in the same set of circumstances. Chronic edema may affect gait by limiting ankle joint motion thereby increasing dorsiflexory demands, extending the midstance phase of gait and reducing propulsion.

Musculoskeletal Disease and Gait

Arthritis affects approximately one in six individuals and is the leading cause of disability in the United States. Any condition affecting the musculoskeletal or neuromotor systems negatively affects gait. It has been estimated that 75% of individuals over 65 years of age have some arthritis of the weightbearing joints with the knee and hip being the most commonly affected[13] (Table 10-6).

The energy cost for locomotion increases in the elderly in the presence of cardiopulmonary and musculoskeletal system changes, reduced tissue tolerance, and the use of gait assistive devices. When systemic musculoskeletal disease is coupled with age-related degeneration, there is a compounded decrease in the maximum manageable stress with a resultant increased chance of failure. It is unlikely that age-related musculoskeletal system degenerative changes alone will immobilize the individual; however, they can and do influence the distance able to be traveled, the time it takes, and the types of terrain that can be traversed.

Musculoskeletal strength decreases with advancing age. By 60 years of age, there is a 25% to 30% loss, and after 70 years of age there is a 30% additional loss of strength per decade.[74] Walking does not require full strength; in fact, the gastroc/soleus requires the greatest strength for propulsion but other muscles may substitute. Cardiopulmonary deterioration negatively affects muscle function. Tendon and ligament changes as a result of musculoskeletal disease and/or compounded by the aging process results in joint stiffness with accompanying decrease in range of motion thereby negatively altering gait. These changes limit the ability of otherwise intact muscles to generate power at various speeds and over varying terrains. Changes in musculoskeletal mass distribution with advancing age present a challenge to balance control systems and increase load on the posterior musculature. These individuals have limited ability to sustain locomotion for extended periods of time.

Table 10-6. Musculoskeletal Disorders Affecting Gait

Osteoarthritis
Rheumatoid arthritis
Psoriatic arthritis
Ankylosing spondylitis
Polyarteritis nodosum
Polymyositis rheumatica
Muscular dystrophy
Systemic lupus erythematosis
Rheumatic fever
Paget disease
Lyme disease
Gout
Reiter syndrome

Rheumatoid Arthritis

Rheumatoid arthritis (RA) affects the feet in 20% of cases at the time of diagnosis, which progresses to 80% with a disease duration of 5 years.[75] The disease leads to functional disability and pathologic gait alterations that substantially and negatively impact the quality of life.[76] Foot pain may have the strongest influence on functional ability regardless of the disease duration.[77] The forefoot is affected in 90% to 97% of patients and the midfoot and ankle in 50%.[78,79] Typical forefoot deformities include severe hallux abducto valgus, hammer and claw toe deformities, subluxated metatarsal and phalangeal articulations with anterior displacement, and atrophy of the plantar fat pad. Forefoot deformity is associated with reduced toe contact, increased forefoot pressures, and delayed heel lift.[80] RA patients demonstrate higher plantar pressures, and this is especially true in the forefoot region.[81] This fact has been linked to increase joint destruction in these regions thereby creating an additional negative gait impact.[79,82] Forefoot pressure increases with disease in duration.[80] Rear and midfoot deformities include classic pesvalgoplanus, with or without peroneal spasm.[77] Navicular height was normal in RA patients with forefoot deformities but was markedly reduced in those with rearfoot and forefoot deformities.[77] A 50% reduction in hallux dorsiflexion was observed during terminal stance in all RA patient groups studied.[77] This finding is consistent with hallux abducto valgus (HAV) production and attendant joint damage.[77] Studies indicate a complete breakdown of sagittal rocker function and windlass mechanism necessary for load acceptance and stability through midstance and propulsion.[77]

Pathomechanical stresses through the genicular region are dependent on mechanical alignment not solely due to the disease process itself. Valgus deformity of the knee is often seen in RA patients and is frequently the result of RA in the hip thereby increasing pathologic medial genicular stresses and influencing lateral tibial subluxation thereby negatively affecting gait. Accompanying this process are increased pathologic forces on the medial segment of the foot, increasing pronation, valgus position of the rearfoot, and eventual subluxation.[83]

It is no surprise that RA patients tend to walk slower with a longer gait cycle, shorter step length, longer double support, stance phase, time, and lower cadence when compared with normal subjects.[75,84] The classic pattern of morning stiffness with its attendant pathologic gait manifestations improves during the day and has been linked to circadian variation in pro-inflammatory cytokines.[85–87]

Absolute walking speed correlates directly with disease activity and characteristics.[77,80,88] Lowered walking speed results in significantly reduced ankle plantarflexion, medial arch flattening, hallux dorsiflexion, and hallux abduction at propulsion.[87,89] Although it has been reported that temporal and spatial characteristics in RA similarly correlate with the disease process, this has been demonstrated to be more linked to accumulated damage over the course of the disease rather than to current disease activity.[88,90] The RA patient has smaller ranges of motion and reduced joint moments and work across the large joints of the lower limbs during walking than in normal individuals.[91] There is reduced joint moments and power of hip/flexion/extension, hip adduction/abduction, knee flexion/extension, and ankle plantarflexion.[75] In fact, the most evident difference between RA patients and normal individuals is the reduced positive work at the ankle, which may be due to decreased plantarflexor moments during preswing. This may be attributed to decreased speed and decreased plantarflexor power.[91] RA subjects tend to walk with a Trendelenburg gait.[91] There is increased internal tibial rotation, delayed heel rise, decreased plantarflexion at toe off, and marked eversion of the rearfoot all contributing to a loss of normal rocker function of the foot.[75] Loss of functional balance accompanies these changes and imposes another obstacle for the RA patient to contend with during ambulation.[91] It is the rearfoot pathomechanics with resultant marked calcaneal eversion that affects gait more severely in RA than in those individuals with severe forefoot deformity alone.[91] Chronic pain is one of the main causes of disability and loss of function.[91] Gait in RA is determined by avoiding pain. Therefore, these patients walk slower to control the speed and forces associated with heel strike and toe off.[75]

Osteoarthritis

Osteoarthritis (degenerative joint disease) of the lower extremity is the most common cause of gait disorders in older individuals. It affects over 60% of those over 65 years of age, and as a result over 50% become disabled. When degenerative joint disease affects the foot or ankle as it frequently does in the elderly, an antalgic gait ensue.[92] This is a result of compensatory gait changes in an attempt to relieve pain and continue to allow forward movement of the body over the supporting limb. The difficulty pain and difficulty in ambulation are most noticeable poststatically especially upon arising. Gait characteristics include decreased velocity and stride length in an attempt to lessen pathologic pressures. Patients experience difficulty and exacerbation of symptomatology when ambulating on uneven surfaces or climbing or descending stairs. Reduced ranges of foot, ankle, and knee articulations occur in an attempt to limit motion and lessen pressures, which lead to secondary soft tissue contractures, including equinus function.[93]

Musculoskeletal gait disorders may be caused postsurgically as following knee or hip replacement. Gait may be affected following prolonged periods of immobility because it occurs after lower extremity fracture care, illness, or surgical intervention. Musculoskeletal dysfunction caused by disuse or disability results in compensatory small modifications of the locomotor pattern until the most efficient pattern for the individual is obtained. Foot discomfort, deformity, or dysfunction as a result of lower extremity systemic disease especially musculoskeletal will negatively influence gait patterns.

Idiopathic Geriatric Gait

A lifetime of weightbearing inevitably takes its toll on the feet even in the absence of systemic disease. Changes may be due to gradual relaxation of ligaments contributing to longitudinal and transverse metatarsal arch collapse, anterior fat pad displacement and atrophy with secondary increased metatarsal head pressure, progressive contractures and stiffness, increased talonavicular lowering, and increased talocalcaneal angle, increasing early degenerative changes. Idiopathic geriatric gait account for 16% of gait disorders and may manifest itself as early as 60 years of age. It is also referred to as essential gait disorder of the elderly, senile gait, marche à petit pas, or the elderly shuffle. It is a guarded gait whose diagnosis may be made by excluding the presence of systemic disease as its etiology. Gait characteristics are commensurate with decreased strength and diminished ability to process sensory information (**Table 10-7**). Vision disorders further exaggerate these findings. Vision plays a primary role in initial adjustment for changes in surface shape or slope. Over 65% of the population is affected with macular degeneration, which causes a loss of center field vision, which affects environmental input information thereby negatively affecting gait. The incidence rises rapidly in older individuals affecting 10% of those in the 70-to-74-year-old age range,

Table 10-7. Idiopathic Geriatric Gait Characteristics
Decreased
Active propulsion and propulsive power
Ankle extension
Vertical center of pressure excursions
Amplitude of sagittal plane rotations
Ability to re-center
Ability to solve movement problems
Velocity
Step and stride length
Cadence
Pelvic rotation
Swing phase
Limb excursions
Joint range of motion
Increased
Double limb support
Stance
Midstance
Horizontal head excursion
Base of gait
COP movement

14% in the 75-to-79-year-old category, and almost 24% are affected with macular degeneration over 80 years of age.[94]

SUMMARY

Abnormalities in gait may be a manifestation of systemic disease or part of idiopathic gait changes associated with the aging process. Observation of gait abnormalities by the astute clinician may enable early diagnosis of its associated underlying disorder in turn allowing more appropriate, effective, and immediate management to be instituted.

ACKNOWLEDGMENTS

I would like to thank Loretta Cacace DPM, MPH for her excellent assistance in the preparation of this manuscript for publication while a 4th-year student at the New York College of Podiatric Medicine.

REFERENCES

1. Fasano A, Bloem BR. Gait disorders. *Continuum (Minneap Minn)*. 2013;19(5):1344–1382.
2. D'Amico J. Developmental flatfoot. In: Thompson P, Volpe R, eds. *Podopediatrics*. Edinburgh, UK: Churchill Livingstone; 2001:257–273.
3. Studenski S, Perera S, Patel K, et al. Gait speed and survival in older adults. *JAMA*. 2011;305(1):50–58.
4. Williams PT, Thompson PD. The relationship of walking intensity to total and cause-specific mortality. results from the national walkers' health study. *PLoS One*. 2013;8(11):e81098.
5. Wrobel JS, Najafi B. Diabetic foot biomechanics and gait dysfunction. *J Diabetes Sci Technol*. 2010;4(4):833–845.
6. Bohannon RW, Williams Andrews A. Normal walking speed: A descriptive meta-analysis. *Physiotherapy*. 2011;97(3):182–189.
7. Vachranukunkiet T, Esquenazi A. Pathophysiology of gait disturbance in neurologic disorders and clinical presentations. *Phys Med Rehabil Clin N Am*. 2013;24(2):233–246.
8. Dietz V, Duysens J. Significance of load receptor input during locomotion: A review. *Gait Posture*. 2000;11(2):102–110.
9. Salzman B. Gait and balance disorders in older adults. *Am Fam Physician*. 2010;82(1):61–68.
10. Spielberg PI. Walking patterns of old people: psychographic analysis. In: Bernstein NA, ed. *Investigation on the Biodynamics of Walking, Running and Jumping: Part 2*. Moscow, Russia: Central Scientific; 1940:72–76.
11. Napier JR. The evolution of bipedal walking in the hominids. *Arch Biol (Liege)*. 1964;75:673–708.
12. Perry J, ed. *Observational Gait Analysis*. Downey, CA: Los Amigos Research and Education Institute; 2001.
13. Kirtley C. *Clinical Gait Analysis: Theory and Practice*. Amsterdam, Netherlands: Elsevier Health Sciences; 2006.
14. Ilg W, Golla H, Thier P, et al. Specific influences of cerebellar dysfunctions on gait. *Brain*. 2007;130(Pt 3):786–798.
15. Morton SM, Bastian AJ. Cerebellar control of balance and locomotion. *Neuroscientist*. 2004;10(3):247–259.
16. Stolze H, Klebe S, Petersen G, et al. Typical features of cerebellar ataxic gait. *J Neurol Neurosurg Psychiatry*. 2002;73(3):310–312.
17. Hsu AL, Tang PF, Jan MH. Analysis of impairments influencing gait velocity and asymmetry of hemiplegic patients after mild to moderate stroke. *Arch Phys Med Rehabil*. 2003;84(8):1185–1193.
18. Jenkers I, Delp S, Patten C. Capacity to increase walking speed is limited by impaired hip and ankle power generation in lower functioning persons post-stroke. *Gait Posture*. 2009;29(1):129–137.
19. Den Otter AR, Geurts AC, Mulder T, et al. Abnormalities in the temporal patterning of lower extremity muscle activity in hemiparetic gait. *Gait Posture*. 2007;25(3):342–352.
20. Boonstra TA, van Vugt JP, van der Kooij H, et al. Balance asymmetry in Parkinson's disease and its contribution to freezing of gait. *PLoS One*. 2014;9(7):e102493.
21. Morris M, Iansek R, Smithson F, et al. Postural instability in Parkinson's disease: a comparison with and without a concurrent task. *Gait Posture*. 2000;12(3):205–216.
22. Bennett DA, Beckett LA, Murray AM, et al. Prevalence of parkinsonian signs and associated mortality in a community population of older people. *N Engl J Med*. 1996;334(2):71–76.
23. Verghese J, LeValley A, Hall CB, et al. Epidemiology of gait disorders in community-residing older adults. *J Am Geriatr Soc*. 2006;54(2):255–261.
24. Saint S, Wiese J, Bent S. *Clinical Clerkships: The Answer Book*. New York, NY: Lippincott Williams & Wilkins; 2006.
25. Lee SM, Kim M, Lee HM, et al. Differential diagnosis of parkinsonism with visual inspection of posture and gait in the early stage. *Gait Posture*. 2014;39(4):1138–1141.
26. Hughes JR, Bowes SG, Leeman AL, et al. Parkinsonian abnormality of foot strike: a phenomenon of ageing and/or one responsive to levodopa therapy? *Br J Clin Pharmacol*. 1990;29(2):179–186.
27. Murray MP, Sepic SB, Gardner GM, et al. Walking patterns of men with parkinsonism. *Am J Phys Med*. 1978;57(6):278–294.
28. Kimmeskamp S, Hennig EM. Heel to toe motion characteristics in Parkinson patients during free walking. *Clin Biomech (Bristol, Avon)*. 2001;16(9):806–812.
29. Koozekanani SH, Balmaseda MT Jr, Fatehi MT, et al. Ground reaction forces during ambulation in Parkinsonism: pilot study. *Arch Phys Med Rehabil*. 1987;68(1):28–30.
30. Ueno E, Yanagisawa N, Takami M. Gait disorders in Parkinsonism. A study with floor reaction forces and EMG. *Adv Neurol*. 1993;60:414–418.
31. Bloem BR, Hausdorff JM, Visser JE, et al. Falls and freezing of gait in Parkinson's disease: a review of two interconnected, episodic phenomena. *Mov Disord*. 2004;19(8):871–884.
32. Giladi N, Nieuwboer A. Understanding and treating freezing of gait in parkinsonism, proposed working definition, and setting the stage. *Mov Disord*. 2008;23(suppl 2):S423–S425.
33. Plotnik M, Giladi N, Balash Y, et al. Is freezing of gait in Parkinson's disease related to asymmetric motor function? *Ann Neurol*. 2005;57(5):656–663.
34. Plotnik M, Giladi N, Hausdorff JM. Bilateral coordination of walking and freezing of gait in Parkinson's disease. *Eur J Neurosci*. 2008;27(8):1999–2006.
35. Cioni M, Richards CL, Malouin F, et al. Characteristics of the electromyographic patterns of lower limb muscles during gait in patients with Parkinson's disease when OFF and ON L-dopa treatment. *Ital J Neurol Sci*. 1997;18(4):195–208.
36. Robertson LT, Horak FB, Anderson VC, et al. Assessments of axial motor control during deep brain stimulation in Parkinsonian patients. *Neurosurgery*. 2001;48(3):544–551; discussion 551–552.
37. Davis JT, Lyons KE, Pahwa R. Freezing of gait after bilateral subthalamic nucleus stimulation for Parkinson's disease. *Clin Neurol Neurosurg*. 2006;108(5):461–464.

Cerebral Palsy

38. Botte MJ, Frank O. Chapter 3: Neuromuscular disorders. In: Thoradsen D, ed. *Foot & Ankle (Orthopedic Surgery Essentials)*. Philadelphia, PA: Lippincott Williams & Wilkins; 2013:45–54.
39. Richards LD, Whittle MW, eds. *Whittle's Gait Analysis*. New York, NY: Churchill Livingston; 2012.
40. Huisinga JM, Schmid KK, Filipi ML, et al. Gait mechanics are different between healthy controls and patients with multiple sclerosis. *J Appl Biomech*. 2013;29(3):303–311.

41. Socie MJ, Motl RW, Pula JH, et al. Gait variability and disability in multiple sclerosis. *Gait Posture*. 2013;38(1):51–55.

42. Neptune RR, Kautz SA, Zajac FE. Contributions of the individual ankle plantar flexors to support, forward progression and swing initiation during walking. *J Biomech*. 2001;34(11):1387–1398.

43. Morris ME, Cantwell C, Vowels L, et al. Changes in gait and fatigue from morning to afternoon in people with multiple sclerosis. *J Neurol Neurosurg Psychiatry*. 2002;72(3):361–365.

44. Candrilli SD, Davis KL, Kan HJ, et al. Prevalence and the associated burden of illness of symptoms of diabetic peripheral neuropathy and diabetic retinopathy. *J Diabetes Complications*. 2007; 21(5):306–314.

45. Chiles NS, Phillips CL, Volpato S, et al. Diabetes, peripheral neuropathy, and lower-extremity function. *J Diabetes Complications*. 2014;28(1):91–95.

46. Deshpande AD, Harris-Hayes M, Schootman M. Epidemiology of diabetes and diabetes-related complications. *Phys Ther*. 2008;88(11):1254–1264.

47. Fernando M, Crowther R, Lazzarini P, et al. Biomechanical characteristics of peripheral diabetic neuropathy: a systematic review and meta-analysis of findings from the gait cycle, muscle activity and dynamic barefoot plantar pressure. *Clin Biomech (Bristol, Avon)*. 2013;28(8):831–845.

48. Gregg EW, Sorlie P, Paulose-Ram R, et al. Prevalence of lower-extremity disease in the US adult population >=40 years of age with and without diabetes: 1999–2000 national health and nutrition examination survey. *Diabetes Care*. 2004;27(7):1591–1597.

49. Gomes AA, Onodera AN, Otuzi ME, et al. Electromyography and kinematic changes of gait cycle at different cadences in diabetic neuropathic individuals. *Muscle Nerve*. 2011;44(2):258–268.

50. Wrobel JS, Najafi B. Diabetic foot biomechanics and gait dysfunction. *J Diabetes Sci Technol*. 2010;4(4):833–845.

51. Sawacha Z, Spolaor F, Guarneri G, et al. Abnormal muscle activation during gait in diabetes patients with and without neuropathy. *Gait Posture*. 2012;35(1):101–105.

52. Sacco IC, Amadio AC. Influence of the diabetic neuropathy on the behavior of electromyographic and sensorial responses in treadmill gait. *Clin Biomech (Bristol, Avon)*. 2003;18(5):426–434.

53. Bus SA, Maas M, Cavanagh PR, et al. Plantar fat-pad displacement in neuropathic diabetic patients with toe deformity: a magnetic resonance imaging study. *Diabetes Care*. 2004;27(10):2376–2381.

54. Cheung YY, Doyley M, Miller TB, et al. Magnetic resonance elastography of the plantar fat pads: preliminary study in diabetic patients and asymptomatic volunteers. *J Comput Assist Tomogr*. 2006;30(2):321–326.

55. Tajaddini A, Scoffone HM, Botek G, et al. Laser-induced autofluorescence (LIAF) as a method for assessing skin stiffness preceding diabetic ulcer formation. *J Biomech*. 2007;40(4):736–741.

56. Thomas VJ, Patil KM, Radhakrishnan S, et al. The role of skin hardness, thickness, and sensory loss on standing foot power in the development of plantar ulcers in patients with diabetes mellitus—a preliminary study. *Int J Low Extrem Wounds*. 2003;2(3):132–139.

57. Yavuzer G, Yetkin I, Toruner FB, et al. Gait deviations of patients with diabetes mellitus: looking beyond peripheral neuropathy. *Eura Medicophys*. 2006;42(2):127–133.

58. Guiotto A, Sawacha Z, Guarneri G, et al. The role of foot morphology on foot function in diabetic subjects with or without neuropathy. *Gait Posture*. 2013;37(4):603–610.

59. Cavanagh PR, Simoneau GG, Ulbrecht JS. Ulceration, unsteadiness, and uncertainty: the biomechanical consequences of diabetes mellitus. *J Biomech*. 1993;26(suppl 1):23–40.

60. Cowley MS, Boyko EJ, Shofer JB, et al. Foot ulcer risk and location in relation to prospective clinical assessment of foot shape and mobility among persons with diabetes. *Diabetes Res Clin Pract*. 2008;82(2):226–232.

61. Ledoux WR, Shofer JB, Smith DG, et al. Relationship between foot type, foot deformity, and ulcer occurrence in the high-risk diabetic foot. *J Rehabil Res Dev*. 2005;42(5):665–672.

62. Kiernan MC, Vucic S, Cheah BC, et al. Amyotrophic lateral sclerosis. *Lancet*. 2011;377(9769):942–955.

63. Sharma KR, Kent-Braun JA, Majumdar S, et al. Physiology of fatigue in amyotrophic lateral sclerosis. *Neurology*. 1995;45(4):733–740.

64. Wu Y, Shi L. Analysis of altered gait cycle duration in amyotrophic lateral sclerosis based on nonparametric probability density function estimation. *Med Eng Phys*. 2011;33(3):347–355.

65. Hausdorff JM, Lertratanakul A, Cudkowicz ME, et al. Dynamic markers of altered gait rhythm in amyotrophic lateral sclerosis. *J Appl Physiol (1985)*. 2000;88(6):2045–2053.

66. Scafetta N, Marchi D, West BJ. Understanding the complexity of human gait dynamics. *Chaos*. 2009;19(2):026108.

67. Wu Y, Ng SC. A PDF classification of gait cadence patterns in patients with ALS 32nd Annual International Conference of the IEEE EMBS; August 31–September 4, 2010; Buenos Aires, Argentina.

68. Sugavaneswaran L, Umapathy K, Krishnan S. Ambiguity domain-based identification of altered gait pattern in ALS disorder. *J Neural Eng*. 2012;9(4):046004-2560/9/4/046004.

69. Liao F, Wang J, He P. Multi-resolution entropy analysis of gait symmetry in neurological degenerative diseases and amyotrophic lateral sclerosis. *Med Eng Phys*. 2008;30(3):299–310.

70. Eggermont LH, Gavett BE, Volkers KM, et al. Lower-extremity function in cognitively healthy aging, mild cognitive impairment, and Alzheimer's disease. *Arch Phys Med Rehabil*. 2010;91(4):584–588.

71. Gras LZ, Kanaan SF, McDowd JM, et al. Balance and gait of adults with very mild Alzheimer disease. *J Geriatr Phys Ther*. 2015;38(1):1–7.

72. Cedervall Y, Halvorsen K, Aberg AC. A longitudinal study of gait function and characteristics of gait disturbance in individuals with Alzheimer's disease. *Gait Posture*. 2014;39(4):1022–1027.

73. Nadkarni NK, Mawji E, McIlroy WE, et al. Spatial and temporal gait parameters in Alzheimer's disease and aging. *Gait Posture*. 2009;30(4):452–454.

74. English KL, Paddon-Jones D. Protecting muscle mass and function in older adults during bed rest. *Curr Opin Clin Nutr Metab Care*. 2010;13(1):34–39.

75. Baan H, Dubbeldam R, Nene AV, et al. Gait analysis of the lower limb in patients with rheumatoid arthritis: a systematic review. *Semin Arthritis Rheum*. 2012;41(6):768–788.e8.

76. Turner DE, Helliwell PS, Emery P, et al. The impact of rheumatoid arthritis on foot function in the early stages of disease: a clinical case series. *BMC Musculoskelet Disord*. 2006;7:102.

77. Turner DE, Woodburn J, Helliwell PS, et al. Pes planovalgus in RA: a descriptive and analytical study of foot function determined by gait analysis. *Musculoskeletal Care*. 2003;1(1):21-33.

78. Fuhrmann RA. The treatment of rheumatoid foot deformities. *Orthopade*. 2002;31(12):1187–1197.

79. Giacomozzi C, Martelli F, Nagel A, et al. Cluster analysis to classify gait alterations in rheumatoid arthritis using peak pressure curves. *Gait Posture*. 2009;29(2):220–224.

80. Turner DE, Woodburn J. Characterising the clinical and biomechanical features of severely deformed feet in rheumatoid arthritis. *Gait Posture*. 2008;28(4):574–580.

81. Rosenbaum D, Schmiegel A, Meermeier M, et al. Plantar sensitivity, foot loading and walking pain in rheumatoid arthritis. *Rheumatology (Oxford)*. 2006;45(2):212–214.

82. Tuna H, Birtane M, Tastekin N, et al. Pedobarography and its relation to radiologic erosion scores in rheumatoid arthritis. *Rheumatol Int*. 2005;26(1):42–47.

83. Woodburn J, Helliwell PS, Barker S. Three-dimensional kinematics at the ankle joint complex in rheumatoid arthritis patients with painful valgus deformity of the rearfoot. *Rheumatology (Oxford)*. 2002;41(12):1406–1412.

84. Hennessy K, Burns J, Penkala S. Reducing plantar pressure in rheumatoid arthritis: a comparison of running versus off-the-shelf orthopaedic footwear. *Clin Biomech (Bristol, Avon)*. 2007;22(8): 917–923.

85. Cutolo M, Seriolo B, Craviotto C, et al. Circadian rhythms in RA. *Ann Rheum Dis*. 2003;62(7):593–596.

86. Gibbs JE, Ray DW. The role of the circadian clock in rheumatoid arthritis. *Arthritis Res Ther*. 2013;15(1):205.

87. Helliwell P, Reay N, Gilworth G, et al. Development of a foot impact scale for rheumatoid arthritis. *Arthritis Rheum*. 2005;53(3):418–422.

88. Backhouse MR, Pickles DA, Mathieson HR, et al. Diurnal variation of gait in patients with rheumatoid arthritis: the DIVIGN study. *Clin Biomech (Bristol, Avon)*. 2014;29(7):811–814.

89. Dubbeldam R, Nene AV, Buurke JH, et al. Foot and ankle joint kinematics in rheumatoid arthritis cannot only be explained by alteration in walking speed. *Gait Posture*. 2011;33(3):390–395.

90. Aletaha D, Smolen J, Ward MM. Measuring function in rheumatoid arthritis: identifying reversible and irreversible components. *Arthritis Rheum*. 2006;54(9):2784–2792.

91. Weiss RJ, Wretenberg P, Stark A, et al. Gait pattern in rheumatoid arthritis. *Gait Posture*. 2008;28(2):229–234.

92. D'Amico JC. Complexities of hallux limitus dictate treatment. *Biomechanics*. 2004;XI(4):51–91.

93. Kile T, Bouchard M. Degenerative joint disease of the ankle and hindfoot. In: Thoradsen D, ed. *Foot & Ankle (Orthopedic Surgery Essentials)*. Philadelphia, PA: Lippincott, Williams & Wilkins; 2013.

CHAPTER 11

Tumors of the Lower Extremity

HENRY DEGROOT

Soft Tissue Tumors of the Foot and Ankle

Soft tissue tumors of the foot and ankle are different from those of the rest of the musculoskeletal system in terms of type, risk of malignancy, age, treatment, and prognosis. Tumors of the foot and ankle may be degenerative, reactive, posttraumatic, or neoplastic in origin, or they may arise from an unknown cause. The treatment varies widely depending on the type of tumor. To select the appropriate treatment, the surgeon must begin with an accurate diagnosis. The ultimate goals of treatment are to eliminate the tumor and restore the patient's long-term mobility and function.

According to the most recent World Health Organization definitions, soft tissue tumors should be described as benign, intermediate (locally aggressive), intermediate (rarely metastasizing), and malignant. These terms have been introduced to eliminate confusion arising from outdated descriptions such as "intermediate malignancy." According to this terminology, benign tumors grow locally, do not infiltrate, do not recur, or recur in a nondestructive fashion. Schwannoma is an example of a benign tumor. Intermediate (locally aggressive) tumors may grow in an infiltrative fashion and may recur locally unless excised with a wide margin of normal tissue. Plantar fibroma is an example. Intermediate (rarely metastasizing) tumors are locally aggressive, grow in an infiltrative fashion, and are likely to recur locally, and also have a demonstrated ability to metastasize to distant sites. An example of this type of tumor is angiomatoid fibrous histiocytoma. Malignant tumors such as synovial sarcoma (SS) and clear cell sarcoma (CCS) grow in an aggressive, infiltrative, and locally destructive manner, and carry a high risk of regional and distant metastasis.

The most common benign soft tissue tumors in the foot and ankle include ganglion cyst, plantar fibroma, hemangioma, schwannoma, neurofibroma, pigmented villonodular synovitis (PVNS), and giant cell tumor of tendon sheath. Lipoma is rare in the foot and ankle. Tumor mimics are benign non-neoplastic soft tissue masses whose behavior is similar to that of true tumors. Examples include gouty tophi,

synovial cysts, synovial masses from degenerative tendinopathy, rheumatoid nodules, and epidermal cysts.[1] More than 100 other types of benign and malignant soft tissue tumors may occur in the foot, but a comprehensive description of them is outside the scope of this chapter. Instead, a strategy for evaluation and management is presented that applies to any tumor.

A larger proportion of soft tissue tumors in the foot and ankle are malignant than elsewhere in the body. Each individual surgeon's chance of encountering a malignant tumor will vary depending on practice profile and referral sources. In some published reports, as many as 20% to 62% of soft tissue tumors in the foot and ankle are malignant, although the true incidence is not known.[1-3] All foot and ankle surgeons should be vigilant. The risk of malignancy increases with age. Malignant melanoma is the most common soft tissue malignancy in the foot. Pleomorphic sarcoma (PS; previously named malignant fibrous histiocytoma [MFH]), SS, and CCS are the most common soft tissue sarcomas in the foot and ankle.

Surgery is the primary form of local control for foot and ankle sarcomas. The surgeon must achieve an appropriate margin around the tumor to minimize the risk of local recurrence. Surgical margins are defined by the terms intralesional, marginal, wide, and radical. The term en bloc, meaning the tumor is removed in one piece, has no oncologic significance and is not by itself an adequate description. Opening, entering, or spilling the tumor by design or by accident such as during a curettage of a bone cyst always creates an intralesional margin. A marginal margin is created when the surgeon dissects outside the tumor adjacent to the capsule or pseudocapsule, even if the tumor is never entered or exposed. A wide margin is created when the surgeon dissects completely outside the pseudocapsule and all reactive or abnormal appearing tissues. By definition, a wide margin includes a continuous unbroken cuff of normal tissue surrounding the entire surgical specimen. A radical margin is achieved when the entire compartment or compartments containing the tumor are resected, along with any and all bone, nerve, vessel, or tendon in the compartment. To achieve a radical margin in the foot and ankle at least a partial amputation is required.

For benign tumors, simple removal with an intralesional or wide margin is adequate. There is no adverse effect if the surgeon spills tumor cells into the nearby tissues, or leaves a portion of the tumor behind. For intermediate tumors, the risk of local recurrence and the debility associated with multiple surgeries demands a more thorough surgical approach. A wide margin is the goal, but a marginal margin is the most likely outcome. The surgical resection must encompass the entire tumor, any pseudocapsule, and the thickest possible cuff of normal tissue around the mass. The surgeon can adjust the size of the margins according to the propensity of the tumor to recur. For example, plantar fibroma is a benign tumor, but it carries a very high risk of local recurrence, and a margin of 1 to 2 cm is optimal. A schwannoma can be resected with a marginal margin.

Local control of malignant tumors requires an uncompromised wide margin. Wide resections are more likely to compromise the skeletal stability, neurovascular status, and soft tissue integrity of the limb. Surgeons seek to balance and optimize the oncologic and functional outcomes, and may accept marginal margins in order to facilitate limb salvage.[4] The goal of surgery is to resect the entire tumor en bloc, with an uncontaminated margin of 5 to 10 mm of normal tissue surrounding all aspects of the mass. A true wide margin requires that no part of the tumor, its capsule, or the reactive zone around the tumor is ever seen in the surgical field. All parts of the dissection take place through uninvolved, nonreactive normal tissues, and these normal tissues completely envelop all parts of the excised specimen. Spilling or exposure of any part of the actual tumor is unacceptable. Surgeons who are unprepared for the degree of collateral damage to the foot that is required to achieve a true wide margin around a sarcoma should not attempt these resections.

Adjuvant chemotherapy and radiation therapy are given routinely for osteosarcoma and Ewing sarcoma, and are used for other high-grade sarcomas on a case-by-case basis. There is strong evidence that conservative surgery combined with radiation therapy result in effective local control. Postoperative radiation can be administered by external beam in fractionated doses or by brachytherapy using surgically implanted radiation sources with a shorter duration of treatment. No strong evidence favors one method over the other. There is increasing interest in preoperative radiation therapy, which more precisely targets the tumor and damages less normal tissue. However, a definite survival benefit has not yet been demonstrated.[5] Preoperative radiation results in higher rates of major wound complications, which may have devastating effects in the foot and ankle.

EVALUATION OF A SOFT TISSUE MASS

History and Physical

The initial evaluation should include a complete history, a comprehensive regional examination, and plain radiographs of the affected area. This information is then used by the clinician to determine the likelihood of malignancy, to decide on the best type of advanced imaging to employ, and to evaluate the

Table 11-1. Clinical Features That Help Distinguish Benign Soft Tissue Masses from Malignant Soft Tissue Tumors

	Good	Bad
Pain history	Pain was present from the beginning	No pain or pain developed later
Growth history	Grows and shrinks	Grows progressively
Size	Small (<2 cm)	Large (>3 cm)
Location	Superficial	Deep
Findings on exam	An indistinct mass	A definite mass

The likelihood of malignancy increases as the number of "bad features" increases.[6]

need for a diagnostic biopsy. For soft tissue tumors, history and physical examination findings can be used to determine the potential for malignancy, based on the presence or absence of five specific "good" or "bad" clinical findings. This assessment is made based solely on the clinical features of the tumor; no advanced imaging is necessary. Factors included in the assessment include pain, growth, size, location, and examination findings (Table 11-1). Benign tumors are more likely to be painful, not progressively growing, small, superficial to the fascia, and difficult to palpate as a distinct mass. Malignant tumors tend to be painless, progressively growing, large, deep to the fascia, and well defined on exam. The risk of malignancy increases with the number of "bad" features the tumor has.

Certain physical examination findings might point toward a specific diagnosis. For example, hemangiomas have a characteristic blue-purple color that may be visible in the overlying skin. These lesions are typically painful to palpation. Ganglion cysts can be transilluminated with a penlight or a laser pointer and, when transillumination is demonstrated, aspirated to confirm the diagnosis.

Laboratory tests are not generally useful in the initial management of tumors of the foot and ankle, unless there is clinical evidence of infection, an inflammatory condition such as rheumatoid arthritis, or gout. Nonspecific laboratory screening tests are not recommended.

Imaging Evaluation of Soft Tissue Tumors

The history and physical examination may be adequate to confirm the diagnosis of many common soft tissue masses in the foot and ankle, such as ganglion cyst and plantar fibroma. In these cases, imaging of the lesion may not be clinically indicated. For soft tissue tumors that cannot be readily diagnosed, two orthogonal high-quality plain radiographs are recommended as the initial imaging study. The radiographic findings may point to a possible diagnosis. For example, intramuscular hemangiomas (IMHs) may contain small rounded pebble-like calcifications called phleboliths, whereas 30% of SSs contain amorphous calcifications. Soft tissue sarcomas and metastatic cancers in the foot may invade a nearby bone, a worrisome sign associated with malignancy. Advanced imaging other than MRI, such as CT scans, positron emission tomography (PET) scans, and bone scans, is not commonly useful in the evaluation of soft tissue lesions.[7]

The malignant potential of some soft tissue tumors may be difficult to determine with confidence. The history and physical examination findings can be unhelpful or even misleading. A contrast-enhanced MRI examination with a dedicated extremity coil is recommended for lesions larger than 2 or 3 cm and for all soft tissue tumors with worrisome clinical features. The MRI signal characteristics may in some cases be adequate to identify the exact nature of the lesion, or for the differential to be narrowed, but in other cases the MRI findings are nonspecific. Nevertheless, MRI is very helpful in determining the size and extent of the tumor as well as its relationship to the neurovascular elements. MRI is an essential tool for clinical staging, biopsy placement, surgical planning, and evaluation of response to therapy.

Determinate versus Indeterminate Soft Tissue Tumors

A systematic approach to assessment of the potential for malignancy of soft tissue masses has been proposed whereby soft tissue tumors are divided into two groups: "determinate" and "indeterminate" based on the clinical and radiographic findings. The subsequent management plan follows directly from this assessment.[8,9]

Soft tissue tumors for which a specific diagnosis can be made based on a combination of history, the physical examination, and analysis of the MRI findings are called determinate lesions. Determinate lesions that may occur in the foot and ankle include lipoma, hemangioma, ganglion cyst, some plantar fibromas, and PVNS. Determinate lesions are treated with observation or by excisional biopsy, depending on the clinical situation.

Soft tissue tumors for which no specific diagnosis is confirmed by the exam, X-ray, and MRI findings are called indeterminate lesions. These lesions are typically isointense with muscle (dark) on T1-weighted imaging and hyperintense (bright) on T2-weighted imaging. In the foot and ankle, this group of tumors includes all soft tissue sarcomas such as SS, CCS, and liposarcoma, as well as a number of benign tumors, such as giant cell tumor of tendon sheath, peripheral nerve sheath tumors, and some plantar fibromas. Indeterminate lesions are treated with incisional or needle biopsy, along with appropriate referral to an orthopedic oncologist. If there is any doubt, it is best to defer the biopsy to the specialist team. Definitive surgical removal of indeterminate lesions is always performed as a separate procedure after the final pathologic diagnosis and staging are completed.

BIOPSY PLANNING AND TECHNIQUES

Some foot and ankle surgeons refer extremity tumors to a specialist for biopsy and definitive treatment, whereas others feel comfortable managing soft tissue lesions within their scope of practice. A systematic approach to the performance of the biopsy is recommended because improper timing, technique, or management of the biopsy process increases the risk of complications. The biopsy technique should be chosen with care so that an accurate diagnosis is made with minimal risk. Complications of improperly planned or executed biopsies include errors in diagnosis, inadequate or nondiagnostic biopsy material, surgical site infection, hematoma, and contamination of nearby tissues. Biopsy complications have been shown to increase the risk of an otherwise avoidable amputation. These problems may be avoided by early referral to an orthopedic oncologist or tumor specialist prior to the biopsy.

The surgeon is responsible for consulting with the pathologist prior to performing a biopsy in cases where malignancy is possible (for all indeterminate lesions). Direct communication by telephone is highly recommended as a means of insuring that the surgeon and pathologist collaborate in an optimal fashion to maximize the diagnostic yield of the biopsy and minimize potentially devastating errors. Because the biopsy will alter the imaging appearance of the tumor, all diagnostic scans should be completed prior to biopsy.

The most appropriate biopsy technique should been selected according to the clinical and anatomic situation. Options include needle aspiration, tru-cut or large-bore needle biopsy, incisional biopsy, and excisional biopsy.

Fine needle aspiration (FNA) and core needle techniques have the advantage of being well tolerated by the patient and causing few complications. FNA is an appropriate choice for patients with a known cancer diagnosis who are suspected to have a recurrence or a metastasis in the foot or ankle. FNA is also useful for other lesions where there is little doubt about the diagnosis and the biopsy is only needed to confirm what is already known. However, FNA is inadequate to evaluate the tissue cytoarchitecture, and the amount of material obtained may be inadequate for tissue banking and ancillary studies. FNA and core needle biopsy is the first-line biopsy technique for soft tissue tumors in some cancer centers. In those centers, a dedicated and experienced team manages all soft tissue tumors. This approach can minimize or eliminate the shortcomings of needle techniques.

In settings where an experienced biopsy team and an experienced solid tumor cytopathologist are not available, needle biopsy may be inadequate or inconclusive. Open (incisional) biopsy techniques are preferred in these cases. Open biopsy is a safe and effective technique when properly planned and executed. More tissue allows for better understanding of the cytoarchitecture of the lesion and reduces the risk of a nondiagnostic result. Essential material for ancillary studies and tissue banking can be obtained.

Excision of the tumor immediately after open biopsy is possible for a small group of tumors where the frozen section features of the tumor are highly diagnostic. This group includes giant cell tumor of tendon sheath, plantar fibroma, schwannoma, and other tumors depending on the experience and confidence of the pathologist. The surgeon and pathologist should both be highly experienced in managing tumors. If sufficient doubt about the final diagnosis exists or the pathologist is not comfortable making a decision based on frozen section alone, the definitive surgery should be delayed until the final pathologic analysis has been completed. Most indeterminate tumors will require immunohistochemical stains and other specialized examinations for diagnosis. Definitive surgery can take place 7 to 14 days after the biopsy.

The success of an incisional biopsy depends on careful prebiopsy planning, proper biopsy execution, and adequate postbiopsy care of the patient (Table 11-2). All imaging studies must be completed prior to biopsy. The pathologist and the surgeon should discuss the case prior to the biopsy or they may do so in the operating room. A tourniquet is applied after elevation but without exsanguination. Tumor sampling is accomplished through adequate longitudinal incisions that approach the lesion most directly. The incision should be long enough to allow visualization of the procedure, confirmation of appropriate sampling, and hemostasis. Small "key hole" biopsy incisions are not recommended. Contamination of uninvolved structures and the neurovascular bundles especially

near the medial malleolus should be carefully avoided. The tourniquet should be released after the tumor is sampled, and measures should be taken to insure that the wound is completely dry. Unintentional spread of the tumor may occur because of postbiopsy bleeding. A hematoma may track under subcutaneous tissues or through intramuscular spaces, causing a wide zone of contamination. During open biopsy, the pathologist should examine a frozen section of the biopsy material to verify that an adequate amount of viable tumor has been obtained. Cultures should be performed unless the potential for infection has been definitively ruled out. A moderately compressive dressing should be applied and the patient is made nonweight-bearing with the extremity elevated for 3 or 4 days. The surgeon who performs the biopsy should schedule a face-to-face encounter with the patient in 7 to 10 days to discuss the results of the procedure and the future treatment plan. It is best to avoid delivering biopsy results over the telephone or via an intermediary.

Excisional biopsy is appropriate for the determination of soft tissue tumors in the foot or ankle as discussed earlier, and may be advisable for small and superficial indeterminate tumors. During excisional biopsy, care should be taken that the tumor is not exposed or entered. The entire tumor, the surrounding capsule, and a small amount of surrounding normal soft tissue are taken en bloc. Excisional biopsy is never appropriate for large or deep soft tissue tumors.

MANAGEMENT OF A PATIENT WITH AN UNPLANNED EXCISION OF A SOFT TISSUE SARCOMA

Soft tissue sarcomas are rare and may have an indolent presentation. As a result, unplanned excision of soft tissue sarcoma in the foot and ankle is common.[10] Unplanned surgery is defined as excisional biopsy or unplanned resection of a malignant sarcoma without an adequate margin. Outcomes after unplanned excision in all body sites are inferior to those after planned surgery.[11] The implications of unplanned treatment of sarcomas in the foot may be more serious than elsewhere in the body. The potential for contamination of uninvolved structures is higher, and unplanned surgeries make the subsequent wide excision surgery more difficult.[12]

Management following unplanned resection of a sarcoma typically requires complete excision of the entire tumor bed and any surgically contaminated tissues to achieve a wide margin. Unplanned surgery results in additional soft tissue reconstruction compared with planned surgery.[13] If the initial surgery resulted in extensive contamination of surrounding structures, amputation may be necessary to achieve local control. Following repeat excision in cases without clinically palpable residual tumor, 50% of the cases were found to have microscopic residual tumor. Following repeat excision, 85% of the patients were alive and disease free at 5 years.

Table 11-2. Checklist of Tasks Required for a Successful Biopsy
Prebiopsy
■ All imaging studies completed
■ Appropriate biopsy technique selected
■ Imaging reviewed to plan approach and tumor sampling strategy
■ Pathologist consulted by telephone or directly in operating room
■ Operating room aware of a frozen section planned
During the Biopsy
■ Adequate longitudinal incisions
■ Direct approach with minimal dissection, no flaps or undermining
■ Do not expose the neurovascular bundle
■ Do not biopsy the pseudocapsule
■ Biopsy the most cellular area of the tumor—usually the outermost part
■ Pathologist performs frozen section to verify biopsy is adequate
■ Perform cultures if indicated or if no evidence of a neoplasm seen on frozen section
Postbiopsy
■ Meticulous hemostasis with tourniquet released
■ Avoid drains
■ Mildly compressive bandage or splint applied
■ Strict activity restriction and elevation written in orders
■ Schedule a face-to-face follow-up visit to share biopsy result

BENIGN SOFT TISSUE TUMORS

Ganglion Cyst

Clinical Presentation

Ganglion cysts tend to present in young to middle age adults, more commonly women, and are very rare in children. The most common location is around the ankle joint or midfoot, especially on the dorsolateral surface. The lesions may arise in association with peripheral nerves, joints, fascia, and bone. In the author's experience, simple, superficial ganglion cysts rarely affect the forefoot. In these cases, examination reveals a palpable, well-defined mass, usually 1 to 3 cm, with no pain or very mild pain. The lesion occurs near the joint or along a tendon sheath. The mass may grow and shrink according to the activity level. In some cases, loading or flexing the tendon or joint will make the mass feel noticeably more firm. The ganglion cysts are typically not associated with significant degenerative pathology of the nearby tendon or joint.

Ganglion cyst may present in a patient with nonlocalized pain, in whom an MRI scan of the foot reveals a small periarticular cystic mass, often adjacent to a joint in the hindfoot, sinus tarsi, or midtarsal joint. These cysts can be aspirated and injected with ultrasound guidance, or excised. In addition, lesions that have MRI features consistent with ganglion cyst are occasionally found in the plantar aspect of the forefoot adjacent to the metatarsal phalangeal joints. In the author's experience, these lesions are caused by plantar plate degeneration associated with aging and overuse. Treatment of these lesions is analogous to the treatment of metatarsalgia and plantar plate–related pain.

Clinical Exam

A typical ganglion cyst is superficial, firm, somewhat compressible, and usually painless. The cyst will transilluminate with a penlight or a laser pointer. Transillumination is the extended transmission of light through the lesion due to the semitransparent material in the cyst. The room lights may need to be dimmed and the area should be shielded from external light sources to maximize the effect. The surgeon should illuminate a nearby area to observe the expected amount of light transmission through normal tissue.

Diagnostic Procedure

The combination of transillumination and needle aspiration confirms the diagnosis of ganglion cyst. Once transillumination is confirmed, aspiration should follow. Lesions that do not transilluminate should not be aspirated. Aspiration of ganglion cysts is simple, safe, and well tolerated in an office setting. A single puncture into the center of the cystic mass with a 22-gauge or larger needle should be performed. The diagnosis is confirmed if slightly yellow/clear, nonturbid, viscous or jelly-like material is aspirated from the cyst. This material can be identified by its characteristic appearance

and material properties, and thus laboratory analysis is not required. If unexpected material, crystals, pus, or blood is encountered, cultures and laboratory and/or pathologic analysis is recommended. If aspiration is negative, the needle should be withdrawn. Additional punctures and multiple passes should not be made. An MRI is recommended to characterize the lesion.

Transillumination and aspiration may lead to a conclusive diagnosis and further workup can thus be avoided. MRI is unnecessary and treatment is at the discretion of the surgeon. The aspiration may be curative. If the lesion recurs after aspiration, surgical removal can proceed without further workup.

Plantar Fascial Fibroma and Fibromatosis

Clinical Presentation

Plantar fibromatosis (also known as Ledderhose disease) is a nonencapsulated thickening and proliferation of the central and medial bands of the plantar fascia. The lesions may also occur in atypical locations, such as in the distal or proximal plantar fascia and in subcutaneous tissues. The cause is unknown. One-third to one-half of patients also present with bilateral nodules. Approximately one-third to two-thirds of patients will also have fibromas in the palmar fascia, the knuckle pads, or elsewhere. Patients with Dupuytren contracture have an increased risk for plantar fibromas. Most patients are asymptomatic, but some have activity-related pain or shoe irritation. When the lesions are large enough to press on the plantar nerves, there may also be numbness or dysesthesia in the distal portions of the foot.

Differential diagnosis for this tumor is SS.[14]

Diagnostic Procedure

Plain radiographs are recommended to rule out the presence of intralesional calcifications that are seen in SS but not in plantar fibroma. No laboratory exams are recommended. MRI is not necessary for small, stable, and typically located lesions. MRI is strongly recommended if the lesion is large or enlarging, or atypical in any way.

Initial management should consist of shoe modifications, custom or readymade orthotics, and pain medication. Numerous nonsurgical treatments have been recommended or published in low-quality clinical studies, including external beam radiation,[15] extracorporeal shockwave therapy,[16] injections of corticosteroids, collagenase clostridium histolyticum injections,[17] and transdermal therapy with 15% verapamil gel. None of these treatments can be recommended due to the low quality or total absence of any supporting data.

Surgical removal is reserved for large lesions that are causing significant disability that have failed a well-documented course of nonoperative care. Surgeons treating this lesion should be prepared to undertake an aggressive and comprehensive resection of the lesion, because recurrences after surgical treatment are inversely proportional to the quality of the margin.[14,18]

Local fasciectomy has a 100% recurrence rate. The presence of multiple fascial nodules, bilateral nodules, and family history is associated with increased risk of recurrence.[14,19] Aggressive resection with a wide margin (subtotal fasciectomy) is necessary and carries a recurrence rate of 25%. Radical fasciectomy is a misnomer because the resection does not achieve a radical margin. The surgeon should achieve a minimum of a 1 cm margin at the fascial boundaries and the widest possible margin at the skin surface that will still permit primary closure. A marginal margin must be accepted at the deep surface of the lesion to allow preservation of the medial and lateral neurovascular bundles. In cases of recurrence after local excision, a subtotal fasciectomy can be expected to be successful in 75% of cases. Skin grafts and tissue transfers may be required to facilitate coverage and closure in reoperated cases. Fibromas that recur after subtotal fasciectomy should be observed.

Pigmented Villonodular Synovitis

Clinical Presentation

PVNS is a locally aggressive synovial proliferation of unknown origin. The tumor cells consistently overexpress colony-stimulating factor-1 (CSF1) that has been implicated in tumor growth.[20] In addition, DNA aneuploidy, chromosomal translocations, and tumor expression of *p63* and *nm23* have been reported in a variable proportion of cases.

Various clinical presentations of this benign tumor exist, including giant cell tumor of tendon sheath/tenosynovial giant cell tumor, which are described later, and PVNS. Most patients are in their thirties and forties. This lesion is rare in children. Approximately 2% to 10% of cases occur in the foot and ankle.[21] There are two forms of PVNS: diffuse and nodular. Nodular PVNS occurs most commonly in the forefoot.[22] Diffuse PVNS is found more commonly in the hindfoot and presents with osteoarthritis. PVNS may also occur in the ankle and often presents as a mildly painful joint with swelling.

Diagnostic Procedure

X-ray imaging is often used in identifying PVNS. The radiologic appearance of PVNS depends on the location. A nodule in the forefoot may have soft tissue swelling and bone erosion on plain X-ray. The ankle usually only has a soft tissue mass, but bone erosion or cysts may be present. The joint space is usually preserved and there may be an effusion. MRI scan is able to identify the hemosiderin contained in the lesion and can demonstrate the extent of the synovial involvement as well as bone erosion and cysts. Hemosiderin appears as low or absent signal (signal dropout) on both T1- and T2-weighted images.

On gross examination, the diffuse form of PVNS is a tan mass of villi and folds of synovium. The lesion may be sessile or have several pedunculated nodules. Bony invasion through the joint capsule is possible. The local form of PVNS is a pedunculated firm nodule. Microscopically, PVNS is characterized by synovial cell hyperplasia both on the surface and below the synovium. Also present are scattered giant cells, hemosiderin, and foam cells. The location of the polyhedral cells below the synovial membrane suggests that perhaps the cell of origin is a fibrohistiocyte. The pathologic differential includes hemosiderotic synovitis, rheumatoid arthritis, and synovial chondromatosis.

Treatment of mild cases of diffuse PVNS is by nonoperative means with clinical and radiologic follow-up. Symptomatic relief can be obtained with a combination of moderate activity restriction, offloading the joint with a removable fracture boot, and daily administration of ibuprofen or naproxen. Complete resolution of symptoms may take 12 to 24 months. Patients are at risk for recurrence of symptoms if they return to high activity levels too soon.

Nodular PVNS is treated by simple excision with a marginal margin. Nodular lesions rarely recur after complete excision, but will almost always recur if macroscopic amounts of the lesion are left behind after surgery. Surgical treatment of diffuse PVNS is indicated for bulky or painful lesions and cases with bone or joint damage, in order to prevent progression. Treatment is by aggressive means, either open or arthroscopic, without adjuvant therapy. There is a 10% to 15% risk of recurrence.[23] Adjuvant treatments including radiation[21] have been used in severe and recurrent cases. In the ankle, arthrodesis or total arthroplasty with a prosthetic implant may be necessary in cases with severe joint damage.[24]

Giant Cell Tumor of Tendon Sheath

Clinical Presentation

Giant cell tumor of tendon sheath is a rare, solitary benign variant of PVNS that may arise in the tendon sheath tissues of the hand and wrist as well as the ankle and foot. Most cases occur in the hand, where local recurrence after excision has been reported in up to 40% of cases. The tumor cells show consistent overexpression of CSF1, the ligand of the tyrosine kinase receptor, as well as frequent chromosomal translocations at 1p13, the locus of the *CSF1* gene.

Clinically, the patients report a slow-growing, painless, firm solitary mass adjacent to the dorsal or plantar tendons, the midfoot joints, or the ankle joint, which has been present for 1 to 2 years on average. There may be a history of trauma, and neurologic symptoms occur rarely. In one study, lesions in the forefoot occurred in the first, second, and fifth rays exclusively, indicating that there may be some relationship between weight-bearing and this tumor. The tumor may cause or accentuate an angular deformity such as hallux valgus.

Diagnostic Procedure

On plain radiographs, there may be a visible soft tissue swelling, sometimes completely encasing the bony elements of the involved digit, and the tumor may invade the adjacent bone and cause cystic lesions that are clearly visible on X-ray.

Approximately 10% involve the bone. The bone involvement and destruction leads to concern for primary bone malignancy, and inappropriately aggressive treatments can result. CT scan will show the extent of the tumor, and clearly delineate any bony involvement. Some of these tumors have small calcifications, a feature shared with SS. MRI scans are helpful to define the extent of the lesion, and can be helpful in the preoperative diagnosis. Hemosiderin in the lesion may result in very low signal intensities on some sequences, and the lesions enhance on T1 sequences after administration of gadopentetate contrast agent, and these features help identify the tumor. Treatment is by complete, meticulous excision of the entire lesion. A wide or radical margin is not necessary. Intralesional margins are acceptable, as long as complete excision is not compromised. Recurrence has been reported in up to 45% of cases, but with careful removal, recurrence can be reduced to 10% to 20%. In the lesser toes, where the lesion has extensively invaded the soft tissues and bone, amputation may be preferable to excision. In the great toe, efforts should be made to preserve the mechanical integrity of the first ray, including complete meticulous excision of the lesion, followed by bone grafts, skin grafts, and fusions as necessary.

A separate, staged biopsy is recommended. The lesion cannot always be characterized by preoperative studies, and aggressive or destructive features may be present that are also consistent with malignancy. Open surgical biopsy with frozen section analysis is preferred, performed through a well-planned longitudinal incision that avoids any involvement of nearby neurovascular structures. If the lesion can be characterized by MRI, and the level of confidence in the preoperative diagnosis is very high, then excisional biopsy is appropriate.

Schwannoma/Nerve Sheath Tumors

Clinical Presentation

Schwannomas/neurilemmomas and neurofibromas are part of a large group of tumors believed to arise from Schwann cells. Schwann cells produce myelin and may also produce collagen, thus the neoplasms that arise from them have a range of histologic features. These tumors may arise in bone as well as in soft tissues. Neurofibromas are more likely to occur in younger individuals, are associated with neurofibromatosis, and carry a significant risk of malignant degeneration. Schwannomas/neurilemmomas occur in middle-aged and older individuals, are rarely associated with neurofibromatosis, and carry an extremely small risk of malignant degeneration. Numerous subtypes of nerve sheath tumors have been described, but an exhaustive review is outside the scope of this chapter. Morton neuroma is not a part of this group of tumors. Morton neuroma is not a true tumor, but rather a fibrotic and degenerative thickening of the plantar digital nerve.

Benign schwannoma/benign neurilemmoma is a slow-growing solitary nerve sheath tumor that typically presents in adults between age 20 and 50. Schwannomatosis/multifocal neurilemmoma has been observed in the foot and ankle and knee.[25,26] The typical solitary tumor presents as a slow-growing painless mass that may have been present for 1 to 2 years or more. Some of these tumors are exquisitely painful and may cause severe radiating neurogenic pain, but others are completely painless. Schwannomas have been reported as a cause of tarsal tunnel syndrome.[27]

Because of prolonged growth of these tumors, there may be local bony impingement and bone remodeling due to pressure from the tumor. However, these benign tumors do not invade the bone. MRI scans show typical features for an indeterminate tumor, with low signal intensity on T1-weighted sequences and high signal intensity on T2-weighted sequences. The anatomical relationship of the tumor to the nerve of origin may be obvious or so subtle as to be impossible to determine.

Because of the indeterminate MRI appearance of this tumor, a complete evaluation and staged biopsy is recommended before definitive surgical removal is planned. A small number of tumors can be definitively identified based on clinical findings and MRI examination. In a patient who does not have neurofibromatosis, the combination of a tumor causing significant neurogenic pain and an MRI demonstrating a clear anatomical relationship between the tumor and a peripheral nerve is diagnostic for benign schwannoma/neurilemmoma.

Treatment is by excision with a marginal margin. Some of these tumors have no obvious relationship to a peripheral nerve. Others occur inside the epineurium of a large nerve such as the posterior tibial nerve.[28] Intraneural schwannomas can usually be separated from the surrounding normal nerve fibers without significant damage. Incomplete excision or intralesional excision is acceptable for tumors that cannot be separated from a major peripheral nerve and where complete excision would cause significant morbidity and permanent nerve damage. Recurrence following resection with a marginal margin is rare.

Intramuscular Hemangioma

Clinical Presentation

IMHs typically present in the lower extremities of children and young adults. These vascular lesions are divided into several types, according to their histologic features. Capillary hemangioma is the most common type, consisting of small capillaries that have normal size and diameter, but that are excessive in number. Cavernous hemangioma is made up of larger dilated blood vessels. Compound hemangiomas have features of both the capillary and cavernous types. Lobular capillary hemangiomas are small, red bumps often occurring on the hands, face, and arms, especially during pregnancy. Most IMHs in the extremities are the capillary type. IMH is a benign lesion with a very low risk of malignant degeneration.

IMH occurs in the leg more commonly than the foot. Patients present with activity-related pain, night pain, and localized tenderness over the lesion. The tumor can cause equinus, toe-walking, and unilateral pes planus.[29] Lesions in the heel may mimic plantar fasciitis. IMHs near the skin or dermis have a visible blue color.

Diagnostic Procedure

The appropriate age, location, history, and examination findings should lead the clinician to suspect a hemangioma. Phleboliths, which are small, rounded calcified intravascular thrombi, are seen on plain films in 50% of hemangiomas.

MRI scans are usually adequate to confirm the diagnosis. On MRI, IMH is a well-defined lobular heterogeneous intramuscular mass, isointense on T1 and hyperintense on T2, with fat and serpentine blood vessels, containing signal voids associated with the phleboliths. The MRI appearance has been described as a "bag of worms." These lesions are usually definite as previously described, and may be treated without biopsy when the diagnosis is certain. It is not unusual for IMH to infiltrate both muscle and nearby structures, including skin, bone, and neurovascular bundles.

In most cases, nonoperative treatment should be attempted. Activity restriction, compression garments, nonsteroidal medications or acetaminophen are usually adequate to control the symptoms. Ultrasound-guided or fluoroscopically guided sclerotherapy using absolute alcohol or ethanolamine oleate has been successfully employed to treat IMH in the foot and ankle.[30] Complications of sclerotherapy include tendon contracture, skin breakdown, reversible nerve injury, and deep venous thrombosis.[31]

Localized, painful IMH that does not infiltrate critical structures can be treated with surgery. Excision with an intralesional or marginal margin is effective for symptomatic control.[32] In pediatric patients, IMH has a high risk of recurrence. More ample margins should be used to lower the rate of recurrence and reoperations.[33] IMH may extend into nearby tissues such as bone, skin, and vascular structures. Resection of the accessible portions of the lesion combined with sclerotherapy, compressive garments, and medications is more suitable for complex lesions.

Tumor Mimics

Tumor mimics are non-neoplastic lesions (not true tumors) that may look and act like tumors. Gouty tophi, enlarged degenerated tendons, and focal collections of subcutaneous fat can sometimes be mistaken for tumors.

Gouty Tophi

Gout is an inflammatory arthropathy that occurs as a result of hyperuricemia. Gouty tophi represent the accumulation of calcium urate crystals within soft tissue and bone. Tophi may occur within the subcutaneous tissues, synovium, subchondral bone, and tendons, resulting in soft tissue masses, osseous erosion, tendon rupture, and tarsal tunnel syndrome. Tophi typically occur adjacent to the metatarsal phalangeal joints and along the lateral border of the foot. The patient may not carry an established diagnosis of gout. In severe cases, there is usually a history of skin breakdown and white pasty material draining from the mass. Treatment for gout is largely medical. Colchicine inhibits the phagocytosis of urate crystals by polymorphonuclear cells and blocks the release of chemotactic factors. Nonsteroidal anti-inflammatory drugs (NSAIDs) such as indomethacin can give patients relief from pain in 2 to 4 hours. Intra-articular steroid injections can also give relief of acute gout symptoms. Extremely bulky gouty tophi can be debulked, but the extensive infiltration of calcium urate crystals within the soft tissues makes it impossible to resect all the abnormal material.

Runner's Bump

Older runners who average more than 30 miles per week may develop a mass on the tibialis anterior tendon sheath that may be mistaken for a tumor. This lesion is because of degeneration of the tibialis anterior tendon and a focal tenosynovial mass at the location of the damage. On examination, a soft, mobile lesion surrounds the tibialis anterior tendon at the level where the top of the shoelace rubs on the tendon. The tendon itself may retain normal caliber and function, depending on the severity. In some cases, the lesion can be partially eliminated by compressive massage, but recurs promptly. MRI shows a mild to moderate degree of tendon disease along with an intimately associated synovial mass. Treatment involves recognition of the origin of the problem, education of the runner, and padding, changing, or repositioning the laces and the tongue of the shoe to minimize the forces on the area. Surgical debulking of the excess synovium and tendon repair should be reserved for severe cases.

Localized Sinus Tarsi Fat Collection

In some overweight or obese individuals, a localized, well-defined subcutaneous collection of fat may occur anterior to the distal fibula in the area of the sinus tarsi. The patient is asymptomatic, but may be displeased with the appearance of the fatty collection. The mass typically measures 3 or 4 cm in proximal distal dimension and 2 or 3 cm in medial lateral dimension, and consists of soft compressible nontender subcutaneous fat. If there are atypical features or clinical suspicion, an MRI is recommended. The lesion consists entirely of fatty tissue that has identical signal characteristics to that of nearby normal subcutaneous fat. This collection of subcutaneous fat is not a lipoma, and surgical removal is not recommended.

SOFT TISSUE SARCOMA IN THE FOOT AND ANKLE

Introduction

Soft tissue sarcomas are a heterogeneous group of malignancies that arise from mesenchymal tissues. These rare tumors comprise less than 1% of all malignancies. Most sarcomas are caused by molecular anomalies in the cellular DNA, such as chromosomal translocations and mutations that activate, inhibit, or amplify the expression of the genetic material. Environmental factors, familial cancer syndromes, herbicides such as dioxin, radiation, and immune deficiency are rare causes of sarcomas.[34]

Approximately 8,700 soft tissue sarcomas are diagnosed per year in the United States, with an estimated 10% of these occurring in the distal lower extremity.[35] Soft tissue sarcomas are more common in older individuals. Approximately one-third of these tumors are superficial, and three-quarters are histologically of high grade. When these tumors recur, it is more often a distal metastasis than a local recurrence.[36] At least one-third of patients with soft tissue sarcomas will die of their disease.

The American Joint Committee on Cancer (AJCC) staging system for soft tissue tumors has been shown to have a significant relationship to the prognosis. The staging system incorporates tumor size, depth, the presence or absence of nodal or distant metastasis, and histologic grade (Table 11-3). Staging is based on data from the CT or MRI of the tumor as well as a CT of the chest. This information is combined with the histologic grade, size, and the intracompartmental or extracompartmental extent of the tumor. Prognosis is strongly related to grade, size, and histologic subtype of sarcoma.

Treatment of soft tissue sarcomas is determined by the histologic diagnosis and stage of the tumor. With rare exceptions, surgical resection with a wide margin is the most effective method of primary tumor control. Wide margins reduce the chance of local recurrence, which has a strong negative impact on survival. Limb-sparing surgery is preferable to amputation when a durable, functional, and pain-free extremity can be achieved. Because of the anatomical constraints of the foot and ankle, it may be difficult to achieve a wide margin without resorting to at least a partial amputation. Approximately 15% to 20% of patients with distal lower extremity sarcomas require some kind of amputation.

In adults with foot and ankle sarcoma, limb-sparing surgery has not been proven to be better than amputation in terms of functional, psychosocial, or quality of life outcomes.[37] Limb salvage is functionally superior to amputation in pediatric sarcoma patients. The soft tissue coverage of the foot and ankle is scant and subjected to high loads and repetitive shear stresses. The bony and articular elements must provide durable support and flexibility while withstanding the stresses of weight-bearing. Limb-sparing surgery must be carefully weighed against other options for tumors of the foot and ankle.[38] Ten percent of patients treated with limb-sparing surgery are ultimately amputated for reasons other than cancer.[39] Limb salvage for sarcomas in the forefoot using free vascularized osteomyocutaneous fibular and scapular grafts has been reported to be successful. All patients required multiple procedures due to complications.[40] In some series, less than half the patients treated with limb salvage regain normal functional status.[38]

Pleomorphic Sarcoma (Previously Identified as Malignant Fibrous Histiocytoma)

Introduction and Definition

PS is a term that recently replaced MFH. MFH was introduced as a diagnosis in 1963, and prior to that time, tumors of this type were classified as rhabdomyosarcoma or fibrosarcoma. The classification continues to evolve, and this fact makes it difficult to interpret the epidemiologic, clinical, and outcomes data from the past. This tumor is a pleomorphic high-grade tumor of unknown origin composed of fibroblasts, myofibroblasts, and histiocytes. PS/MFH is the most frequent soft tissue tumor in adults in some series. PS/MFH is found in the extremities 70% to 75% of the time, and 50% of all cases are in the lower extremity. Other less common sites include the retroperitoneum, and the head and neck. The highest incidence is during the fifth decade of life, and there is a male to female ratio of 1.5:1.

Incidence and Demographics

PS/MFH is secondary to another process such as radiation, surgery, fracture, osteonecrosis, Paget disease, nonossifying fibroma, or fibrous dysplasia 20% of the time. PS/MFH arising from a previous abnormality is usually more aggressive and has a poorer prognosis than primary PS/MFH.

Table 11-3. The American Joint Committee on Cancer Staging System					
Stage	**Size**	**Depth**	**Node**	**Metastasis**	**Grade**
I	Any	Any	None	None	G1–G2 (low)
II	<5 cm	Any	None	None	G2–G3/G3–G4 (high)
	>5 cm	Superficial	None	None	G2–G3/G3–G4 (high)
III	Any	Deep	None	None	G2–G3/G3–G4 (high)
IV	Any	Any	Present	None	Any (high or low)
	Any	Any	None	Present	Any

AJCC, The American Joint Committee on Cancer; Superficial, above the fascia; Deep, deep to fascia; G1, well differentiated; G2, moderately well differentiated; G3, poorly differentiated; G4, undifferentiated. (Adapted from Green FL, Page DL, Fleming ID, et al. *AJCC Cancer Staging Handbook.* 6th ed. New York, NY: Springer-Verlag; 2002:221–225.)

Symptoms and Presentation

Clinically, PS/MFH presents with local pain and swelling. There is often a history of a rapidly enlarging mass. It usually presents with a soft tissue mass with or without nearby bone erosion.

X-ray Appearance and Advanced Imaging Findings

Calcifications may be seen at the periphery of the mass on plain X-ray. CT scan is helpful in determining any intraosseus extension. MRI findings in PS/MFH are intermediate signal intensity on T1-weighted images and high-intensity signal on T2-weighted images. MRI helps define the soft tissue mass, marrow involvement, neurovascular structures, and joint invasion. PS/MFH has increased uptake on bone scan, which helps demonstrate any metastases.

Differential Diagnosis

The radiologic differential includes metastatic cancer, plasmacytoma, lymphoma, and fibrosarcoma.

Histopathology Findings

On gross examination, MFH is a lobulated, fleshy, gray-white mass. There may be yellow areas of lipid or darker areas of hemorrhage. The mass may be all soft tissue or have intraosseus extension. The margins of the tumor are normally ill-defined and destructive. Under the microscope, there are plump spindle cells in a storiform pattern in fascicles. A pinwheel pattern is found especially around vessels. The tumor stains positive for histiocytic markers CD68 and lysozyme. Like other sarcomas, PS/MFH is graded from 1 to 4, with a higher grade having a worse prognosis. The classification and identification of PS continues to evolve. Some pathologists believe that many of the tumors now classified as PS/MFH should be reclassified with a more specific diagnosis such as synovial cell sarcoma or leiomyosarcoma, based on careful study of cellular markers.

Treatment Options for This Tumor

Treatment of PS/MFH depends on grade, stage, and site. Local tumor control is almost always accomplished with surgical resection with a wide margin. Radiation may be given preoperatively or postoperatively. Preoperative chemotherapy can sometimes reduce the tumor bulk and may increase the chances of a limb-sparing procedure. Selective transcatheter intra-arterial chemotherapy has been employed to reduce systemic toxicity. Local recurrences are common

Outcomes of Treatment and Prognosis

The prognosis of PS/MFH becomes worse as the lesion is larger and deeper in the soft tissue. PS/MFH metastasizes to the lungs, lymph nodes, liver, and bone.

Synovial Sarcoma

Introduction and Definition

SS is the most common malignant soft tissue sarcoma in the foot, accounting for 18% to 22% of all such tumors. In some series, it is the single most common sarcoma of any type in the distal lower extremity. This tumor deserves the full attention of every foot and ankle specialist for several reasons. Among these is the slow, painless growth pattern that mimics a benign process, its peak incidence in young patients, and the serious consequences of delay in diagnosis.

SS was named in 1934 by Sabrazes based on what appeared to be synovial tissue on light microscopy. However, the name is misleading and bears no relation to the origin of the tumor. The inaccurate name continues to lead to mistaken assumptions about the location and behavior of the tumor. Recent complementary DNA microarray-based studies found that the gene expression profile of SS is closely related to neural crest–derived malignant peripheral nerve sheath tumor. SS displays two distinct types of chromosomal translocations t(X;18;p11;q11), named fusion type SYT-SSX1 and SYT-SSX2.

Incidence and Demographics

Most patients with SS are in their second through fifth decades, with the average age of incidence around 28 years, but SS can occur at any age. SS may occur anywhere in the leg, ankle, or foot.

Symptoms and Presentation

This tumor can exhibit slow, painless growth, and there are serious consequences due to the delay in diagnosis. The most common location is the leg, ankle, or foot. The presentation of SS is variable and may mimic a benign process such as ganglion cyst. The lesion is usually deeply seated, firm, and painless, but small subcentimeter lesions are also seen. The tumor is firm to examination and does not transilluminate. Metastasis may occur to regional lymph nodes and these should be included in the physical examination. The patient may have a mass that has been present for months, years, or even decades, with slow growth and little or no symptoms. There may have been recent rapid growth of a lesion that has been present for years without apparent change. Conversely, some SS may be very painful from the outset. The average duration of symptoms before diagnosis is 21 months.

X-ray Appearance and Advanced Imaging Findings

Imaging studies are not adequate to distinguish this tumor from benign soft tissue masses. Plain radiographs are still useful and may show the invasiveness and the stippled calcification some SSs have. MRI findings are "indeterminate" as defined previously, with intermediate or low signal intensity on T1 sequences and high signal intensity on T2 sequences. Axial imaging may reveal this lesion's potential to invade and destroy adjacent bones or soft tissues, but the tumor may appear well circumscribed. Most lesions present in stage II, which indicates it has spread beyond the compartment of origin. Imaging of regional lymph nodes should be included in the MRI examination.

Differential Diagnosis

Plantar fibroma can be surprisingly large and aggressive, and its appearance and location overlap with SS. Biopsy is recommended for all soft tissue tumors greater than 2 or 3 cm in the foot unless the diagnosis is otherwise established with certainty.

Histopathology Findings

High-grade, monophasic, poorly differentiated SS may appear to be a "small round blue cell tumor," a group of tumors that includes Ewing/primitive neuroectodermal tumor (PNET), rhabdomyosarcoma, lymphoma, and others. Final diagnosis requires immunohistochemical staining analysis. However, immunohistochemical markers such as epithelial membrane antigen (EMA) and cytokeratin that are considered to be the most specific for SS may be absent. Vimentin is typically positive in SS. EMA and cytokeratin are usually positive in SS. S-100 may be positive or negative in SS. On light microscopy, SS may be monophasic fibrous and biphasic. The monophasic type may appear to be a mass of small round blue cells, or more fibrous with spindle-shaped cells. The biphasic type is of fibrous areas with clefts or spaces or areas with epithelial cells.

Treatment Options for This Tumor

Surgical resection with a wide margin remains the cornerstone of treatment. Both chemotherapy and radiotherapy have been shown to have a positive effect on survival. In one series, 10 of 12 patients who had surgical treatment for SS in the foot required either a below-knee or a Chopart amputation.

Outcomes of Treatment and Prognosis

Overall prognosis of SS is only fair. Approximately 50% to 60% of patients will be free of disease at 5 years. There is an inverse correlation between prognosis and age at presentation. Distal lower extremity location may be a positive prognostic factor. Negative prognostic factors include large tumor size, high histologic grade, and metastasis at presentation.

Special and Unusual Features

Recent data have shown that SS displays two distinct types of chromosomal translocations t(X;18;p11;q11), named fusion type SYT-SSX1 and SYT-SSX2. Fusion type seems to have a significant impact on disease course and survival. In one study, median and 5-year overall survival for the SYT-SSX1 and SYT-SSX2 groups were 6.1 years and 53%, and 13.7 years and 73%, respectively.

Diagnostic Procedure

Imaging studies are not adequate to distinguish this tumor from benign soft tissue masses. Plain radiographs are recommended and may show the invasiveness of the lesion or the stippled calcification 30% of SSs have. MRI findings are indeterminate as defined previously, with intermediate or low signal intensity on T1 sequences and high signal intensity on T2 sequences. Axial imaging may reveal this lesion's potential to invade and destroy adjacent bones or soft tissues, but the tumor may appear well circumscribed.

Clear Cell Sarcoma

CCS, also known as malignant melanoma of soft parts, is an aggressive malignant sarcoma arising from melanoblasts that occur in tendons, aponeuroses, and subcutaneous tissues of the foot and ankle. This tumor is one of a group of rare malignancies associated with the gene fusion product EWSR1/ATF1 or EWSR1/CREB1, which includes CCS of the salivary gland, CCS of the gastrointestinal tract, and others. More than 90% of CCS have a reciprocal translocation t(12;22)(q13;q12). This rare tumor differs from malignant melanoma in both histology and natural history.

Although CCS accounts for only 1% of soft tissue sarcomas, surgeons who treat the foot and ankle should be familiar with its presentation and treatment due to the predilection of CCS for the lower extremity. More than 90% of cases in some series involve the lower extremity.[41] Unlike most sarcomas, CCS has a tendency to metastasize to lymph nodes. Late metastasis to locoregional nodes or lung may occur months or years after treatment. Long-term follow-up and surveillance for metastasis is warranted.

CCS may occur at any age including childhood, but is most likely to occur in adults 20 to 40 years of age. The tumor does not contain melanin pigment. Typical presentation of this tumor is of a benign, indolent appearing slow-growing soft tissue mass that is superficial or adjacent to a tendon or an aponeurosis in the ankle, the heel, or the plantar fascia. Average tumor size is 4 cm.[42]

Treatment depends on early recognition, comprehensive staging, and aggressive surgical extirpation of the tumor. The workup should include CT scan of the chest and MRI of the entire limb and locoregional lymph nodes. The mainstay of treatment is resection with a wide margin. Multiagent chemotherapy has not been shown to have any impact on survival.[43] Overall disease-free survival at 5 years is approximately 68%.[44] Tumor size appears to be a prognostic factor. Prognosis was dismal in cases where metastasis was present.[45]

Other Malignant Soft Tissue Tumors with Benign Clinical Appearance

Two other uncommon malignant soft tissue tumors also have a predilection for the foot. Acral myxoinflammatory fibroblastic sarcoma[46] and aggressive digital capillary adenocarcinoma[47] are indolent, often painless tumors that may mimic a benign process. Because these lesions may be mistaken for a skin condition such as a sebaceous cyst or a wart, it is recommended that all mass lesions removed from the foot be submitted for pathologic analysis to avoid a missed diagnosis in these potentially deadly tumors. Both these malignant tumors require aggressive surgical removal with wide margins, which usually requires at least a partial amputation.[46,48]

SECTION B:
Bone Tumors of the Foot and Ankle

The term "tumor" originates from the Latin tumere "to swell" and denotes any type of mass or swelling of bone or soft tissue. Bone tumors can arise from several causes, including hamartomas (an overgrowth of normal tissues), reactive or posttraumatic processes, and inflammatory lesions, or they may be benign or malignant neoplasms. The foot is comprised of numerous tightly confined and well-vascularized anatomic compartments that predispose to local and distant spread of disease. The clinician examining the patient presenting with a tumor of the foot or ankle must approach the problem in an informed and systematic fashion.

Tumors of the foot and ankle represent a unique subset of all bone and soft tissue tumors, showing variance in type, location, age, prognosis, and treatment from tumors in the rest of the musculoskeletal system. In large series of tumors of the entire skeleton, approximately 3% to 4% of all bone tumors are located in the bones of the foot. Bone tumors in this location are more common in males by a small margin. Most are cartilaginous or cystic, with a minority of tumors being osteoblastic.

Certain tumors are overrepresented in the bones of the foot, likely because of the unique structure and functional demands placed on the bones. For example, aneurysmal bone cyst (ABC), a tumor that may develop following injury or trauma, is more common than expected in the foot.[49] Chondromyxoid fibroma (CMF) and chondroblastoma are generally rare tumors, but for unknown reasons these lesions are relatively common in the foot.

For benign bone tumors, the optimal management strategy involves a careful evaluation and in many cases a preliminary biopsy so that the nature of the lesion is known with certainty before the definitive surgery is performed. After a benign tumor is fully characterized, surgical removal is usually performed by curettage or marginal excision, according to the type and location of the tumor.

Malignant tumors require a completely different and more comprehensive management strategy. Primary malignant tumors of mesenchymal origin are termed sarcomas. Although sarcomas in the foot and ankle are rare, there is a significant likelihood that foot and ankle surgeons will encounter one or more malignant foot and ankle tumors over the course of their practice. Treatment of bone sarcomas in the foot and ankle requires a timely and complete workup and staging of the tumor, as well as attention to avoidance of errors and delays in diagnosis and initial management. Surgery for sarcomas usually involves resection with a wide margin, and may include adjuvant chemotherapy and/or radiotherapy depending on tumor type. In the foot and ankle, adequate resection with a wide margin may require partial or complete amputation of the part.

Limb salvage for lower extremity sarcomas is preferred to amputation when it can be accomplished without compromising the oncologic outcome of the surgery. It has been shown to be equivalent to amputation in terms of functional outcome and overall patient survival.[50,51] Limb salvage following removal of tumors in the foot and ankle is complicated by the loads on the skeletal elements and the generally scant soft tissue coverage. These factors make the salvage of a viable, durable foot with useful function a major challenge in some instances. The goal of treatment in sarcomas is not necessarily preservation of the foot, but rather the elimination of the tumor and prompt restoration of the patient's quality of life, long-term mobility, and function.

PRESENTATION AND INITIAL ASSESSMENT

The patient presenting with a mass in the foot and ankle should have a complete history and physical examination. It is important to precisely determine the time of onset of the pain as well as the rate of progression and precise location. This will allow the clinician to determine whether the pain is actually coming from the tumor or from some nearby less worrisome abnormality.

Tumor pain, although variable, is usually a gradually progressive pain, well localized, that grows more persistent over many weeks or months. In many cases, the patient will ascribe the pain to some minor traumatic event. The examining physician is cautioned not to take these red-herring stories at face value. Careful questioning may reveal that the pain clearly predated the event.

For bone tumors, the physical examination can provide useful information pertaining to the diagnosis of the lesion. The examiner should note the palpable size, local extent, and the presence and dimensions of a palpable mass in the chart. The examination should also focus on the nearby structures of the foot or ankle to reveal possible pathology that may be causing the pain or disability. Any angular or positional deformity should be noted.

Patients beyond the age of 40 are at increased risk for metastatic cancer in the foot and ankle, and thus adults over 40 should be questioned about their personal history of cancer and cancer screening. The status of cancer screening examinations such as the prostate exam and prostate-specific antigen level in men, mammography in women, and low-dose CT scans of the chest in high-risk smokers should be noted. Risk factors for the five most common tumors that contribute to bone metastasis, which are lung, breast, prostate, kidney, and thyroid, should be enumerated. These include immediate family members with lung or breast cancer; known *BRCA1* and *BRCA2* genes; Von Hippel–Lindau disease; a history of smoking, radiation to the chest, or thyroid; exposure to radon and trichloroethylene; and obesity.

Some tumors and tumorlike lesions in the foot and ankle present simultaneously in multiple bones. This finding immediately limits the differential diagnosis to a small number of entities (Table 11-4). Combining this finding with other information from the history, images, and labs, the clinician may be able to easily confirm the correct diagnosis without the need for biopsy. The clinician should carefully inspect the X-rays and imaging studies for additional lesions. The multiple lesions that present in the foot and ankle are shown in Table 11-4.

Recommended Imaging Modalities

The initial screening examination of a bone tumor should always include two high-quality orthogonal plain radiographs. MRI is indicated in cases where a tumor is suspected due to positive local or systemic symptoms, but the initial X-rays are negative or where the X-ray findings do not explain the symptoms. No other imaging modalities are useful or recommended in the initial evaluation of a suspected bone tumor. Ultrasound, CT, and PET/CT are not recommended as part of a screening evaluation for a bone lesion of any type.[52]

Advanced imaging should not be ordered without careful consideration of the appropriateness of the study. Some bone lesions can be definitively diagnosed based on the history and plain radiographs, for example, intraosseous lipoma in the calcaneus, osteochondroma of the metatarsal, and enchondroma in the phalanges. In these cases, advanced imaging is unnecessary, and may incur a substantial and avoidable cost to the patient and to the health care system. Inappropriate imaging studies should be minimized. When advanced imaging studies are ordered, the single best study should be selected, rather than a multitude of studies. The diagnostic value of an MRI scan with and without contrast is generally somewhat superior to the value of a CT scan without contrast except in the evaluation of osteoid osteoma. Therefore, in most cases, the first advanced imaging modality selected should be MRI scan.

The indications for the use of CT scans in bone tumors of the foot and ankle include a bone lesion with possible cortical disruption or bone fragility, a calcific matrix that requires further evaluation, a suspected osteoid osteoma, or a bone lesion where previous metallic implants preclude the use of MRI. For the purpose of surgical planning, CT scans are very useful in evaluating the extent of bony involvement in the tarsal bones and hindfoot. CT imaging of bone is complementary and in some ways superior to MRI and is essential for the evaluation of mechanical integrity and fracture risk.

Appropriate criteria for the use of MRI for bone tumors of the foot and ankle include a destructive bone lesion, a biopsy suggestive of sarcoma or malignancy with no previous MRI, or an interosseous lesion of significant size or documented growth with uncertain etiology. The diagnostic usefulness of MRI scans with and without contrast is

Table 11-4. Tumors and Tumorlike Lesions That Present Simultaneously in Multiple Bones

Diagnosis	X-ray Appearance	Typical Presentation	Helpful Studies	Frequency
Gout	Multiple punched-out lesions at margins of joints	Older, male, admitted for "cellulitis of foot"	Serum uric acid CT or MRI shows multiple typical lesions	Common
PVNS	Cysts in bone on both sides of the involved joint	Younger person, ankle most common	MRI shows thick synovium and cysts, MRI "signal void" in synovium due to iron in tissues	Infrequent
Synovial chondromatosis	Multiple lobules of calcified cartilage in joint	Young to middle age adult, ankle and midfoot	MRI findings are diagnostic	Uncommon
Metastatic adenocarcinoma	Multiple adjacent bones with aggressive lytic lesions	Older person, usually has known history of carcinoma	Bone scan usually will show multiple bone lesions	Uncommon
Multiple myeloma	Multiple small punched-out lesions	Age 50–70	Serum protein electrophoresis	Rare in the bones of the foot
Multiple cartilaginous exostoses	Multiple sessile or pedunculated exostoses in ankle and metatarsal lesions	Young adult	X-rays are diagnostic	Rare
Enchondromatosis (Ollier disease)	Multiple expansile lucent lesions in metatarsals and phalanges	Young adult	Skeletal survey and X-rays of hands confirm diagnosis	Rare

CT, computed tomography; MRI, magnetic resonance imaging; PVNS, pigmented villonodular synovitis.

somewhat higher than noncontrast scans; therefore, MRI scans should be performed with contrast if possible. Bone scans are indicated when the differential diagnosis or biopsy is highly consistent or conclusive for malignancy, metastatic disease, or multifocal systemic disease, and for the evaluation of a possible stress fracture. Indications for PET/CT scans include staging of cancers involving the breast, colon and rectum, esophagus, head and neck, lung, lymphoma, melanoma, and sarcoma.[53]

BENIGN BONE TUMORS

Giant Cell Tumor

Introduction, Incidence, and Demographics

Giant cell tumor accounts for 5% to 9% of all primary bony tumors[54,55]: It is the most common benign bone tumor in adults aged 25 to 40. Giant cell tumor is found more commonly in women than in men, and occurs most often during the third decade.[56] This tumor is most commonly found in the distal femur, proximal tibia, and distal radius, and is uncommon in the foot. Approximately 3% of giant cell tumors affect the bones of the foot. Giant cell tumor is one of the most common primary bone lesions in the distal phalanx. Whether that tumor arises in the epiphysis or distal metaphysis is a matter of controversy, but giant cell tumors only occur after the epiphyseal plates have closed. A diagnosis of giant cell tumor in a patient with open growth plates should be questioned. Giant cell tumor of bone is a benign lesion that is usually solitary and locally aggressive (**Fig. 11-1**).

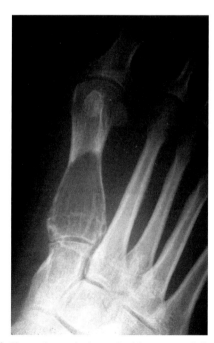

FIGURE 11-1. Giant cell tumor in the proximal 1st metatarsal of a 36-year-old female. The tumor is characteristically a lytic lesion in the metaphysis extending to the joint level but preserving the subchondral bone.

It is believed by some to be potentially malignant. In very rare instances, this lesion has the potential for metastasis to the lungs. In these cases, the lung lesions may behave in an indolent fashion and even require no treatment. The authors recommend a chest CT scan for all patients newly diagnosed with giant cell tumor.

Symptoms and Presentation

Most patients present with slowly progressive pain, with or without a mass. Symptoms arise when the lesion begins to destroy the cortex and irritate the periosteum or when the weakening of the bone causes pain due to pathologic fracture. Some giant cell tumors present after a pathologic fracture.

X-ray Appearance and Advanced Imaging Findings

The lesion originates in the metaphyseal segment of the bone adjacent to the physeal scar, and expands proximally and distally into the diaphysis and epiphysis. The tumor will grow until it reaches the subchondral surface of the joint, which forms a partial barrier against further tumor extension. The adjacent cortex may be expanded, thin, or destroyed, and the tumor can extend into the nearby soft tissues. There may be numerous septae or longitudinal striations in the involved bone. The zone of transition is a few millimeters wide, there is no permeation, and there is no matrix mineralization. These tumors often thin the cortex, and may expand into the soft tissues surrounding the bone, or they may expand the bone extensively, remaining within an eggshell-thin rim of periosteal new bone. If the lesion has been present long enough, the involved bone can become expanded to many times its original volume. CT scan will define the local extent of the tumor and help confirm the absence of matrix mineralization. MRI findings are nondiagnostic, although the lesions tend to be highly heterogeneous if they are large enough. There may be cystic loculated blood-filled internal spaces. Bone scan findings are nonspecific.

Histopathology Findings

The gross appearance of the giant cell tumor is firm and homogeneous, with foci of hemorrhage or necrosis. Microscopically, there are numerous multinucleated giant cells. The stromal cells are homogeneous mononuclear cells with round or ovoid shapes, large nuclei, and indistinct nucleoli. The nuclei of the stromal cells are identical to the nuclei in the giant cells, a feature that distinguishes giant cell tumors from other lesions that also contain giant cells. Another feature of giant cell tumor is that the giant cells may contain very large numbers of nuclei, often several hundred. In some tumors, the giant cells can be seen to be engulfing more nuclei from the stroma.

Differential Diagnosis

Other aggressive tumors in this age group and location include ABC, sarcomas in bone such as MFH, and desmoplastic fibroma.

Treatment Options and Outcomes

Treatment of giant cell tumors is by intralesional excision by "extended" curettage. Curettage alone is associated with a high recurrence rate. Recurrence can be decreased by "extended" curettage that involves the application of a local adjuvant treatment to the tumor cavity after mechanical curettage is complete. This treatment is designed to eliminate any viable tumor cells that remain in the walls of the tumor cavity after mechanical curettage. Available local adjuvant treatment choices include chemical cautery using phenol; multiple freeze–thaw cycles using liquid nitrogen; and/or treating the walls of the cavity with a high-speed rotary burr. All of these have been shown to decrease the risk of local recurrence. The author's preference is the high-speed burr, because of availability, ease, and precision of application. Local recurrence after curettage alone may be as high as 50%. Recurrence after extended curettage is 10%.[57]

The tumor cavity may be filled with polymethylmethacrylate cement (PMMA) or bone graft, according to the surgeon's preference. Some believe that PMMA lowers the risk of a local recurrence due to the large amount of heat given off during hardening. Recurrences are normally treated with a second interlesional surgery. The use of bone graft to fill the tumor cavity instead of PMMA may allow for more favorable biomechanical loads on the nearby joint and decrease the risk of late arthrosis. However, the recurrence rate is higher when bone graft is used instead of PMMA.[58] The early signs of local recurrence may be more difficult to detect in cases treated with bone graft.

Lesions that are highly expansile and destructive or lesions that occur in "expendable" bones such as the proximal fibula may be excised with a wide margin. Multiply recurrent giant cell tumors are also treated with wide resection. Giant cell tumors may occur in the sacrum, a site where complete surgical excision is very difficult. Intralesional removal of as much of the lesion as possible followed by radiation to the tumor site has been associated with acceptable tumor control. There is concern about secondary malignancy arising in irradiated giant cell tumors. A variety of reconstructive methods are utilized depending on the extent of bony defect, or no reconstruction may be necessary. Chemotherapy is not used.

Outcomes of Treatment and Prognosis

Following surgery, patients should be made aware of the ongoing risk of local recurrence. Patients should be followed on a regular basis for the first 2 years at least. Metastasis to the lungs is more common in axial lesions, locally aggressive lesions, and recurrent lesions. Local recurrence of giant cell tumor should trigger a complete workup for metastasis for the lung including CT scan of the chest.

Osteochondroma

Introduction and Definition

Osteochondroma, or osteocartilaginous exostosis, is the most common skeletal neoplasm. This cartilage-capped subperiosteal bone projection accounts for 20% to 50% of

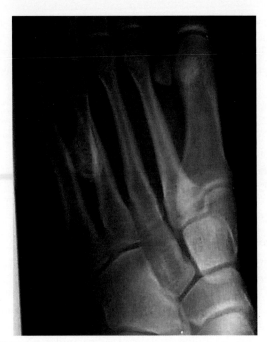

FIGURE 11-2. A solitary pedunculated osteochondroma on the metatarsal of a 17-year-old girl. There had been an injury to the area at age 12.

benign bone tumors and 10% to 15% of all bone tumors. The cause of solitary osteochondromas is unknown. Hereditary multiple osteochondroma (HMO), also termed hereditary multiple exostoses, is an autosomal dominant bone disorder in which most individuals show mutations of the *EXT1* or *EXT2* genes on chromosomes 8 and 11. The disease manifestations encompass multiple benign cartilage-capped tumors, short stature, growth disturbance and deformity, joint dysfunction, premature osteoarthritis, and malignant degeneration of the osteochondromas in 1% to 4% of individuals.[59,60] Osteochondromas can be either flattened (sessile) or stalk-like (exostosis) and appear in a juxta-epiphyseal location. Osteochondromas can occur as a result of radiation therapy in children. After the closure of the growth plate in late adolescence, there is normally no further growth of the osteochondroma (**Fig. 11-2**).

Incidence and Demographics

The lesions occur only in bones that develop from cartilage (endochondral ossification). Osteochondromas are found most often in long bones, especially the distal femur and proximal tibia, with 40% of the tumors occurring around the knee. The distal tibia and fibula are a relatively common site. Osteochondroma is uncommon in the bones of the foot. It usually occurs in the forefoot on a metatarsal. Osteochondromas occur most frequently in the first two decades of life, with a ratio of males to females of 1.5:1.

Symptoms and Presentation

Clinically, osteochondromas present with pain due to mechanical irritation or a painless mass. A fracture can occur through the stalk of the lesion, which also causes pain. Osteochondromas are relatively common on the distal fibula and tibia, where they can cause growth disturbance, mechanical impingement, recurrent sprains, ankle stiffness, subluxation of the ankle tendons, or a palpable mass. In HMO, differential longitudinal growth of the tibia and fibula leads to valgus deformity of the ankle. Patients with HMO may present in early adulthood with ankle pain, instability, and valgus.

X-ray Appearance and Advanced Imaging Findings

Plain films are normally enough to diagnose osteochondromas. Sessile lesions cover a wide area and as a result cause metaphyseal widening or a "trumpet-shaped deformity" on X-ray. Lesions with stalks are often found more distally. The lesion appears as a pedunculated or sessile mature bony mass on the surface of the metaphyseal portion of the bone. The cortex of the lesion is continuous with the nearby normal cortex. CT scans can be helpful, because the pathognomonic appearance of the lesion can be verified. The CT scan should show that the cortex and medullary cavity of the underlying bone are continuous with the cortex and medullary cavity of the lesion. MRI scans are helpful in evaluating the thickness of the cartilage cap. Growth of the cartilage cap or growth of the lesion after skeletal maturity is a worrisome finding and should be investigated as a potential sign of malignant degeneration. The relationship of the lesion to other structures and the thickness of the cartilage cap is best delineated with MRI.

Histopathology Findings

On gross examination, an osteochondroma is an irregular bony mass with a bluish-gray cap of cartilage. Opaque yellow cartilage has calcification within the matrix. The base of the lesion has a rim of cortical bone and central cancellous bone. Occasionally, a bursa develops over an osteochondroma. Normally, the cartilage cap ranges from 1 to 6 mm thick. Over 2 cm of cartilage thickness or renewed growth of a dormant lesion is a sign of possible malignant transformation. Under the microscope, an osteochondroma has endochondral ossification on the basal surface of hyaline cartilage so it resembles a normal, albeit disorganized growth plate. The benign cartilage is less spatially organized, has binucleate chondrocytes in lacunae, and is covered with a thin layer of periosteum.

Treatment Options for This Tumor

There is no treatment necessary for asymptomatic osteochondromas. Symptomatic lesions may be treated with simple excision by osteotomy through the base of the lesion. The surgeon does not need to remove every vestige of the lesion to achieve resolution of the symptoms. Treatment should be delayed until skeletal maturity in all cases. At that time the lesions are better defined and easier to remove, and the active cartilaginous portion of the lesion is located farther from the underlying bone. If the entire active cartilaginous portion of the lesion is not removed, recurrence may follow. Distal fibular and tibial lesions often impinge on the adjacent tibia or fibula and require removal.

In HMO, multiple lesions in the distal leg result in differential longitudinal growth of the tibia and fibula leading to ankle

valgus.[61] Epiphysiodesis of the medial malleolus is performed to reduce or correct valgus. Supramalleolar osteotomy of the tibia for correction of ankle valgus is performed in severe or neglected cases. After tibial epiphysiodesis for correction of ankle valgus, removal of hardware prior to skeletal maturity has been associated with rebound of valgus deformity.[62]

Outcomes of Treatment and Prognosis

As long as the entire cartilage cap is removed, there should be no recurrence. Patients with many, especially large, osteochondromas should have regular screening exams and radiographs to detect malignant transformation early.

Enchondroma

Introduction and Definition

Enchondroma is a solitary, benign, intramedullary cartilage tumor that is often found in the short tubular bones of the hands and feet, distal femur, and proximal humerus. The peak incidence is in the third decade and is equal between men and women.

Multiple enchondromatosis is a nonheritable condition also known as Ollier disease. Multiple enchondromas and hemangiomas of soft tissue constitute a condition known as Maffucci syndrome (**Fig. 11-3**).

Incidence and Demographics

The peak incidence is in the third decade and is equal between men and women. It is the most common primary tumor in the hand and is normally found in the diaphysis. The mature hyaline cartilage located centrally within short tubular bones usually presents clinically as a fracture due to an enlarging lesion. Enchondromas are also found incidentally in long

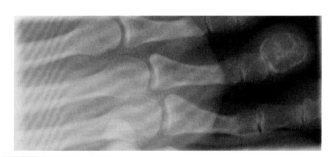

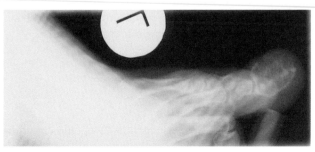

FIGURE 11-3. AP and lateral radiographs showing an expansile enchondroma of the distal phalanx in a 34-year-old woman with mild activity-related pain and enlargement of the toe.

bones and undergo malignant transformation in less than 1% of cases. Approximately 8% of these tumors occur in the bones of the foot. The peak age at diagnosis is around the middle of the fourth decade, but the tumor may present at virtually any age. Enchondroma usually occurs in the metatarsals or phalanges of the lesser toes. The hindfoot is rarely involved.

Symptoms and Presentation

Most patients have no symptoms. The most common presentation is a patient who has injured their ankle or foot and who has an X-ray, leading to the discovery of the previously asymptomatic lesion. Lesions in the hands and the feet may weaken the bone and cause pain, swelling, and small pathologic fractures during activities. Patients present with pain during activities or after an injury, but there is rarely any mass palpable on physical examination. Occasionally, pathologic fracture through the lesion will cause the patient to seek medical care.

X-ray Appearance and Advanced Imaging Findings

Enchondromas are usually elongated, oval with well-defined margins, and may have punctate or ring and arc-like calcifications. In larger lesions or in smaller bones, the lucent defect has endosteal scalloping and the cortex is expanded and thinned. Calcifications throughout the lesion can range from punctate to rings. In the small bones of the foot, particularly the phalanges, benign enchondromas may have worrisome X-ray features that are associated with chondrosarcoma in other locations. In the phalanges, enchondroma may cause dramatic bone expansion, bone deformation, cortical destruction, or a soft tissue mass outside the bone. In a large bone, these X-ray findings would indicate that the tumor is likely to be malignant chondrosarcoma, but in small bones these behaviors are consistent with a benign tumor.

CT is useful for detecting matrix mineralization and cortex integrity. MRI is helpful for describing the nonmineralized portion of the lesion and visualizing any aggressive or destructive features. Radiographic and imaging features of enchondroma that are considered worrisome because of an observed higher incidence of malignancy include large size, a large unmineralized component, significant thinning of the adjacent cortex, and bone scan activity greater than that of the anterior superior iliac spine. Features of enchondroma that are very strongly associated with malignant transformation are progressive destruction of the chondroid matrix by an expanding, nonmineralized component, an enlarging lesion associated with pain, or an expansile soft tissue mass.

Laboratory Findings

No laboratory examination is helpful.

Differential Diagnosis

Other cartilaginous lesions, such as low-grade chondrosarcoma, CMF, and chondroblastoma, and lesions with scattered densification such as fibrous dysplasia should be considered. If there is definite growth of the lesion, a definite pain from the lesion, or a lesion in a large bone is acting in an aggressive manner, such as damaging the cortex or breaking out into the soft tissues, a different diagnosis should be considered.

Preferred Biopsy Technique for This Tumor

Minimally invasive techniques are sufficient in lesions that are documented to be latent by radiologic examination.

Histopathology Findings

On gross examination, an enchondroma consists of bluish-gray lobules of fine translucent tissue. The degree of calcification of the lesion determines if the consistency is gritty. Under the microscope, a thin layer of lamellar bone surrounding the cartilage nodules is a positive sign that the lesion is benign. At low power, there are lobules of different sizes. Blood vessels are surrounded by osteoid. Enchondromas have chondrocytes without atypia inside hyaline cartilage. The nuclei are small, round, and pyknotic. The cellularity varies between lesions and within the same lesion. Each potential enchondroma needs to be evaluated for cellularity, nuclear atypia, double nucleated chondrocytes, and mitotic activity in a viable area without calcifications to distinguish it from low-grade chondrosarcoma. Small peripheral lesions are more likely to be benign than large axial lesions. The pathologic diagnosis is so difficult that it always needs to be made in conjunction with the radiologist and the surgeon.

Treatment Options for This Tumor

Asymptomatic, latent lesions that do not cause bone fragility may be observed without biopsy. This type is commonly encountered in the distal femur and proximal humerus. In the small bones of the foot, enchondromas are more likely to become symptomatic due to expansion and weakening of the cortex and pathologic fracture. Painful or problematic enchondromas can be treated with simple curettage and packing with bone graft. Recurrence is rare. Extremely expansile lesions may require complete excision and substitution of a structural allograft. Large lesions in the distal phalanges that have dramatically expanded the bone should be considered for partial amputation of the toe, because the functional and cosmetic result of curettage and bone grafting may be unacceptable.

All specimens must be analyzed carefully for malignancy. Small, peripheral cartilage tumors tend to be benign, whereas large central cartilage lesions are more likely to be malignant. Reliable differentiation of benign from malignant cartilage tumors is difficult. Tumors that are larger, tumors located in the hindfoot or midfoot, or new tumors presenting in a patient with a known history of enchondromatosis (Ollier disease) have an increased risk of malignancy.

Preferred Margin for This Tumor

Intralesional.

Outcomes of Treatment and Prognosis

Removal of enchondroma is curative. The lesions do not grow; therefore, recurrence is not expected. Recurrence of the lesions considered to be an enchondroma may be a sign that the lesion is actually a low-grade chondrosarcoma.

Special and Unusual Features

Multiple enchondromatosis is a nonheritable condition also known as Ollier disease. Multiple enchondromas and hemangiomas of soft tissue are otherwise known as Maffucci syndrome. In both conditions, men are affected more than women, and the disease process often only affects one side of the body. In both diseases, there is a 30% risk of malignant transformation of the enchondromas.[63] Chondrosarcoma is much more common in older patients, so large enchondromas in older individuals demand a careful workup.

Chondromyxoid Fibroma

CMF is a rare benign cartilage tumor that also has myxoid and fibrous elements. It is extremely uncommon and accounts for less that 1% of all bone tumors. CMF has a predilection for the bones of the lower extremity and the foot.[64] CMF is found most often in the metaphysis around the knee in the proximal tibia, proximal fibula, or distal femur. Recent studies have pointed to anomalies in chromosome 6 as a possible genetic factor in CMF. The breakpoint on the long arm of chromosome 6 appears to involve *COL12A1* gene, a collagen gene that may play a role in another tumor, subungual exostosis (**Fig. 11-4**).

Incidence and Demographics

It presents in the second to third decade and has a male to female ratio of 2:1. This rare benign tumor has a predilection for the bones of the tibia and the foot. Most patients are younger than 30. It is more common in males, typically in the second or third decade of life. About one-quarter of all of these tumors involve the foot, with the metatarsals the most common location.

Symptoms and Presentation

The clinical presentation is usually chronic pain, swelling, and possibly a palpable soft tissue mass or restriction of movement. Only 5% of patients with CMF present with a pathologic fracture.

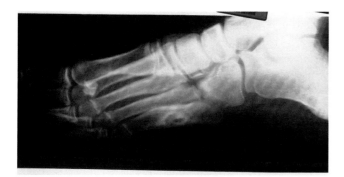

FIGURE 11-4. Chondromyxoid fibroma in the 5th metatarsal of a 15-year-old boy.

X-ray Appearance and Advanced Imaging Findings

Radiologic findings demonstrate an eccentrically placed lytic lesion with well-defined margins. It is an expansile, lobulated, lytic lesion in the metaphysis with partial cortical erosion and local extension into the soft tissue. There may be a sclerotic margin, and the long axis is typically parallel to the bone. The lesion usually has a sclerotic margin of bone and a lobulated contour. Ridges and grooves that appear in the margins secondary to scalloping falsely appear to be trabeculae. CT helps define cortical integrity and confirms that there is no mineralization of the matrix, unlike other cartilage tumors. CMF has the same appearance on MRI as other cartilage tumors, which is decreased signal on T1-weighted images and increased signal on T2-weighted images. MRI is helpful in preoperative planning and staging.

Differential Diagnosis

Giant cell tumor, ABC, unicameral bone cyst (UBC), chondroblastoma, fibrous dysplasia, osteosarcoma.

Preferred Biopsy Technique for This Tumor

Open incisional.

Histopathology Findings

CMF resembles fibrocartilage grossly. It has a sharp border often with an outer surface of thin bone or periosteum. The glistening grayish-white lesion is firm and lobulated. It may also have small cystic foci or areas of hemorrhage. Histologically, CMF appears very similar to chondrosarcoma. They are so close in histology that often radiology helps to make the final diagnosis. The predominant features of CMF are the zonal architecture and lobular pattern. Nodules of cartilage are found in between fibromyxoid areas. In some fields, the loose myxoid dominates and in others the dense chondroid dominates. The chondrocytes are plump to spindly in shape and have indistinct cell borders in sparsely cellular lobules of myxoid or chondroid matrix. There are also more cellular zones of the tumor, with some giant cells at the edges. The sharp borders of each lobule and the lesion itself help to differentiate it from chondrosarcoma.

Treatment Options for This Tumor

Curettage may be adequate, but may result in local recurrence in as many as a quarter to one-third of patients. Unlike giant cell tumor, this tumor has a propensity to recur due to seeding of the soft tissues during curettage. Local recurrence can be treated with meticulous repeat curettage and excision of the entire soft tissue mass. Marginal or wide excision and substitution of the involved bone with a structural bone graft is usually curative. If possible, the initial treatment of CMF should favor en bloc excision.

Osteoid Osteoma

Introduction and Definition

Osteoid osteoma is a benign bone lesion with a nidus of less than 2 cm surrounded by a zone of reactive bone. This lesion accounts for approximately 10% of benign bone tumors (**Fig. 11-5**).

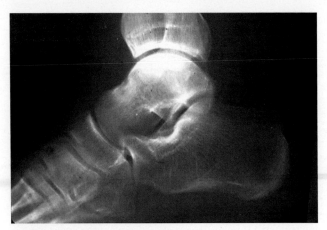

FIGURE 11-5. Osteoid osteoma of the talar neck.

Incidence and Demographics

The tumor occurs most frequently in the second decade, with a peak age in the early twenties, and affects males twice as often as females. The proximal femur is the most common location followed by the tibia, posterior elements of the spine, and the humerus. Osteoid osteoma is found in the diaphysis or the metaphysis of the proximal end of the bone more often than the distal end. Approximately 11% of these painful, benign tumors occur in the bones of the foot. The neck of the talus is the most common location.

Symptoms and Presentation

Patients present with persistent pain and swelling, which is unrelated to activity. The pain may be more intense at night. In most cases, NSAIDs give substantial relief, and any history of taking these medicines should be carefully reviewed. The pain is often described as dull and decreases within 20 to 30 minutes of treatment with NSAIDs. If there is absolutely no relief of pain from taking NSAIDs, the diagnosis of osteoid osteoma is less likely. Lesions adjacent to a joint may cause ankylosis or mimic a pauciarticular inflammatory arthritis, such as Reiter disease. Local symptoms can include an increase in skin temperature and increased sweating and tenderness. Epiphyseal lesions can cause abnormal growth. The local swelling, erythema, and tenderness can mimic infection. When there is significant involvement of a nearby joint, the relief from NSAIDs can be less dramatic.

X-ray Appearance and Advanced Imaging Findings

The classic radiologic presentation of an osteoid osteoma is a radiolucent nidus surrounded by a dramatic reactive sclerosis in the cortex of the bone. The center can range from partially mineralized to osteolytic to entirely calcified. The lesion can occur only in the cortex, in both the cortex and medulla, or only the medulla. The reactive sclerosis may be present or absent. The four diagnostic features include (1) a sharp round or oval lesion that (2) is less than 2 cm in diameter, (3) has a homogeneous dense center, and (4) has a 1 to 2 mm peripheral radiolucent zone. Bone scan shows a small, very intense focus of abnormal uptake. MRI findings

are nonspecific. CT is the preferred method of evaluation, especially if the lesion is in the cortex or obscured by reactive sclerosis. Characteristic plain radiograph, CT scan, and bone scan findings are sufficient to confirm the diagnosis of this tumor.

Differential Diagnosis

Osteoblastoma, osteomyelitis (Brodie abscess), arthritis, stress fracture and enostosis/bone island.

Histopathology Findings

On gross examination, osteoid osteoma is a brownish-red, mottled, and gritty lesion that is distinct from the surrounding bone. It can be present in the cortex or medullary canal. Osteoclasts are present. The nidus is surrounded by sclerotic bone with thickened trabeculae. Microscopically, the nidus consists of a combination of osteoid and woven bone surrounded by osteoblasts. The oval-shaped nidus is well vascularized and clearly separate from the reactive woven or lamellar bone.

Treatment Options for This Tumor

Surgical removal is not mandatory for this lesion. Patients whose pain and dysfunction respond well to NSAIDs and aspirin may be successfully treated with these medications until the lesion disappears. The average time to resolution is 22 months. Some patients will not be able to tolerate medical treatment, and request surgical removal. For these cases, the goal is complete removal of the lesion by the least invasive means possible. Occasionally, the tumor is an unexpected finding during an arthroscopy of the ankle. Juxta-articular and subperiosteal lesions of the talus have been treated with unplanned arthroscopic excision using a motorized shaver, with variable results.

For lesions in the distal tibia and fibula, hindfoot, and midfoot, radiothermal ablation by CT-guided needle is the recommended technique.[65] During radiothermal ablation, the tip of a radiofrequency generator electrode is placed into the center of the lesion under CT guidance and general anesthesia. A radiofrequency generator forms an alternating high-frequency radio wave that passes from the electrode tip into the surrounding tissue, where energy is dissipated as heat. The tissue itself is heated, not the radiofrequency probe. A sphere with a diameter of 1 cm can be effectively treated in this manner, making this treatment ideal for osteoid osteoma. In order to be treated with radialthermal ablation, the diagnosis should be confirmed based on the imaging studies with a high degree of confidence. There should be sufficient distance between the lesion and any major neurovascular structure. The lesion should have a clearly formed nidus less than 1 cm in largest dimension. Although radiothermal ablation was previously only available in tertiary medical centers, it is now more widely available. The high success rate combined with the extremely low rate of complications strongly favors this technique. Recurrence of pain can be treated with repeat radiofrequency ablation or open surgical removal of the lesion.

Radiothermal ablation can be difficult in the smaller bones because of difficulties with targeting the lesion in the CT scanner. In addition, when the lesion is in a small bone, there is risk of damage to nearby tendons or neurovascular structures. For superficial lesions in the forefoot, open surgery is still the preferred treatment. The surgeon needs to be able to locate the nidus using radiographs, anatomic landmarks, and direct observation. Other techniques for locating the nidus have been described. The surrounding reactive bone can be extremely dense, and it may also be hypervascular and somewhat porous. It is essential to remove the entire nidus because failure to do so will lead to recurrence. Surgical removal often leads to weakening of the affected bone, and bone grafting, plating, and prolonged nonweight-bearing with activity restrictions may be necessary.

Osteoblastoma

Introduction and Definition

Osteoblastoma is a solitary, benign bone-forming tumor that occurs in the posterior elements of the spine and long bones of young adults. The bones of the foot are the third most common location of this tumor, accounting for 12% of all osteoblastomas in one series.[66] Although osteoblastoma and osteoid osteoma are histologically quite similar, these two tumors are very different in their presentation, localization, radiographic appearance, treatment, and potential for recurrence.

Incidence and Demographics

The tumor most commonly occurs in the dorsal aspect of the vertebrae, the metaphysis or diaphysis of long bones, and rarely in the pelvis. In the spine, the tumor is usually located in the posterior processes while the vertebral bodies are spared. Also, though tumor frequency is lower in the thoracic region of the spine, it has greater and equal occurrence in the cervical and lumbar regions. The foot is the third most common location of osteoblastoma after the spine and the femur; 12.5% of osteoblastomas occur in the bones of the foot. Most occur in the hind foot, and the talus is the most commonly affected bone. Osteoblastoma predominantly affects young adults. The peak age of occurrence is approximately age 20, though the tumor may present as early as age 10 to as late as age 60. The mean age of the patient is about 22 years.

Symptoms and Presentation

Common symptoms are pain of long duration, swelling, and tenderness. Tumors of the spine can cause scoliosis and neurologic symptoms. Spinal lesions may present with myelopathic and/or radicular symptoms.

X-ray Appearance and Advanced Imaging Findings

On X-ray, osteoblastomas appear as a radiolucent defect with a central density due to ossification. The lesion is well circumscribed and may have a surrounding sclerosis. The tumor demonstrates increased isotope uptake on bone scan.

Differential Diagnosis

The differential diagnosis of osteoblastoma includes osteoid osteoma, osteosarcoma, giant cell tumor, and ABC.

Histopathology Findings

On gross examination, osteoblastomas are red to tan in color with hemorrhagic areas. The compact tissue is granular, friable, and gritty. Hyperemia is particularly evident in the spongy bone of vertebrae, ribs, and the pelvis. The classic microscopic finding of osteoblastoma is irregular spicules of mineralized bone and eosinophilic osteoid rimmed by osteoblasts. The vascular stroma is characterized by pleomorphic spindle cells. The tumor cells differentiate into osteoblasts, which make varying amounts of osteoid and woven bone. Cartilage production is a very rare finding in an osteoblastoma and should raise the suspicion of osteosarcoma.

Treatment Options for This Tumor

Usually, a biopsy is performed to confirm the diagnosis. Surgical resection by curettage, intralesional excision, or en bloc excision are all treatment options depending on the site. Recurrence after surgery is approximately 10% to 15%. Bone grafting is commonly used after curettage of these lesions, but complete healing may still occur without bone grafting.

There remains some concern for malignant degeneration of osteoblastoma because of a few published reports of malignant sarcomas arising in osteoblastoma. In addition, a subset of these tumors can behave in a much more locally aggressive fashion. These tumors have been found to be larger and occur in slightly older individuals. Microscopically, this more aggressive variant of osteoblastoma may have a distinct appearance, including epithelioid features and larger osteoblasts with abundant eosinophilic cytoplasm and vesicular nuclei. There is a lack of consensus as to what histologic characteristics are associated with more or less aggressive behavior.[66] These tumors have been variously termed "aggressive osteoblastoma" or "malignant osteoblastoma." The radiographic and pathologic features of these tumors overlap with osteosarcoma. In one review of 41 osteoblastomas in the foot, 2 evolved into malignant sarcomas.

Preferred Margin for This Tumor

Margins should be as wide as possible without functional sacrifice.

Special and Unusual Features

Osteoid osteoma and osteoblastoma can be differentiated because the former causes persistent nocturnal pain and the latter causes inconsistent pain. The former is less than 1 cm and the latter greater than 2 cm.

Chondroblastoma

Introduction and Definition

Chondroblastoma is a rare, benign tumor derived from chondroblasts. It is found in the epiphysis of long bones, usually of the lower extremity. The most common site is the distal femur followed by the proximal femur, proximal humerus, and proximal tibia. This is one of a very few lesions that occur primarily in the epiphysis. Others include clear cell chondrosarcoma and osteomyelitis. In addition, very rare cases of metastasis of chondroblastoma to the lungs have been reported.

Incidence and Demographics

Chondroblastoma accounts for approximately 1% of benign bone tumors, but around 10% to 15% of these rare tumors occur in the bones of the foot. The tumor is much more common in males than females, and the mean age of presentation is approximately 20 years. Males are affected five to six times as commonly as females. The average age at presentation in the foot is around 25 years, significantly older than the average age in other parts of the skeleton. In the foot, chondroblastoma is most commonly located in the posterior subchondral surfaces of the talus and calcaneus, in the calcaneal apophysis, and in the midtarsal bones.

Symptoms and Presentation

Patients complain of pain with or without a mass near a joint. The pain can be severe. The nearby joint may be locally inflamed. There is poor response to NSAIDs. Eventually, a mass appears.

X-ray Appearance and Advanced Imaging Findings

The diagnosis of chondroblastoma can usually be made by radiograph when the age of the patient and location of the lesion are considered. The most common site for chondroblastoma is the epiphysis. The lesion is lytic with well-defined margins and can be from 1 to 6 cm in size. Scalloping or expansion of cortical bone may be present. Fine calcifications, either punctate or in rings, may be visible. In the foot and ankle, the lesion is located exclusively in the epiphysis, although in the small bones of the foot the location of the epiphysis may not be obvious. The lesions appear well defined, expansile, and lucent, and there may be stippled calcification or there may be no matrix mineralization. Cystic features are seen in approximately half the chondroblastomas of the foot bones. The tumor is adjacent to an articular surface or an apophysis. Chondroblastoma in the foot most commonly occurs in subchondral areas of the talus and calcaneus as well as the calcaneal apophysis.

CT scan is useful for defining the relationship of the tumor to the joint and the integrity of the underlying bone and to identify intralesional calcifications. Cysts are present about 20% of the time, and both MRI and CT can define the fluid levels.

Differential Diagnosis

The differential diagnosis includes enchondroma, central chondrosarcoma, and ABC.

Preferred Biopsy Technique for This Tumor

Incisional, may be combined with excision in selected cases.

Histopathology Findings

On gross examination, a chondroblastoma has a lobulated, round form and is made up of friable, soft, grayish-pink tissue that may be gritty. If present, the cystic fluid is rust or straw colored. Chondroblastoma is made up of uniform, polygonal cells that are closely packed. These primitive cells are derived from the epiphyseal cartilage plate and have abundant cytoplasm. These cells have oval-shaped nuclei with a prominent groove that has been likened to a coffee bean. There is little mitotic activity. A scant chondroid matrix may be superimposed by a pericellular deposit of calcification that appears like "chicken wire." The rapid proliferation of immature chondrocytes does not create lacunae or formal cartilage matrix. Giant cells are often present.

Treatment Options for This Tumor

Treatment of the primary lesion consists of complete curettage and bone grafting. Extending the zone of the curettage by removing two or three additional millimeters of bone using a mechanical burr, or by placing phenol or liquid nitrogen in the tumor cavity has been proposed as a method to reduce the risk of local recurrence. Because of the risk of recurrence and associated functional loss, the initial curettage should be as meticulous as necessary to ensure complete removal of the lesion. The surgical approach chosen and bone window created should allow complete visualization of the entire extent of the lesion. Minimally invasive techniques that provide restricted access to the lesion should be used with caution due to the elevated risk of recurrence. It may be necessary to reconstruct articular surfaces due to subchondral erosion. Any joint invasion is usually secondary to previous instrumentation.

Recurrence is common, and recurrent lesions should be treated with repeat curettage. If a recurrent lesion is located in a readily reconstructable location, marginal resection with structural allograft or autograft reconstruction is preferable. Recurrence and severe destruction of bone integrity in the foot and ankle may necessitate ankle arthrodesis or en bloc resection with associated functional loss. Chondroblastoma can behave aggressively and invade soft tissue, and metastasize to the lungs. Patients with recurrent lesions should have follow-up CT scans of the chest to detect pulmonary nodules. Benign pulmonary metastases have been treated with observation as well as excision via thoracoscopy.

Preferred Margin for This Tumor

Intralesional.

Outcomes of Treatment and Prognosis

Functional outcomes of surgical treatment of chondroblastoma are generally good, provided the tumor is not discovered very late and that the tumor does not recur. For lesions located in the proximal part of the femur and in the foot and ankle, recurrence is common, and outcomes are generally worse than in other locations in the skeleton. The risk of recurrence appears to be highest for lesions located only in the epiphysis, as opposed to lesions in the apophysis or those that extend into the metaphysis or diaphysis. Recurrence is not definitely related to patient age, sex, or demographic data, but it is generally held that patients with open physes are at increased risk.

Unicameral Bone Cyst

Introduction and Definition

UBCs, also known as simple bone cysts, are lesions that consist of a fluid-filled cavity lined by a thin membrane. They are found in the metaphysis of long bones, with the most common site being the proximal humerus, followed by the proximal femur. "Active" cysts are located near the epiphysis (such as in the top two images), and as they move farther away (such as in the third image) as the child grows they become inactive. The lesion may be found in unusual sites such as the calcaneus and pelvis in patients more than 17 years old. The etiology of UBCs is unknown. Several etiologies have been proposed, including expansion of synovial tissue trapped in the bone during development, local failure of ossification, or obstruction of the venous outflow of the bone. It is possible the lesion is a reaction to trauma. The most popular theory is that local venous obstruction causes an increase in pressure that leads to reactive bone resorption. The cyst fluid contains prostaglandin and interleukin Iβ, which independently can cause bone resorption.

Incidence and Demographics

UBCs are found most commonly in children between the ages of 5 and 20 years, and the ratio of males to females is 2:1.

Symptoms and Presentation

Most UBCs are asymptomatic and only present when a pathologic fracture occurs. These lesions usually heal when the patient is skeletally mature, but a few persist into adulthood. The lesions grow in proportion to the growth of the bone they are in. Once the bone is finished growing, the UBC should also stop growing. In the foot, UBC occurs almost exclusively in the calcaneus, and presents in teenagers or young adults as an incidental finding or with mild aching pain during sports or running. The location and appearance is characteristic and biopsy may not be needed to confirm the diagnosis.

X-ray Appearance and Advanced Imaging Findings

The plain film is usually enough to make a diagnosis of an UBC, once the observer is thoroughly familiar with the appearance of this lesion. The lesion appears as a well-defined osteolytic area with a thin sclerotic margin. It fills and perhaps slightly expands the juxta-epiphyseal metaphysis of the bone. The lesion is relatively symmetrical with respect to the midline axis of the bone. The lesion is not eccentric and does not break out through the cortex or form any extraosseous mass. There is no periosteal reaction visible unless there has been a previous fracture. A fragment of cortex that has fallen into a dependent position inside the cyst is known as the "fallen leaf" or "fallen fragment" sign.

In the foot, UBC occurs almost exclusively in the calcaneus. The location and appearance is characteristic and biopsy may not be needed to confirm the diagnosis. The location is very specific. The lesion is in the lateral portion of the calcaneus subadjacent to the middle facet. The apex of the lesion is toward the forefoot. The margin of the lesion is sharply defined, sometimes with a sclerotic rim. There is no matrix mineralization, central calcification, or periosteal reaction. Central calcification is a feature of lipomas of the calcaneus.

MRI is useful to differentiate UBC from lipoma of bone, which may have nearly identical location and appearance. MRI demonstrates that the UBC is filled with fluid that has low signal intensity on T1-weighted images and high signal on T2 images. In lipoma of bone, the MRI signal intensity will be identical to nearby normal fat. CT scan is not especially helpful unless the UBC is in the pelvis. On bone scan, UBCs have light peripheral uptake with a cold center. However, the use of bone scans to characterize UBCs is not recommended.

Laboratory Findings

There are no helpful laboratory tests for this tumor.

Histopathology Findings

Microscopically, the UBC has a membrane made up of a layer of flattened or cuboidal cells that resemble endothelium. The cyst fluid resembles synovial fluid. If a fracture has occurred, there may be a hemorrhage, granulation tissue, calcifications, or giant cells that may confuse the diagnosis.

Treatment Options for This Tumor

Treatment of UBCs can take several forms. The mere presence of a UBC in the calcaneus does not mandate treatment. The physician should be extremely confident of the diagnosis prior to selecting treatment. A consultation is recommended if the surgeon sees bone tumors infrequently. When the lesion presents with a pathologic fracture, closed treatment of the fracture is the first priority. Sometimes, the trauma and subsequent healing process of a pathologic fracture can be enough to cause resolution of the UBC.

UBCs are relatively common in the calcaneus, but fractures through UBC in the calcaneus are uncommon. The mere presence of a UBC in the calcaneus does not mandate treatment for the cyst or for possible pathologic fracture. Treatment for asymptomatic cases consists of observation and follow-up radiographs to insure the lesion is not growing or changing. Painful cysts can be treated with a wide variety of more or less invasive techniques. There is a lack of consensus as to the optimum choice of treatment. There is some evidence to suggest that open curettage with allografting is most likely to lead to clinical and radiographic resolution of the cyst.

Published treatment techniques include aspiration and injection with methylprednisolone acetate (steroids), bone marrow injections, percutaneous grafting with autogenous or allogenous bone graft or bone graft substitutes, or a combination of these. Surgical techniques include curettage with and without grafting, creating multiple drill holes, and "continuous decompression" using a percutaneous cannulated screw. All of these techniques have been shown to be effective for some cysts, although the quality of the supporting evidence is universally low.[67] Surgical interventions should be reserved for difficult cases. The author recommends a fluoroscopically guided injection of methylprednisolone acetate as the initial treatment for symptomatic lesions in the calcaneus. UBCs that persist after a trial of one or two steroid injections should be curetted through a lateral approach and densely packed with allograft bone chips. There is no good evidence favoring commercial bone graft substitutes over morselized autograft or allograft bone used to fill UBCs. UBCs in young children should be approached with great care due to the high risk of recurrence and the potential for growth plate damage from surgery. Open curettage and bone graft for UBCs in children carry a recurrence rate of 40% to 45% due to difficulty of complete excision of the lesion. Damage to the nearby growth plate may result in growth arrest. Referral to a musculoskeletal tumor specialist is recommended.

Various technical factors have been proposed that may increase the success rate of steroid injections, including wide spacing of the needles to ensure complete treatment of the lesion and using radiologic dye to insure complete filling of the lesion. These techniques may decrease the need for multiple injections. A recent Cochrane review[68] concluded that the quality of the data was insufficient to demonstrate that injections of methylprednisolone were more or less effective than injections of bone marrow. The biologic mode of action of the injections remains unknown.

Preferred Margin for This Tumor

Intralesional.

Aneurysmal Bone Cyst

Introduction and Definition

This lesion is not a true neoplasm, but rather is thought to be a reactive lesion that may be caused by a local arteriovenous malformation or vascular injury. One theory of the etiology of primary ABCs is that these lesions are secondary to increased venous pressure that leads to hemorrhage and osteolysis. This osteolysis can in turn promote more hemorrhage causing amplification of the cyst. Another theory is that these lesions do not arise de novo but rather develop secondarily within another primary tumor such as osteoblastoma, and subsequently enlarge and destroy all or most of the primary tumor. The true cause is unknown. There is a definite relationship to local trauma in some cases, and other cases are associated with another tumor such as osteoblastoma, chondroblastoma, or fibrous dysplasia. A proportion of these lesions arise de novo without any definite traumatic or neoplastic cause.

A solid variant of ABC has been described. This variant consists of a nonaneurysmal tumor with identical histologic findings, which affects the axial skeleton and the short tubular bones of the hands and feet. This variant was described by Sanerkin et al.[69] The solid variant is associated with perilesional edema and cyclooxygenase 2 expression in the lesional giant cells and spindle cells.

Incidence and Demographics

ABC is found most commonly during the second decade, and the ratio of females to males is 2:1. ABCs can be found in any bone in the body. Approximately 6% of ABCs occur in the feet. The most common location is the metaphysis of the lower extremity long bones, more so than the upper extremity. The vertebral bodies or arches of the spine also may be involved. Approximately one-half of lesions in flat bones occur in the pelvis. In the foot and ankle, the metatarsals are the most commonly affected bones. Some patients have a history of trauma to the area of the lesion. Patients complain of pain and a slow-growing mass. The authors have seen the solid variant of ABC in the short tubular bones of the forefoot and in the tarsal bones of the midfoot.

Symptoms and Presentation

Symptoms are gradually increasing pain, a mass, or a pathologic fracture through the lesion. Rapid increase is lesion size has been reported in a few cases.

X-ray Appearance and Advanced Imaging Findings

Lesions are located on the surface of the bone as well as in the metaphysis or epiphysis. Plain radiographs show an expansile lesion with internal septae or longitudinal striations. The expansile nature of this lesion may be very striking, and the bone may be many times larger than normal. Even in highly expanded lesions, there is a thin eggshell layer of reactive bone on the surface of the lesion. This layer may be poorly mineralized in active lesions that are still growing and become more apparent as the lesion matures. The radiographic appearance may be strikingly aggressive in the early phase of growth, but after a few weeks the margin of the lesion becomes better defined and the appearance is less worrisome. The highly expansile lesion perched at the end of the bone has been described with the catchphrase "finger in a balloon." Most patients in the United States will receive treatment well before the tumor reaches this stage, so the catchphrase may be of historical value only.

MRI of aneurysmal lesions may show fluid–fluid levels within the lesion, which may demonstrate multiple separate loculations or one large loculated cavity, and these can be highly suggestive of the diagnosis, but are not diagnostic. ABC appears on both T1 and T2 MRI, with a low signal rim encircling the cystic lesion. CT and bone scan are not helpful in diagnosis, but may help define the lesion or rule out multiple lesions. CT scan can also help delineate lesions in the pelvis or spine where plain film imaging may be inadequate. A careful search for radiologic signs of the precursor lesion, if any, is recommended. Some of these precursor lesions may have a flocculent chondroid matrix that may be a clue to their pathogenesis.

Laboratory Findings

No relevant findings.

Differential Diagnosis

Giant cell tumor, UBC, telangiectatic osteosarcoma.

Preferred Biopsy Technique for This Tumor

Incisional/combined with curettage if certainty of diagnosis is high.

Histopathology Findings

On gross examination, an ABC is like a blood-filled sponge with a thin periosteal membrane. Soft, fibrous walls separate spaces filled with friable blood clot. Microscopically, the ABC has cystic spaces filled with blood. The fibrous septae have immature woven bone trabeculae as well as macrophages filled with hemosiderin, fibroblasts, capillaries, and giant cells. The treatment approach will vary depending on the location and aggressiveness of the lesion. A slow-growing, indolent ABC has been observed to regress spontaneously. Selective embolectomy of nutrient vessels and percutaneous injection of a fibrosing agent are newer treatment modalities. Percutaneous injection of methylmethacrylate was used successfully by Herve Deramond for an aggressive ABC lesion in the second cervical vertebra.

Treatment Options for This Tumor

Treatment for most lesions can be accomplished by curettage and application of a high-speed burr to remove an additional 2 mm of bone. Recurrence is common, approximately 20%. The cyst can be packed with bone chips or PMMA cement. Bone fragility must be addressed with plates, screws, or rods as indicated. During surgical treatment, these lesions may bleed profusely until removal is complete. Where appropriate, the lesions may be resected with a marginal or wide margin, such as in the fibula. Large lesions in the pelvis or long bones may require other treatments, such as embolization. Percutaneous transvascular treatments have been used with good results, and are especially useful in difficult to access lesions of the spine and skull base.

Local recurrence rates vary widely, with one recent report having 4 recurrences in 40 patients.[70] Recurrence rates may be as high as 20%. Recurrence was statistically related to young age and open growth plates, and may be less likely following wide excision than following intralesional treatment by curettage. If a recurrence is detected, a thorough examination of the original radiographs and pathology specimens should be performed to insure that the primary lesion, if any, is discovered, because this may radically alter the treatment plan. Once the precise diagnosis is known, local recurrences may be retreated by appropriate methods.

Preferred Margin for This Tumor

Intralesional.

Lipoma of Bone

Introduction and Definition

This is a rare benign bone tumor. If present in adults, often as an incidental finding, it is rarely symptomatic. The most common site is the calcaneus, followed by the femur. This lesion has also been found in multiple bones, including the tibia, fibula ulna, and skull.

Incidence and Demographics

The true incidence is unknown. It is thought to represent 0.1% of bone tumors, but because these tumors do not create symptoms, most may be missed. The mean age at presentation is 43 years; males and females are equally affected.

Symptoms and Presentation

Most of these tumors are not symptomatic and are discovered as an incidental lesion. Some patients may present with pain, and pathologic fracture can occur.

X-ray Appearance and Advanced Imaging Findings

Lipoma of bone and UBC in the calcaneus have very similar radiologic appearance. On X-rays, lipoma of bone is located within Ward triangle, and is well defined with a latent, non-aggressive appearance, a narrow zone of transition, a partial sclerotic rim, and a central calcific density. Not all lipomas of bone have calcifications. When present, the calcification is amorphous and without detectable patterns such as rings and arcs or popcorn (chondroid pattern) or ground glass (fibrous dysplasia pattern). The calcification is typically relatively dense, limited, and central. UBCs do not contain calcifications of any type. Lipoma of bone typically forms a single rounded or roughly ovoid lytic lesion, rather than a loculated "soap bubble" appearance such as might be seen in ABCs, or nonossifying fibroma. Mild expansion of the bone may be present. A sclerotic rim is present in three-quarters of these tumors. In the calcaneus, all these features are shared to some degree by UBC. Both occupy the same region of the calcaneus. Lipoma of bone is distinguished principally by the presence of a central calcific density and by MRI.

The tumor has a low CT attenuation coefficient consistent with fat, with high attenuation in areas of calcification, when present. On MRI, the tumor has signal intensity identical to that of nearby normal fat on all sequences. Some intraosseous lipomas undergo cystic change, which is best seen on MRI. Calcifications appear as areas of low signal intensity.

Laboratory Findings

No laboratory findings are useful in diagnosis.

Differential Diagnosis

UBC, nonossifying fibroma, ABC, chondrosarcoma, fibrous dysplasia.

Preferred Biopsy Technique for This Tumor

Tru-cut needle, open.

Histopathology Findings

Grossly, the tumor may be yellow or tan fatty material, soft or semiliquid, with a gritty texture. Squeezing the tissue will cause oil droplets to be produced. There may be oily liquid within the tumor cavity. The tumor is comprised of mature fat cells and varying amounts of fibrous and vascular tissue.

Based on a large case series, lipoma of bone has been divided into three stages, according to the histopathology findings, which also correspond with the radiologic findings. Stage I lesions are radiolucent with fine trabecular bone. Stage II lesions have partial fat necrosis and some fat calcification. Stage III lesions have a reactive ossified rim and more central calcification and ossification. Stage III lesions show more extensive necrosis on histologic examination. It is not clear whether this staging system has any value for diagnosis, treatment, or prognosis.[71]

Treatment Options for This Tumor

The mere presence of a lipoma in the calcaneus does not mandate treatment for the tumor or for possible pathologic fracture. Many patients can be treated with observation and follow-up only. Because the lesion can be diagnosed with certainty based on imaging studies, biopsy is not always necessary. Curettage and bone grafting should be reserved for large, worrisome, or symptomatic lesions, or lesions where there has been documented radiographic change, or definite increase in symptomatology. Lesions in weight-bearing bones that require treatment may require additional bone stabilization procedures, such as internal fixation or intramedullary rodding. This lesion is not expected to recur following curettage. However, curettage does not always result in complete relief of symptoms related to the tumor. In the calcaneus, the author's preferred treatment is curettage and packing of the bone defect with corticocancellous allograft chips.

Preferred Margin for This Tumor

Intralesional.

PRIMARY MALIGNANT BONE TUMORS

Introduction

Chondrosarcoma, Ewing sarcoma, and osteosarcoma are the most common bone sarcomas in the foot and ankle. Epithelioid hemangioma (epithelioid hemangioendothelioma), a low-grade vascular tumor that is intermediate between benign hemangioma and highly malignant angiosarcoma, also seems to have a predilection for the foot bones. The proportion of tumors in reported series of foot and ankle tumors that exhibit malignant behavior varies from 5% to 45%. Malignancies appear to comprise a larger proportion of tumors in the foot and ankle than elsewhere in the body. However, patient survival is significantly better in distal lower extremity tumors than for sarcomas in other musculoskeletal sites. A larger than usual proportion of the osteosarcomas in

the foot are low-grade tumors. Taken together, the metatarsals are the most common location of malignant tumors in the foot, whereas the calcaneus is the most common single bone affected.[49]

Bone and soft tissue sarcomas are thought to arise from alterations in the structure or expression of the cellular DNA. A few are caused by exposure to radiation or by an underlying genetic abnormality such as the *RB-1* gene in hereditary retinoblastoma, or the *p53* gene in Li–Fraumeni syndrome. A minority of sarcomas have a simple karyotype and carry defined genetic alterations or translocations, whereas most have a complex karyotype and show a variety of such alterations. Sarcomas with defined translocations may express an oncogenic fusion gene, such as SS, CCS, dermatofibrosarcoma protuberans, and myxoid liposarcoma. These sarcomas are relatively frequent in the foot. The presence of specific fusion proteins in these malignant tumors represents a pathway for future targeted treatments.[72]

The discovery of a potentially malignant tumor in the foot and ankle can overwhelm the patient and the family with fear and worry. The behavior of the clinician at the time of the initial discovery of the tumor has a strong impact on the patient's psychological well-being. The best way to manage anxiety is through directed action. The clinician should steer the focus away from worry and speculation and instead lay out a course toward an accurate diagnosis, a comprehensive treatment plan, and a prospect for recovery. Minimization of the problem, false assurances, and uninformed conjecture should be avoided, as these contribute to diagnostic delay. The surgeon should promptly seek assistance from the radiologist, the pathologist, an orthopedic tumor specialist, and other colleagues. It is important to document any advice or recommendations received from other physicians in the patient's chart. The information gathered should be shared fully with the patient and the patient's family, and presented in an understandable and emotionally sensitive way. Even when presenting very bad news, the surgeon should always leave room for hope.

The mainstay of treatment of sarcoma in the foot and ankle is by surgical resection with a wide margin. Adjuvant chemotherapy and radiation therapy are given for osteosarcoma, Ewing sarcoma, and other high-grade sarcomas on a case-by-case basis. The goals of the surgery include an en bloc excision of the entire tumor with an uncontaminated margin of 5 to 10 mm of normal tissue surrounding all aspects of the mass. Optimally, there is no spilling or exposure of any part of the actual tumor. A true wide margin requires that no part of the tumor, its capsule, or the reactive zone around the tumor is ever seen in the surgical field. All parts of the dissection take place through uninvolved, nonreactive normal tissues, and these normal tissues completely envelop all parts of the excised specimen. Many foot and ankle surgeons are unprepared for the degree of collateral damage to the foot that is required to achieve a true wide margin around a sarcoma. As a result, surgeons who infrequently treat sarcoma may be more likely to fail to achieve an optimal margin.

Chondrosarcoma

Introduction and Definition

Chondrosarcoma is a malignant tumor that produces cartilage matrix. Primary chondrosarcoma is very uncommon, arises centrally in the bone, and is found in children. Secondary chondrosarcoma arises from benign cartilage tumors such as osteochondroma or enchondroma. Chondrosarcomas can also be classified as intramedullary, which generally arise from enchondromas, and surface which arise from osteochondromas (**Fig. 11-6**).

Incidence and Demographics

Chondrosarcoma most commonly affects adults aged 30 to 70 years, with the peak age of incidence being sometime around 40 to 60 years. Chondrosarcoma has a male to female ratio of 1.5:1. It is most common in the femur, humerus, ribs, and on the surface of the pelvis. Patients with Ollier disease (multiple enchondromatosis) or Maffucci syndrome (multiple enchondromas and hemangiomas) are at much higher risk of chondrosarcoma than the normal population and often present in the third and fourth decade.

Chondrosarcoma is relatively rare in the bones of the foot, with this location accounting for approximately 2% of all such tumors. The tumors may be primary or develop as a secondary malignancy in an enchondroma or osteochondroma. Because enchondroma occurs frequently in the foot, it is essential to properly differentiate between benign and malignant cartilage tumors. Benign enchondromas in the small bones of the foot may have X-ray features that are suggestive of chondrosarcoma in larger bones.

Symptoms and Presentation

The presentation of chondrosarcoma depends on the grade of the tumor. A high-grade, fast-growing tumor can present with excruciating pain. A low-grade, more indolent tumor is more likely to present in an older patient complaining of hip pain and swelling. Pelvic tumors present with urinary frequency or obstruction or may masquerade as "groin muscle pulls."

X-ray Appearance and Advanced Imaging Findings

On plain radiographs, chondrosarcoma is a fusiform, lucent defect in bone with scalloping of the inner cortex and minimal periosteal reaction. Extension of the lesion into the soft tissue may be present as well as punctate or stippled calcification of the cartilage matrix. CT is helpful in defining the integrity of the cortex and distribution of calcification. MRI is invaluable in surgical planning as it demonstrates the intraosseus and soft tissue involvement of the tumor. MRI is also helpful in evaluating possible malignant degeneration of osteochondromas by allowing accurate measurements of the cartilage cap, which should be less than 2 cm thick.

In the foot, the radiographic appearance of chondrosarcoma may overlap considerably with that of enchondroma. Both types of tumors are lytic and may expand, damage, and weaken the bone significantly. Matrix mineralization, in the form of rings and arcs, occurs in about two-thirds of both benign and malignant lesions. The presence of scalloping, expansion, and cortical destruction is not a reliable way to discriminate benign from malignant lesions in the foot. In a recent study, size greater than 5 cm and location in the hindfoot were found to be associated with potential for malignancy.[73]

Differential Diagnosis

Osteosarcoma, benign cartilage lesions.

Preferred Biopsy Technique for This Tumor

Incisional.

Histopathology Findings

On gross examination, chondrosarcoma is a grayish-white, lobulated mass. It may have focal calcification, mucoid I degeneration, or necrosis. Histologically, chondrosarcoma is differentiated from benign cartilage growths by enlarged plump nuclei, multiple cells per lacunae, binucleated cells, and hyperchromic nuclear pleomorphism. Chondrosarcoma is graded from 1 (low) to 3 (high). Low-grade chondrosarcoma is very close in appearance to enchondromas and osteochondromas and has occasional binucleated cells. High-grade chondrosarcomas have increased cellularity, atypia, and mitoses. There is an inverse relationship between histologic grade and prognosis, with higher grades having a worse prognosis and early metastases.

Treatment Options for This Tumor

Treatment of chondrosarcoma is wide surgical excision. There is a very limited role for chemotherapy or radiation. Biopsies must be planned with future tumor excision in mind. Patients with adequately resected low-grade chondrosarcomas have an excellent survival rate. The survival of patients with high-grade tumors depends on the location, size, and stage of the tumor.

Preferred Margin for This Tumor

Wide.

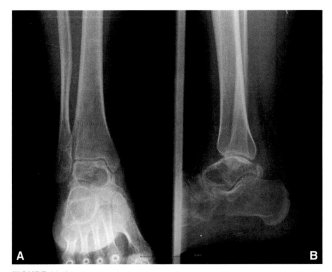

FIGURE 11-6. AP and lateral radiographs showing a mesenchymal chondrosarcoma of the talus. Location in the hindfoot is a sign of potential malignancy.

Treatment

Treatment of high-grade chondrosarcoma is by surgical resection with a wide margin.

Innovative limb salvage procedures, such as replacement of the entire calcaneus with a fresh osteoarticular allograft, have been reported. Maximum restoration of mobility in a timely fashion and with minimal complications is the goal of surgery. If conservation of a durable, minimally painful plantigrade foot is impossible to achieve without compromising the surgical margin, amputation should be considered.

Chemotherapy and radiation therapy are used in cases where surgical control is inadequate or impossible. Chemotherapy is given for high-grade chondrosarcoma in some cancer centers where experimental protocols are being investigated.

Outcomes of Treatment and Prognosis

Survival of chondrosarcoma is difficult to precisely define because of the large number of subtypes, varying histologic grades of the tumor, and a wide variety of treatments that are given depending on tumor extent than location. Recent data from a relatively homogeneous group of patients with primary central chondrosarcoma who presented with localized disease are available.[74] Overall survival at 5 years was 72% and at 10 years was 69%. Event-free survival at 5 and 10 years was 57% and 53%, respectively.

One of the most striking findings in the data concerns the development of local recurrence and distant metastasis. The authors found that both local recurrence and distant metastasis lead to a significant decrease in overall survival regardless of tumor grade and localization. In this group of patients, long-term survival was only possible if the recurrence or metastasis was completely resected with wide margins.

Factors associated with improved overall survival for chondrosarcoma located in the extremity included low-grade tumors, age under 40 years, and tumor size less than 100 cm³. Factors that did not affect long-term survival included male sex, AJCC stage, and quality of surgical margins. However, multiple other studies have shown that inadequate surgical margins are associated with poor prognosis.

Special and Unusual Features

There are three additional types of chondrosarcoma. Mesenchymal chondrosarcoma is a rare variant with a bimorphic histologic picture of low-grade cartilaginous cells and hypercellular small, uniform, and undifferentiated cells that resemble Ewing sarcoma. Mesenchymal chondrosarcoma has a predilection for the spine, ribs, and jaw and presents in the third decade. It is more common in females and can grow exceptionally large. It is very likely to metastasize to lungs, lymph nodes, and other bones. Clear cell chondrosarcoma is a malignant cartilage tumor that may be the adult variant of chondroblastoma. It is a rare, low-grade tumor with an improved prognosis over other chondrosarcomas. Like chondroblastoma, it is found in the epiphysis of the femur and humerus. Histologically, soft tissue invasion is rare. Clear cell chondrosarcoma has clear cells with vacuolated cytoplasm.

The cartilage matrix has significantly calcified trabeculae and giant cells. Dedifferentiated chondrosarcoma is the most malignant form of chondrosarcoma. This tumor is a mix of low-grade chondrosarcoma and high-grade spindle cell sarcoma where the spindle cells are no longer identifiable as having a cartilage origin. The dedifferentiated portion of the lesion may have histologic features of MFH, osteosarcoma, or undifferentiated sarcoma. This biphasic quality is evident on X-ray, with areas of endosteal scalloping and cortical thickening contrasting with areas of cortical destruction and soft tissue invasion. Dedifferentiated chondrosarcoma has a 5-year survival of 10%.

Osteosarcoma

Introduction and Definition

Osteosarcoma (osteogenic sarcoma) is the most common primary sarcoma of bone. In its most common form, it is an aggressive sarcoma that occurs in teenagers and young adults. Osteosarcoma is more common in males than in females. Current treatment results in excellent chances for survival for patients with manageable tumors who do not have metastasis. Although patients experience lingering negative effects following treatment, these are readily accepted due to the aggressive and potentially deadly nature of the tumor. Osteosarcoma is not caused by injury, fluoride, vaccines, or exposure to chemicals. The exact cause is unknown. In most cases, an abnormality in the chromosomal DNA (the genes) of a primitive bone cell or bone precursor cell can be detected. Current research is focused on the role of the Notch signaling pathway, which controls many crucial aspects of cell proliferation, migration, invasiveness, and angiogenesis, as well as the ability of cancer cells to break away from the original tumor and metastasize to distant sites within the body.

Incidence and Demographics

Approximately 1,000 new cases of osteosarcoma occur in the United States each year, including about 600 in children. About 85% of osteosarcoma cases are of the "conventional intramedullary" type, and the other 15% consists of several other subtypes, including telangiectatic, low-grade intramedullary, and small cell, as well as the surface subtypes parosteal, periosteal, and high-grade surface osteosarcoma. Osteosarcoma can occur at any age. The most common site is the distal femur and proximal tibia. Osteosarcoma can occur in any bone of the foot.

Symptoms and Presentation

The most common presentation is pain and eventually a mass, which occurs near a joint. The pain may initially accompany activity, gradually becomes more constant, and may be severe at night. Patients otherwise may have few or no symptoms. Initially, the pain may be intermittent and related to a minor injury or exercise activity, and thus the problem is misdiagnosed as a common sprain or strain.

X-ray Appearance and Advanced Imaging Findings

The most common form of osteogenic sarcoma is conventional osteosarcoma, which accounts for 75% to 85% of all osteosarcomas. On radiographs, conventional osteosarcoma occurs predominately in the metaphysis, and appears as a mixed sclerotic and lytic lesion, that may permeate the bone and the nearby cortex, causing a soft tissue mass and a periosteal reaction. Bone formation within the tumor is characteristic of osteosarcoma and is usually visible on the X-rays. Radiographs will initially reveal a subtle mixed lysis and sclerosis, followed by increasing sclerosis, permeation, destruction, and expansion into the adjacent soft tissues with bone formation in the soft tissue mass.

Laboratory Findings

Laboratory tests do not aid in the diagnosis, but a link between alkaline phosphatase levels in the blood and prognosis of the disease has been established.

Preferred Biopsy Technique for This Tumor

Biopsy must be carefully planned so that subsequent definitive surgical removal of the tumor is not compromised. Most authors strongly recommend that the biopsy be performed by the surgeon who will be doing the final tumor resection. An increased rate of avoidable amputations has been attributed to errors in biopsy technique. In some centers, tru-cut needle biopsy is used, but a well-planned and meticulously executed open biopsy remains the mainstay of diagnosis in osteosarcoma.

Differential Diagnosis

The differential diagnosis should include infection, lymphoma, chondrosarcoma, Ewing sarcoma, and pleomorphic undifferentiated sarcoma (previously termed MFH).

Treatment Options for This Tumor

Before treatment can be planned, a complete oncologic staging workup must be completed. This includes assessment of any potential for metastasis to the chest, to nearby bones or the rest of the extremity, or to other areas as indicated. Most patients have CT scans of the chest, whole-body bone scan, and MRI of the extremity including the lesion. Additional scans such as PET scan may have a role in the staging workup.

For most types of osteosarcoma, treatment is multimodal. Neoadjuvant multiagent chemotherapy is given prior to surgery. Surgical resection with a wide margin follows. The majority of patients can have limb-sparing surgery rather than amputation. In the foot and ankle, the tumor is removed and the foot is reconstructed with a fusion, an allograft, or a combination of these. Following surgery, postoperative chemotherapy is usually given, and may be modified depending on the response of the tumor to the preoperative chemotherapy. Radiation is usually not used. Low-grade osteosarcoma is treated by surgery only.

Preferred Margin for This Tumor

Wide.

Outcomes of Treatment and Prognosis

The prognosis of osteogenic sarcoma depends very largely on the extent of the tumor. Localized, nonmetastatic tumors in relatively accessible sites such as the knee, hip, and shoulder generally have a very good to excellent prognosis. Very large tumors and tumors in difficult sites such as the pelvis and spine have a less favorable prognosis due to the difficulty with completely removing the tumor by surgical techniques. Once clinically evident metastasis occurs, the prognosis is substantially diminished. Tumors that present with metastasis already present or tumors where metastasis is discovered after the initial treatment have a poor prognosis. Surgical removal of metastasis coupled with chemotherapy may lead to improved survival.

Special and Unusual Features

It is estimated that 80% of patients with osteosarcoma have metastasis at presentation, although only 15% of these are clinically apparent. The most common site of metastasis is the lungs. Systemic chemotherapy is given to all patients. Following treatment of osteosarcoma, patients continue to experience lingering effects. The functional capacity and quality of life are impaired to an extent that depends on the extent of the tumor and the success of the limb-sparing surgery. Lingering effects and toxic effects of the chemotherapy require ongoing observation and sometimes treatment.

Ewing Sarcoma

Introduction and Definition

Ewing sarcoma is a highly malignant small, round, blue cell tumor that occurs mainly in the second decade of life. Ewing sarcoma, along with PNET, comprises the Ewing sarcoma family of tumors. The tumor commonly stains for CD99 and has translocations of the EWS gene *EWSR1-FLI1*. Ewing sarcoma is found in the lower extremity more than the upper extremity, but any bone may be affected. The most common sites are the metaphysis and diaphysis of the femur followed by the tibia and humerus.

Incidence and Demographics

Ewing sarcoma is most common in the first and second decade but may affect persons from age 2 to 80. This tumor preferentially affects whites more than blacks and Asians. The ratio of males to females is 3:2. Ewing sarcoma is relatively rare in the bones of the foot. The calcaneus is the most commonly involved site, but this tumor may also present in any bone or as a mass in the soft tissues.

Symptoms and Presentation

The clinical presentation of Ewing sarcoma includes pain and swelling of weeks' or months' duration. Erythema and warmth of the local area are sometimes seen. Osteomyelitis is often the initial diagnosis based on intermittent fevers, leukocytosis, anemia, and an increased erythrocyte sedimentation rate (ESR).

Patients with Ewing sarcoma in the foot frequently suffer delays in diagnosis. The mean age at presentation for lesions in the foot is 17 years, and the average duration of symptoms is 14 months. Patients with forefoot tumors had an average of 7 months of symptoms prior to diagnosis, whereas patients with hindfoot tumors had an average of 22 months of symptoms prior to diagnosis. In many cases, patients are treated for osteomyelitis before the correct diagnosis is made. The lesion presents with pain, which initially will follow some minor sporting activity or injury. The patient appears entirely healthy other than the foot and ankle symptoms. Poor prognostic signs include increased age, increased ESR, and leukocytosis at presentation.

X-ray Appearance and Advanced Imaging Finding

Radiologically, Ewing sarcoma is often associated with a lamellated or "onion skin" periosteal reaction. This appearance is caused by splitting and thickening of the cortex by tumor cells. The lesion is usually lytic and central. Endosteal scalloping is often present. The "onion skin" appearance is often followed with a "moth-eaten" or mottled appearance and extension into soft tissue. Bone marrow infiltration is not obvious on plain X-ray. Although Ewing sarcoma is usually lytic, it may present as a sclerotic lesion with bone expansion.

CT is helpful in defining bone destruction. MRI is essential to elucidate the soft tissue involvement; T1-weighted images the tumor has low intensity compared to the normal high intensity of bone marrow. On T2-weighted images the tumor is hyper intense compared to muscle. Ewing sarcoma has increased uptake on bone scan. A complete radiologic workup should consist of plain radiographs of the part, CT scan and MRI scan of the primary tumor, whole-body bone scan, and CT scan of the chest.

In the foot and ankle, the initial radiographs will show very minor, unimpressive changes, with focal lysis and permeation of the involved bone. If the diagnosis is delayed, extensive permeation, bony destruction, and a soft tissue mass will develop. The characteristic "onion scanning" or lamellar periosteal reaction is not usually seen because of the anatomy of the foot.

Differential Diagnosis

Infection, neuroblastoma metastasis, lymphoma, leukemia, osteosarcoma.

Preferred Biopsy Technique for This Tumor

Open biopsy is recommended for bone lesions. Core or trucut is adequate for soft tissue lesions if the pathologist has significant experience with sarcomas.

Histopathology Findings

Grossly, the tumor is gray to white in color and poorly demarcated. The consistency is soft and gray and sometimes semiliquid, especially after breaking through the cortex. Areas of hemorrhage and necrosis are common. The destruction is often greater on gross appearance than was visible on radiographs. Under the microscope, Ewing sarcoma consists of densely packed uniform small cells in sheets. The cells have scant cytoplasm without distinct borders. The cells are two to three times as big as lymphocytes and have a single oval or round nucleus without prominent nucleoli. The tumor spreads through Haversian canals, which cause the appearance of permeative margins on X-ray. Glycogen is present within the cells, causing a positive reaction to periodic acid-Schiff stain. Most Ewing sarcomas are positive with HBA-71 or 0-13 stain, which is an antibody to the protein product of myc 2. The microscopic differential includes lymphoma and metastatic neuroblastoma, which must be excluded by reticulin stain and urine vanillylmandelic acid and homovanillic acid, respectively. Rhabdomyosarcoma is ruled out if the specimen stains negatively with desmin, myoglobin, and actin stains. A neural origin is supported by electron microscope findings of pseudorosettes. This is further supported by the common finding in Ewing sarcoma and PNETs of choline acetyltransferase and the translocation t(11:22)(q24;ql2). It is thought that Ewing sarcoma with its few organelles is the poorly differentiated end of the spectrum of PNET. Neuroepithelioma is an example of well-differentiated PNET and has neurosecretory granules and neuritic processes.

Treatment Options for This Tumor

Treatment for Ewing sarcoma includes surgery, radiation, and multidrug chemotherapy. Radiation or chemotherapy with vincristine, dactinomycin, and cyclophosphamide is used preoperatively. Adjuvant chemotherapy follows surgery and decreases recurrences. The tumor can metastasize to the lungs and lymph nodes. Poor prognostic signs include increased age, increased ESR, and leukocytosis at presentation.

Ewing sarcoma that occurs in the forefoot has an overall survival of 70%, whereas Ewing sarcoma in the hindfoot has an overall survival of only 33%. The survival of patients with metastasis at the time of presentation is 0%.[75] Treatment depends on the stage and local extent of the tumor. Localized tumors are treated with chemotherapy and wide surgical excision with or without radiation. Radiation may be avoided if adequate margins can be achieved at the time of surgery. Radiation carries the risk of secondary sarcoma in the radiated field. For this reason, amputation may be the procedure of choice for this tumor in the foot.

Lymphoma

Introduction and Definition

Primary lymphoma of bone (PLB) is a rare tumor that comprises approximately 5% to 7% of malignant bone tumors. Secondary bone involvement is seen in about 16% to 20% of patients with widespread lymphoma. Most cases of PLB are non-Hodgkin, diffuse large B-cell lymphomas. There is a lack of consensus on the optimal treatment, which generally includes combined radiation and multiagent chemotherapy. Overall prognosis for PLB is generally good. Surgery is not used to cure PLB, but only to stabilize weakened bones or treat pathologic fractures. Approximately two-thirds of patients with PLB require surgery, most because of pathologic fractures.[76]

Lymphoma involving bone can be separated into four groups:

1. A single skeletal site, with or without regional lymph node involvement;
2. Multiple bones are involved, but there is no visceral or lymph node involvement;
3. Patients present with a bone tumor, but work up shows involvement of other visceral sites or multiple lymph nodes at multiple sites;
4. The patient has a known lymphoma and a bone biopsy is done to rule out involvement of bone.

Groups 1 and 2 are considered by many to be PLB, but there is a lack of consensus.[77]

Incidence and Demographics

The median age at presentation for single-bone PLB is 44, and for polyostotic PLB the median age is 64. The most common location is the appendicular skeleton, especially the femur and tibia. PLB in the foot is rare, but has been reported in the calcaneus, metatarsal, and talus.

X-ray Appearance and Advanced Imaging Findings

Radiographic findings in lymphoma of bone are variable and nonspecific. Early on, the most common appearance is a vague, mottled lucency in the metadiaphysis of a long bone. The intraosseous lesion usually has permeative pattern of lysis, but may appear blastic or sclerotic. Periosteal reaction and cortical destruction are generally not seen on the initial X-rays, but will develop with time. Plain radiographs often substantially underestimate the anatomic extent of the lesion.

Findings on MRI are nonspecific, with low signal intensity on T1-weighted sequences and high signal intensity on T2-weighted sequences. The tumor enhances in a homogeneous fashion after administration of gadolinium. Approximately three out of four tumors have an associated soft tissue mass. MRI findings that are indicative of PLB include an extensive marrow-replacing lesion and associated soft tissue mass with little or no cortical destruction. Lymphoma has an increased uptake on bone scan.

Differential Diagnosis

The radiographic differential diagnosis of PLB includes osteosarcoma, small round cell tumors like leukemia, myeloma, Langerhans cell histiocytosis, Ewing sarcoma ,and osteomyelitis.

Preferred Biopsy Technique for This Tumor

Open. In disseminated lymphoma, tru-cut needle biopsy is more than adequate for diagnosis. Because PLB is an unusual variant of lymphoma, small biopsy specimens leave room for uncertainty. Lymphoma may be difficult to differentiate from Ewing sarcoma, chronic osteomyelitis, Langerhans cell histiocytosis, and small cell undifferentiated carcinoma with insufficient biopsy specimens. A larger biopsy specimen helps "prove" to all concerned that the lesion is truly a lymphoma.

Histopathology Findings

On gross examination, primary non-Hodgkin lymphoma of the bone is a gray-white tumor that diffusely infiltrates bone. Pathologic diagnosis requires clinical suspicion of lymphoma for good tissue handling. It is essential to get tissue without crush artifact or decalcification to preserve cell morphology. Needle biopsy is not adequate. Non-Hodgkin lymphoma appears most commonly with large cells with irregular cleaved nuclei and prominent nucleoli surrounded by reticulin fibers. The most common subtype is diffuse histiocytic lymphoma. Hodgkin lymphoma has a mixed cell population with plasma cells, lymphocytes, histiocytes, and eosinophils. Reed–Sternberg are large cells with a bilobed nucleus or multiple nuclei and prominent eosinophilic nuceoli. Their presence is essential to the diagnosis of Hodgkin lymphoma. The pathologic differential includes Ewing sarcoma, chronic osteomyelitis, and eosinophilic granuloma.

Treatment Options for This Tumor

No definitive treatment guidelines have been established for the treatment of PLB. Traditionally, treatment has been based on radiation therapy alone. Improved survival rates were reported with the advent of combined treatment with chemotherapy and radiation. Other than diagnostic biopsy, surgery is used for treatment or prevention of pathologic fractures. Avascular necrosis and extensive destruction of bone may also require surgery. Although wide resection is rarely indicated in lymphoma of bone, extensive bone destruction especially in weight-bearing bones of the lower extremities may necessitate resection and reconstruction with structural allografts and/or endoprosthesis. In the foot and ankle, PLB is generally treated with radiation, systemic chemotherapy, restriction of weight-bearing, and protection of the foot with a fracture boot. The tumor generally responds well to treatment, and this results in significant reversal of the damage to the affected bones. Full weight-bearing can be resumed in many cases once medical and radiation treatments have been underway for a few months.

Preferred Margin for This Tumor

Any margin is appropriate, surgery is done for bone fragility, not tumor resection.

Outcomes of Treatment and Prognosis

Prognosis of PLB is controversial. There are a wide range of prognoses reported in the literature. Variations in the definition and the treatment of the PLB may be some of the reasons for this. In one large report of PLB,[76] the overall 5-year survival was 91%. Overall 5-year survival for systemic lymphoma patients with bone involvement was 79%. Combined modality treatment is reported to yield better survival. Younger age and localized disease are positive prognostic factors.

Special and Unusual Features

Pathologic fractures from lymphoma may occur at the time of diagnosis, during treatment, and months or years after treatment is concluded. Fractures after treatment were attributed to radiation doses of 50 Gy or higher, chemotherapy containing prednisolone, and other risk factors such as old age, female sex, surgical infection, and Paget disease.[76]

METASTATIC TUMORS AND TUMOR MIMICS

Metastatic Bone Tumors in the Foot

Introduction and Demographics

Metastases distal to the knee are unusual, and metastases to the bones of the foot (acrometastases) are even more rare.[56] Metastases to the bone develop in 30% of all patients with cancer, with only 0.007% to 0.3% having acrometastases.[78] Libson et al.[79] found that the most common sources were the colorectal, renal, and lung carcinomas, with bladder, uterus, and breast cancers also contributing metastases to the foot. Zindrick et al.[56] found the main sources of metastases to the bones of the feet to be the genitourinary tract and colon.[80] The talus is most commonly affected, then the calcaneus.[49] The tarsal bones are involved in 50% of cases, the metatarsals in 23%, whereas the phalanges account for only 17% of the reported cases[80] (**Fig. 11-7**).

Symptoms and Presentation

Common complaints include foot pain, localized or diffuse swelling and progressive enlargement, subungual lesion, or an ulcerated discharging lesion. Many cases present to the surgeon mimicking other benign processes, and a delay in diagnosis may result. Patients may have pain for weeks or months before radiographic changes can be detected.[81] Clinical features of metastasis to the phalanges include redness, warmth, swelling, ulceration, or tenderness.[80]

X-ray Appearance and Advanced Imaging Findings

Radiologic signs on plain X-rays will vary depending on the type and aggressiveness of the tumor and the time elapsed until presentation. These include soft tissue swelling, moderate to marked bone destruction, and in some cases complete bone lysis.[80] Bone destruction is not accompanied by a distinct periosteal reaction.[56,82] When the distal phalanx of the big toe is the site of the lesion, the joint is rarely involved or crossed by the lesion,[56] and a thin margin of subchondral bone usually remains, even with extreme destruction.[56,80] The subchondral bone plate as well as the joint space is usually preserved.[80] The neoplasm may cause ballooning of the thinned cortical shell as it enlarges.[56]

Differential Diagnosis

The radiographic differential diagnosis of metastasis includes osteosarcoma, small round cell tumors like lymphoma, myeloma, Ewing sarcoma, and also osteomyelitis. Tuberculosis sepsis located in a joint of the foot or ankle can present with an aggressive destructive appearance and mimic a malignancy.

Recommended Biopsy Technique for Metastatic Bone Tumors in the Foot

Patients with metastatic lesions in the foot require surgery for biopsy only. Biopsy may also be easily accomplished via CT-guided tru-cut needle. If the patient already has a known cancer diagnosis, only a small sample of the tumor in the foot is required to confirm the diagnosis of metastasis. In some cases where there are widespread bone metastasis from a known primary tumor, a biopsy of a newly discovered bone lesion in the foot is completely unnecessary. Unusual lesions and lesions located in joints should be comprehensively cultured at the time of biopsy.

Surgical Treatment for Metastatic Bone Tumors in the Foot

Reconstructive surgical intervention for these tumors is almost never necessary. Immobilization with a removable fracture boot, offloading and restricted weight-bearing to prevent fracture, and pain control are warranted. Radiation treatment is almost always needed, and prompt administration of antiresorptive bisphosphonate medications is strongly recommended to prevent further bone damage.

Tumor Mimics

Introduction and Definition

Tumor mimics are non-neoplastic lesions that mimic the appearance and behavior of a true bone neoplasm. Because of the overlap in presentation between these lesions and true

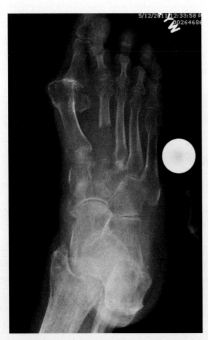

FIGURE 11-7. A metatarsal lesion in a 90-year-old woman with history of nephrectomy for renal cancer 6 years previous.

bone tumors, a similar systematic approach to diagnosis is necessary. The imaging, workup, and biopsy techniques are identical to those appropriate or potentially malignant bone lesions in a similar location. Because bone tumors are relatively rare, tumor mimics may be equally as likely in patient groups. Treatment of tumor mimics depends on the diagnosis.

Stress Fracture

Introduction and Definition

Most stress fractures can be readily identified based on the clinical history, plain X-ray findings, and MRI findings when necessary. However, in some cases, there is a lack of an appropriate history, or the imaging findings are equivocal. Stress fractures may be difficult to differentiate from infection, bone infarction, or malignant neoplasm. Stress fractures are caused by repetitive episodes of mechanical loading, which result in bone strain. Strain is a unitless value that represents a change in the unit length per unit length of bone. The amount of injury caused by a given amount of strain increases with both magnitude and rate of application. During normal activities, a healthy bone is capable of targeted remodeling of injured areas. Both large loads applied over short periods and small loads applied repetitively without sufficient time for bone remodeling can cause stress fractures.

Stress fractures can be caused by extrinsic and intrinsic factors. Intrinsic factors include the type of activity or sport, training program, environmental factors, shoe characteristics, and surface characteristics. Intrinsic factors include bone structure, muscle dysfunction, joint flexibility, and foot shape. A cavus foot is associated with an increase of tibial stress fractures, whereas a planus foot is associated with metatarsal stress fractures.[83]

Incidence and Demographics

Stress fractures may occur at any age and in any patient. Females, athletes, and military recruits have increased risk. Among male and female athletes, the incidence is approximately 3% and approximately 9.2%, respectively. The typical presentation is activity-related bone pain of insidious onset following a burst of physical activity. Some patients lack any history of increased activity or walking. Children may not be able to give a history that is sufficient for the clinician to consider stress fracture in the differential.

Common locations of stress fracture include the tibia, tarsal navicular, metatarsals, and fibula. Stress fracture location is based partly on the type of sport or activity. Endurance athletes are at increased risk of stress fractures in the proximal skeleton such as the femur, whereas power athletes such as sprinters and weight lifters are more likely to have distal stress fractures in the tarsal bones or metatarsals.

Risk factors include repetitive, high-intensity training, recreational runners averaging more than 25 miles per week, and participation in track, dance, basketball, and soccer. Women are at higher risk than men. Patients with low 25-hydroxyvitamin D levels are more prone to stress factors. Other risk factors include eating disorders, amenorrhea, osteoporosis, smoking, and consuming more than 10 alcoholic drinks per week.

X-ray Appearance and Advanced Imaging Findings

In the early stages, the typical radiographic features of stress fracture are not present. There may be a vague, partially mineralized mass that can be mistaken for a tumor. An MRI at this early stage further confounds the diagnosis, because the edema and early callus around the lesion have signal characteristics identical to tumor. A bone scan at the early stage may or may not demonstrate the characteristic narrow, transverse band of intense tracer uptake. An MRI may lack the characteristic transverse line of low signal intensity at the site of the fracture.

Low-quality MRI scans, scans degraded by motion artifact, and low field strength MRIs should be repeated. For maximum diagnostic value, MRIs should combine T1- and T2-weighted images as well as short tau inversion recovery and fat-suppressed T2-weighted images. High-resolution multislice CT scan imaging focused on the area of interest can be very helpful in revealing fracture lines. Limiting the CT scan to a narrow area of interest is recommended to reduce radiation exposure. Bone scan does not appear to increase diagnostic accuracy over the combination of plain X-ray, MRI, and CT scan. The correct diagnosis can sometimes be made by reanalysis of the available imaging findings. Low-quality X-rays should be repeated. Comparing new X-rays with old ones will often reveal useful findings. Over time, stress fractures evolve toward healing, maturation, and consolidation, whereas true bone tumors evolve toward growth, bone destruction, and a larger soft tissue mass.[84]

Treatment for This Tumor Mimic

Biopsy is only rarely necessary. Careful attention to the interpretation of the biopsy is necessary due to the overlap between stress fracture histology and the histology of malignant bone tumors such as osteosarcoma. Treatment of stress fracture is by conventional means.

Gout

Introduction

Gout has been known to mimic many diseases since the time of Hippocrates. The association of gout with pain, redness, and warmth in the big toe is so pervasive that a patient with gout in any other location is at risk of a delay in diagnosis even when the clinical picture is typical. Destructive bone lesions from gout may present in a teenaged patient or in a patient with normal uric acid; with minimal redness, warmth, or pain; or in an atypical location in the foot. Gout can mimic both a soft tissue tumor and an aggressive bone lesion. Clinical examples include a painful, expansile bone lesion in the medial hallux sesamoid in a teenager with no prior history, a cystic tumor in the talus of an obese teenager with concurrent diagnosis of juvenile rheumatoid arthritis, and a destructive lesion at a bone–prosthesis interface of a total ankle.

Symptoms and Presentation

The intensity of the pain is the hallmark of gout, and a careful history is usually sufficient to make the diagnosis. At some point during the evolution of the lesion, the patient will have had severe pain in the area of the lesion, a few days or a week when the pain was so severe that normal function was impossible. A comparable degree of pain and sensitivity to pressure is not seen in benign or malignant bone tumors. Patients may present after the acute phase has passed, but the bone lesion remains.

X-ray Appearance and Advanced Imaging Findings

The radiologic appearance of bone lesions from gout may mimic an aggressive or malignant tumor, with poorly marginated bone lysis, cortical destruction, and an associated soft tissue mass. The MRI scan may overstate the worrisome features of the lesion and add to the confusion. It is often sufficient to realize that the "tumor" may simply be gout presenting in an unusual location.

The classic X-ray appearance of gout in bone is a well-defined eccentric, periarticular lytic erosive "punched-out" lesion with an overhanging edge. The cortical destruction and associated soft tissue inflammation contribute to the appearance of an aggressive tumor. In contrast to rheumatoid arthritis, the joint space is typically preserved until late, and there is no associated periarticular osteopenia. Tophaceous deposits do not contain calcifications but are plainly visible on the X-rays.

MRI of gout bone lesions is nonspecific. MRI may be helpful in differentiating soft tissue masses (tophi) from a true neoplasm. The MRI appearance of tophi is characteristically low-intermediate signal intensity on T1-weighted images, with heterogeneous signal intensity on T2-weighted images. The edematous tissue surrounding the tophus enhances with gadolinium.

There have been recent developments in the ultrasound imaging of gout. The so-called double contour sign is a specific ultrasonographic feature of gout, best seen with high-resolution equipment. This finding has also been described as "urate icing." This finding arises from a hyperechoic layer of urate crystals deposited on the cartilage surface. This finding is present in both symptomatic and "silent" joints of patients with elevated serum uric acid with or without full-blown gout. This new modality may potentially contribute to noninvasive methods for early diagnosis and better management of the skeletal damage that gout can cause. The role of ultrasound in the diagnosis and management of gout is being reassessed in light of these new findings.

Osteoarthritis-Related Cysts of Bone

The origin of osteoarthritis-related cysts (ganglion cysts) is unclear, but they are commonly associated with degenerative conditions of soft tissue or bone. They may occur adjacent to joints, tendons, fascial planes, and within bone. Most ganglion cysts can be definitively diagnosed based on a careful history and physical examination. By history, the lesion has a tendency to both increase and decrease in size over time.

On exam, ganglion cyst typically has superficial location, and may be adjacent to a joint. When these lesions occur near a joint, there is often osteoarthritis seen on the X-ray. The mass is soft when the nearby joint is relaxed, and becomes firm when the nearby joint or muscle is tensed. A penlight or a small laser pointer will transilluminate the cyst. When these lesions occur near a joint, there is often osteoarthritis seen on the X-ray. An MRI should be obtained to further delineate the mass. Aspiration of the characteristic clear viscous material from the mass confirms the diagnosis. If the characteristic fluid is not obtained, no further attempts should be made. Treatment includes further aspiration and injection with cortisone, which should lead to resolution in about half the cases. Surgical removal is indicated for persistent, large, or troublesome cysts.

PVNS of Bone

PVNS is an uncommon proliferative condition of the synovium that can invade the bone. PVNS was first described by Chassaignac in 1852. He described a nodular lesion that arose within the flexor tendon sheaths of the hand. Simon in 1864 recorded the localized form of the disease. Moserin in 1909 noted the diffuse form. It was Jaffe in 1941 who coined the term "pigmented villonodular synovitis" in a case series.[78] It is generally believed to be a benign neoplastic process; however, some believe that it can occur secondary to inflammation or trauma. A few cases of metastasis have been reported in the literature. It most commonly occurs in the synovial lining of joints, and it can also occur in tendon sheaths, where it is called giant cell tumor of the tendon sheath. These tumors have also been found within synovial bursae. The ankle is the third most common location for diffuse intra-articular PVNS. Lesions in the ankle may invade the distal tibia or talus, or both. The ankle and hindfoot are affected approximately twice as often as the forefoot. PVNS has distinctive characteristics, which allow it to be identified on imaging studies.

On plain radiographs, PVNS may present as a sharply defined cystic lesion adjacent to the involved joint. Because the lesion is synovial in origin, bone cysts may form on both sides of the joint, which differentiates this lesion from all other benign bone tumors. Other than PVNS, lytic lesions on both sides of the joint may be caused by severe untreated osteoarthritis and septic tuberculosis of the ankle. On MRI, PVNS has a unique and diagnostic appearance due to the hemosiderin contained within the tumor.

REFERENCES

1. Bousson V, Hamzé B, Wybier M, et al. Soft tissue tumors and pseudotumors of the foot and ankle. *J Radiol.* 2008;89(1 pt 1):21–34.
2. Hofstaetter SG, Huber M, Trieb K, et al. Tumors and tumor-like lesions of the foot and ankle—a retrospective analysis of 22 years. *Wien Med Wochenschr.* 2010;160(11–12):297–304.
3. Bakotic BW, Borkowski P. Primary soft-tissue neoplasms of the foot: the clinicopathologic features of 401 cases. *J Foot Ankle Surg.* 2001;40(1):28–35.

4. Cribb GL, Loo SC, Dickinson I. Limb salvage for soft-tissue sarcomas of the foot and ankle. *J Bone Joint Surg Br*. 2010;92(3):424–429.

5. Strander H, Turesson I, Cavallin-Ståhl E. A systematic overview of radiation therapy effects in soft tissue sarcomas. *Acta Oncol*. 2003;42(5–6):516–531.

6. Datir A, James SL, Ali K, et al. MRI of soft-tissue masses: the relationship between lesion size, depth, and diagnosis. *Clin Radiol*. 2008;63(4):373–378; discussion 379–380.

7. Miller BJ, Avedian RS, Rajani R, et al. What is the use of imaging before referral to an orthopaedic oncologist? A prospective, multicenter investigation. *Clin Orthop Relat Res*. 2015;473(3):868–874.

8. Frassica FJ, Khanna JA, McCarthy EF. The role of MR imaging in soft tissue tumor evaluation: perspective of the orthopedic oncologist and musculoskeletal pathologist. *Magn Reson Imaging Clin N Am*. 2000;8(4):915–927.

9. Papp DF, Khanna AJ, McCarthy EF, et al. Magnetic resonance imaging of soft-tissue tumors: determinate and indeterminate lesions. *J Bone Joint Surg Am*. 2007;89(suppl 3):103–115.

10. Thacker MM, Potter BK, Pitcher JD, et al. Soft tissue sarcomas of the foot and ankle: impact of unplanned excision, limb salvage, and multimodality therapy. *Foot Ankle Int*. 2008;29(7):690–698.

11. Umer HM, Umer M, Qadir I, et al. Impact of unplanned excision on prognosis of patients with extremity soft tissue sarcoma. *Sarcoma*. 2013;2013:498604.

12. Noria S, Davis A, Kandel R, et al. Residual disease following unplanned excision of soft-tissue sarcoma of an extremity. *J Bone Joint Surg Am*. 1996;78(5):650–655.

13. Arai E, Nishida Y, Tsukushi S, et al. Clinical and treatment outcomes of planned and unplanned excisions of soft tissue sarcomas. *Clin Orthop Relat Res*. 2010;468(11):3028–3034.

14. van der Veer WM, Hamburg SM, de Gast A, et al. Recurrence of plantar fibromatosis after plantar fasciectomy: single center long-term results. *Plast Reconstr Surg*. 2008;122:486–491.

15. Heyd R, Dorn AP, Herkströter M, et al. Radiation therapy for early stages of morbus Ledderhose. *Strahlenther Onkol*. 2010;186(1):24–29.

16. Knobloch K, Vogt PM. High-energy focussed extracorporeal shockwave therapy reduces pain in plantar fibromatosis (Ledderhose's disease). *BMC Res Notes*. 2012;5:542.

17. Hammoudeh ZS. Collagenase Clostridium histolyticum injection for plantar fibromatosis (Ledderhose disease). *Plast Reconstr Surg*. 2014;134(3):497e–498e.

18. Dürr HR, Krödel A, Trouillier H, et al. Fibromatosis of the plantar fascia: diagnosis and indications for surgical treatment. *Foot Ankle Int*. 1999;20(1):13–17.

19. Aluisio FV, Mair SD, Hall RL. Plantar fibromatosis: treatment of primary and recurrent lesions and factors associated with recurrence. *Foot Ankle Int*. 1996;17(11):672–678.

20. Cupp JS, Miller MA, Montgomery KD, et al. Translocation and expression of CSF1 in pigmented villonodular synovitis, tenosynovial giant cell tumor, rheumatoid arthritis and other reactive synovitides. *Am J Surg Pathol*. 2007;31(6):970–976.

21. Schnirring-Judge M, Lin B. Pigmented villonodular synovitis of the ankle-radiation therapy as a primary treatment to reduce recurrence: a case report with 8-year follow-up. *J Foot Ankle Surg*. 2011;50(1):108–116.

22. Korim MT, Clarke DR, Allen PE, et al. Clinical and oncological outcomes after surgical excision of pigmented villonodular synovitis at the foot and ankle. *Foot Ankle Surg*. 2014;20(2):130–134.

23. Sung KS, Ko KR. Surgical outcomes after excision of pigmented villonodular synovitis localized to the ankle and hindfoot without adjuvant therapy. *J Foot Ankle Surg*. 2015;54(2):160–163.

24. Mori H, Nabeshima Y, Mitani M, et al. Diffuse pigmented villonodular synovitis of the ankle with severe bony destruction: treatment of a case by surgical excision with limited arthrodesis. *Am J Orthop (Belle Mead NJ)*. 2009;38(12):E187–E189.

25. Maceroli M, Uglialoro AD, Beebe KS, et al. Recurrent knee pain in an athletic adult: multiple schwannomas secondary to schwannomatosis: a case report. *Am J Orthop (Belle Mead NJ)*. 2010;39(11):E119–E122.

26. Kim DH, Hwang JH, Park ST, et al. Schwannomatosis involving peripheral nerves: a case report. *J Korean Med Sci*. 2006;21(6):1136–1138.

27. Milnes HL, Pavier JC. Schwannoma of the tibial nerve sheath as a cause of tarsal tunnel syndrome—a case study. *Foot (Edinb)*. 2012;22(3):243–246.

28. Graviet S, Sinclair G, Kajani N. Ancient schwannoma of the foot. *J Foot Ankle Surg*. 1995;34(1):46–50.

29. Kryzak TJ Jr, DeGroot H 3rd. Adult onset flatfoot associated with an intramuscular hemangioma of the posterior tibialis muscle. *Orthopedics*. 2008;31(3):280.

30. Uslu M, Beşir H, Turan H, et al. Two different treatment options for intramuscular plantar hemangioma: surgery versus percutaneous sclerotherapy. *J Foot Ankle Surg*. 2014;53(6):759–762.

31. Crawford EA, Slotcavage RL, King JJ, et al. Ethanol sclerotherapy reduces pain in symptomatic musculoskeletal hemangiomas. *Clin Orthop Relat Res*. 2009;467(11):2955–2961.

32. Tang P, Hornicek FJ, Gebhardt MC, et al. Surgical treatment of hemangiomas of soft tissue. *Clin Orthop Relat Res*. 2002;399:205–210.

33. Canavese F, Soo BC, Chia SK, et al. Surgical outcome in patients treated for hemangioma during infancy, childhood, and adolescence: a retrospective review of 44 consecutive patients. *J Pediatr Orthop*. 2008;28(3):381–386.

34. Fletcher CDM, Sundaram M, Rydholm A, et al. WHO classification of soft tissue tumours. http://www.iarc.fr/en/publications/pdfs-online/pat-gen/bb5/bb5-classifsofttissue.pdf.

35. Brennan MF, Antonescu CR, Moraco N, et al. Lessons learned from the study of 10,000 patients with soft tissue sarcoma. *Ann Surg*. 2014;260(3):416–421; discussion 421–422.

36. Johnstone PA, Wexler LH, Venzon DJ, et al. Sarcomas of the hand and foot: analysis of local control and functional result with combined modality therapy in extremity preservation. *Int J Radiat Oncol Biol Phys*. 1994;29(4):735–745.

37. Ottaviani G, Robert RS, Huh WW, et al. Functional, psychosocial and professional outcomes in long-term survivors of lower-extremity osteosarcomas: amputation versus limb salvage. *Cancer Treat Res*. 2009;152:421–436.

38. Ferguson PC. Surgical considerations for management of distal extremity soft tissue sarcomas. *Curr Opin Oncol*. 2005;17(4):366–369.

39. Cassidy RJ, Indelicato DJ, Gibbs CP, et al. Function preservation after conservative resection and radiotherapy for soft-tissue sarcoma of the distal extremity: utility and application of the Toronto Extremity Salvage Score (TESS). *Am J Clin Oncol*. 2016;39(6):600–603.

40. Toma CD, Dominkus M, Pfeiffer M, et al. Metatarsal reconstruction with use of free vascularized osteomyocutaneous fibular grafts following resection of malignant tumors of the midfoot. A series of six cases. *J Bone Joint Surg Am*. 2007;89(7):1553–1564.

41. Mavrogenis A, Bianchi G, Stavropoulos N, et al. Clinicopathological features, diagnosis and treatment of clear cell sarcoma/melanoma of soft parts. *Hippokratia*. 2013;17(4):298–302.

42. Kawai A, Hosono A, Nakayama R, et al. Clear cell sarcoma of tendons and aponeuroses: a study of 75 patients. *Cancer*. 2007;109(1):109–116.

43. Finley JW, Hanypsiak B, McGrath B, et al. Clear cell sarcoma: the Roswell Park experience. *J Surg Oncol*. 2001;77(1):16–20.

44. Jacobs IA, Chang CK, Guzman G, et al. Clear cell sarcoma: an institutional review. *Am Surg*. 2004;70(4):300–303.

45. Bianchi G, Charoenlap C, Cocchi S, et al. Clear cell sarcoma of soft tissue: a retrospective review and analysis of 31 cases treated at Istituto Ortopedico Rizzoli. *Eur J Surg Oncol*. 2014;40(5):505–510.

46. Meis-Kindblom JM, Kindblom LG. Acral myxoinflammatory fibroblastic sarcoma: a low-grade tumor of the hands and feet. *Am J Surg Pathol*. 1998;22(8):911–924.

47. Altmann S, Damert HG, Klausenitz S, et al. Aggressive digital papillary adenocarcinoma—a rare malignant tumor of the sweat glands: two case reports and a review of the literature. *Clin Cosmet Investig Dermatol*. 2015;8:143–146.

48. Duke WH, Sherrod TT, Lupton GP. Aggressive digital papillary adenocarcinoma (aggressive digital papillary adenoma and adenocarcinoma revisited). *Am J Surg Pathol*. 2000;24(6):775–784.

49. Bakotic B, Huvos AG. Tumors of the bones of the feet: the clinicopathologic features of 150 cases. *J Foot Ankle Surg*. 2001;40(5):277–286.

50. Ottaviani G, Robert RS, Huh WW, et al. Functional, psychosocial and professional outcomes in long-term survivors of lower-extremity osteosarcomas: amputation versus limb salvage. *Cancer Treat Res*. 2009;152:421–436.

51. Mei J, Zhu XZ, Wang ZY, et al. Functional outcomes and quality of life in patients with osteosarcoma treated with amputation versus limb-salvage surgery: a systematic review and meta-analysis. *Arch Orthop Trauma Surg*. 2014;134(11):1507–1516.

52. American College of Radiology (ACR). ACR Appropriateness Criteria—Primary bone tumors. 1995. https://acsearch.acr.org/docs/69421/Narrative. Accessed January 11, 2017.

53. Nystrom LM, Reimer NB, Dean CW, et al. Evaluation of imaging utilization prior to referral of musculoskeletal tumors: a prospective study. *J Bone Joint Surg Am*. 2015;97(1):10–15.

54. Turcotte RE. Giant cell tumor of bone. *Orthop Clin North Am*. 2006;37(1):35–51.

55. O'Keefe RJ, O'Donnell RJ, Temple HT, et al. Giant cell tumor of bone in the foot and ankle. *Foot Ankle Int*. 1995;16(10):617–623.

56. Zindrick MR, Young MP, Daley RJ, et al. Metastatic tumors of the foot: case report and literature review. *Clin Orthop Relat Res*. 1982;170:219–225.

57. Oliveira VC, van der Heijden L, van der Geest IC, et al. Giant cell tumours of the small bones of the hands and feet: long-term results of 30 patients and a systematic literature review. *Bone Joint J*. 2013;95-B(6):838–845.

58. Zuo D, Zheng L, Sun W, et al. Contemporary adjuvant polymethyl methacrylate cementation optimally limits recurrence in primary giant cell tumor of bone patients compared to bone grafting: a systematic review and meta-analysis. *World J Surg Oncol*. 2013;11:156.

59. Porter DE, Lonie L, Fraser M, et al. Severity of disease and risk of malignant change in hereditary multiple exostoses. A genotype-phenotype study. *J Bone Joint Surg Br*. 2004;86(7):1041–1046.

60. Qasem SA, DeYoung BR. Cartilage-forming tumors. *Semin Diagn Pathol*. 2014;31(1):10–20.

61. Driscoll M, Linton J, Sullivan E, et al. Correction and recurrence of ankle valgus in skeletally immature patients with multiple hereditary exostoses. *Foot Ankle Int*. 2013;34(9):1267–1273.

62. Rupprecht M, Spiro AS, Schlickewei C, et al. Rebound of ankle valgus deformity in patients with hereditary multiple exostosis. *J Pediatr Orthop*. 2015;35(1):94–99.

63. Gajewski DA, Burnette JB, Murphey MD, et al. Differentiating clinical and radiographic features of enchondroma and secondary chondrosarcoma in the foot. *Foot Ankle Int*. 2006;27(4):240–244.

64. Roberts EJ, Meier MJ, Hild G, et al. Chondromyxoid fibroma of the calcaneus: two case reports and literature review. *J Foot Ankle Surg*. 2013;52(5):643–649.

65. Daniilidis K, Martinelli N, Gosheger G, et al. Percutaneous CT-guided radio-frequency ablation of osteoid osteoma of the foot and ankle. *Arch Orthop Trauma Surg*. 2012;132(12):1707–1710.

66. Temple HT, Mizel MS, Murphey MD, et al. Osteoblastoma of the foot and ankle. *Foot Ankle Int*. 1998;19(10):698–704.

67. Levy, DM, Gross, CE, Garras, DN. Treatment of unicameral bone cysts of the calcaneus: a systematic review. *J Foot Ankle Surg*. 2015;54(4):652–656.

68. Zhao J, Ding N, Huang W, et al. Treatments for simple bone cysts in the long bones of children. *Cochrane Libr*. 2014. http://www.cochrane.org/CD010847/MUSKINJ_treatments-for-simple-bone-cysts-in-the-long-bones-of-children.

69. Sanerkin NG, Mott MG, Roylance J. An unusual intraosseous lesion with fibroblastic, osteoclastic, osteoblastic, aneurysmal and fibromyxoid elements. "Solid" variant of aneurysmal bone cyst. *Cancer*. 1983;51(12):2278–2286.

70. Gibbs CP Jr, Hefele MC, Peabody TD, et al. Aneurysmal bone cyst of the extremities. Factors related to local recurrence after curettage with a high-speed burr. *J Bone Joint Surg Am*. 1999;81(12):1671–1678.

71. Milgram JW. Intraosseous lipomas: radiologic and pathologic manifestations. *Radiology*. 1988;167(1). http://pubs.rsna.org/doi/citedby/10.1148/radiology.167.1.3347718.

72. Toguchida J, Nakayama T. Molecular genetics of sarcomas: applications to diagnoses and therapy. *Cancer Sci*. 2009;100(9):1573–1580.

73. Desmanet E, Amrani M, Fievez R, et al. Les Acrometastases. Apropos of 2 cases. Review of the literature. *Ann Chir Main Memb Super*. 1991;10(2):154–157.

74. Andreou D, Ruppin S, Fehlberg S. Survival and prognostic factors in chondrosarcoma: results in 115 patients with long-term follow-up. *Acta Orthop*. 2011;82(6):749–755.

75. Adkins CD, Kitaoka HB, Seide RK, et al. Ewing's sarcoma of the foot. *Clin Orthop Relat Res*. 1997;343:173–182.

76. Demircay E, Hornicek FJ Jr, Mankin HJ, et al. Malignant lymphoma of bone: a review of 119 patients. *Clin Orthop Relat Res*. 2013;471(8):2684–2690.

77. Fletcher C, Unni K, Mertens F. *WHO Classification of Tumours. Pathology and Genetics of Tumours of Soft Tissue and Bone*. Lyon, France: IARC Press; 2002.

78. Healey JH, Turnbull AD, Miedema B, et al. Acrometastases. A study of twenty nine patients with osseous involvement of the hands and feet. *J Bone Joint Surg Am*. 1986;68:743–746.

79. Libson E, Bloom RA, Husband JE, et al. Metastatic tumors of bones of the hand and foot: a comparative review and report of 43 additional cases. *Skeletal Radiol*. 1987;16:387–392.

80. Kaplansky DB, Kademian ME, Vancourt RB. Metastatic squamous cell carcinoma resembling cellulitis and osteomyelitis of the fifth toe. *J Foot Ankle Surg*. 2006;45(3):182–184.

81. Ramkumar U, Munshi NI, El-Jabbour JN. Occult carcinoma of the lung presenting as pain in the hallux: a case report. *J Foot Ankle Surg*. 2005;44(6):483–486.

82. Sundberg SB, Carlson WO, Johnson KA. Metastatic lesions of the foot and ankle. *Foot Ankle*. 1982;3:167–169.

83. Simkin A, Leichter I, Giladi M, et al. Combined effect of foot arch structure and an orthotic device on stress fractures. *Foot Ankle*. 1989;10(1):25–29.

84. Fottner A, Baur-Melnyk A, Birkenmaier C. Stress fractures presenting as tumours: a retrospective analysis of 22 cases. *Int Orthop*. 2009;33(2):489–492.

CHAPTER 12

Regional Pain Syndromes That Present in the Foot, Ankle, and Lower Extremity

JEFFREY Y. F. NGEOW • MINYI TAN

Case Illustration

Patient A

S.A. is a 59-year-old woman who had a nondisplaced right 5th metatarsal fracture in October 1997. She was treated with cast stabilization for 8 weeks. She was referred to pain management consultation 5 months after the injury. S.A. reported that she had suffered from throbbing, aching, and occasional shooting pain while wearing the cast. Symptoms escalated since cast removal. Movements and weather changes aggravated the pain. She could not tolerate wearing sock and walked with a cane. Her pain score on visual analog score was 8/10. Bone scan revealed diffuse increased vascularity and uptake in the right lower leg, ankle, and foot (**Fig. 12-1**). The right plantar skin temperature was 29.7°C versus 28.7°C on the left. The patient's history, symptoms, and signs were consistent with early-stage complex regional pain syndrome (CRPS). Diagnostic lumbar sympathetic nerve block (LSB) resulted in 2 to 3 days of significant pain relief. Thereafter, three more LSBs were performed with concomitant physical therapy. Gabapentin (Neurontin) was also prescribed. Within 3 weeks, she reported improvement of 70% to 80%. She could wear shoes and walk without a cane.

Patient B

D.C. is a 30-year-old man who suffered a right foot and ankle injury after falling through an improperly covered manhole. There was no fracture, but he had progressive debilitation and pain in the right lower extremity. He described his pain as constant, sharp, and burning, from the tips of the toes to the groin. Physical findings included cold skin with atrophic changes, limited range of motion, and inability to bear weight. He could not tolerate wearing a shoe on the injured side. He had undergone treatments, including several kinds of medication (amitriptyline, tramadol, and gabapentin), physical therapy, and invasive treatments with LSB as well as 5 days of local anesthetic infusion with an epidural catheter. He had no long-term relief. About 20 months after the injury, a spinal cord stimulation trial (**Fig. 12-2**) produced immediate improvement. One week later, the permanent stimulator was implanted. D.C. continues to do well at 5-month follow-up with 70% less pain medication, and he could tolerate aggressive physical therapy.

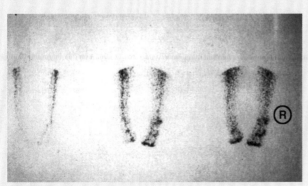

FIGURE 12-1. Bone scan from a patient 4 months after right 5th metatarsal fracture. Clinical CRPS developed within 8 weeks of injury.

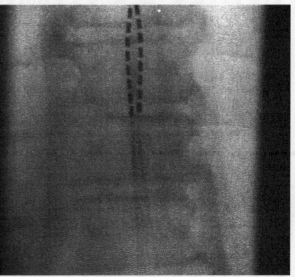

FIGURE 12-2. Spinal cord stimulator inserted at T10–T11 with eight electrodes.

INTRODUCTION

CRPS is difficult to diagnose and treat. So it has perplexed many physicians throughout medical history. Patients with such a condition invariably complained of severe disabling pain, yet their history of present illness may often only amount to trivial injuries. Routine or even extensive investigations usually fail to reveal significant underlying causes. The baffled physicians understandably think these patients exaggerated their symptoms and sufferings. Such complainers were labeled neurotics and promptly referred to psychologists for "pain management." Patients with CRPS affecting their lower extremities have often suffered such fates, and never had their condition treated appropriately.

Recent animal and human studies have shed light on the pathophysiology of the CRPS-related group of conditions. It is our intention to discuss some of the foot and ankle conditions that we have seen in a pain unit at an orthopedic center that have been associated with CRPS and to review their treatment in light of current understanding.

Brief Historic Review

In 1864, Mitchell and colleagues[1] first described, in victims of the American Civil War who sustained bullet injuries to their peripheral nerves, the syndrome of severe lancinating, burning pain in a limb that showed features of dystrophy. Later, Mitchell also named the condition "causalgia," from the Greek kausis (burning) and algos (pain).[2] Since then, several similar conditions, not necessarily the result of penetrating injuries but sharing the common features of burning pain with dystrophy, have been recognized. In many of them, evidence of sympathetic hyperactivity such as vasospasm, hyperhidrosis, and decreased skin temperature is also present. These causalgia-like conditions were given different names such as posttraumatic pain dysfunction syndrome, shoulder-hand syndrome, reflex neurovascular dystrophy, neuroalgodystrophy, Sudeck atrophy, and others. These labels make long, interesting lists, but they merely served to emphasize differences and reflect the disagreement regarding their underlying mechanisms. There was general agreement, however, that the sympathetic nervous system was somehow involved, and excessive activity in this autonomic system brought about the dystrophic changes. This led to the gradual adoption of the term "reflex sympathetic dystrophy (RSD)."

As RSD implies, physicians are apt to believe that blocking the sympathetic pathway would result in resolution of the neuropathic symptoms and dystrophy. Sympathetic blockade, either with local anesthetics or with other means, became the preferred treatment modality. Disappointment soon set in, however, when it was found that many of the RSD cases simply did not respond to sympatholysis and, therefore, could not have been sympathetically mediated.

By 1986, the term sympathetically maintained pain (SMP) as proposed by Roberts[3] was accepted for those cases labeled RSD that responded to sympathetic blockade. True RSD was naturally a member of SMP. Other cases that might not show much sympathetic overactivity but yet responded to sympathetic blockade were also included here. Conversely, pain conditions that showed features of sympathetic overactivity and even dystrophy but yet failed to respond to sympathetic blocks were labeled sympathetic independent pain (SIP). It was later recognized that SMP and SIP could represent the two ends of the spectrum for a single disease process.[4] Despite improved nomenclature, much debate still continued as more underlying mechanisms were proposed for the SMP–SIP syndromes. Further attempts to reduce the confusion brought forth another revision in the terminology. A special Consensus Workshop in 1993 chose the umbrella name complex regional pain syndrome.[4] To emphasize the distinction of the original causalgia, CRPS was subdivided into two categories:

1. **CRPS-I** covers a syndrome that develops after an initiating noxious event. Spontaneous pain or allodynia–hyperalgesia occurs. It is not limited to the territory of a single peripheral nerve and is disproportionate to the inciting event. There is or has been evidence of edema, skin blood flow abnormality, or abnormal sudomotor activity in the region of the pain since the inciting event. This diagnosis is excluded by the existence of conditions that would otherwise account for the degree of pain and dysfunction. RSD thus falls into this category.

2. **CRPS-II** is a syndrome similar to CRPS-I except that it develops after a known nerve injury. Traditionally, these injuries involve large nerves, such as the median or sciatic nerve.

CLINICAL FEATURES

History of Present Illness

CRPS may present at the time of the initial injury or be delayed for weeks. CRPS-I occurs without any known nerve injury, whereas CRPS-II has an identifiable nerve lesion. CRPS-I may be associated with minor (e.g., sprains or bruises, skin irritation) or major (e.g., fractures, thermal or chemical burns, wound or joint infections, ischemic necrosis) injuries. In these conditions, involvement of peripheral nerves is common. Its association with other diseases in which direct nerve damage is not so apparent has also been reported. Such conditions include metastatic malignancy, Lyme borreliosis, diabetes, hyperthyroidism, hyperlipoproteinemia, lumbar radiculopathy resulting from lateral disc fragment, previous lumbar laminectomy, tarsal tunnel syndrome, and so on.

Without history of significant trauma, the patient may appear disproportionately disabled, frequently with startling loss of range of motion if an extremity is affected. If the patient has undergone an operation, a protracted recovery period during which the patient poorly tolerated all rehabilitative efforts is a common feature. Stories such as these when elicited should raise a high index of suspicion and should prompt the search for more specific CRPS features.

Symptoms and Signs

The outstanding feature of CRPS pain is a spontaneous superficial burning sensation superimposed on a continuous deep, often described as crushing, tearing, or throbbing pain. Exacerbation with movement is usual, but many patients notice worse pain when resting at night. There is often increased pain with weather changes as well as heat or cold intolerance. Patients usually shy away from bright sunshine and cold wind or even air conditioners. Peculiar signs in the affected parts include allodynia (pain resulting from nonpainful stimuli such as light pressure), dysesthesia (unpleasant abnormal sensation such as stinging when lightly scratched), and hyperesthesia (increased pain sensation to mild noxious stimuli such as a pinprick or a heat lamp). Other findings may be more extensive spread of pain that is not limited to the territory of a single nerve or dermatome. Vasomotor (**Fig. 12-3**) and sudomotor disturbances may be found in more than just the affected limb. In more advanced or chronic cases, structural changes of the skin appendages and deeper tissues may be present.

Varied symptoms and signs may be grouped according to their severity. In 1953, Bonica[5] proposed a continuum of the RSD syndrome using stage I to III. Later, Schwartzman[6] redefined the stages as acute, dystrophic, and atrophic, respectively.

Acute (Stage I)

This stage may occur immediately or within days of the inciting event. It is characterized by spontaneous pain with dysesthesia and warm skin with localized edema. There is a reluctance to touch and move the affected body part as a result of tenderness and muscle spasm. Increased hair and nail growth may be seen. In early stage I, the pain is usually limited to the distribution of the principal nerves involved. The skin is usually warm, dry, and red, sometimes showing vasomotor instability including areas of erythema mixed with blanching. In late stage I, however, the pain spreads beyond the involved dermatomes, and the skin becomes cyanotic or mottled resembling livedo reticularis (**Fig. 12-4**), cold, and clammy. In some patients, friction from clothing or light air movement on the skin may cause excruciating pain. There are usually no radiographic bone changes at this time.

Dystrophic (Stage II)

Dystrophic stage usually sets in 3 to 6 months from the onset but may appear sooner in rapidly progressing cases. This stage is heralded by a gradual increase in the area of pain, extent of the edema, degree of joint stiffness, extent of soft

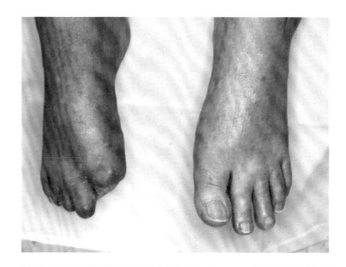

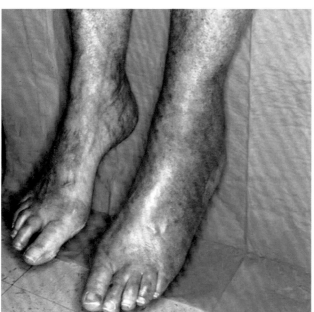

FIGURE 12-3. Patient with history of CRPS caused by blunt trauma to the left foot showing vasomotor instability. Note erythematous patch over dorsum of foot that is distinct from the unaffected right foot.

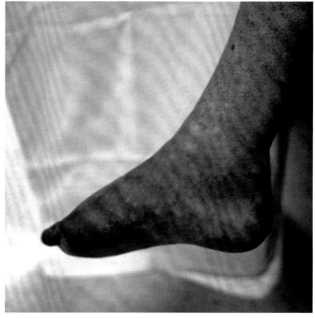

FIGURE 12-4. Patient with CRPS resulting from ischemic necrosis, which required toe amputation. Patchy erythema and pallor produced a mottled appearance.

tissue, and muscle wasting. The edema changes from a soft to a brawny type with glazed overlying skin. More advanced changes in the skin appendages are present. The hair becomes scant, and the nails become brittle, cracked, and grooved. Disturbance of motor functions such as tremors or dystonia may be present. Radiographic changes appear in this stage.

Atrophic (Stage III)

This stage is characterized by advanced trophic changes that are mostly irreversible. The skin is smooth, almost glossy. It may be pale or cyanotic and feels cold as the temperature further decreases. The hair becomes sparse and coarse. Subcutaneous tissue turns brawny as it becomes atrophic with marked loss of fat. The digits are thin with severe atrophy of muscles, particularly the interossei. The interphalangeal and other joints of the extremity become stiff with decreased range of motion. They eventually result in ankylosis. Pain symptoms may have spread proximally or to other parts of the body. The affected parts are almost always aggravated by passive motion or touching. Emotional disturbance and visual or auditory stimuli can also cause marked sudden aggravation.

It should be noted that in any individual case, there is usually some overlapping of the features described in the different stages because the changes are seldom clear-cut. For example, when the initial injury includes bone or joint trauma, osteoporotic changes may appear within a few weeks in a limb that otherwise appears completely normal. Furthermore, vasomotor instability and trophic changes, disparate though they may seem, are thought to be manifestations of a progressive pathophysiologic process.[7]

SYSTEMIC SPREAD OF CRPS

Long-standing CRPS patients suffer pain that spreads beyond the area of initial injury. It often spreads spontaneously to the contralateral or ipsilateral limb. Diagonal pattern of spread is often associated with new trauma.[8] It was postulated that the "pathologic impulse" of CRPS is spread through the chain of sympathetic ganglia.[9] CRPS patients often have constitutional symptoms such as lethargy, tiredness, or weakness. CRPS is a proinflammatory state where the body initiates nonspecific immune response following injury. The constitutional symptoms experienced by these patients maybe in part because of this response. Studies have shown that these patients have increased heart rate and decreased heart rate variability due to generalized autonomic imbalance related to disease duration, but not pain intensity.[10] CRPS patients can develop dystonia, affecting chest wall muscles leading to restrictive lung disease.[11] These patients can also feel chest discomfort that may be because of irritation of the intercostobrachial nerve that innervates pectoral and intercostal muscles. This chest discomfort may be mistaken for cardiac pain or gallbladder disease.[12] These patients often suffered from bone and joint pain. It is thought that release of substance P results in activation of osteoclasts, thus forming

intracortical excavation due to bone demineralization and resorption.[13] Pathologic fractures are common and often occur in the 5th metatarsal bone. In addition to skin color changes, dermatologic manifestations include development of morbilliform rash, punched-out ulcer-like lesions, and recurrent bullous lesions, to name a few.

PATHOPHYSIOLOGY

Despite advancement in our understanding of CRPS, its pathophysiology remains uncertain. As more knowledge is gained from the clinical observations and experimental studies, there is less agreement in a single common mechanism. The manifestation of somatosensory and motor disorders, autonomic dysfunction, and tissue structural changes makes it even more difficult for clinicians and scientists to accept a single animal model or hypothesis as the sole cause for this disorder.[14]

What is now generally accepted is that there is experimental evidence that suggests partial injury to a mixed peripheral nerve may be responsible for at least some of the features found in CRPS. Under normal conditions, sympathetic nerve stimulation does not excite the nociceptors (pain receptors) at the ending of an uninjured somatic nerve. Within days after partial nerve injury, however, changes occur that render the nociceptors excitable by sympathetic stimulation. The nociceptors now also respond to intra-arterially injected norepinephrine. If tissue injury and inflammation have already sensitized these nociceptors, their responses can be further augmented by sympathetic activities. Some of the proposed hypotheses that link this local event of nociceptor sensitization to the generalized manifestation of sympathetic hyperactivity are as follows.

Inflammation

Tissue and nerve injury causes the release of proinflammatory cytokines and neuropeptides, such as interleukin 6, tumor necrosis factor alpha, and substance P, in the affected area. An exaggerated localized inflammatory response is found in patients with CRPS. Studies have shown that CRPS patients have elevated levels of proinflammatory cytokines in their cerebrospinal fluid compared to healthy controls as well as those with different types of pain.[15]

Sympathetic Dysfunction

Local tissue factors, including sensitized nociceptors as well as neurotransmitter mediators, may activate the sympathetic system. In a vicious cycle, the noxious stimuli activate segmental and suprasegmental sympathetic discharges, producing vasoconstriction, ischemia, and further nociceptor activation. These result in impaired perfusion, which eventually leads to dystrophic changes.[16] After tissue injury, abnormal connections between the sympathetic and somatic nervous systems are established. The resulting cross-talk (called ephapses) between sympathetic efferent and somatosensory afferent nerves explains the sympathetic component of the pain in causalgia.[17] In 1983, Devor[18] presented finding showing that inflamed or damaged peripheral nerve twigs formed abnormal synapses in the same manner as injured nerve trunks. Such abnormal connections allowed cross-talk between the two systems, leading to increased signal input into the spinal cord, increased activity of the internuncial neuronal pool, and further stimulation of the sympathetic efferent and sensory afferents.

Spinal Mechanism

The neuronal turbulence hypothesis proposed by Sunderland[19] in 1976 suggested that injury to the postganglionic sympathetic ganglia and trans-synaptic degeneration in the spinal cord would impair the function of spinal neuron groups. These groups of neurons could then form self-sustaining reverberating circuits.

Central Mechanism

In 1965, when Melzack and Wall[20] proposed the gate control theory of pain transmission in the spine, they also suggested a central biasing mechanism mediated through a system of descending fibers. These descending fibers arise from the brain stem reticular system, and they exert a tonic inhibition on the somatic sensory system at all levels. Reduced sensory input after somatic nerve injury (especially when the nerve is severed) would result in a decrease in the descending tonic inhibition and thus allow an increase in the transmission of the self-sustaining neuronal activities generated either in the periphery or within the spinal cord. In this situation, they postulated that prolonged pain may leave "memory traces" in the somatosensory system, making an individual more susceptible to recurrent pain. The practical application of this theory becomes relevant in the treatment of patients with phantom limb pain.[21,22]

Neuronal Plasticity Mechanism

This proposed theory, which has become more commonly accepted, suggests that the perpetuation of abnormal firing pattern in the internuncial neuron pool in the spinal cord is responsible for abnormal pain perception. At the spinal cord level, a class of dorsal horn neurons that are multireceptive, the so-called wide dynamic range (WDR) neurons, usually do not contribute to painful sensations under normal conditions.[23] Sustained stimulation of the WDR by nociceptors, however, causes hyperexcitability and plasticity of the WDR by nociceptors, resulting in expansion of their receptive fields. This may explain why innocuous stimulations are now perceived as painful (hyperalgesia).[22] Roberts and Foglesong[24] demonstrated that WDR neurons are the only spinal nociceptive neurons activated by sympathetic efferent activity. Therefore, WDR neurons (i.e., the high-threshold neurons) are most likely to mediate the spinal component of

SMP. Sympathetic activation of WDR neurons is abolished by subcutaneous injection of local anesthetic, cooling the receptive field with ice, and intravenous injection of the α-adrenergic blocker phentolamine.

Glial Cell Activation

It has recently been hypothesized that CRPS is associated with activation of glial cells following tissue injury or inflammation. Glial cell, such as microglia and astrocytes, secretes substances that enhance pain transmission in the central nervous system once they are activated. These substances include proinflammatory cytokines, nitric oxide, and glutamate, to name a few. Animal studies have shown that activation of glial cells augments nociception. Human autopsy study of CRPS showed that long-standing CRPS patients had significant glial cell activation as well as neuronal loss in the posterior horn, predominantly at the level of the original injury.[25]

Psychological Predisposition

Because none of the previously proposed mechanisms offer any predictability on who is more susceptible to CRPS, it is not surprising that some suggested that particular personality traits indicated predisposition toward developing CRPS. The patients' seemingly exaggerated response to innocuous stimulations naturally led the physician to suspect psychological disorders. There is literature on both adults and children that hypothesize the presence of psychological disorders, particularly anxiety and depression, which predispose one to CRPS. Conversely, others believe that any chronic pain and suffering, in and of itself, will produce a host of psychological complications.

DIAGNOSIS

A complete history and physical examination with high index of suspicion is crucial for diagnosis of CRPS in the early stages when disproportionate pain may be the only abnormal feature. Differentiation from other conditions may be difficult. Neuropathic pain caused by an injured or entrapped peripheral nerve or a neuroma anywhere from its root to the terminal branches may present similar symptoms, such as burning pain with hyperpathia. They are, however, usually limited to the territory of the involved nerve and associated with little sympathetic activities. Inflammatory processes not involving nerves, such as tenosynovitis and bursitis, may produce burning pain, which persists for months.[7] They do not typically show Tinel sign, which is specific to nerves. Vascular diseases that cause decreased circulation such as Raynaud phenomenon or disseminated lupus erythematosus may mimic CRPS, although they usually affect more than one extremity at once. Therefore, the diagnosis is not infrequently made by exclusion, especially in the early stages of CRPS. For such reasons, some clinicians still do not accept CRPS as a distinctive pathologic disorder.

Several investigative tools may help to consolidate the diagnosis of CRPS:

1. Quantitative sweat test may show excessive sweating.
2. Thermography can demonstrate a disorder in heat regulation. Heat loss from the skin surface is mainly regulated by sudomotor activity on the sweat glands and the dermal microcirculation.[26] An affected hand or foot may at times be hyperthermic, but relative coldness is the most common finding. These changes produce the observation of vasomotor instability. They are related to sympathetic vasoconstriction and to compensatory or rebound vasodilatation of skin capillaries, which are, in turn, influenced by irritation of peripheral nerve fibers.[27]
3. Radiographic studies may reveal characteristic though not pathognomonic changes. Patchy osteoporosis is the primary roentgenographic manifestation of early dystrophic CRPS.[28] Other features such as patchy epiphyseal demineralization of the short bones with soft tissue swelling; subperiosteal resorption; striation and tunneling in the cortex; as well as large excavation and tunneling of the endosteal surfaces may also be present. One must be aware, however, that similar pictures may also be seen in hyperparathyroidism, thyrotoxicosis, and other conditions with increased bone turnover.[29] In later dystrophic stage, when dystrophy borders on atrophy, severe and diffuse osteoporosis is the usual finding.
4. Triple-phase bone scan using technetium-99 may demonstrate increased periarticular uptake in the involved extremity (**Fig. 12-1**).[28] A positive bone scan in a patient with clinical signs and symptoms of CRPS helps to confirm the diagnosis. Conversely, a negative scan in a patient with clinical CRPS does not rule out the condition because some patients will present with initial negative scans that become positive later.[30]

Each finding, be it thermographic, radiographic, or scintigraphic, despite their sensitivity, when present in isolation, tends to be nonspecific and impossible to distinguish from other metabolic or inflammatory conditions. Taken together, they greatly strengthen the diagnosis.

The diagnostic "gold standard" has been pain relief from a sympathetic nerve block. When evaluating the result of a sympathetic nerve block, care must be taken that somatic nerves are not anesthetized during the sympathetic block, or the outcome cannot be interpreted. Even when done properly, there is still the unavoidable confounding placebo effect. To circumvent this, it has been recommended that an α-adrenergic receptor blocker such as phentolamine be used intravenously as a predictor agent before invasive LSB.[31,32] Of course, a negative response to sympathetic blocks does not rule out CRPS.

Since the nomenclature conversion of RSD to CRPS, there have been multiple consensus meetings convened to derive the diagnostic criteria for CRPS. In 1994, the International Association for the Study of Pain (IASP) came up with the first consensus-driven diagnostic criteria. In subsequent years, the IASP criteria was found to be adequately sensitive, but had problems with specificity, resulting in overdiagnosis of CRPS. As a result, updated criteria called the Budapest Criteria were recommended in 2003 when an international group of researchers and clinician experts in CRPS met in Budapest, Hungary. The Budapest consensus statement for CRPS is as follows:[33]

General definition of the syndrome: CRPS describes an array of painful conditions that are characterized by a continuing (spontaneous and/or evoked) regional pain that is seemingly disproportionate in time or degree to the usual course of any known trauma or other lesion. The pain is regional (not in a specific nerve territory or dermatome) and usually has a distal predominance of abnormal sensory, motor, sudomotor, vasomotor, and/or trophic findings. The syndrome shows variable progression over time.

To make the clinical diagnosis, the following criteria must be met:

1. Continuing pain, which is disproportionate to any inciting event
2. Must report at least one symptom in three of the four following categories:
   Sensory: Reports of hyperesthesia and/or allodynia
   Vasomotor: Reports of temperature asymmetry and/or skin color changes and/or skin color asymmetry
   Sudomotor/Edema: Evidence of edema and/or sweating changes and/or sweating asymmetry
   Motor/Trophic: Reports of decreased range of motion and/or motor dysfunction (weakness, tremor, dystonia) and/or trophic changes (hair, nail, skin)
3. Must display at least one sign at time of evaluation in two or more of the following categories:
   Sensory: Evidence of hyperalgesia (to pinprick) and/or allodynia (to light touch and/or temperature sensation and/or deep somatic pressure and/or joint movement)
   Vasomotor: Evidence of temperature asymmetry (1°C) and/or skin color changes and/or asymmetry
   Sudomotor/Edema: Evidence of edema and/or sweating changes and/or sweating asymmetry
   Motor/Trophic: Evidence of decreased range of motion and/or motor dysfunction (weakness, tremor, dystonia) and/or trophic changes (hair, nail, skin)
4. There is no other diagnosis that better explains the signs and symptoms

TREATMENT

Any treatment must be targeted toward relief of pain, avoidance of disuse atrophy, and ultimately a return to normal function. Many patients, especially those with early stages of CRPS, do recover gradually with physiotherapy and analgesic drugs alone. In more advanced or chronic cases, more aggressive treatments are needed to break the vicious cycle of pain, immobility, disuse atrophy, and more pain. For any patient, treatment should follow a preplanned algorithm to effect minimum time loss between each chosen method. Psychological evaluation with ongoing counseling for the patients and their immediate family members should be an integral part of the treatment regimen. The emphasis is toward a multidisciplinary approach, which ensures that important aspects of the patient's care are not overlooked.

NONINVASIVE MODALITIES

Physical Therapy

Physical therapy is the mainstay of overcoming disuse atrophy. To minimize fear of painful motion, patients should be given only active or actively assisted therapy within limits of tolerance. Aggressive physical therapy without adequate pain management usually leads to patient noncompliance with the treatment program and delayed recovery. Therefore, passive exercise may be undertaken only when both the patient and the therapist thoroughly understand and accept the risk of more pain, swelling, and stiffness by forcing motions beyond the point of discomfort.[34]

Transcutaneous Electrical Nerve Stimulation

Transcutaneous electrical nerve stimulation became popular after the gate theory, proposed by Melzack and Wall, became generally accepted. When delivered at levels that produce skin tingling, it has been postulated to activate both large ($A\beta$, B) and small ($A\delta$, C) fibers.[35] The large-fiber signals "close the gate" and block the small-fiber signals. Alternatively, activation of small fibers may facilitate the descending inhibitory system.[35,36] Using this modality, Robaina and colleagues reported excellent results in 25% and good results in 45% of RSD patients.[37]

Nonsteroidal Anti-Inflammatory Drugs

Although often used as the first-line analgesic for most chronic conditions, nonsteroidal anti-inflammatory drugs may be helpful during the acute stage when inflammatory changes and tissue edema are present. Their efficacy in established CRPS has not been established.

Tricyclic Antidepressants

Tricyclic antidepressants block norepinephrine and serotonin reuptake. They also block the α1-adrenergic receptors, hence reducing sympathetic efferent activity. In animal models, they have been shown to block the hyperalgesia induced by intrathecally injected N-methyl-D-aspartate (NMDA).[38,39] They have been shown effective in reducing some of the neuropathic symptoms such as burning sensation. The popularity of this group of drugs has been limited by their significant side effects.

Opioids

Opioid analgesics have been shown to block neuropathic pain less effectively than nociceptive pain. Although opioids are not very effective in treating CRPS pain symptoms, they do improve the quality of pain control. They are especially helpful to patients getting over severe acute episodes. Because tolerance inevitably builds up, chronic use will result in escalating doses, with increasing potential for side effects. These medications should, therefore, be given judiciously.

Corticosteroids

Steroids have been used since 1953, when favorable results were reported in the treatment of shoulder-hand syndrome.[40] The pharmacodynamics remains largely unknown. Kozin and coworkers[41] observed a chronic perivascular inflammatory infiltrate in synovial biopsy specimens from involved extremities. Hence, the potent anti-inflammatory properties of the corticosteroids may partially account for their therapeutic effects. By stabilizing basement membranes, they reduce capillary permeability and decrease plasma extravasation commonly associated with early stages of CRPS.[36] One potential advantage of systemic corticosteroids over the beneficial effects of sympathetic block becomes apparent when multiple body parts are involved. A 1997 review by Kingery[39] confirmed consistent support in the literature for use of corticosteroids, which showed long-term effectiveness.

Gabapentin

Gabapentin, an anticonvulsant, was initially used for partial seizures with or without secondary generalization. Recently, it has been used for neuropathic pain with notably good results, as reported by Rosner and associates.[42] When given to patients with CRPS, dramatic pain relief was observed and, in some cases, reversal of early trophic changes. Mellick and Mellicy[43] reported corrections in skin temperature and color and lessening of and eventual relief from allodynia, hyperalgesia, and hyperpathia. A major advantage of gabapentin is its low toxicity and side effect profile. It is generally well tolerated by most patients.

Carbocalcitonin

When bone scans show increases in blood flow and uptake of the tracer in the involved area, both porcine and salmon calcitonin have been reported to reduce local blood flow and decrease local clinical signs with relief from pain.[44] Nuti and others[34] demonstrated similar improvements in the feet of CRPS patients. Salmon calcitonin is now available as a nasal spray, which significantly increases patient acceptance over the older injectable formulation.

Clonidine Transdermal Application

Clonidine has a dual mode of action. In the central nervous system, it acts as an α2 agonist. In the peripheral nervous

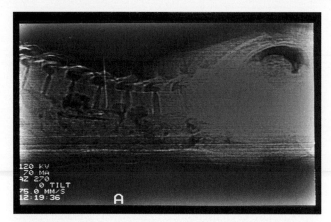

FIGURE 12-5. Lumbar sympathetic block under fluoroscopy showing the tip of the needle is at anterior body of the L2 vertebra to block the lumbar sympathetic pain with local anesthetic.

system, it inhibits the release of norepinephrine from sympathetic terminals. Thus, centrally, it has analgesic effects, whereas peripherally it reduces the ongoing activity of nociceptors, hence decreasing the central sensitization and relieving hyperalgesia.[45] It is available as a transdermal patch, which is easy to use. In some patients, however, it may cause unacceptable hypotension or sedation.

INVASIVE MODALITIES

Intermittent sympathetic nerve blocks done in the early stages can be effective in achieving remission. Even in established cases, they are valuable as an option in offering to the patients periodic "breaks" from the vicious cycle of pain and

dysfunction. The procedure is not without risk, and repeated blocks tend to lose efficacy. When judiciously done at the crest of periods of exacerbation, intermittent sympathetic nerve block can usually abort the need to resort to opioid medication. Of course, this is applicable only to those who respond to sympathetic blockade. Sympathetic nerve blocks with local anesthetics can either be done at the lumbar sympathetic chain or as a regional perfusion in the limb.

Lumbar Sympathetic Block

The purpose of sympathetic blockade in patients with CRPS is to interrupt the abnormal reflexes mediated by the autonomic nervous system. Sympathetic blockade can be both diagnostic and therapeutic.[36] In the early stage of CRPS, a prolonged remission may be obtained from a single sympathetic block (**Figs. 12-5** and **12-6**). Far more commonly, however, repeated nerve blocks are required for prolonged pain control.[14] Typically, blocks are done closely, up to three times per week for 2 weeks in early cases, and then are tapered off to once weekly or less when symptoms subside or responses are stabilized.[46] When the condition is bilateral, LSB can be achieved bilaterally with an epidural infusion for inpatients.[47] To maximize benefit from the nerve block, it should be followed by a course of physical therapy to improve range of motion.

Neurolytic LSB with Injectable Chemicals

Chemical agents such as concentrated alcohol or phenol can produce longer duration nerve blocks lasting from a few weeks

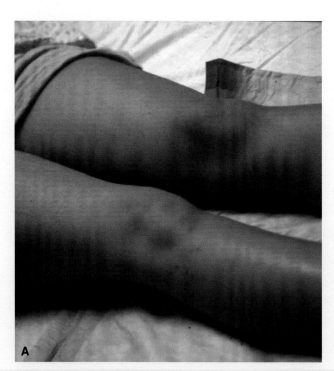
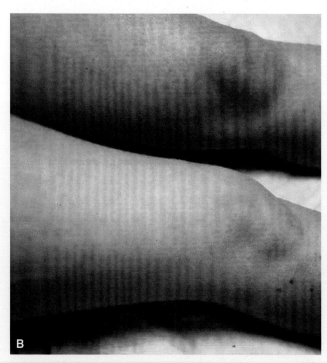

FIGURE 12-6. Patient with CRPS of left lower extremity **(A)** with increased vascular flow and temperature after lumbar sympathetic block **(B)**.

to several months. Haynsworth and Noe[48] reported that 89% of patients in the phenol group showed signs of sympathetic blockade after 8 weeks. Some controversy surrounds the use of these agents, however, such as a high incidence (5% to 40%) of postsympathectomy neuralgia resulting from inadvertent damage to somatic nerves (e.g., genitofemoral neuralgia).[49,50]

Surgical Lumbar Sympathectomy

Because of the relative extensive area involved, surgical lumbar sympathectomy is usually not recommended, except when definitely indicated. The sympatholytic effect can be transient as a result of incomplete denervation.

Intravenous Regional Sympatholysis

Done with guanethidine and reserpine as described by Hannington-Kiff[51] in 1977, intravenous regional sympatholysis is essentially a modification of the Bier block procedure for regional anesthesia. Pharmacologically, guanethidine acts as a false transmitter. It is taken up by sympathetic nerve endings and displaces norepinephrine from its storage sites. Thus, there is an initial release of norepinephrine followed by depletion. Excellent pain relief lasts from 12 to 36 hours but may be as long as a few weeks. Wahren and colleagues demonstrated that patients with SMP benefited considerably for 2 weeks or more, whereas no significant pain relief was achieved in patients with SIP.[52] Reserpine acts by reducing reuptake of catecholamines, thereby slowly depleting norepinephrine stores in sympathetic nerve endings. Pain relief lasting from weeks up to a few months has been reported.[53] Although reported complications from these drugs have been few, prolonged orthostatic hypotension with dizziness, somnolence, nausea, and vomiting can occur. Neither of these two agents was approved by the U.S. Food and Drug Administration for intravenous infusion. Studies such as that by Blanchard and associates[54] have thrown doubt on the efficacy of these drugs when used in this fashion. Saline infusion was observed to produce comparable results. This led to some to contend that tourniquet ischemia was actually the active ingredient.

Ketamine Infusion

CRPS patients that have refractory pain despite conventional treatment are likely to have central sensitization of pain due to release of the magnesium blockade of the NMDA receptor. Ketamine is an NMDA receptor antagonist that can be used to treat neuropathic pain in these patients. Double blind, randomized, placebo-controlled studies have shown that patients treated with ketamine infusion have significant pain relief.[55,56] Furthermore, retrospective study by Correll et al.[57] showed that patients have prolonged period of pain relief with repeat ketamine infusion compared to single infusion. Some potential side effects of ketamine infusion are diuresis, elevated liver enzyme, tachyarrhythmia, hallucination, flashbacks, and erratic behavior. Thus, urine output, liver enzyme

level, and EKG should be monitored during the infusion. Clonidine and benzodiazepine should be used to prevent tachyarrhythmia and psychological effects of ketamine.

Electroacupuncture

Electroacupuncture is claimed to release endogenous opioids, endorphins, and enkephalins in the central nervous system, thereby achieving pain reduction. The electric current during electroacupuncture may also act locally to relax the postcapillary sphincters, thus reducing the local edema and swelling.[58] Needle stimulation may also increase large-fiber transmission and "close the gate" to small-fiber pain signals according to the gate control theory of Melzack and Wall.[20]

New Invasive Modalities

Radiofrequency Lumbar Sympathectomy

This technique uses a heat-generating radiofrequency directed through an insulated wire at the nerve or ganglion. It offers a limited, controlled thermal lesion, thus avoiding significant neurologic deficits that may occur with injected chemicals. Also, less scar is produced, making repeated procedures possible.[59] Sri Kantha[60] reported that the duration of relief from radiofrequency sympathectomy appears to be longer than that from chemical neurolytic agents and may be as long as that from open surgery. On the other hand, Rocco concluded that despite early successful LSB, long-lasting pain relief was difficult to obtain.[61] Comparing incidence of postsympathectomy neuralgia, Haynsworth and Noe's[48] study showed 11% in the radiofrequency group versus 33% in the phenol group.

Epidural Clonidine

Clonidine is an α2-adrenoceptor agonist, which binds both pre- and postsynaptic neurons. It decreases anesthetic requirement during surgery[62,63] and postoperative morphine requirement.[64] Clonidine administered epidurally produces analgesia that is not reversed by opiate antagonist. Rauck and colleagues[65] demonstrated extensive analgesia with epidural clonidine. The proposed mechanisms include reduced norepinephrine release peripherally, reduction of sympathetic outflow centrally, and the postsynaptic action of hyperpolarization of dorsal horn WDR neurons.[65]

Neuromodulation

Neuromodulation is based on the gate control theory proposed by Melzack and Wall,[20] whereby electrical stimulation of non-nociceptive Aβ nerve fibers inhibits dorsal horn interneurons and interrupts the transmission of pain signals. These investigators were able to suppress pain with electrical stimulation of infraorbital nerves using peripheral nerve stimulation (PNS). Peripheral stimulation may augment blood flow, decrease excitability of peripheral nerve fibers as well as changing the local concentration of neurotransmitters that produce chronic pain.[66,67] Case studies have shown that implantation of peripheral nerve stimulator proximal to the lesion was able to provide long-lasting reduction of pain score in patients with CRPS.[68,69]

Because of the initial complexity of PNS procedure and unpredictability of its outcome, electrical stimulation of the spinal cord for analgesia was proposed soon after publication of the gate control therapy. Technically simplistic, it involves insertion of an electrode-tipped catheter into the epidural space at the appropriate spinal segment. This allows a variety of currents to stimulate the spinal cord directly (**Fig. 12-2**). Many different theories have been proposed to explain how it works.[70] Experience has shown that, in addition to pain relief, spinal cord stimulation has been successful to some degree in reversing the "inability" to move injured extremities.[71] It was also found helpful in patients who suffer recurrent pain after surgical sympathectomy.[72]

PERIOPERATIVE MANAGEMENT

The general goals of perioperative management of CRPS patients are aggressive pain control as well as preventing exacerbation of this condition. Surgery can precipitate development of CRPS. Preoperative factors that precipitate CRPS include preoperative anxiety, preoperative pain intensity, and intraoperative factors. Intraoperative factors include prolonged tourniquet time and motor nerve injury. Asaad and Glass[73] have reviewed studies for different perioperative approaches of these patients. They found three components that are critical to management of these patients. Those include preventive measures, anesthetic and intraoperative management, and postoperative pain management.

Elective surgery should be performed when symptoms are well controlled. Marx et al.[74] reported that administering calcitonin 2 to 4 days preoperatively and up to 4 weeks postoperatively may prevent recurrence of CRPS. Studies also found that three daily doses of vitamin C preoperatively can decrease the incidence of postoperative CRPS.[75–77]

The anesthetic plan of CRPS is not limited to the choice between regional anesthesia and general anesthesia. In a prospective, controlled study, it found no difference in the development of CRPS in patients who received general anesthesia, intravenous regional anesthesia with lidocaine, or intravenous anesthesia with lidocaine and clonidine, in comparison with patients who received a brachial plexus block. The same study also found a positive correlation between tourniquet time and the development of CRPS.[78]

A multimodal approach is important in decreasing flare-up of CRPS symptoms postoperatively. Patients should resume their oral medication as early as possible. An early mobilization and rehabilitation should also be taking place.[74] In addition to continuous regional anesthesia, adjuvant medication such as clonidine may be added to the infusion. Subanesthetic dose (10 to 20 mg per hour) of ketamine intravenous infusion in the immediate postoperative period could also be helpful.[73] Other adjuvant pain medications such as gabapentin could be part of the multimodal pain management.[79]

PROGNOSIS

Two important factors that influence long-term patient outcome regardless of etiology are (1) early recognition with appropriate treatments and (2) vigorous rehabilitation therapies. If diagnosed early, the majority of patients with CRPS will respond to a course of prudent physical therapy and adequate analgesia. With delayed treatment, the CRPS syndrome may spread proximally from one extremity or even to the other extremities. It is potentially devastating to patients in whom the disease progresses to the dystrophic–atrophic stages. Evaluation of any particular treatment regimen must be tempered by the awareness that a certain number of cases will show spontaneous resolution, whereas certain others will continue to progress despite appropriate therapeutic efforts.

Any surgery performed in or close to the CRPS affected area may lead to acute and prolonged exacerbation of preexisting symptoms. In other words, to a CRPS patient, there is no minor surgery. Therefore, adequate pain control by regional anesthetic and/or opiate infusion for a period of time postoperatively to create a pain-free window for regaining or maintaining range of motion is of utmost importance.

SUMMARY

Despite voluminous literature, many aspects of the treatment of these disorders are still based on empiricism. For example, it is not yet clear why sympathetic interruption in a warm, edematous, and vasodilated extremity does not produce further relaxation of arteriolar smooth muscle and subsequently an increase in swelling and pain.[36] Hypotheses have been proposed, but they lack experimental support.[80] The precise role of steroids also remains to be settled. There is no explanation either for the phenomenon that LSBs become less effective with repetition. Part of the difficulty in studying these patients has been the ubiquitous confounding effect of the placebo response.[81] Establishing a rationale for the treatments requires further careful investigation.

To the physician, the ultimate goal is restoration of complete functional and anatomic integrity of the extremities at the earliest possible time and by the simplest therapeutic procedure. Selecting the treatment best suited to the individual at the earliest moment will increase the chances of remission and reduce intractability. Long, continued vascular disturbances and disuse because of pain are the major causes of permanent disability.[45] Early diagnosis and specific, goal-directed treatments buttressed by a supportive social structure offer the best chance of returning the patient to a meaningful existence.

REFERENCES

1. Mitchell SW, Morehouse GR, Kean WW. *Gunshot Wounds and Other Injuries of Nerves.* Philadelphia, PA: J.B. Lippincott; 1864:164.
2. Mitchell SW. On the diseases of nerves, resulting from injuries. In: Flint A, ed. *Contributions Relating to the Causation and Presentation*

of Disease, and to Camp Diseases. New York, NY: U.S. Sanitary Commission Memoirs; 1867:412–468.

3. Roberts W. A hypothesis on the physiological basis for causalgia and related pains. *Pain.* 1986;24:297–311.

4. Stanton-Hicks M, Janig W, Hassenbusch S, et al. Reflex sympathetic dystrophy: changing concepts and taxonomy. *Pain.* 1995;63:127–133.

5. Bonica J. *The Management of Pain.* Philadelphia, PA: Lea & Febiger; 1953.

6. Schwartzman RJ. Reflex sympathetic dystrophy. *Arch Neurol.* 1987;44:555–559.

7. Butler SH. Reflex sympathetic dystrophy: clinical features. In: Stanton-Hicks M, Janig W, Boas RA, eds. *Reflex Sympathetic Dystrophy.* Boston, MA: Kluwer Academic Publishers; 1990:1–8.

8. van Rijin M, Marinus J, Putter H, et al. Spreading of complex regional pain syndrome: not a random process. *J Neural Transm.* 2011;118:1301–1309.

9. Hooshmand H. *Chronic Pain: Reflex Sympathetic Dystrophy. Prevention and Management.* Boca Raton, FL: CRC Press; 993:1–202.

10. Terkelsen AJ, Molgaard H, Hansen J, et al. Heart rate variability in complex regional pain syndrome during rest and mental and orthostatic stress. *Anesthesiology.* 2012;116(1):133–146.

11. Irwin DJ, Schwartzman RJ. Complex regional pain syndrome with associated chest wall dystonia: a case report. *J Brachial Plex Peripher Nerve Inj.* 2011;6:6.

12. Rasmussen JW, Grothusen JR, Rosso AL, et al. Atypical chest pain: evidence of intercostobrachial nerve sensitization in Complex Regional Pain Syndrome. *Pain Physician.* 2009;12(5):329–334.

13. Kingery WS, Offley SC, Guo TZ, et al. A substance P receptor (NK1) antagonist enhances the widespread osteoporotic effects of sciatic nerve section. *Bone.* 2003;33(6):927–936.

14. Ngeow J. Reflex sympathetic dystrophy of the knee. In: Scuderi G, ed. *The Patella.* New York, NY: Springer-Verlag; 1995:333–339.

15. Huygen FJ, De Bruijn AG, De Bruin MT, et al. Evidence for local inflammation in complex regional pain syndrome type 1. *Mediators Inflamm.* 2002;11(1):47–51.

16. Kuntz A. Afferent innervation of blood vessels through sympathetic trunks. *JAMA.* 1951,44.673–678.

17. Doupe J, Cullen CR, Chance CQ. Post-traumatic pain and the causalgia syndrome. *J Neurol Neurosurg Psychiatr.* 1944;7:33–38.

18. Devor M. Nerve pathophysiology and mechanism of pain in causalgia. *J Auton Nerv Syst.* 1983;7:371–384.

19. Sunderland S. Pain mechanism: a new theory. *Science.* 1976;39:441–448.

20. Melzack R, Wall PD. Pain mechanisms: a new theory. *Science.* 1965;150:971–979.

21. Melzack R. Phantom limb pain: implication for treatment of pathologic pain. *Anesthesiology.* 1971;35:405–419.

22. Melzack R, Leser J. Phantom body pain in paraplegics: evidence for a central "pattern-generating mechanism" for pain. *Pain.* 1978;4:195–210.

23. Woolf C, King A. Dynamic alterations in the cutaneous mechanoreceptive fields of dorsal horn neurons in the rat spinal cord. *J Neurosci.* 1990;10:2717–2726.

24. Roberts W, Foglesong M. Spinal recordings suggest that wide-dynamic range neurons mediate sympathetically maintained pain. *Pain.* 1988;34:289–304.

25. Del Valle L, Schwartzman RJ, Alexander G. Spinal cord histopathological alterations in a patient with longstanding complex regional pain syndrome. *Brain Behav Immun.* 2009;23:85–91.

26. Brelsford K, Uematsu S. Thermographic presentation of cutaneous sensory and vasomotor activity in the injured peripheral nerve. *J Neurosurg.* 1985;62:711–715.

27. Pochaczevsky R. Thermography in posttraumatic pain. *Am J Sports Med.* 1987;15:243–250.

28. Kozin F, Genant H, Berkerman C, et al. The reflex sympathetic dystrophy syndrome: roentgenographic and scintigraphic

evidence of bilaterality and periarticular accentuation. *Am J Med.* 1976;60:332–338.

29. Genant HK, Kozin JS, Bekerman C, et al. The reflex sympathetic dystrophy syndrome. *Radiology.* 1957;117:21–32.

30. Holder LE, Cole LA, Myerson MS. Reflex sympathetic dystrophy in the foot: clinical and scintigraphic criteria. *Radiology.* 1992;184:531–535.

31. Arner S. Intravenous phentolamine test: diagnostic and prognostic use in reflex sympathetic dystrophy. *Pain.* 1991;46:17–22.

32. Raja S, Treede R-D, Davis K, et al. Systemic alpha-adrenergic blockade with phentolamine: a diagnostic test for sympathetically maintained pain. *Anesthesiology.* 1991;74:691–698.

33. Harden RN, Bruehl S, Stanton-Hicks M, et al. Proposed new diagnostic criteria for complex regional pain syndrome. *Pain Med.* 2007;8(4):326–331.

34. Nuti R, Vattimo A, Martiini G, et al. Carbocalcitonin treatment in Sudeck's atrophy. *Clin Orthop Relat Res.* 1987;215:217–222.

35. Melzack R. Prolonged relief of pain by brief, intense transcutaneous somatic stimulation. *Pain.* 1975;1:357–373.

36. Schutzer S, Gossling H. Current concepts review—the treatment of reflex sympathetic dystrophy syndrome. *J Bone Joint Surg Am.* 1984;66:625–629.

37. Robaina FJ, Rodriguez JL, de Vera JA, et al. Transcutaneous electrical nerve stimulation and spinal cord stimulation for pain relief in reflex sympathetic dystrophy. *Stereotact Funct Neurosurg.* 1989;52:53–62.

38. Eisenach JC, Gebhart GF. Intrathecal amitriptyline acts as an NMDA receptor antagonist in the presence of inflammatory hyperalgesia in rats. *Anesthesiology.* 1995;83:1046–1054.

39. Kingery W. A critical review of controlled clinical trials for peripheral neuropathic pain and complex regional pain syndromes. *Pain.* 1997;73:123–139.

40. Steinbrocker O. The shoulder-hand syndrome: present perspective. *Arch Phys Med Rehabil.* 1968;49:388–395.

41. Kozin F, Ryan LM, Carerra GF, et al. The reflex sympathetic dystrophy syndrome (RSDS): III. Scintigraphic studies, further evidence of the therapeutic efficacy of systemic corticosteroids, and proposed diagnosis criteria. *Am J Med.* 1981;70:23–30.

42. Rosner H, Rubin L, Kestenbaum A. Gabapentin adjunctive therapy in neuropathic pain states. *Clin J Pain.* 1996;12:56–58.

43. Mellick G, Mellick L. Gabapentin in the management of reflex sympathetic dystrophy (letter). *J Pain Symptom Manage.* 1995;10:265–266.

44. Caniggia A, Gennari C, Vattimo A, et al. Effottitorapeutici della calcitonina sintetica di salmonenel morgo di Paget e nelle osteoporosi. *Clin Terap.* 1981;82:213.

45. Davis KD, Treede RD, Raja SN, et al. Topical application of clonidine relieves hyperalgesia in patients with sympathetically maintained pain. *Pain.* 1991;4:309–317.

46. O'Brien S, Ngeow J, Gibney M, et al. Reflex sympathetic dystrophy of the knee: etiology, diagnosis and treatment (abstract). *Orthop Trans.* 1991;15:747.

47. Betcher A, Casten D. Reflex sympathetic dystrophy: criteria for diagnosis and treatment. *Anesthesiology.* 1995;16:994–1003.

48. Haynsworth R, Noe C. Percutaneous lumbar sympathectomy: a comparison of radiofrequency denervation versus phenol neurolysis. *Anesthesiology.* 1991;74:459–463.

49. Cousins MJ, Reeve TS, Glynn JA, et al. Neurolytic lumbar sympathetic blockade: duration and relief of rest pain. *Anesth Intensive Care.* 1979;7:121–133.

50. Sayson SC, Ramamurthy S, Hoffman J. Incidence of genitofemoral nerve block during lumbar sympathetic block: comparison of two lumbar injection sites. *Reg Anesth.* 1997;22:569–574.

51. Hannington-Kiff JG. Relief of Sudeck's atrophy by regional intravenous guanethidine. *Lancet.* 1977;1:1132–1133.

52. Wahren L, Torebjork E, Nystrom B. Quantitative sensory testing before and after regional guanethidine block in patients with neuralgia in the hand. *Pain.* 1991;46:23–30.

53. Benzon H, Chomka C, Brunner E. Treatment of reflex sympathetic dystrophy with regional intravenous reserpine. *Anesth Analg.* 1980;59:500–502.

54. Blanchard J, Ramamurthy S, Walsh N, et al. Intravenous regional sympatholysis: a double-blind comparison of guanethidine, reserpine, and normal saline. *J Pain Symptom Manage.* 1990;5:357–361.

55. Sigtermans MJ, van Hilten JJ, Bauer MC, et al. Ketamine produces effective and long term pain relief in patients with complex regional pain syndrome type 1. *Pain.* 2009;145:304–311.

56. Schwartzman RJ, Alexander GM, Grothusen JR, et al. Outpatient intravenous ketamine for the treatment of complex regional pain syndrome: a double-blind placebo controlled study. *Pain.* 2009;147:107–115.

57. Correll GE, Maleki J, Gracely EJ, et al. Subanesthetic ketamine infusion therapy: a retrospective analysis of a novel therapeutic approach to complex regional pain syndrome. *Pain Med.* 2004;5:263–275.

58. Chan CS, Chow SP. Electroacupuncture in the treatment of post-traumatic sympathetic block (Sudeck's atrophy). *Br J Anaesth.* 1981;53:899.

59. Kline M. *Stereotactic Radiofrequency Lesions as Part of the Management of Pain.* Delray Beach, FL: St. Lucie Press; 1996:75.

60. Sri Kantha R. *Techniques of Neurolysis.* Boston, MA: Kluwer Academic Publishers; 1989.

61. Rocco A. Radiofrequency lumbar sympatholysis: the evolution of a technique for managing sympathetically maintained pain. *Reg Anesth.* 1995;20:3–12.

62. Bloor BC, Flacke WE. Reduction in halothane anesthetic requirement by clonidine, an alpha-adrenergic agonist. *Anesth Analg.* 1982;61:741–745.

63. Richard MJ, Skues MA, Jarvis AP, et al. Total IV anesthesia with propofol and alfentanil: dose requirements for propofol and the effect of premedication with clonidine. *Br J Anesth.* 1990;65:157–163.

64. Park J, Forrest J, Kolesar R, et al. Oral clonidine reduces postoperative PCA morphine requirements. *Can J Anest.* 1996;43:900–906.

65. Rauck R, Eisenach J, Jackson K, et al. Epidural clonidine treatment for refractory reflex sympathetic dystrophy. *Anesthesiology.* 1993;79:1163–1169.

66. Ellrich J, Lamp S, Peripheral nerve stimulation inhibits nociceptive processing: an electrophysiological study in human volunteers. *Neuromodulation.* 2005;8:225–232.

67. Bartsch T, Goadsby PJ. Central mechanisms of peripheral nerve stimulation in headache disorders. In: Slavin KV, ed. *Peripheral Nerve Stimulation.* Basel, Switzerland: Karger; 2011:16–26.

68. Buschmann D, Oppel F. Peripheral stimulation for pain relief in CRPSII and phantom limb pain. *Schmerz.* 2014;13(2):113–120.

69. Mione G, Natale M, Rotondo M. Peripheral median nerve stimulation for the treatment of iatrogenic complex regional pain syndrome type II after carpal tunnel surgery. *J Clin Neurosci.* 2009;16(6):825–827.

70. Krames E. Mechanism of action of spinal cord stimulation. In: Waldman S, Winnie A, eds. *Interventional Pain Management.* Philadelphia, PA: W. B. Saunders Company; 1996:407–411.

71. Barolat G. Current status of epidural spinal cord stimulation. *Neurosurg Qu.* 1995;5.

72. Kumar K, Nath RK, Toth C. Spinal cord stimulation is effective in the management of reflex sympathetic dystrophy. *Neurosurgery.* 1997;40:503–508.

73. Asaad B, Glass P. Perioperative management for patients with complex regional pain syndrome. *Pain Manag.* 2012;2(6):561–567.

74. Marx C, Wiedersheim P, Michel BA, et al. Preventing recurrence of reflex sympathetic dystrophy in patients requiring an operative intervention at the site of dystrophy after surgery. *Clin Rheumatol.* 2001;20(2):114–118.

75. Rogers BA, Ricketts DM. Can vitamin C prevent complex regional pain syndrome in patients with wrist fractures? *J Bone Joint Surg Am.* 2008;90(2):447–448.

76. Shah AS, Verma MK, Jebson PJ. Use of oral vitamin C after fractures of the distal radius. *J Hand Surg Am.* 2009;34(9):1736–1738.

77. Frölke JP. Can vitamin C prevent complex regional pain syndrome in patients with wrist fractures? *J Bone Joint Surg Am.* 2007;89(11):2550–2551.

78. Da Costa VV, De Oliveira SB, Fernandes Mdo C, et al. Incidence of regional pain syndrome after carpal tunnel release. Is there a correlation with the anesthetic technique? *Rev Bras Anesthesiol.* 2011;61(4):425–433.

79. Gilron I, Bailey JM, Tu D, et al. Morphine, gabapentin, or their combination for neuropathic pain. *N Engl J Med.* 2005;352(13):1324–1334.

80. Blumberg H, Hoffmann U, Mohadjer M, et al. Clinical phenomenology and mechanisms of reflex sympathetic dystrophy: emphasis on edema. In: Gebhart GF, Hammond DL, Jensen TS, eds. *Proceedings of the 7th World Congress on Pain, Progress in Pain Research and Management.* Vol 2. Seattle, WA: IASP Press; 1994:455–481.

81. Ochoa JL, Verdugo RJ, Campero M. Pathophysiological spectrum of organic and psychogenic disorders in neuropathic pain patients fitting the description of causalgia or reflex sympathetic dystrophy. In: Gebhart GF, Hammond DL, Jensen TS, eds. *Proceedings of the 7th World Congress on Pain, Progress in Pain Research and Management.* Vol 2. Seattle, WA: IASP Press; 1994:483–494.

Congenital Foot, Ankle, and Lower Extremity Conditions

TYLER A. GONZALEZ • RAYMOND HSU

Congenital foot and ankle conditions are common problems that pediatricians and orthopedic surgeons see throughout their careers. Pediatric foot and ankle surgery is becoming its own unique field within orthopedics, and knowledge of these conditions is a key component in orthopedic education. In general, pediatric foot and ankle conditions can be seen at birth, progress over time, or develop in adolescence. Many of these resolve spontaneously, but others may require operative management in order to improve ambulation, create a plantigrade foot, or even permit shoe wear. Congenital disorders of the foot and ankle can occur in isolation; however, many occur as sequela of genetic syndromes or neuromuscular diseases. Orthopedic surgeons, podiatrists, and other musculoskeletal clinicians should be cognizant of the potential underlying systemic implications of these congenital manifestations. Just as critical is an awareness among other clinicians of what foot and ankle deformities may be attributed to congenital etiologies. This chapter discusses the most common congenital foot, ankle, and lower extremity conditions, their etiology, associated conditions, and treatment options.

KNEE DISLOCATIONS

Congenital Dislocation of the Knee

Congenital anterior dislocation of the tibia relative to the femur is a rare condition, with an estimated incidence of less than 1 per 100,000.[1] Examination findings range from a hyperextension deformity of the knee or genu recurvatum to the most severe form demonstrating frank dislocation. Radiographs confirm a fixed anterior subluxation or dislocation of the tibia on the distal femur. Although it may occur in isolation, there is an association with arthrogryposis, Larsen syndrome, and myelomeningocele.[2,3] There is also an increased incidence with breech delivery and other "packaging disorders" including clubfeet, congenital vertical talus (CVT), and developmental hip dysplasia.[2–5]

Simple hyperextension deformities and dislocations not associated with other disorders can generally be treated early with gentle stretching, serial casting, or splinting in a Pavlik harness.[2,5,6] Frank dislocations or cases that fail conservative management may need surgical treatment with either (1) quadriceps lengthening and anterior capsulotomy or (2) femoral shortening and variable anterior releases.[7] With appropriate early treatment, conservative or surgical, patients can generally expect to have functional range of motion and ambulate without a brace, but may have a stiff-knee gait pattern.[2,7] There are only a few case reports of congenital dislocations identified and treated in adolescence.[8–10] All required surgical treatment with some combination of quadricepsplasty, open reduction, frame distraction, and femoral shortening to reconstruct an extremity that allowed ambulation.

Congenital Dislocation of the Patella

Congenital dislocation of the patella is characterized by irreducible lateral dislocation of the patella, flexion contracture of the knee, knock-knee deformity (genu valgum), and rotation deformity of external tibial torsion. The fixed deformity is not to be confused with patellar instability or recurrent patella dislocation, more often seen later in development, which can often be treated conservatively.[11–13] The congenital disorder is almost if not always associated with systemic disorders such as arthrogryposis and chondrodysplasia punctata. In addition, at least two published series have found that all patients have associated foot deformities.[11,14]

Although the knee deformity is not subtle and generally recognized at birth, the diagnosis may be delayed because the patella does not ossify and is not visible on radiographs until 3 to 5 years of age. Palpation, however, should identify the patella laterally and demonstrate the absence of the patella anteriorly. Ultrasound may confirm the diagnosis early. By definition, conservative measures are ineffective, and early surgical correction involves quadriceps lengthening, lateral release, and medial tightening. Without early surgical correction, significant disability results including compromised ambulation. If surgery is delayed until adolescence or early adulthood, treatment requires bony reconstruction with distal femoral and tibial tubercle osteotomies combined with soft tissue reconstruction.[15] Treatment even later in life after the development of arthritis may be addressed with arthroplasty and concurrent soft tissue reconstruction.[16,17]

TIBIAL BOWING

Anterolateral Bowing

Congenital bowing at the middle and distal third junction of the tibia with the apex in the anterolateral direction and with a high risk of progressing to pathologic fracture is characteristic of neurofibromatosis type 1 (NF1). Although the bowing is often noted at birth, there may be a delay in recognition of the fracture risk and the underlying systemic syndrome. The bowing in combination with any one of the other seven diagnostic criteria for the syndrome is sufficient to make the clinical diagnosis of NF1.[18] Patients with NF1 present with wide clinical variability, however, and less than 5% have tibial pathology.[19] Radiographs of anterolateral bowing associated with NF1 will confirm the direction of bowing and demonstrate cortical thickening, particularly on the posteromedial aspect, and a narrower medullary canal.[20] Pathologic fractures, however, frequently occur at the apex, which heal abnormally leading to nonunion or pseudoarthrosis (**Fig. 13-1**). Although typical of anterolateral bowing, tibial pseudoarthrosis may also be seen with amniotic bands, fibrous dysplasia, intrauterine trauma, osteogenesis imperfecta, or any endocrine process that weakens the bone.[18]

Although the entire entity is often referred to as congenital pseudoarthrosis of the tibia, this is a misnomer as the bowing is congenital, but the fracture and subsequent pseudoarthrosis are almost always seen only later.[21] Unlike the early stages with cortical thickening, later radiographs will demonstrate cystic changes, frank fracture, or tapered thin cortices of a pseudoarthrosis. Even when fractures heal, healing is usually abnormal, and the risk of refracture is high.

The goal of treatment in children identified with anterolateral bowing is prevention of fracture. The conservative approach involves casting in young children and bracing in older children until skeletal maturity, with obvious compliance difficulties. Success with purely conservative measures, at least in patients with NF1, appears to be rare.[21,22] Surgically, prophylactic bypass strut grafting has been shown to be successful in several series.[21,22] Simple osteotomy of the bowed segment with local bone grafting and intramedullary rod fixation appears to inevitably fail and only hasten the development of a pseudoarthrosis. In patients who have already fractured and developed a pseudoarthrosis, options include intramedullary nailing with bone graft, vascularized fibular grafting, and thin-wire external framing.[2,21,23]

Refracture even after bone grafting and fixation is relatively common, and skeletal maturity is believed but not proven to be a milestone for diminished risk.[23,24] Other long-term functional issues include leg length discrepancy, ankle stiffness if intramedullary rods crossed the ankle joint, and valgus ankle deformity if there was a concurrent fibular pseudoarthrosis.[21–24]

There also exists a separate subset of anterolateral tibial bowing associated with ipsilateral hallux duplication.[25–30] Recognizing these patients as a different cohort from patients with NF1 is important as this "benign" form is not associated with the development of pseudoarthrosis. Although some may still benefit from operative correction, many of these resolve spontaneously, with only a subclinical leg length difference. Additionally, fractures and osteotomies tend to heal normally in these patients in contrast to NF1-associated bowing. Other than the obvious duplication of the hallux, the bowing also tends to be more proximal and mid-tibial, and there may be a duplication of the medullary canal at the apex of the tibial bow.

FIGURE 13-1. Anteroposterior and lateral radiograph of anterolateral tibial bowing with pseudoarthrosis.

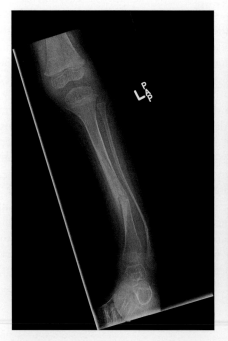
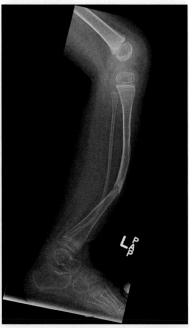

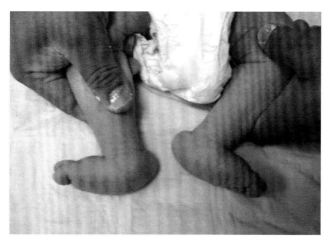

FIGURE 13-3. Clinical photograph of congenital vertical talus showing rocker bottom deformity. (Courtesy of Gleeson Rebello, MD, Boston, MA.)

foot can also be involved and causes dorsal subluxation of the cuboid on the calcaneus.

■ Forefoot abduction and dorsiflexion—Contracture of tibialis anterior and peroneals

After a thorough exam and assessment, radiographic imaging is used to confirm the diagnosis. Standard 3 views of the foot should be obtained. Anteroposterior (AP) radiographs will show an increased talocalcaneal angle usually greater than 40°. Radiographs in the lateral position will show increased Meary angle usually over 20°. Forced plantarflexion lateral views are used to confirm the diagnosis, which will demonstrate an irreducible talonavicular joint. These fully plantarflexed lateral radiographs differentiate CVT from congenital oblique talus. Radiographically, the navicular is assessed by the location of the first ray as the navicular does not ossify until age 3. The first ray will remain dorsally displaced in CVT and reduce in an oblique talus on the plantarflexed lateral view.[36,38,47]

Without treatment, CVT will develop into a painful rigid flatfoot deformity. Both nonoperative and operative treatments have been described, but a combination is usually necessary to adequately address this condition.

Nonoperative management begins with serial casting to place the foot in plantar flexion and inversion to stretch out the dorsal soft tissues. Despite possible large improvements with serial casting, however, complete correction is rarely obtained.[48] After serial casting, many authors recommend minimally invasive single-stage surgical correction to reduce and temporarily fix the talonavicular joint and if needed the calcaneocuboid joint. Extensive release of the dorsolateral tendons was historically performed but associated with major complications. Achilles tendon lengthening is also performed. Surgical treatment is usually done at 6 to 18 months of age. Common complications include wound breakdown, stiffness, talar avascular necrosis, and recurrence.[37,46]

Calcaneovalgus Foot

Calcaneovalgus foot deformity is a common congenital foot deformity and occurs at a rate of 1 in 1,000 live births.[49] It is often caused by intrauterine packaging and is unrelated to neuromuscular or genetic disorders. It is more common in females and the breech position. Calcaneovalgus deformity should be differentiated from posteromedial tibial bowing, CVT, and paralytic foot deformities, which can have similar presentations.[38,47,50]

On exam, the foot is dorsiflexed and lying on the anterior tibia. Unlike CVT, the foot is passively corrected to neutral and there is no Achilles contracture (**Fig. 13-4**).[41] Complete and thorough neurovascular exam must be performed as a L5 myelomeningocele, with intact dorsiflexors and evertors and weak plantar flexors and inverters can produce the same clinical deformity. Radiographs are obtained to rule out CVT, and on forced plantar flexion views, there is no evidence of dislocation of the navicular on the talus. At this age, the ossification nucleus is not seen, but the first ray will be in line with the talus in a calcaneovalgus foot, ruling out a CVT. Oftentimes, calcaneovalgus is associated with posteromedial bowing, which can be seen on radiographs. Also, patients with

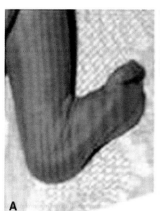
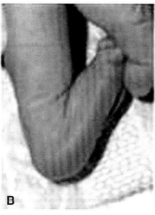
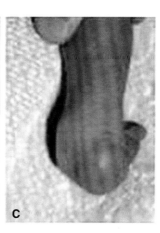

A   B   C

FIGURE 13-4. Clinical photographs showing flexibility of calcaneovalgus deformity. (Courtesy of Gleeson Rebello, MD, Boston, MA.)

calcaneovalgus deformity are more likely to have associated developmental dysplasia of the hip, so a thorough exam of the hips and pelvis is needed.[36,37,41]

Treatment is usually observation and passive stretching by the parents as the condition usually resolves spontaneously at 3 to 6 months of age. In severe cases, casting in plantarflexion and inversion can be done.[37,51]

Tarsal Coalitions

Tarsal coalitions are fusions between the tarsal bones resulting in rigid flatfoot deformity. The coalition can be a bony, cartilaginous, or fibrous connection and is an often isolated finding. Conditions that have been associated with tarsal coalitions, however, include fibular hemimelia, Apert syndrome and Nievergelt–Pearlman syndrome.[36,52]

Tarsal coalition results from failure of mesenchymal segmentation in the developing fetus. The most common forms are calcaneonavicular and talocalcaneal coalitions usually presenting in 8- to 12-year-olds and 12- to 15-year-olds.[52,53] These coalitions are congenital but present later in life as further ossification of the tarsal bones occur.

Patients often present in their early teens with lateral ankle pain, recurrent ankle sprains, calf pain, and rigid flatfoot deformity. The coalition leads to a rigid flatfoot deformity causing tight Achilles and peroneal spasticity. Physical examination shows hindfoot valgus, forefoot abduction, limited subtalar motion, positive Silfverskiold test, and no inversion of the heel or reconstitution of the foot arch on toe rise. Radiographs are necessary but may not fully visualize the coalitions. One should obtain weight-bearing AP, lateral, 45° oblique views, and Harris heel views. The 45° oblique view is very helpful to see calcaneonavicular coalitions, which may demonstrate elongation of the anterior process of the calcaneus often referred to as the "anteater" sign (**Fig. 13-5**). Talonavicular coalitions may show talar beaking on lateral radiographs as well as an abnormal medial facet on the Harris heel view. CT scan should be performed to assess the size of the coalition as well as assess for additional coalitions for surgical planning. An MRI can be performed to assess for fibrous or cartilaginous coalitions if the CT scan is nondiagnostic.[36,52–54]

Treatment consists of both nonoperative and operative management. For asymptomatic coalitions, observation is appropriate. Initial treatment for painful coalitions involves immobilization in a short leg cast for 4 weeks or orthotics, such as a University of California Biomechanics Laboratory orthosis, which are useful to limit eversion and inversion stress.[54] In patients with persistent pain after casting or trial of orthotics, surgical management is recommended. In subtalar coalitions that involve less than 50% of the middle facet or only an isolated bar, resection with fat interposition is performed. If there are multiple bars or more than 50% joint involvement, then subtalar fusion is usually performed.[55] For calcaneonavicular coalitions, resection with extensor digitorum brevis or fat interposition is the preferred treatment.[56,57]

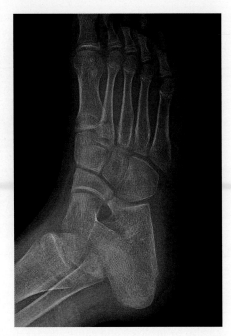

FIGURE 13-5. 45° oblique radiograph of the foot showing calcaneonavicular coalitions with elongation of the anterior process of the calcaneus, often referred to as the "anteater" sign.

CONGENITAL TOE CONDITIONS

Syndactyly

Syndactyly is a condition characterized by fusion of the bones or the soft tissue of the toes. Syndactyly occurs in 1 in 2,000 births and is most common between the second and third digits. Syndactyly is often inherited in an autosomal dominant pattern and is because of incomplete or absent apoptosis during gestation. Syndactyly can be isolated or associated with syndromes such as Klippel–Feil syndrome, Apert syndrome, and Down syndrome. It occurs bilaterally in 50% of the cases.[35]

Syndactyly can be characterized as either simple or complex. Simple syndactyly does not involve bony or nail structures, whereas complex syndactyly does. Differentiation generally requires radiographs.[36,37]

Simple syndactyly in the foot does not often cause footwear problems or pain, and therefore, surgical management is not recommended unless symptomatic. Complex syndactyly can cause problems with shoe wear and pain as the foot grows; therefore, it should be treated surgically. In these situations, surgical management should be performed at 9 to 12 months of age.[35–37]

Polydactyly

Polydactyly occurs in approximately 2 in 1,000 newborns, and there is usually a strong positive family history, with reports as high as 30% within the family. Eighty percent of the cases have a postaxial (lateral border of foot) duplication of the fifth digit, and it is more common in African Americans. Preaxial polydactyly occurs in 15% of the patients, with central duplication occurring in the remaining 5%.[35] Inheritance is thought to be autosomal dominant with variable penetrance. Polydactyly is caused by failure of differentiation in the apical ectodermal ridge during the first trimester of pregnancy and usually occurs in isolation but can be associated with Down syndrome, Apert syndrome, tibial hemimelia, or trisomy 13.[36,41]

Examination reveals whether digits are well-formed articulated digits or rudimentary digits. Radiographs should be obtained to identify the degree of involvement of the bony structures. Duplications can involve all levels from the metatarsal to the distal phalanx. Polydactyly can cause problems with shoe wear and angular deformity of the toes and therefore usually requires surgical removal.

Options for treatment include both nonoperative and operative management. In patients with central or postaxial polydactyly with good alignment and a narrow foot, observation is reasonable. Surgical resection, however, should be considered if shoe wear is a problem or the extra digit causes angular deformity. There are several guiding principles in resection including saving the digit with the best axial alignment, resecting the projecting symptomatic toe, repairing the capsule, balancing the soft tissues, and removing any metatarsal prominence.[36] Rudimentary digits can often be ligated in the newborn nursery, whereas more complex forms will be removed around 9 to 12 months of age. Most often, the border digit and metatarsal should be removed in order to narrow the forefoot. If the outer toes are better developed than the inner toes, however, the inner toes should be removed. Without surgical treatment, 75% of patients will experience shoe fitting problems and 25% will have persistent pain.[36,37,58]

Oligodactyly

Oligodactyly is a failure of formation and usually results in loss of one or more rays of the foot. The lateral rays are more often affected than the hallux. There may be a strong family history, but most cases occur sporadically. Oligodactyly results from improper differentiation in the apical ectodermal ridge and can be caused by teratogenic agents, amniotic bands, or impaired blood flow. Oligodactyly can be associated with many other musculoskeletal or systemic conditions including fibular hemimelia, proximal femoral focal deficiency, tarsal coalition, polydactyly, syndactyly, constriction rings, brachydactyly, VACTERL syndrome, and Fanconi anemia.[36]

A thorough musculoskeletal exam along with cardiovascular, gastrointestinal, and genitourinary assessments is crucial. Radiographs of the foot, leg, and hip should be obtained. If Fanconi anemia is suspected, a complete blood count should be done.

Surgical treatment is rarely indicated unlike with polydactyly and syndactyly as this condition usually does not cause problems with shoe wear or function. Shoe inserts or modifications may be needed to accommodate a narrowed foot. If there are several rays absent, however, then a shoeable balanced foot may not be achievable and amputation may need to be considered.[36]

Brachymetatarsia

Brachymetatarsia is a congenital hypoplasia or shortening of one or more metatarsals. This condition is often bilateral, occurs in a female:male ratio of 25:1, and the 4th metatarsal is most commonly involved. It occurs because of premature closure of the epiphysis of the metatarsal or dissolution of the apical ectodermal ridge. Brachymetatarsia is often isolated but can be associated with many other syndromes including Down syndrome, multiple hereditary exostoses, diastrophic dwarfism, Albright osteodystrophy, Turner syndrome, and Larsen disease.[36,41]

On exam, there is a short ray relative to the others as well as a loss of the normal cascade of the toes. Sometimes, the involved toe resides on the dorsum of the foot due to extension at the metatarsal phalangeal joint. Weight-bearing AP and lateral views of the feet should be obtained.

Treatment consists of both operative and nonoperative management. Depending on the extent of the disease, nonoperative interventions usually involve extra depth and extra width shoes to accommodate the deformity. This usually is successful to help manage symptoms. Taping and/or splinting is usually ineffective. In patients with recalcitrant symptoms, surgery is indicated. There are several surgical procedures described including extensor tenotomy and capsulotomy, metatarsal lengthening, and amputation.[35,36,41]

CONCLUSION

Congenital disorders of the lower extremity span the spectrum from easily managed with conservative stretching and bracing to possibly benefiting from complex surgical reconstructions. Almost all diagnoses can be made by examination and basic radiographs. The detailed diagnosis and management of the more complex conditions is likely best left to the purview of dedicated pediatric orthopedic surgeons. Any clinician who cares for patients with lower extremity complaints, however, should be familiar with the general spectrum of disease and associated systemic conditions.

REFERENCES

1. Jacobsen K, Vopalecky F. Congenital dislocation of the knee. *Acta Orthop Scand.* 1985;56(1):1–7.
2. Shah NR, Limpaphayom N, Dobbs MB. A minimally invasive treatment protocol for the congenital dislocation of the knee. *J Pediatr Orthop.* 2009;29(7):720–725. doi:10.1097/BPO.0b013e3181b7694d.
3. Weinstein SL. *Lovell & Winter's Pediatric Orthopaedics.* 7th ed. Philadelphia, PA: LWW; 2013.
4. Johnson E, Audell R, Oppenheim WL. Congenital dislocation of the knee. *J Pediatr Orthop.* 1987;7(2):194–200.
5. Nogi J, MacEwen GD. Congenital dislocation of the knee. *J Pediatr Orthop.* 1982;2(5):509–513.
6. Haga N, Nakamura S, Sakaguchi R, et al. Congenital dislocation of the knee reduced spontaneously or with minimal treatment. *J Pediatr Orthop.* 1997;17(1):59–62.
7. Oetgen ME, Walick KS, Tulchin K, et al. Functional results after surgical treatment for congenital knee dislocation. *J Pediatr Orthop.* 2010;30(3):216–223. doi:10.1097/BPO.0b013e3181d48375.

8. Sudesh P, Singh D, Goni V, et al. Late presentation of congenital dislocation of the knee: a case report. *J Knee Surg.* 2013;26(Suppl 1):S1–S5. doi:10.1055/s-0031-1275396.

9. Kumar J, Dhammi IK, Jain AK. Neglected surgically intervened bilateral congenital dislocation of knee in an adolescent. *Indian J Orthop.* 2014;48(1):96–99. doi:10.4103/0019-5413.125524.

10. Kazemi SM, Abbasian MR, Hosseinzadeh HRS, et al. Congenital dislocation of the knee in a 16-year-old girl. *Orthopedics.* 2010;33(5). doi:10.3928/01477447-20100329-22.

11. Wada A, Fujii T, Takamura K, et al. Congenital dislocation of the patella. *J Child Orthop.* 2008;2(2):119–123. doi:10.1007/s11832-008-0090-4.

12. Ghanem I, Wattincourt L, Seringe R. Congenital dislocation of the patella. Part I: pathologic anatomy. *J Pediatr Orthop.* 2000;20(6):812–816.

13. Eilert RE. Congenital dislocation of the patella. *Clin Orthop.* 2001;(389):22–29.

14. Ghanem I, Wattincourt L, Seringe R. Congenital dislocation of the patella. Part II: orthopaedic management. *J Pediatr Orthop.* 2000;20(6):817–822.

15. Yoshvin S, Southern EP, Wang Y. Surgical treatment of congenital patellar dislocation in skeletally mature patients: surgical technique and case series. *Eur J Orthop Surg Traumatol.* 2015;25(6):1081–1086. doi:10.1007/s00590-015-1619-0.

16. Bergquist PE, Baumann PA, Finn HA. Total knee arthroplasty in an adult with congenital dislocation of the patella. *J Arthroplasty.* 2001;16(3):384–388. doi:10.1054/arth.2001.20545.

17. Kumagi M, Ikeda S, Uchida K, et al. Total knee replacement for osteoarthritis of the knee with congenital dislocation of the patella. *J Bone Joint Surg Br.* 2007;89(11):1522–1524. doi:10.1302/0301-620X.89B11.19598.

18. Stevenson DA, Viskochil DH, Schorry EK, et al. The use of anterolateral bowing of the lower leg in the diagnostic criteria for neurofibromatosis type 1. *Genet Med.* 2007;9(7):409–412. doi:10.1097GIM.0b013e3180986e05.

19. Szudek J, Birch P, Riccardi VM, et al. Associations of clinical features in neurofibromatosis 1 (NF1). *Genet Epidemiol.* 2000;19(4):429–439. doi:10.1002/1098-2272(200012)19:4<429::AID-GEPI13>3.0.CO;2-N.

20. Stevenson DA, Carey JC, Viskochil DH, et al. Analysis of radiographic characteristics of anterolateral bowing of the leg before fracture in neurofibromatosis type 1. *J Pediatr Orthop.* 2009;29(4):385–392. doi:10.1097/BPO.0b013e3181a567e3.

21. Khan T, Joseph B. Controversies in the management of congenital pseudarthrosis of the tibia and fibula. *Bone Joint J.* 2013;95-B(8):1027–1034. doi:10.1302/0301-620X.95B8.31434.

22. Ofluoglu O, Davidson RS, Dormans JP. Prophylactic bypass grafting and long-term bracing in the management of anterolateral bowing of the tibia and neurofibromatosis-1. *J Bone Joint Surg Am.* 2008;90(10):2126–2134. doi:10.2106/JBJS.G.00272.

23. Johnston CE. Congenital pseudarthrosis of the tibia: results of technical variations in the Charnley-Williams procedure. *J Bone Joint Surg Am.* 2002;84-A(10):1799–1810.

24. Dobbs MB, Rich MM, Gordon JE, et al. Use of an intramedullary rod for treatment of congenital pseudarthrosis of the tibia. A long-term follow-up study. *J Bone Joint Surg Am.* 2004;86-A(6):1186–1197.

25. Breckpot J, Thienpont B, Vanhole C, et al. Congenital anterolateral bowing of the tibia with ipsilateral polydactyly of the great toe associated with cerebral cyst: a new entity? *Clin Dysmorphol.* 2009;18(4):195–200. doi:10.1097/MCD.0b013e32832d06d7.

26. Bressers MM, Castelein RM. Anterolateral tibial bowing and duplication of the hallux: a rare but distinct entity with good prognosis. *J Pediatr Orthop B.* 2001;10(2):153–157.

27. Han J, Qu L, Li Y, et al. A benign form of congenital anterolateral bowing of the tibia associated with ipsilateral polydactyly of the hallux: case report and literature review. *Am J Med Genet A.* 2012;158A(7):1742–1749. doi:10.1002/ajmg.a.35417.

28. Lemire EG. Congenital anterolateral tibial bowing and polydactyly: a case report. *J Med Case Rep.* 2007;1:54. doi:10.1186/1752-1947-1-54.

29. Manner HM, Radler C, Ganger R, et al. Pathomorphology and treatment of congenital anterolateral bowing of the tibia associated with duplication of the hallux. *J Bone Joint Surg Br.* 2005;87(2):226–230.

30. Weaver KM, Henry GW, Reinker KA. Unilateral duplication of the great toe with anterolateral tibial bowing. *J Pediatr Orthop.* 1996;16(1):73–77.

31. De Maio F, Corsi A, Roggini M, et al. Congenital unilateral posteromedial bowing of the tibia and fibula: insights regarding pathogenesis from prenatal pathology. A case report. *J Bone Joint Surg Am.* 2005;87(7):1601–1605. doi:10.2106/JBJS.D.02551.

32. Shah HH, Doddabasappa SN, Joseph B. Congenital posteromedial bowing of the tibia: a retrospective analysis of growth abnormalities in the leg. *J Pediatr Orthop B.* 2009;18(3):120–128. doi:10.1097/BPB.0b013e328329dc86.

33. Napiontek M, Shadi M. Congenital posteromedial bowing of the tibia and fibula: treatment option by multilevel osteotomy. *J Pediatr Orthop B.* 2014;23(2):130–134. doi:10.1097/BPB.0000000000000024.

34. Bedoya MA, Chauvin NA, Jaramillo D, et al. Common patterns of congenital lower extremity shortening: diagnosis, classification, and follow-up. *Radiographics.* 35(4):1191–1207. doi:10.1148/rg.2015140196.

35. Herring JA. *Tachdjian's Pediatric Orthopaedics.* Philadelphia, PA: W. B. Saunders Company; 2002.

36. McCarthy JJ, Drennan JC. *Drennan's The Child's Foot and Ankle.* 2nd ed. Philadelphia, PA: Lippincott Williams and Wilkins; 2010.

37. Hart ES, Grottkau BE, Rebello GN, et al. The newborn foot: diagnosis and management of common conditions. *Orthop Nurs.* 24(5):313–321; quiz 322–323.

38. Churgay CA. Diagnosis and treatment of pediatric foot deformities. *Am Fam Physician.* 1993;47(4):883–889.

39. Wenger DR, Leach J. Foot deformities in infants and children. *Pediatr Clin North Am.* 1986;33(6):1411–1427.

40. Dietz F. The genetics of idiopathic clubfoot. *Clin Orthop.* 2002;(401):39–48.

41. Jay R. *Pediatric Foot and Ankle Surgery.* Philadelphia, PA: Saunders Company; 1999.

42. Treadwell MC, Stanitski CL, King M. Prenatal sonographic diagnosis of clubfoot: implications for patient counseling. *J Pediatr Orthop.* 19(1):8–10.

43. Colburn M, Williams M. Evaluation of the treatment of idiopathic clubfoot by using the Ponseti method. *J Foot Ankle Surg.* 42(5):259–267.

44. Gray K, Pacey V, Gibbons P, et al. Interventions for congenital talipes equinovarus (clubfoot). *Cochrane Database Syst Rev.* 2012;4:CD008602. doi:10.1002/14651858.CD008602.pub2.

45. Heilig MR, Matern RV, Rosenzweig SD, et al. Current management of idiopathic clubfoot questionnaire: a multicentric study. *J Pediatr Orthop.* 23(6):780–787.

46. Drennan JC. Congenital vertical talus. *Instr Course Lect.* 1996; 45:315–322.

47. Greenberg AJ. Congenital vertical talus and congenital calcaneovalgus deformity: a comparison. *J Foot Surg.* 1981;20(4):189–193.

48. Chalayon O, Adams A, Dobbs MB. Minimally invasive approach for the treatment of non-isolated congenital vertical talus. *J Bone Joint Surg Am.* 2012;94(11):e73. doi:10.2106/JBJS.K.00164.

49. Nunes D, Dutra MG. Epidemiological study of congenital talipes calcaneovalgus. *Braz J Med Biol Res.* 1986;19(1):59–62.

50. Sankar WN, Weiss J, Skaggs DL. Orthopaedic conditions in the newborn. *J Am Acad Orthop Surg.* 2009;17(2):112–122.

51. Sullivan JA. Pediatric flatfoot: evaluation and management. *J Am Acad Orthop Surg.* 1999;7(1):44–53.

52. Mosier KM, Asher M. Tarsal coalitions and peroneal spastic flat foot. A review. *J Bone Joint Surg Am.* 1984;66(7):976–984.

53. Cass AD, Camasta CA. A review of tarsal coalition and pes planovalgus: clinical examination, diagnostic imaging, and surgical planning. *J Foot Ankle Surg.* 49(3):274–293. doi:10.1053/j .jfas.2010.02.003.

54. Vincent KA. Tarsal coalition and painful flatfoot. *J Am Acad Orthop Surg.* 6(5):274–281.

55. Swiontkowski MF, Scranton PE, Hansen S. Tarsal coalitions: long-term results of surgical treatment. *J Pediatr Orthop.* 1983;3(3):287–292.

56. Mubarak SJ, Patel PN, Upasani VV, et al. Calcaneonavicular coalition: treatment by excision and fat graft. *J Pediatr Orthop.* 29(5):418–426. doi:10.1097/BPO.0b013e3181aa24c0.

57. Khoshbin A, Law PW, Caspi L, et al. Long-term functional outcomes of resected tarsal coalitions. *Foot Ankle Int.* 2013;34(10):1370–1375. doi:10.1177/1071100713489122.

58. Phelps DA, Grogan DP. Polydactyly of the foot. *J Pediatr Orthop.* 5(4):446–451.

CHAPTER 14

Endocrine Disorders Presenting in the Lower Extremity

DANIEL GUSS

Although hormone secretion is necessarily systemic in nature, many of the effects of hormones extend to the lower extremities. This becomes especially true during derangements of the endocrine system.

GROWTH HORMONE DISORDERS

Critical for normal growth to adult stature, growth hormone (GH) is secreted by the anterior pituitary under the influence of hypothalamic hormones.[1] Growth hormone–releasing hormone and somatostatin secreted by the hypothalamus stimulate and inhibit GH secretion, respectively, at the level of the pituitary gland. GH in turn acts peripherally, either directly on its target tissues or through its intermediary so-matomedins (insulin-like growth factors), whose production it induces in the liver. The normal response to GH includes accelerated linear growth, increased lean body mass, and increased organ size.

GH hypersecretion occurs in the context of somatotropic adenomas, the second most common pituitary tumor after prolactinomas.[2] If such an adenoma develops before physeal closure, it results in excess linear growth known as gigantism. More commonly, however, such adenomas occur after physeal closure, leading to acromegaly whose constellation of symptoms includes expansion of the jaw and brow, enlargement of the hand and feet, and internal derangements such as organ swelling, hyperglycemia, hypertension, and osteoporosis.[3] In addition to the increased size of the hands and feet, patients also frequently note an associated sponginess in the feet, especially in the heel pad, and may describe erythematous spots on the skin of the extremities.[4]

CUSHING SYNDROME

Cushing syndrome refers to elevated levels of glucocorti-coids, primarily cortisol. Most commonly, this is because of exogenous administration of steroids, but other etiologies also exist.[5,6] Cortisol is normally produced by the adrenal cortex under the influence of adrenocorticotropic hormone (ACTH) secreted by the pituitary gland. Hypersecretion of ACTH by a pituitary adenoma or, more rarely, via ectopic production of ACTH by a nonpituitary carcinoma such as small cell lung cancer can lead to elevated levels of cortisol.[7] Similarly, direct production of cortisol by an adrenal cortical adenoma or carcinoma can also rarely lead to elevated cortisol levels.

The clinical manifestations of Cushing syndrome include central weight gain with a characteristic round moon face and buffalo hump.[8] Thinning of the skin with easy bruising, as well as reddish-purple striations on the trunk and legs, is also seen. Other features include proximal muscle weakness, acne, hirsutism, hypertension, hyperglycemia, and bone loss. Notably, in contrast to the observed truncal weight gain, the extremities may become quite thin secondary to associated muscle wasting, and slow healing of cuts and bruises may also occur. Matched cohort studies also underscore an elevated risk of thromboembolic disease and infections.[9]

ADDISON DISEASE

Addison disease or primary adrenocortical deficiency is de-fined by loss of adrenal cortical function, most commonly because of autoimmune destruction.[10] The resultant loss of glucocorticoid and mineralocorticoid production by the adrenal cortex can precipitate a life-threatening adrenal crisis marked by hypotension and volume depletion.[11] Many of the preceding symptoms are subtle, and include fatigue, nausea, orthostasis, salt craving, and muscle and joint pain. Notably, patients may also manifest skin hyperpigmentation due to the fact that both ACTH, which is elevated in the setting of low glucocorticoids, and melanocyte-stimulating hormone share the same hormone precursor.[12] Skin darkening occurs in sun-exposed areas, but also characteristically in palmar creases, recent scars, and pressure points such as the knees and knuckles.

DIABETES

Diabetes is generally divided into insulin-dependent and non–insulin-dependent varieties, or Type I and Type II, re-spectively. Type I, also known as juvenile onset, has a peak incidence in patients younger than age 14, but can also occur in adults.[13] It is caused by selective autoimmune destruction of the pancreas' islets of Langerhans (beta cells), with resultant inability to produce insulin.[14] In contrast, Type II occurs most often in middle age and is hallmarked by peripheral tissue resistance to insulin, particularly skeletal muscle but also hepatic and adipose cells.[15] In the long run, Type II diabetes can also lead to loss of beta cells and hyperglycemia.

Elevated serum glucose can lead to blood vessel atherosclerosis through a number of mechanisms. Nonenzymatic glycosylation of critical proteins and lipids occurs in vessel wall endothelial cells, smooth muscle cells, and macrophages, which can lead to their dysfunction.[16,17] In turn, receptor activation by glycosylated proteins can lead to oxidative stress and alterations in growth factor expression. Peripheral artery disease is a contributing component of an estimated 25% to 30% of diabetic ulcerations.[18]

Distal symmetric polyneuropathy also characterizes diabetes and is a significant source of morbidity. At least 50% of diabetics will develop neuropathy, which can be marked not only by decreased sensation, but also by "positive" symptoms such as burning and tingling.[19] Its causes include a combination of direct nerve injury from hyperglycemia and ischemic insult from microvascular dysfunction. The loss of protective sensation contributes to almost all diabetic ulcerations, and over 60% of ulcerations result from a triad of neuropathy, minor foot trauma, and foot deformity.[18,20]

Furthermore, decreased joint mobility occurs in both large and small joints due to stiffening of collagen-containing tissues.[21,22] Decreased mobility of the ankle or 1st metatarsophalangeal joint directly correlates with the severity of diabetic neuropathy. This in turn increases plantar pressure, which can contribute to ulcerations.

Notably, a small portion of patients who have poorly controlled diabetes develop an acute and painful "insulin neuritis" upon initiating insulin for glycemic control.[19] It is more common among Type I diabetics, but can also occur in those with Type II. The pain is self-limited in duration but can be quite severe, and can recur with subsequent lapses in glycemic control followed by reinitiation of insulin therapy.

THYROID HORMONE

The hormones thyroxine (T_4) and triiodothyronine (T_3) are produced by the thyroid gland under an axis of hypothalamic and pituitary control. Target tissues in turn convert T_4 to T_3, which is the more biologically active form. These hormones play an important role in reaching adult stature and act in concert with GH to promote bone formation.[23] They also affect physeal closure, wherein patients with juvenile thyrotoxicosis have accelerated growth and early skeletal development, whereas those with hypothyroidism frequently have a bone age that lags behind chronologic age.[24]

Excess or a deficiency of thyroid hormone in adults can lead to osteoporosis and fractures.[24,25] Studies have found a significantly increased risk of fracture upon diagnosis of hyperthyroidism (incidence rate ratio [IRR] between 1.26 and 2.29), with a concomitant decreased risk after surgical treatment (relative risk = 0.66, 95% confidence interval [CI]: 0.55 to 0.78) or initiation of antithyroid medication.[26,27] Similarly, an increased risk is also found in patients with hypothyroidism (IRR between 2.17 and 2.35), but this risk abates 10 years after diagnosis.

Hypothyroidism may also increase the risk of wound dehiscence after surgical procedures.[28] Among patients undergoing foot and ankle procedures, a threefold increase in the rate of wound dehiscence has been observed after correcting for age, gender, hypertension, and peripheral vascular disease (odds ratio = 3.7; 95% CI: 1.3 to 11.4; $P = 0.01$).[29] Proposed mechanisms include alterations in keratin gene expression and the effect of hypothyroidism on collagen type predominance.[30,31]

PARATHYROID HORMONE

Parathyroid hormone (PTH) is the major regulator of serum calcium, synthesized by the chief cells of the parathyroid glands.[32] A decrease in serum calcium stimulates the secretion of PTH through a negative feedback loop. In turn, PTH increases serum calcium by triggering bone resorption, increased renal tubule absorption of calcium, and an increase in intestinal absorption of calcium via PTH's effects on vitamin D.

The most common cause of hyperparathyroidism is because of chronic renal failure, whereby a decreased ability of the kidneys to secrete phosphate results in ionic binding of serum calcium.[33] Furthermore, renal activation of vitamin D is also impaired, leading to decreased intestinal absorption of calcium. The resultant decrease in serum calcium concentrations stimulates PTH secretion. Primary hyperparathyroidism can also be caused by a parathyroid adenoma, which results in oversecretion of the hormone independent of serum calcium concentrations.[34]

Regardless of its cause, hyperparathyroidism stimulates osteoclastic resorption of bone, causing cystic changes to the bone. When severe, fibrous replacement of these cystic areas may lead to non-neoplastic, tumor-like masses known as brown tumors, named for the color of their hemosiderin deposits.[35,36] Pathologic fractures through brown tumors have been described, and treatment ultimately includes ameliorating the underlying cause of hyperparathyroidism.[37]

Hyperparathyroidism can also be associated with the deposition of calcium pyrophosphate crystals in joints and other soft tissues, known as pseudogout.[38] Although the vast majority of patients with pseudogout do not have hyperparathyroidism, perhaps 20% of patients with hyperparathyroidism develop pyrophosphate arthropathy.[39] Interestingly, surgical parathyroidectomy can itself precipitate pseudogout attacks.[40] Furthermore, over half of patients with pseudogout in the knee will also demonstrate ultrasonographic features of pyrophosphate crystals in the Achilles tendon and a quarter in the plantar fascia.[41]

Interestingly, although chronically high levels of PTH can lead to bone resorption, intermittent, low doses of PTH are anabolic in nature, resulting in an increased bone density and decreased rate of osteoporotic fractures.[42] This may be partly through a direct effect on osteoblast lineage cells, but also through indirect effects on skeletal growth factors. PTH therapies have therefore increasingly become a mainstay of osteoporotic management.

Hypoparathyroidism is most commonly caused by accidental removal during surgical excision of the thyroid gland.[43] Hypocalcemia may in turn lead to neuromuscular excitability and, in severe cases, tetany.[44]

SUMMARY

In addition to their diffuse effects across numerous organ systems, hormones frequently directly impact normal musculoskeletal function. Derangements in the endocrine system often unveil the delicate equilibrium under which hormone levels must be maintained.

REFERENCES

1. Meinhardt U, Nelson AE, Hansen JL, et al. The effects of growth hormone on body composition and physical performance in recreational athletes: a randomized trial. *Ann Intern Med.* 2010;152(9):568–577. doi:10.7326/0003-4819-152-9-201005040-00007.

2. Ezzat S, Asa SL, Couldwell WT, et al. The prevalence of pituitary adenomas: a systematic review. *Cancer.* 2004;101(3):613–619. doi:10.1002/cncr.20412.

3. Reid TJ, Post KD, Bruce JN, et al. Features at diagnosis of 324 patients with acromegaly did not change from 1981 to 2006: acromegaly remains under-recognized and under-diagnosed. *Clin Endocrinol (Oxf).* 2010;72(2):203–208. doi:10.1111/j.1365-2265.2009.03626.x.

4. Mankin HJ, Jupiter J, Trahan CA. Hand and foot abnormalities associated with genetic diseases. *Hand (NY).* 2011;6(1):18–26. doi:10.1007/s11552-010-9302-8.

5. Carroll TB, Findling JW. Cushing's syndrome of nonpituitary causes. *Curr Opin Endocrinol Diabetes Obes.* 2009;16(4):308–315. doi:10.1097/MED.0b013e32832d8950.

6. Prague JK, May S, Whitelaw BC. Cushing's syndrome. *BMJ.* 2013;346:f945. http://www.ncbi.nlm.nih.gov/pubmed/23535464. Accessed September 14, 2014.

7. Mazzone PJ, Arroliga AC. Endocrine paraneoplastic syndromes in lung cancer. *Curr Opin Pulm Med.* 2003;9(4):313–320. http://www.ncbi.nlm.nih.gov/pubmed/12806246. Accessed September 14, 2014.

8. Kirk LF, Hash RB, Katner HP, et al. Cushing's disease: clinical manifestations and diagnostic evaluation. *Am Fam Physician.* 2000;62(5):1119–1127, 1133–1134. http://www.ncbi.nlm.nih.gov/pubmed/10997535. Accessed September 14, 2014.

9. Dekkers OM, Horváth-Puhó E, Jørgensen JOL, et al. Multisystem morbidity and mortality in Cushing's syndrome: a cohort study. *J Clin Endocrinol Metab.* 2013;98(6):2277–2284. doi:10.1210/jc.2012-3582.

10. Michels A, Michels N. Addison disease: early detection and treatment principles. *Am Fam Physician.* 2014;89(7):563–568. http://www.ncbi.nlm.nih.gov/pubmed/24695602. Accessed September 14, 2014.

11. Chakera AJ, Vaidya B. Addison disease in adults: diagnosis and management. *Am J Med.* 2010;123(5):409–413. doi:10.1016/j.amjmed.2009.12.017.

12. Pritchard LE, Turnbull A V, White A. Pro-opiomelanocortin processing in the hypothalamus: impact on melanocortin signalling and obesity. *J Endocrinol.* 2002;172(3):411–421. http://www.ncbi.nlm.nih.gov/pubmed/11874690. Accessed September 14, 2014.

13. Dabelea D, Bell RA, D'Agostino RB, et al. Incidence of diabetes in youth in the United States. *JAMA.* 2007;297(24):2716–2724. doi:10.1001/jama.297.24.2716.

14. Willcox A, Richardson SJ, Bone AJ, et al. Analysis of islet inflammation in human type 1 diabetes. *Clin Exp Immunol.* 2009;155(2):173–181. doi:10.1111/j.1365-2249.2008.03860.x.

15. DeFronzo RA, Tripathy D. Skeletal muscle insulin resistance is the primary defect in type 2 diabetes. *Diabetes Care.* 2009;32(suppl 2):S157–S163. doi:10.2337/dc09-S302.

16. Aronson D. Hyperglycemia and the pathobiology of diabetic complications. *Adv Cardiol.* 2008;45:1–16. doi:10.1159/0000115118.

17. Chait A, Bornfeldt KE. Diabetes and atherosclerosis: is there a role for hyperglycemia? *J Lipid Res.* 2009;50(Suppl):S335–S339. doi:10.1194/jlr.R800059-JLR200.

18. Wu SC, Driver VR, Wrobel JS, et al. Foot ulcers in the diabetic patient, prevention and treatment. *Vasc Health Risk Manag.* 2007;3(1):65–76. http://www.pubmedcentral.nih.gov/articlerender.fcgi?artid=1994045&tool=pmcentrez&rendertype=abstract. Accessed September 16, 2014.

19. Smith AG, Singleton JR. Diabetic neuropathy. *Continuum (Minneap Minn).* 2012;18(1):60–84. doi:10.1212/01.CON.0000411568.34085.3e.

20. Reiber GE, Vileikyte L, Boyko EJ, et al. Causal pathways for incident lower-extremity ulcers in patients with diabetes from two settings. *Diabetes Care.* 1999;22(1):157–162. http://www.ncbi.nlm.nih.gov/pubmed/10333919. Accessed September 16, 2014.

21. Singh N, Armstrong DG, Lipsky BA. Preventing foot ulcers in patients with diabetes. *JAMA.* 2005;293(2):217–228. doi:10.1001/jama.293.2.217.

22. Zimny S, Schatz H, Pfohl M. The role of limited joint mobility in diabetic patients with an at-risk foot. *Diabetes Care.* 2004;27(4):942–946. http://www.ncbi.nlm.nih.gov/pubmed/15047653. Accessed September 16, 2014.

23. Nilsson O, Marino R, De Luca F, et al. Endocrine regulation of the growth plate. *Horm Res.* 2005;64(4):157–165. doi:10.1159/000088791.

24. Bassett JHD, Williams GR. Critical role of the hypothalamic-pituitary-thyroid axis in bone. *Bone.* 2008;43(3):418–426. doi:10.1016/j.bone.2008.05.007.

25. Wirth CD, Blum MR, da Costa BR, et al. Subclinical thyroid dysfunction and the risk for fractures: a systematic review and meta-analysis. *Ann Intern Med.* 2014;161(3):189–199. doi:10.7326/M14-0125.

26. Vestergaard P, Mosekilde L. Fractures in patients with hyperthyroidism and hypothyroidism: a nationwide follow-up study in 16,249 patients. *Thyroid.* 2002;12(5):411–419. doi:10.1089/105072502760043503.

27. Vestergaard P, Rejnmark L, Mosekilde L. Influence of hyper- and hypothyroidism, and the effects of treatment with antithyroid drugs and levothyroxine on fracture risk. *Calcif Tissue Int.* 2005;77(3):139–144. doi:10.1007/s00223-005-0068-x.

28. Shermak MA, Chang D, Magnuson TH, et al. An outcomes analysis of patients undergoing body contouring surgery after massive weight loss. *Plast Reconstr Surg.* 2006;118(4):1026–1031. doi:10.1097/01.prs.0000232417.05081.db.

29. Grunfeld R, Kunselman A, Bustillo J, et al. Wound complications in thyroxine-supplemented patients following foot and ankle surgery. *Foot Ankle Int.* 2011;32(1):38–46. doi:10.3113/FAI.2011.0038.

30. Safer JD, Crawford TM, Holick MF. A role for thyroid hormone in wound healing through keratin gene expression. *Endocrinology.* 2004;145(5):2357–2361. doi:10.1210/en.2003-1696.

31. Thá Nassif AC, Hintz Greca F, Graf H, et al. Wound healing in colonic anastomosis in hypothyroidism. *Eur Surg Res.* 2009;42(4):209–215. doi:10.1159/000208519.

32. Lee M, Partridge NC. Parathyroid hormone signaling in bone and kidney. *Curr Opin Nephrol Hypertens.* 2009;18(4):298–302. doi:10.1097/MNH.0b013e32832c2264.

33. Goodman WG. Medical management of secondary hyperparathyroidism in chronic renal failure. *Nephrol Dial Transplant.* 2003;18(Suppl 3):iii2–iii8. http://www.ncbi.nlm.nih.gov/pubmed/12771290. Accessed March 31, 2015.

34. Wieneke JA, Smith A. Parathyroid adenoma. *Head Neck Pathol.* 2008;2(4):305–308. doi:10.1007/s12105-008-0088-8.

35. Nassar GM, Ayus JC. Images in clinical medicine. Brown tumor in end-stage renal disease. *N Engl J Med.* 1999;341(22):1652. doi:10.1056/NEJM199911253412204.

36. Quinn CE, Healy J, Lebastchi AH, et al. Modern experience with aggressive parathyroid tumors in a high-volume New England referral center. *J Am Coll Surg.* 2014. doi:10.1016/j.jamcollsurg .2014.10.007.

37. Vernace N, Bancroft LW. Multiple brown tumors and pathologic patellar fracture in a patient with secondary hyperparathyroidism. *Orthopedics.* 2014;37(8):564–567. doi:10.3928/01477447-20140728-01.

38. Richette P, Bardin T, Doherty M. An update on the epidemiology of calcium pyrophosphate dihydrate crystal deposition disease. *Rheumatology (Oxford).* 2009;48(7):711–715. doi:10.1093 /rheumatology/kep081.

39. Huaux JP, Geubel A, Koch MC, et al. The arthritis of hemochromatosis. A review of 25 cases with special reference to chondrocalcinosis, and a comparison with patients with primary hyperparathyroidism and controls. *Clin Rheumatol.* 1986;5(3):317–324. http://www .ncbi.nlm.nih.gov/pubmed/3490947. Accessed March 31, 2015.

40. Rubin MR, Silverberg SJ. Rheumatic manifestations of primary hyperparathyroidism and parathyroid hormone therapy. *Curr Rheumatol Rep.* 2002;4(2):179–185. http://www .ncbi.nlm.nih.gov/pubmed/11890884. Accessed March 31, 2015.

41. Filippou G, Filippucci E, Tardella M, et al. Extent and distribution of CPP deposits in patients affected by calcium pyrophosphate dihydrate deposition disease: an ultrasonographic study. *Ann Rheum Dis.* 2013;72(11):1836–1839. doi:10.1136/annrheumdis-2012-202748.

42. Canalis E, Giustina A, Bilezikian JP. Mechanisms of anabolic therapies for osteoporosis. *N Engl J Med.* 2007;357(9):905–916. doi:10.1056/NEJMra067395.

43. Lin DT, Patel SG, Shaha AR, et al. Incidence of inadvertent parathyroid removal during thyroidectomy. *Laryngoscope.* 2002;112(4):608–611. doi:10.1097/00005537-200204000-00003.

44. De Sanctis V, Soliman A, Fiscina B. Hypoparathyroidism: from diagnosis to treatment. *Curr Opin Endocrinol Diabetes Obes.* 2012;19(6):435–442. doi:10.1097/MED.0b013e3283591502.

CHAPTER 15

Dermatologic Manifestations of Systemic Disease in the Lower Extremity

SHARON R. BARLIZO • THOMAS M. DELAURO • MARK LEBWOHL

As the body's point of contact with the weight-bearing surface, the foot is constantly bombarded with dermatologic insults. It resists abrasive forces for a lifetime, yet requires little care in return. It is the site of a wide variety of local and systemic afflictions, some even portending a state of relative emergency. This chapter hopes to present an algorithmic approach useful in a clinical setting, paying careful attention to the consideration and exclusion of serious or systemic conditions.

DERMATOLOGIC SYMPTOMS AND SIGNS

The primary dermatologic symptom is pruritus, and its discovery helps to support the notion that a dermatologic change is indeed the result of skin disease as opposed to alteration caused by affliction of another organ system. This is best illustrated by the scaling and hyperpigmentation observed approximately 2 weeks after acute gouty arthritis. On initial examination, these findings might suggest tinea pedis or other primary skin disease; however, the changes are in fact the result of a rheumatologic rather than dermatologic illness.

Dermatologic signs consist of the lesions themselves: macule, papule, vesicle, etc. In this regard, the clinician's powers of observation and description are acutely challenged. Patients often present for care only after multiple attempts at self-cure using a variety of over-the-counter products. The effects of those medicinals, as well as the chronicity of the condition, commonly combine to form a dermatosis that defies recognition and description. In these situations, foot care providers should look to the periphery of a dermatosis for an early, representative primary lesion. Identification of the primary lesion is key to accurate diagnosis and successful treatment, and provides the foundation for the algorithm that follows. The reader is asked to use this chapter as a starting point, adding and modifying the algorithm as new conditions are reported and older ones clarified.

MACULAR DISEASES

Macules are identified by their color or pigmentary contrast to adjacent skin, and should be flat and nonpalpable. Macular diseases affecting the feet can be subdivided on the basis of color: brown, red, white, and blue. Of course, one should apply this scheme to account for expected variations in shading (e.g., lesions lighter than adjacent skin would fall in the "white" category, violaceous lesions within the "blue" category, and so on).

Erythematous

Rocky Mountain Spotted Fever

Rocky Mountain spotted fever (RMSF) typically presents as a triad with fever, rash, and headache. It presents dermatologically as a maculopapular rash on the hands and feet along with a late petechial rash on the forearm and hands. The exanthema consists of small blanching pink macules, located in the arches, wrists, and forearms, eventually expanding to the proximal extremities and torso.[1–3]

This disease has its greatest incidence during the late spring and early summer months, when ticks are most active and act as arthropod vectors for the organism *Rickettsia rickettsii*. Usually 1 week following a tick bite, RMSF presents with an abrupt onset characterized by severe headache, fever, chills, nausea, and generalized myalgia. The fourth febrile day is joined by the onset of erythematous macules that start on the hands and feet and then spread centrally to the trunk and face. Two to three days later, the macules become papular and then purpuric, consistent with vasculitis. These same changes occur within viscera, potentially resulting in shock or renal failure.

The diagnostic tools used to confirm RMSF are serologic testing and skin biopsy. The best serologic test is immunofluorescent antibody assays. Also available are enzyme-linked immunosorbent assays and latex agglutination assays. If RMSF is suspected, treatment should not be delayed while awaiting confirmatory test results. The drug of choice used to treat RMSF is doxycycline. It is a broad spectrum antibiotic, in the tetracycline family. When doxycycline is administered for short courses and under strict guidelines, it has not been found to discolor teeth in children <8 years old; however, use in pediatric patients is usually the contraindication.

Meningococcemia

Although presenting in a fashion similar to RMSF, the rash of meningococcemia occurs very rapidly after the onset of constitutional changes. In addition, nuchal rigidity and pain on passive flexion of the neck (secondary to stretching of painful meninges) provide additional differentiating clues.

The widespread ecchymosis and limb ischemia is usually preceded by a petechial or purpuric rash that is rapidly spreading.[4] The process involves a number of factors that are initiated by a bacterial infection invading the soft tissue, causing swelling, hypoperfusion, and hypoxia, ultimately resulting in disseminated intravascular coagulation.[5]

It is recommended to have blood cultures drawn prior to the start of treatment, and if the patient is stable, a lumbar puncture is also recommended. Having said that, therapy should not be delayed if the suspicion is high and the diagnostic procedures are not performed.[5]

The following are the current treatment options[5]: ceftriaxone 100 mg/kg/d in one to two divided doses, cefotaxime 200 mg/kg/d in three divided doses, and penicillin G 500,000 units/kg/d in six divided doses.

Prophylaxis against meningococcus is recommended for those who have been in close contact with the patient. In this case, the drug of choice is rifampin, which is administered every 12 hours for 2 days or, alternatively, a single dose of ciprofloxacin or ceftriaxone.[5]

Patients who present with a chronic meningococcemia pose a diagnostic challenge. They usually present with prolonged periods of intermittent fever, arthritis that is migratory, as well as disseminated skin lesions in the form of macules or nodules that are erythematous.[6] Patients with chronic meningococcemia may fail to reveal its identity with routine microbiologic testing. It has been suggested in these cases that polymerase chain reaction (PCR) testing of the skin biopsy be performed along with an immunohistochemical approach, sometimes using silver staining of the lesions.[6]

Secondary Syphilis

The ham-colored maculopapular rash of secondary syphilis usually presents within 3 to 6 weeks after the appearance of the primary chancre. The rash is always painless, and never hemorrhagic or vesiculobullous. Plaques, nodules, and ulcerated lesions are rare but can also occur. Lesions develop slowly in crops rather than abruptly. Constitutional symptoms are absent. The reader is reminded that guttate palmoplantar keratoses also exist in this stage.

Diagnostic procedures may include HIV, hepatitis B/C, Venereal Disease Research Laboratory (VDRL), *Treponema pallidum* particle agglutination test, and anti–*T. pallidum*

immunoglobulin M enzyme-linked immunosorbent assay (ELISA) index.[7,8] The serologic tests are also combined with immunohistochemical staining of the lesional and nonlesional skin using PCR and Ziehl–Neelsen stain.[7]

The treatment involves giving the patient a prophylactic dose of prednisone to avoid a Jarisch–Herxheimer reaction. Then treatment would follow with weekly injections of 2.4 million units of benzathine penicillin (PCN) for three consecutive weeks. It can also be dosed at 1 million units for 21 days, depending on the specific guidelines being followed.[8]

Familial Mediterranean Fever

Often considered a familial form of amyloidosis with childhood onset, familial Mediterranean fever (FMF) presents with hot, tender, erythematous patches on the calves, ankles, or the dorsa of the feet. FMF is a condition that results in recurrent episodes of fever and polyserositis, which does not involve infection or autoantibodies.[9,10] It is an autoinflammatory condition that results from a mutation in the MEFV gene, which usually starts during childhood.[9,10] Laboratory tests may include elevations in serum amyloid A, erythrocyte sedimentation rate, C-reactive protein, leukocytosis, and fibrinogen during febrile episodes. Definitive diagnosis is made with genetic testing and confirmed when a mutation of the MEFV gene is established.[1] The mainstay of treatment is colchicine, but in cases where there are patients resistant to the drug, interferon-α may be a treatment option.[9,10]

Mucocutaneous Lymph Node Syndrome (Kawasaki Disease)

Kawasaki disease is a condition that typically affects infants and young children. It is known as a self-limiting disease causing systemic vasculitis, resulting in coronary artery aneurysms, myocardial infarctions, and death if not promptly diagnosed and treated.[11] The diagnosis is based on both clinical and laboratory findings. The following is required to make the diagnosis, persistent fever >101°F for a minimum of 5 days along with at least four of the following characteristics: edema and erythema of the extremities; bilateral bulbar conjunctival injection without exudate; edema of the oropharynx with lips that become cracked or red, a "strawberry tongue"; erythematous rash; and cervical lymphadenopathy.[11] This disease demonstrates palmoplantar erythema and pedal edema, followed by a course of marked desquamation of the palms and soles. These patients often have fevers that continue to spike despite being treated with antipyretics and antibiotics. The diagnosis may also be made if fever is persistent for a minimum of 5 days, and less than four of the respective criteria are met, if there are coronary abnormalities found on 2D echo, or if four or more of the critical criteria have been established.[12] The drug of choice for Kawasaki disease is intravenous immunoglobulin and acetylsalicylic acid (aspirin) (ASA); steroids and immunosuppressive therapy may also be a treatment option for those patients who fail to respond to the initial therapy.[11]

Graves' Disease

In addition to palmoplantar erythema and onycholysis, patients may present with a combination of diffuse goiter, exophthalmos, pretibial myxedema, nail clubbing, and periosteal new bone formation (the combination is often referred to as "thyroid acropachy").

Glucagonoma Syndrome

In this disorder, an α-cell tumor of the pancreas results in increased serum glucagon levels coupled with erythematous macules and patches that transform into flaccid bullae (**Fig. 15-1**). The blisters subsequently rupture to leave a collarette of desquamating skin. Lesions have a predilection for the abdomen, groin, thighs, hands, periorificial areas, legs, and feet. Although the dermatosis responds to oral diiodohydroxyquin, removal of the tumor leads to resolution of the skin changes.

Leukocytoclastic Vasculitis

The lesions may begin as erythematous macules and therefore are included for the sake of completeness. They rapidly progress to purpuric macules and papules; a more complete discussion may be found in the section on purpuric lesions.

Nonerythematous

Peutz–Jeghers Syndrome

Brown macules may be found on the palms, soles, and mouth (lips) (**Fig. 15-2**). These outward signs are associated with gastrointestinal polyposis. Historically, treatment options involved cryotherapy, surgical removal, dermabrasion, electric cautery, and the use of carbon dioxide and argon lasers.[13]

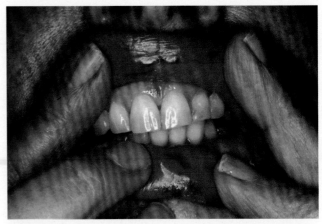

FIGURE 15-2. Brown macules of the oral mucosa associated with Peutz–Jeghers syndrome (borrowed from the Mount Sinai Collection photographs).

Alternatively, Li et al.[13] have studied the use of a Q-switched alexandrite laser in the treatment of both labial and facial lentigines associated with Peutz–Jeghers syndrome. Their results revealed that after three treatments, 55.8% (24/43) of their patients had excellent results and 44% (19/43) had good results.[13] They did not document any serious complications related to the use of the laser.

Kaposi Sarcoma

Although more fully discussed in other chapters of this text, Kaposi sarcoma (KS) is included because it may present with violaceous macules and papules that coalesce (**Fig. 15-3**). Four types of KS are generally recognized: classic, African, allograft associated, and epidemic (AIDS related). It is imperative that AIDS-associated KS be treated with highly active antiretroviral therapy.[14] Other treatments include intralesional chemotherapy or radiation therapy, with systemic chemotherapy reserved for advanced cases of the disease and AIDS-associated KS.[14]

Patients with KS secondary to the classic type may do well using laser and photodynamic therapy.[13] It has also been shown that the classic type as well as patients who

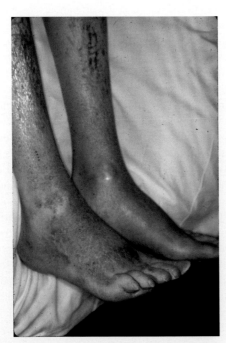

FIGURE 15-1. Erythematous macules and patches transform into flaccid bullae in patients with the α-cell pancreatic tumor associated with the glucagonoma syndrome (borrowed from the Mount Sinai Collection photographs).

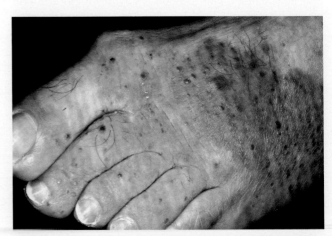

FIGURE 15-3. Classic Kaposi sarcoma affecting the dorsum of the foot (borrowed from the Mount Sinai Collection photographs).

are elderly and immunocompromised have responded well to the use of topical immune response modifiers.[15] The use of intralesional 3% sodium tetradecyl sulfate has also been proposed, especially in cases where KS presents as nodular lesions, ultimately resulting is sclerotization of the vessels.[15]

KERATOTIC LESIONS OF THE FOOT

Foot care practitioners and their patients readily admit to the prevalence of keratotic skin disorders. Over-the-counter remedies abound, each attempting to thin and/or accommodate the area(s) of chief complaint. What goes unrecognized, however, is the relation of keratosis to truly neoplastic or systemic disease. The most useful algorithmic approach to this commonplace identity would allow rapid categorization of disease entities, with each category representing nonoverlapping diagnostic and therapeutic interventions. The algorithm should also arrange these categories in terms of their clinical urgency.

The algorithm presented here, therefore, attempts to answer the following questions: (1) is the presenting keratosis or keratoses a sign of a more widespread systemic illness, or (2) is the keratotic change associated with a cutaneous neoplasm? The reader is reminded that diffuse keratoses are those that extend over most or all of the plantar surface. Guttate keratoses are drop-like lesions such as heloma miliare, and geographic keratoses have a morphology that falls somewhere in between, such as in a tyloma. The categories of systemic and neoplastic disease will be discussed without subclassifying keratotic lesions into diffuse, guttate, or geographic groups.

This section is meant only to augment preexisting comprehensive works that describe, in detail, each of the entities mentioned later. Because the palms share the same ontogenic development of the soles, an examination of the hands is always in order. Abnormalities of dentition, the cornea, and other ectodermally derived tissues may also occur.

Keratotic Diseases Associated with Systemic Illness

In this category, clinicians should exclude Howel–Evans syndrome, hypothyroidism, chronic arsenic intoxication, secondary syphilis, Bazex syndrome, and the basal cell nevus (BCN) syndrome.

Howel–Evans Syndrome

Patients present with diffuse keratoses of their palms and soles bilaterally, in association with a past or present history of esophageal carcinoma. At times, suspecting clinicians may first make the diagnosis solely on the basis of diffuse palmoplantar keratoses in a patient with symptoms of dysphagia and/or hematemesis.

Hypothyroidism

Diffuse plantar keratoses, thick and brittle nails, and easy bruisability of the legs (manifested as purpura or ecchymoses) suggest the diagnosis. Confirmation is aided by finding the cardinal symptoms and signs of weight gain, constipation, cold intolerance, and mental or physical sluggishness. The hypothyroid foot can closely resemble one with the dry, scaly form of tinea pedis. This diagnosis might therefore be considered in patients who are unresponsive to standard antifungal therapy.

Chronic Arsenic Intoxication

Acute intoxication does not fall into this category because it presents with nausea, vomiting, and other signs of gastrointestinal upset rather than skin change. Ingestion of contaminated groundwater is considered to be the most common cause of chronic arsenic poisoning, especially endemic in regions such as Bangladesh, Inner Mongolia, China, and the West Bengal province of India.[16–18] Inorganic arsenic sulfide was also found in Chinese proprietary medicines as well as in American tobacco in the 1950s.[19] There appears to be a dose–response relationship or rather a dose and frequency relationship, with skin manifestations being the most common adverse effect; furthermore, chronic exposure has been known to increase the risk of cancer affecting multiple organs and not limited to the skin.[16–18] The most common initial skin manifestations are melanosis, keratosis, leukomelanosis, and hyperkeratosis[16–18] (Fig. 15-4). There are a number of treatment options for the skin manifestations secondary to chronic arsenic exposure; however, the effects may be irreversible, though worth exploring, and may involve phototherapy, topical keratolytics, and chemotherapeutic agents along with surgical excision and cryotherapy.[17]

Secondary Syphilis

Guttate keratoses of the palms and soles are also found in patients with secondary syphilis. Concomitantly, they also exhibit a generalized, ham-colored, maculopapular rash (Fig. 15-5). Questions should be posed regarding sexual history, and the spontaneous resolution of a genital "sore" (the primary chancre).

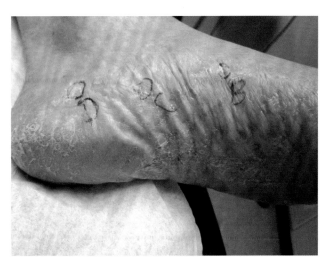

FIGURE 15-4. Arsenical keratoses predilecting for the skin creases (borrowed from the Mount Sinai Collection photographs).

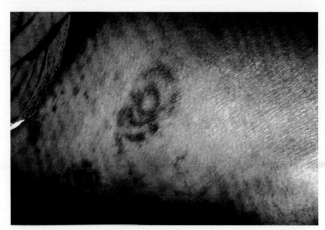

FIGURE 15-5. The ham-colored maculopapular dermatosis of secondary syphilis (borrowed from the Mount Sinai Collection photographs).

Bazex Syndrome

Bazex syndrome (acrokeratosis paraneoplastica) occurs in association with carcinoma of the upper respiratory and gastrointestinal tracts. Symmetrical, well-defined psoriasiform nails, palmoplantar hyperkeratoses, and keratosis of the ears, nose, and cheeks comprise the syndrome's major clinical features.[20–22] This condition may manifest with recent onset of nail dystrophy, nail atrophy, localized erythema, and edema of the digit without improvement with usual topical antifungals or keratolytics.[20]

The keratoses generally precede tumor symptoms or diagnosis by almost 1 year, with the eruption being resistant to topical therapy. Clearing of the tumor usually results in a clearing of all cutaneous changes except for nail involvement, with exacerbation of dermatologic disease heralding recurrence or metastasis. An immune reaction to the presence of an antigen common to both the tumor and normal skin, or tumor production of a keratinocyte growth factor has been proposed as a potential etiology. The diagnosis is based on establishing a thorough history, physical findings, and histologic findings.

Basal Cell Nevus Syndrome

BCN syndrome is an autosomal dominant disorder caused by a mutation in the Patched 1 gene or G protein–coupled receptor Smoothened (SMO).[23,24] It involves a triad of cerebral calcifications, basal cell carcinomas, and keratocysts.[23] Multiple basal cell tumors and mandibular cysts typify this disorder. In contrast to the conditions previously described, keratotic pits or depressions are found on the palms and soles. Keratotic pits may also be found in patients with other diseases unrelated to BCN syndrome. For example, pitted keratolysis, caused by a corynebacterial infection, is manifested by pits on the plantar aspect of the foot. These pits trap dirt and debris that cause the pits to become hyperpigmented. In the case of BCN syndrome, the pigment is easily removed with an alcohol sponge. In pitted keratolysis, the pigmentation cannot be removed, because it is a genuine discoloration produced by bacterial diphtheroids believed to cause the

disease. Although pitted keratolysis is often asymptomatic, painful variants in adult males during military service and in children can occur. In pediatric cases, topical erythromycin can cure the disorder. BCN syndrome is associated with a number of neurologic findings. Medulloblastomas and calcification of the falx cerebri and dura occur.

Diagnosis is based on major and minor criteria established by Evans et al., and modified by Kimonis et al. and Bree et al.[23] Early clinical features along with a family history of BCN syndrome should warrant the need for standard imaging tests such as panorex of the jaw, MRI of the brain, CT, PET scan, along with biopsies of lesions and genetic testing.[24,25] Definitive therapy involves surgical excision or the use of Mohs, and radiation therapy. Palliative therapy includes the use of retinoids, photodynamic therapy, vitamin D supplements, topical chemotherapeutic agents, cryotherapy, and laser therapy.[23–25] Emerging therapy has been developed targeting the genetic deficiencies, such as SMO inhibitors which have shown great promise in inhibiting the Hedgehog signaling pathway known to drive the development of BCC.[23–26]

Keratotic Change Associated with Cutaneous Neoplasm

A discussion of cutaneous neoplastic disease is certainly beyond the scope of this chapter; however, there are a number of clinical clues to suggest that a keratotic lesion is in fact neoplastic. First, it is safe to assume that many cutaneous neoplasms lose their classic morphologic appearance when affecting the sole, some becoming as nondescript as a localized area of hyperkeratosis.

Second, clinicians have come to expect that isolated keratoses form around sites of pressure, friction, or invasive events. Keratoses that form de novo in foot areas that are typically nonweight-bearing and relatively free from trauma (i.e., the midsole, the phalangeal or metatarsal shafts, etc.), or those that do not respond to accommodative measures are, as a result, also suggestive of neoplasm.

Last, keratoses that harbor neoplastic change often exhibit an erythematous rim, probably an indicator of the metabolic and inflammatory events occurring at the margin of the lesion. This erythematous rim has also been described in heritable keratotic diseases, known collectively as the genokeratoses. The family history, however, should readily distinguish neoplasm from genokeratosis.

Treatment of the Keratotic Diseases

The standard treatments for keratotic diseases have always included paring, abrasive tools (e.g., pumice stones, loofah pads, etc.), accommodative insoles, pads, and/or shoes, emollients (including urea), keratolytics, and antiproliferation agents. At times, surgical resection of bony prominences and local skin flaps have been advocated. Retinoids are also used, and will be discussed separately.

Emollients

These drugs function by adding moisture and lubrication to the skin when applied topically. Major categories include urea preparations, topical vitamins A, D, and E, and a final grouping that contains various mixtures of the above ingredients with mineral oil, glycerin, petrolatum, and any one of a large number of vehicles. Of special note is the widespread use of parabens in these mixtures, because parabens are known skin sensitizers capable of initiating a marked dermatitis. Patients who are paraben sensitive should beware, because 44 of the 93 (almost 50%!) prescription and over-the-counter emollients recently listed contained parabens.

Keratolytics, Antiproliferative and Desmolytic Agents

Anthralin, salicylic acid (SA), podophyllin, and cantharidin have been the best known keratolytic and antiproliferative preparations. However, research has shown that vitamin D_3 helps to regulate growth and differentiation of many cell types including epidermal cells[27]; it also enhances the cornified envelop formation as well as exhibits anti-inflammatory effects by inhibiting neutrophil function.[6] Vitamin D_3 and its analogs have been commercially available since the mid-1990s in the United States as a topical treatment for psoriasis and has proven to have moderate efficacy. Additionally, vitamin D_3 (calcipotriol, calcitriol, and tacalcitol) has definite potential in treating ichthyoses and other diseases resulting in excessive epidermal proliferation.[28] Calcipotriol has been used in treating chronic plaque psoriasis, and found to be as potent as corticosteroids and more effective than using coal tar, short-term dithranol, as well as tacalcitol.[29]

Most importantly, patient education of the basics in skin hygiene and in preventive care including maintaining a certain level of humidity in the home, using mild and unscented soaps/detergents, and avoiding long hot showers or baths is crucial.[4] If the areas show signs of localized inflammation, one may include a mild topical steroid, which may be discontinued after 7 to 14 days.[30]

SA was once categorized as a keratolytic agent; however, it is now considered as a desmolytic agent, due to its mechanism of action, which involves disrupting intercellular junctions.[12] SA has the ability to alter the underlying dermal tissue without directly wounding the skin.[12] In effect, SA results in exfoliation due to its ability to extract desmosomal proteins causing a loss of cohesion between epidermal cells. It has antihyperplastic effects, which have been studied in the guinea pig epidermis, and a reduction in hyperplasia of viable epidermal cells. Loden et al.[31] studied SA on human skin and concluded that it does not affect the thickness of the epidermis, rather resulting in thinning of the corneal layer.[12]

Contraindications to using SA include contact allergies, active infection, pregnancy, skin malignancy, and concurrent use of topical retinoids. Retinoids should be discontinued 1 to 2 weeks prior to use, in order to avoid complications such as postinflammatory hyperpigmentation, excessive erythema, and desquamation.[12]

Table 15-1. Various Uses of SA Based on Its Concentration	
SA Concentration (30) (%)	**Uses**
0.5–10	Acne
3–6	Hyperkeratosis, psoriasis, ichthyoses, keratosis pilaris
5–40	Warts, corns
50	Actinic damage and pigmented lesions
20–30	Superficial chemical peeling of the face

SA, salicylic acid.

Salicylism, secondary to cutaneous absorption, is a rare phenomenon. SA is a lipid-soluble agent that is readily absorbed by the skin; its rate of absorption can be enhanced when combined with a hydrophilic base or under occlusion.[30] SA toxicity has been reported by dermatologists when 20% of SA is applied to 50% of the body surface and at 40% and 50% SA paste preparations (Table 15-1).[12]

Anthralin is a naturally occurring substance known as Goa powder derived from the araroba tree; it inhibits DNA synthesis and cell mitosis, which in turn inhibits epidermal cell proliferation.[32,33] Common side effects include staining and pigmentation of the skin and clothing and contact dermatitis. Extreme caution must be used with children and pregnant or lactating females.

Coal tar works along the same mechanism as anthralin, and its actions are enhanced with the use of ultraviolet light; when combined, it results in a phototoxic reaction resulting in the inhibition of epidermal DNA synthesis.[33]

Cantharidin is a keratolytic agent and topical vesicant resulting in selective acantholysis that occurs intraepidermally.[16,34] A progressive degeneration of desmosomal dense plaques results from the activation of neutral serine proteases when absorbed by the lipids in the keratinocyte.[35,36] When applied, cantharidin causes blister formation in 24 to 48 hours. Primary indications have been for verruca vulgaris and molluscum contagiosum.[36] The off-label uses for cantharidin include callus removal, perforating collagenosis, postherpetic neuralgia, and leishmaniasis lesions.[36] The most common adverse reactions are blistering, localized erythema, and pain.

Podophyllin is locally cytotoxic, causing mitotic arrest. Unfortunately, it can lead to ulceration of the skin or severe neuropathy, especially when applied to large areas of skin. Although the total cross-sectional area of the soles is relatively small, patients should be warned of and monitored for these changes.

When these medicaments are used singly or in combination, noninvolved areas of skin must be protected. Application under occlusion will enhance penetration and, therefore, effect. Coupling these therapies with mechanical debridement (paring) is time-consuming but offers a speedy reward for the suffering patient.

Retinoids

Retinoids, both topical and systemic, can inhibit keratin formation and function as morphogens capable of altering growth and differentiation of the epidermis.[29] Retinoids, vitamin A derivatives, its analogs and synthetics, exert an antiproliferative effect acting at the molecular level, with some inhibiting the expression of keratinocyte enzyme transglutaminase.[29] By inhibiting the expression of this enzyme, it directly results in a decrease in proliferation and cohesion of cornified cells,[29] ultimately normalizing keratinization and decelerating the process of desquamation. Tretinoin, the first topical retinoid on the market, continues to have secondary antimicrobial and anti-inflammatory activity.[29] Newer synthetics (adapalene, tazarotene) have more selective receptor binding and anti-inflammatory activity.[37] Currently, in the United States, the topical retinoids available include tretinoin, second-generation tretinoin, and third-generation *retinoids* (adapalene and tazarotene).[34,37]

Accutane (isotretinoin) was taken off the market in the summer of 2009, due to the expiration of its patents and also because of thousands of litigation issues. Roche, its manufacturer, has stood by their product's safety; however, it has been linked to serious birth defects, bowel disorders, depression, and suicidal ideation. Accutane's generic equivalent continues to be available. According to Davis et al.,[38] in its generic form, isotretinoin continues to be the leading medication used by dermatologists in teens with acne. Although there has been a decline in trend due to the safety concerns and strict requirements of federal monitoring programs, acitretin, a second-generation retinoid, continues to be available on the market. However, etretinate, also a second-generation retinoid, has been discontinued due to its narrow therapeutic index as well as its long elimination half-life, making dosing difficult. FDA-approved indications for retinoids have been acne vulgaris, mitigation of fine wrinkles, mottled hyperpigmentation, and tactile roughness of facial skin and plaque psoriasis. Off-label uses include photoaging, intrinsic aging, actinic keratosis, and actinic lentigines.[34]

Isotretinoin and acitretin are administered orally and share similar adverse effects: hypertriglyceridemia, hair loss and skin fragility, hyperostoses, tendinous and ligamentous calcifications (especially in patients on long-term therapy, i.e., five or more years), and marked teratogenicity. For the latter reason, pregnancy is an absolute contraindication to the use of these drugs.

VESICULOBULLOUS DISEASES

Vesicles are palpable, fluid-filled skin lesions less than 1 cm in diameter. Bullae are similarly defined except that they demonstrate larger dimensions.

Vesiculobullous lesions can be localized as to whether they are intraepidermal or subepidermal. Erythema multiforme is one example of a subepidermal reaction. This condition is characterized by large bullae which dissect and extend along the epidermal–dermal interface.

Diseases of the skin demonstrating intraepidermal vesicle or bulla formation include disorders as varied as herpes simplex or herpes zoster.

Mechanobullous Diseases

As a group, each of these diseases is inherited with traumatically induced vesiculobullae appearing in characteristic pressure areas, that is, feet, knees, hands, and elbows. Epidermolysis bullosa is often considered the prototype for the mechanobullous disorders.

The dermatoses are subdivided into scarring and nonscarring types, with the former usually having their onset in infancy and resulting in mutilating pseudosyndactyly and contractures, with generalized disease resulting in early mortality (**Fig. 15-6**).

Weber–Cockayne disease, also referred to as recurrent bullous dermatosis of the feet, is an example of the nonscarring variety. Prolonged marching during summer months exacerbates the condition. Although this presentation is reminiscent of skin changes in healthy individuals, the family history points to the ultimate diagnosis.

Paraneoplastic Pemphigus

Vesiculobullous eruptions associated with internal carcinoma have been reported in patterns resembling dermatitis herpetiformis, bullous pemphigoid, erythema multiforme, and in leukemias and lymphomas. In one report, the development of palmoplantar blisters heralded a leukemic crisis. Recently, a bullous disorder resembling pemphigus has been described in patients with underlying neoplasms.

Acrodermatitis Enteropathica

Onset usually occurs before 2 years of age, with vesiculobullae on erythematous bases that collapse to form papulosquamous plaques. The dorsal toes (resembling candidiasis at the proximal nail fold) and periorificial areas are typically affected.

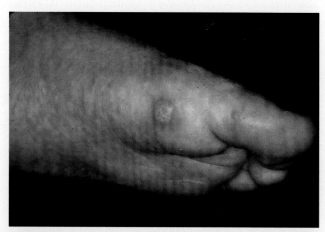

FIGURE 15-6. Trivial injury to the fragile skin of patients with epidermolysis bullosa simplex leads to blister formation (borrowed from the Mount Sinai Collection photographs).

Hemodialysis

Simple vesiculobullae on the dorsum of a foot can develop spontaneously in patients undergoing this therapy.

Hand, Foot, and Mouth Disease

Football-shaped vesicles and bullae on an erythematous base affect the sites listed in this self-limiting disorder (**Fig. 15-7**). The Coxsackie A16 virus is the causative agent, resulting in epidemics among school-aged children.

Herpes Gestationis

Blisters developing during pregnancy or shortly after parturition may result from herpes gestationis, which has been associated with a higher-than-normal incidence of maternal and/or fetal complications (**Fig. 15-8**).

Glucagonoma Syndrome

Repeated for the sake of completeness, the reader is referred to the section on erythematous macules.

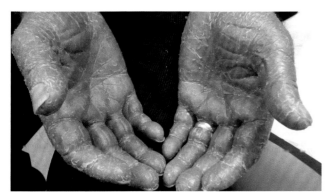

FIGURE 15-7. Palmar desquamation associated with late-stage Coxsackie A6 virus–induced hand, foot, and mouth disease (borrowed from the Mount Sinai Collection photographs).

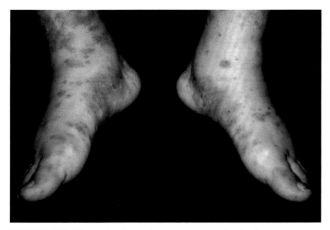

FIGURE 15-8. Blisters develop during pregnancy or shortly after parturition in herpes gestationis (borrowed from the Mount Sinai Collection photographs).

Diagnostic Aids and Treatment

There are five basic laboratory tests that can assist in making the correct diagnosis: (a) the Gram stain; (b) KOH prep; (c) Tzanck smear; (d) the patch test; and of course, (e) biopsy. In addition to the standard tests, there are cases in which one may need to test for yeast, acid-fast bacilli, and other microorganisms. Dark field microscopy for *Treponema pallidum*, VDRL, enzyme immunoassay, HIV, and genetic tests may also play significant roles in establishing a diagnosis.[7,8,39]

When performing the Tzanck smear, an early lesion should be selected, its top removed with a scalpel, and the fluid contents blotted away in order to avoid contact with the base of the lesion. The lesion is then pinched firmly to prevent bleeding while the floor is scraped with a sharp curette. These scrapings are then spread on a clean glass slide, allowed to air dry, and then stained with Giemsa solution. In pemphigus patients, acantholytic cells with pyknotic nuclei will be seen, whereas in cases of herpes zoster or simplex or in varicella, multinucleated giant cells will be noted.

The traditional technique used to biopsy blistering lesions has been a two-punch biopsy approach. It is recommended to first biopsy the perilesional skin for direct immunofluorescence (DIF) and then perform a secondary biopsy from lesional skin for light microscopy using a hematoxylin and eosin (H&E) stain.[40] Braswell et al.[40] recommended marking the blisters to ensure proper orientation, as well as to include at least 75% of perilesional skin at the edge of the blister.

Braswell et al.[40] have also recommended an alternative approach for subepidermal blisters. The technique involves using an 8-mm unit biopsy tool for a single-punch biopsy for both DIF and light microscopy using H&E stain. The first method uses an 8-mm punch biopsy centered over a 1 to 2 mm new lesion. This approach includes approximately 3 mm of perilesional skin. Once the specimen is obtained, half of the specimen is placed in Zeus medium for DIF and the remaining half in formalin for H&E staining. For larger blisters, a second approach is recommended. They suggest marking the roof of the blister along with the surrounding perilesional skin. An 8-mm punch biopsy unit is then used, creating a sample comprised of three-fourths of the perilesional skin and one-fourth of the center of the lesion. Again, half of the tissue would be sent for H&E staining, whereas the remaining portion would be sent for DIF.[40] With the larger blister, it is important to bisect the specimen from the subcutaneous tissue using a #15 blade.[41] The technique also helps to preserve both epithelium and dermis as specimen.

There are two primary advantages to using a single-punch biopsy technique; it is cost-effective and also avoids having to perform a second procedure. The limitation of a single-biopsy approach is that it would require that the pathologist or technician be familiar with the technique.[40] It is also necessary for the portion that includes the cut edge of each half to be included for DIF specimens and H&E staining. This technique is not recommended for blistering disorders found to have a positive Nikolsky sign.[40]

Treatment for all the vesiculobullous diseases that affect the foot includes the prevention of sepsis, soaking to dry the lesions, and incision with drainage of large bullae that interfere with proper function. The entire roof of a vesicle or bulla should probably never be completely removed. General treatment will vary according to the specific disease. It is wise for the podiatrist to seek the aid of a good dermatologist, internist, or oncologist, depending on the underlying disorder.

Steroids are sometimes used to minimize the inflammatory components of vesiculobullous disease, whether the foot alone is involved or other body surfaces are affected.

PURPURIC ERUPTIONS

In contrast to erythematous macules, purpuric lesions are the result of actual bleeding into the skin. Eventually, extravasated red blood cells break down to form the pigment, hemosiderin, and lesions will not blanch upon diascopy. Purpura will assume different configurations based on the dimension of the pathologic vessels. Rupture of small vessels (i.e., arterioles, venules, and capillaries) will result in pinpoint or "petechial" hemorrhages, whereas damage to larger vessels will result in ecchymosis, hematoma, or hemarthrosis. Lastly, the clinician should bear in mind that purpuric eruptions may in fact represent microembolization, vasospastic disease (i.e., pernio, Behçet disease), etc.

Leukocytoclastic Angiitis

This autoimmune disease affects arterioles, capillaries, and venules in skin and internal organs. It differs from other forms of angiitis (i.e., macroscopic polyarteritis nodosa, Wegener granulomatosis) both histologically and in its broader clinical manifestations. Leukocytoclastic angiitis (LCA) derives its name from the characteristic appearance of the leukocytes found in involved segments. These cells exhibit nuclear fragmentation, or "nuclear dust," hence the designation leukocytoclastic angiitis.

The cutaneous changes of LCA are secondary to exudation and hemorrhage rather than to ischemia. Blood vessels within the upper dermis are usually affected, leading initially to the formation of an erythematous macule, as described previously. Edema and subsequent extravascular hemorrhage transform macules into papules and then purpuric papules, respectively. The feet, ankles, and lower legs are characteristically involved in a bilateral fashion (**Fig. 15-9**). Progression of disease leads to thrombosis and therefore ulceration.

LCA may appear in two clinical forms: (a) Henoch–Schönlein or anaphylactoid purpura or (b) a cutaneous-systemic variant. The former affects mainly young boys, is preceded by an upper respiratory infection with mild constitutional symptoms, and has a predilection for the late fall and early spring months. In addition to the cutaneous rash, the vasculitis can affect the kidney, gut, and joints, leading to complaints referable to these areas.

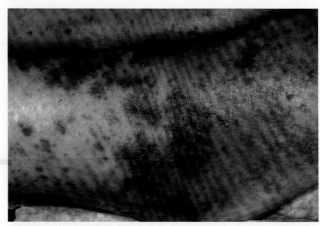

FIGURE 15-9. The palpable purpura associated with leukocytoclastic vasculitis (borrowed from the Mount Sinai Collection photographs).

The cutaneous-systemic form more commonly affects adults; there is no sex predilection. The form represents a spectrum of disease: It may range from pure cutaneous to purely visceral involvement, with a certain percentage exhibiting both cutaneous and visceral involvement. Signs of cutaneous vasculitis are preceded by mild constitutional changes, as in the Henoch–Schönlein form. Death can result from vasculitis-induced renal failure. Fortunately, fatality occurs in only a small percentage of patients (in contrast to the rapidly fatal course of macroscopic polyarteritis nodosa). Early urinalysis in such patients can detect renal involvement, permitting rapid initiation of therapy directed at halting the process.

LCA can therefore exist in a relatively benign form, but it may develop serious complications. It can also occur, for unknown reasons, in association with patients afflicted by rheumatoid arthritis, lupus erythematosus, leukemias, and lymphomas.

Diagnosis depends upon recognition of characteristic lesions and histopathology.

Bacterial Endocarditis

Bacterial endocarditis exists in subacute and acute clinical forms, determined by the infectious organism and the presence of preexisting cardiac disease. The acute type with its rapidly fulminating course results from invasion by true pathogens; a prior cardiopathy is not a prerequisite. Conversely, subacute bacterial endocarditis occurs in patients with congenital or rheumatic heart disease following infection with less pathogenic bacterial species.

In either case, vegetations composed of fibrin and platelets develop at the site of infection. Small fragments may now break free and embolize to any tissue, producing a variable clinical picture. Cutaneous lesions of the extremities are secondary to such vascular change and may be petechial or gangrenous. In the case of petechial lesions, histologic section reveals these to be secondary to an immune vasculitis, and therefore they are probably not embolic in nature.

The combination of fever, cardiac murmurs, and cutaneous lesions of the type to be discussed is a certain indicator of bacterial endocarditis. In the subacute type, subungual splinter hemorrhages are often found. Digital pulps may exhibit tender, purple, or erythematous subcutaneous papules known as Osler nodes. Larger nodules, probably embolic in origin, may develop on the palms and soles. These are known as Janeway lesions. Emboli to larger arteries may create claudication or frank gangrene.

In contrast, acute bacterial endocarditis demonstrates many petechial and embolic changes, but Osler nodes and Janeway lesions are absent.

Early diagnosis of bacterial endocarditis is imperative and known to improve clinical outcome and decrease patient mortality rate. Although new diagnostic biomarkers are emerging and show promise, definitive diagnosis of bacterial endocarditis continues to remain a challenge. The most important diagnostic tools continue to involve high clinical suspicion, blood cultures, and echocardiology.[42] Mestres et al.[43] discuss the importance of preventive measures to avoid infection through proper hand washing techniques, along with an emphasis on patient education. This involves the patient's understanding of the disease process, procedures that may ultimately cause bacteremia, as well as the prophylactic antibiotics involved to prevent the disease.

Papular-Purpuric "Gloves and Socks" Syndrome

The papular-purpuric "gloves and socks" syndrome (PPGSS) is a dermatosis of acute onset in adults, characterized by pruritic, erythematous, papulopurpuric lesions on the hands and feet in a gloves and socks distribution. Oral aphthoid lesions and fever are concomitant findings. PPGSS patients often demonstrate cytomegalovirus or parvovirus infection.[4,12,23,40]

Meningococcemia, leukemia, and rickettsial disease may also manifest with palpable purpura, as described earlier.

NODULAR DISEASES

Nodules represent masses located beneath the skin. When they approach large dimension, they may be called tumors. Nodules may be either soft or firm, solitary or multiple, tender or nontender, and fixed or nonfixed to the overlying skin.

Leukocytoclastic Angiitis

The identical pathologic process may affect vessels more deeply placed within the dermis. In this location, nodules develop, rather than purpuric papules. These nodules are inflammatory in nature, and tender to palpation. When vessels in this cutaneous location are affected, other presentations include livedo reticularis and atrophie blanche.

Churg–Strauss Syndrome

The histologic examination of erythematous nodules occurring on the feet rendered a final diagnosis in a patient with acutely developed bilateral pulmonary infiltrates and marked

eosinophilia. Even a transbronchial biopsy did not reveal the necrotizing extravascular granulomas and dermal eosinophilic infiltrates witnessed in the pedal lesions.[25]

Lesions typically present on the head, trunk, and extremities. They range from a palpable purpura, or nodular lesions along with erythematous maculopapular or pustular in formation. Patients with Churg–Strauss syndrome will present with specific histopathologic characteristics, including eosinophils and flame figures with diffuse necrotizing vasculitis.[44]

There are six criteria in the classification of Churg–Strauss syndrome according to the American College of Rheumatology. Four of the six have a sensitivity of 85% and specificity of 99.7% for Churg–Strauss syndrome: asthma bronchiale, peripheral eosinophilia, paranasal sinusitis, pulmonary infiltration, vasculitis proven by histology, and mononeuropathy.[44] The lesions will often resolve with the use of systemic steroids that will result in its permanent clearing.[32]

Once the diagnosis of Churg–Strauss syndrome has been established, patients usually respond well to corticosteroid therapy. However, for those who fail to respond to corticosteroids or those who present with fulminant multisystem disease, cyclophosphamide can be added, depending on the severity of the disease.[41] Topical corticosteroids may also be added to the regimen to be applied to the skin of the lesions.[45]

Bacterial Endocarditis

The reader should recall that Osler nodes and Janeway lesions may occur in these patients.

Macroscopic Polyarteritis Nodosa

Because of the larger-sized vessels afflicted, this autoimmune disease does not primarily affect the skin. The only valid cutaneous signs include 5- to 10-mm subcutaneous nodules (which are in actuality small aneurysms). These nodules follow the course of arteries, ulcerations that result from infarction, in addition to gangrene of fingers and toes, and ecchymoses secondary to rupture of aneurysms and weakened arterial walls. As in LCA, visceral blood vessels are also affected. As a result, macroscopic polyarteritis nodosa frequently follows a fatal course.

The Panniculitides

The panniculitides represent a group of painful disorders involving subcutaneous fat. Factitial and purulent types result from readily identifiable etiologies. The remaining types form the "nodular nonsuppurative" variety.

Nodular nonsuppurative panniculitis may be associated with fever and a synovitis of the distal articulations, including the metatarsophalangeal joints. Females in the third to fourth decade of life appear to be most commonly affected, although an infant form does exist. Occasionally single, but more often multiple, tender subcutaneous nodules develop in recurrent crops, which is characteristic of these disorders. Necrosis and drainage of the nodules rarely occurs. Histologically, these nodules form secondary to leukocytic invasion. The postinflammatory healing and fibrosis lead to localized fat atrophy, which is manifest clinically as hyperpigmented depressions in the previously nodular areas. Although they occur most commonly over the shins, dorsal foot nodules have been reported in both the adult and infant forms.

Nodular nonsuppurative panniculitis is included because of its association with pancreatic diseases, including carcinoma of the pancreas (particularly that of the body and tail). Such patients usually present with multiple panniculitic areas of the lower extremities, which in theory are the result of circulating lipases released by the diseased pancreas.

Nodular nonsuppurative panniculitis has been found to be associated with trauma, halogen compounds or other drug ingestions, and infections, especially of a tuberculous nature. Association with histoplasmosis, dermatomyositis, systemic lupus erythematosus, and steroid withdrawal can occur. Other conditions, such as ulcerative colitis, jejunoileal bypass surgery, erythema nodosum, sarcoidosis, Hodgkin disease, glomerulonephritis, diabetes mellitus, and α_1-antitrypsin deficiency, have been implicated. This last occurrence, with α_1-antitrypsin deficiency patients, has resulted in terminal disease. These disorders are generally not immediately life-threatening conditions, however.

CONCLUSION

Space limitations and expanding medical knowledge preclude the "all-encompassing" chapter. Nevertheless, it is hoped that the treatment of the material presented is consistent with the algorithm described in the introductory sections. Common sense and experience dictate that histologic diagnosis (i.e., biopsy) be performed in the patient with a pedal dermatosis nonresponsive to standard therapies.

REFERENCES

1. Mays RM, Gordon RA, Durham C, et al. Rocky Mountain spotted fever in a patient treated with anti-TNF-alpha inhibitors. *Dermatol Online J*. 2013;19(3):7.
2. Regan J, Traeger M, Hmupherys D, et al. Risk factors for fatal outcome from rocky mountain spotted Fever in a highly endemic area-Arizona, 2002–2011. *Clin Infect Dis*. 2015;60(11):1659–1666.
3. Woods CR. Rocky Mountain spotted fever in children. *Pediatr Clin North Am*. 2013;60:455–470.
4. Hwang S, Schwartz RA. Keratosis pilaris: a common follicular hyperkeratosis. *Pediatr Dermatol*. 2008;82:177–180.
5. Milonovich L. Meningococcemia: epidemiology, pathophysiology, and management. *J Pediatr Health Care*. 2007;21(2):76–79.
6. Wenzel M, Jakob L, Wieser A, et al. Corticosteroid-induced meningococcal meningitis in a patient with chronic meningococcemia. *JAMA Dermatol*. 2014;150(7):752–755.
7. Glatz M, Achermann Y, Kerl K, et al. Nodular secondary syphilis in a woman. *BMJ Case Rep*. 2013. doi:10.1136/bcr-2013-009130.
8. Kazlouskaya V, Wittmann C, Tsikhanouskaya I. Pustular secondary syphilis: report of three cases and review of the literature. *Int J Dermatol*. 2014;53(10):e428–e431.
9. Ahmadinejad Z, Mansori S, Ziaee V, et al. Periodic Fever: a review on clinical, management and guideline for Iranian patients—part 1. *Iran J Pediatr*. 2014;24(1)1–13.
10. Ozen S, Batu ED. The myths we believed in familial Mediterranean fever: what have we learned in the past years? *Semin Immunopathol*. 2015;37:363–369.
11. Patel R, Shulman S. Kawasaki disease: a comprehensive review of treatment options. *J Clin Pharm Ther*. 2015;40:620–625.
12. Arif T. Salicylic acid as a peeling agent: a comprehensive review. *Clin Cosmet Investig Dermatol*. 2015;8:455–461.
13. Li Y, Tong X, Yang J, et al. Q-switch alexandrite laser treatment of facial and labial lentigines associated with Peutz–Jeghers syndrome. *Photodermatol Photoimmunol Photomed*. 2012;28:196–199.
14. Lee MA, Downing CP, Tyring K. Skin and mouth plus weight loss in an elderly man. *JAMA*. 2015;313(5):514–515.
15. Kim JY, Kim JS, Kim MH, et al. Intralesional 3% sodium tetradecyl sulfate for treatment of cutaneous Kaposi's sarcoma. *Yonsei Med J*. 2015;56(1)307–308.
16. Khan MMH, Sakauchi F, Sonoda T, et al. Magnitude of arsenic toxicity in the tube-well drinking water in Bangladesh and its adverse effects on human health including cancer: evidence from a review of the literature. *Asian Pac J Cancer Prev*. 2003;4:7–14.
17. Pratt M, Wadden P, Gulliver W. Arsenic keratosis in a patient from Newfoundland and Labrador, Canada: case report and review. *J Cutan Med Surg*. 2015:1–5.
18. Yu H, Liao W, Chai C. Arsenic carcinogenesis in the skin. *J Biomed Sci*. 2006;13:657–666.
19. Wong SS, Tan KC, Goh CL. Cutaneous manifestations of chronic arsenicism: review of seventeen cases. *J Am Acad Dermatol*. 1998;38:179–185.
20. Fleming JD, Stefanato CM, Attard NR. Bazex syndrome (acrokeratosis paraneoplastica). *Clin Exp Dermatol*. 2014;39:955–956.
21. Robert M, Gilabert M, Rahal S, et al. Bazex syndrome revealing a gastric cancer. *Case Rep Oncol*. 2014;7:285–287.
22. Sharma V, Sharma NL, Ranjan N, et al. Acrokeratosis paraneoplastica (Bazex syndrome): case report and review of the literature. *Dermatol Online J*. 2006;12(1):11.
23. Athar M, Li C, Kim A, et al. Sonic hedgehog signaling in Basal cell nevus syndrome. *Cancer Res*. 2014;74(18):4967–4975.
24. Fecher L, Sharfman WH. Advanced basal cell carcinoma, the hedgehog pathway, and treatment options-role of smoothened inhibitors. *Biologics*. 2015;9:129–140.
25. John AM, Schwartz RA. Basal cell nevus syndrome: an update on genetics and treatment. *Br J Dermatol*. 2016;174:68–76. doi:10.1111/bjd.14206.
26. Dreier J, Drummer R, Felderer L, et al. Emerging drugs and combination strategies for basal cell carcinoma. *Expert Opin Emerg Drugs*. 2014;19(3):353–365.
27. Kragballe K. Vitamin D3 and skin diseases. *Arch Dermatol Res*. 1992;284(1):S30–S36.
28. Van de Kerkhof P. An update on topical therapies for mild-moderate psoriasis. *Dermatol Clin*. 2015;33:73–77.
29. Millikan L. The rationale for using a topical retinoid for inflammatory acne. *Am J Clin Dermatol*. 2003;4(2):75–80.
30. Veien NK, Menne T. Treatment of hand eczema. *Skin Therapy Lett*. 2003;8(5):1–7.
31. Loden M, Bostrom P, Kneczke M. Distribution and keratolytic effect of salicylic acid and urea in human skin. *Skin Pharmacol*. 1995;8:173–178.
32. Ashton RE, Andre P, Lowe NJ, et al. Anthralin: historical and current perspectives. *J Am Acad Dermatol*. 1983;9(2):173–192.
33. Walter JF, Stoughton RB, De Quoy PR. Suppression of epidermal proliferation by ultraviolet light, coal tar and anthralin. *Br J Dermatol*. 1978;99:90–96.
34. Balkrishnan R, Sansbury J, Shenolikar RA, et al. Prescribing patterns for topical retinoids within NAMCS data. *J Drugs Dermatol*. 2005;4(2):172–179.
35. Haddad V, Costa Cardoso J, Lupi O, et al. Tropical dermatology: venomous arthropods and human skin Part I. Insecta. *J Am Acad Dermatol*. 2012;67:e1–e14.
36. Torbeck R, Pan M, de Moll E, et al. Cantharidin: a comprehensive review of the clinical literature. *Dermatol Online J*. 2014;20(6):3.

37. Weiss J, Shavin J. Topical retinoid and antibiotic combination therapy for acne management. *J Drugs Dermatol*. 2004;3(2):146–154.

38. Davis S, Sandoval L, Gustafson C, et al. Treatment of preadolescent acne in the United States: an analysis of nationally representative data. *Pediatr Dermatol*. 2013;30(6):689–694.

39. Walsh TL, Stalling SS, Natalie AA, et al. Mycobacterium avium-intracellulare pulmonary infection complicated by cutaneous leukocytoclastic vasculitis in a woman with anorexia nervosa. *Infection*. 2014;42:559–563.

40. Braswell MA, McCowan BS, Schulmeier J, et al. High yield biopsy technique for subepidermal blisters. *Cutis*. 2015;95:237–240.

41. Fung TH, Wong C, Ahmed U, et al. An unusual cause of a recurrent painful rash. *Acute Med*. 2012;11(2):89–92.

42. Snipsoyr M, Ludvigsen M, Petersen E, et al. A systemic review of the biomarkers in the diagnosis of infective endocarditis. *Int J Cardiol*. 2015;202:564–570.

43. Mestres CA, Pare JC, Miró JM; Working Group on Infective Endocarditis of the Hospital Clínic de Barcelona. Organization and functioning of a multidisciplinary team for the diagnosis and treatment of infective endocarditis: a 30 year perspective (1985–2014). *Rev Esp Cardiol (Engl Ed)*. 2015;68(5):363–368.

44. Ratzinger G, Zankl J, Zelger B. Wells syndrome and its relationship to Churg–Strauss syndrome. *Int J Dermatol*. 2013;52:949–954.

45. Dinić MŽ, Sekulovic K, Zolotarevski L, et al. Churg–Strauss syndrome: a case report. *Vojnosanit Pregl*. 2013;70(7):700–703.

CHAPTER 16

Laboratory Evaluation of Systemic Rheumatic Diseases in the Lower Extremity

BELLA MEHTA • STEVEN K. MAGID

The clinical laboratory can be of great help in the diagnosis of disorders of the foot. Although laboratory tests are often informative, they are rarely definitive or diagnostic. Laboratory examinations must be used in conjunction with a complete history, physical, and radiographic examinations. Over the past few years, many new tests have been developed, some of which will be discussed later.

Laboratory tests may be used in a number of different ways. For example, they may be used to diagnose a specific illness involving the foot. Examples of this include detecting the presence of intracellular monosodium urate crystals in synovial fluid aspirated from an acutely inflamed joint. This finding is diagnostic of gout. A positive Gram stain or culture from an acutely inflamed joint is diagnostic of infection. Laboratory tests may also be used to diagnose a systemic illness (e.g., a complete blood cell count [CBC] and bone marrow examination may be diagnostic of leukemia in a patient with bone pain or a low platelet count or abnormal coagulation profile with sudden foot swelling may reflect hemarthrosis or a high white count may reflect septic arthritis). The laboratory should always be used with a goal in mind: to arrive at a specific diagnosis; to provide further evidence of a suspected diagnosis, such as a positive rheumatoid factor (RF) in a patient with a systemic polyarthritis; to rule out competing diagnoses; to guide therapy; or to assess prognosis or response to treatment. Treatment decisions are rarely based on one test alone. Clinicians should also be aware about variability between different laboratories and different testing approaches.

Four characteristics of diagnostic tests help determine their usefulness in evaluating patients:

1. Sensitivity, or the likelihood that a test will be positive in a person with the disease.
2. Specificity, or the likelihood that a test will be negative in a person without the disease.
3. Positive predictive value, or the likelihood that a disease will be present in a person with a positive test result.
4. Negative predictive value, or the likelihood that a disease will be absent in a patient with a negative test result.

TESTS ASSOCIATED WITH INFLAMMATION—ACUTE PHASE REACTANTS

When diagnosing a disorder, one of the most important considerations is to determine whether the cause is inflammatory (and frequently systemic) or noninflammatory. Many metabolic changes occur in the setting of inflammatory processes. Together, they are called the acute phase response. The acute phase response occurs after many events, including infections, trauma, immune diseases, crystalline diseases, and malignancy.

C-Reactive Protein

C-reactive protein (CRP) is composed of five identical subunits that are linked together. This protein is present in animals that trace their evolutionary origins for hundreds of millions of years (such as the horseshoe crab). CRP is normally present in plasma in only trace amounts: approximately 0.2 mg per dL. Levels increase dramatically and quickly after a stimulus. Moderate elevations occur in most connective tissue diseases (1 to 10 mg per dL). Very high levels are seen in bacterial infections and systemic vasculitis (15 to 20 mg per dL). Diabetes, obesity, and cigarette smoking can increase CRP levels in variable amounts. CRP is not thought to be altered by age or gender. The CRP levels can increase within 4 to 6 hours and normalize within 1 week in response to a stimulus. These changes occur much more quickly compared to the erythrocyte sedimentation rate (ESR). CRP levels fall when inflammation subsides. Because a substantial stimulus is required for CRP elevation, a normal value does not exclude an inflammatory process. Many clinicians prefer sending ESR concomitantly with CRP. Of interest, in systemic lupus erythematosus (SLE) and other connective tissue diseases, CRP levels are lower than one would expect for the amount of inflammation present. CRP was initially identified by its ability to form a precipitin reaction with pneumococcal polysaccharide. It is now measured by either latex agglutination or rocket electrophoresis. In contrast to the ESR, CRP can be assayed on specimens that have been stored by freezing. This is an advantage compared with ESR, which must be performed on fresh blood. Generally for CRP, the upper limit of the reference range is age/50 in men and age/50 +0.6 in women. Recently, high-sensitivity CRP has become available. This test is much more sensitive, and can detect slight elevations of CRP that are technically within the normal range, but may have clinical relevance with respect to coronary artery disease. However, it has not been proven cost-effective or having additional benefit in routine monitoring of rheumatologic diseases.

Erythrocyte Sedimentation Rate

Although an elevated CRP is highly associated with inflammation, ESR has been the most widely used indicator of inflammation and the acute phase response. ESR is performed by placing anticoagulated blood in a vertical glass tube and measuring the rate of red blood cell (RBC) settling. Normally, RBCs repel each other because the electrical charges on the surface of all RBCs are the same. When inflammation is present, there is an increase in the concentration of asymmetrically charged proteins that bind to the RBCs and thus prevent this repulsion. The RBCs, therefore, tend to aggregate. Aggregated clumps of cells settle more rapidly than individual cells, thus providing a higher ESR. Fibrinogen is the protein that is most responsible for elevations in ESR in acute states of inflammation. However, in chronic inflammation, decreased serum albumin and hematocrit levels also contribute to an increased ESR. An increase in immunoglobulin (Ig) such as that seen with myeloma or monoclonal gammopathies can also lead to an ESR elevation, although such changes may not necessarily indicate an inflammatory state. The ESR is influenced by anemia, polycythemia, and alterations in the size and shape of erythrocytes. Falsely low levels are seen in sickle cell disease, anisocytosis, spherocytosis, polycythemia, and heart failure. Prolonged storage of blood before testing or tilting of the calibrated tube will tend to an increase in the ESR. The Westergren method is thought to be the most reliable. This method measures the fall of RBCs in millimeters per hour in a standardized tube. Normal is considered 0 to 15 for males and 0 to 20 for females. However, the ESR also increases with age; thus, "normal" levels are variable. Levels up to 40 mm per hour are common in healthy elderly people. A rule of thumb is that the age-adjusted upper limit of normal of ESR is age divided by 2 for men and age plus 10 divided by 2 for women. The ESR is probably most helpful if it is normal. Active inflammatory disorders such as acute rheumatic fever, SLE, rheumatoid arthritis (RA), temporal arteritis, and infections tend to have elevated ESRs. Although elevations of the ESR in septic arthritis and crystal-induced arthritis are the rule, a normal ESR does not completely rule out these entities. Joint aspiration is required. From this, it is clear that the ESR and CRP are neither diagnostic nor specific. Nonetheless, they can be helpful in evaluating

patients when RA or other systemic and local inflammatory conditions are being considered. ESR and CRP are a part of the metrics used to measure and follow disease activity in RA patients along with signs and symptoms.

Additional Acute Phase Reactants

Other acute phase reactants include ferritin, fibrinogen, serum amyloid A, etc. Although markers of inflammation, they are not routinely measured because they are nonspecific.

BIOMARKERS

Cytokines like interleukin (IL)-6 increase swiftly and dramatically with inflammation; however, they are not viewed as acute phase reactants. There are several cytokine panels and multiprotein biomarker algorithms now commercially available to monitor disease activity in diseases like RA and SLE. There is a commercially available test used to assess disease activity in RA (Vectra DA). It measures the following biomarkers: adhesion molecules (VCAM-1), growth factors (EGF, VEGF-A), cytokine-related proteins (IL-6 and tumor necrosis factor [TNF]-R1), matrix metalloproteinases (MMP-1, MMP-2), skeletal-related proteins (YKL-40), hormones (leptin and resistin), and acute phase proteins (SAA, CRP). A complex algorithm is then applied, to provide a disease activity scale that ranges from 1 to 100 and categorizes RA into low (1 to 29), moderate (30 to 44), and high disease activity (45 to 100). Diagnostic biomarker panels for SLE are also available. The "AVISE" SLE diagnostic panel measures cell-bound complement activation products (CB-CAPs). The current panel, which will likely evolve with future study, includes antinuclear antibody (ANA), anti–double-stranded deoxyribonucleic acid (dsDNA), anti–mutated citrullinated vimentin (anti-MCV) antibody, and the CB-CAPs erythrocyte-bound C4d (E-C4d) and B-cell C4d (B-C4d). Larger studies are required to confirm the validity of these panels.

Rheumatoid Factor

Rheumatoid factors (RFs) are autoantibodies that are directed against the Fc fragment of immunoglobulin G. It is believed that they are synthesized in response to immunoglobulins (Igs) that have been conformationally altered after reaction with antigen. They are most commonly associated with RA but are also found in other disorders.

Historically, the test was performed by coating sheep red blood cells or latex particles with human IgG and measuring the dilution of patient serum that will still aggregate the particle. Newer methods include radioimmunoassay, enzyme-linked immunoassay (ELISA), and nephelometry. These methods increase sensitivity and specificity.

RF is one of the laboratory tests most frequently ordered in the evaluation of patients with joint complaints. The test is positive in 75% to 90% of patients with RA. In early RA, only 50% of patients may have a positive RF. However, these data are taken from highly selected populations and might be subject to referral bias. The high specificity that is also reported in studies from these populations may not be observed in patients who have weak indications for the test, who may be elderly, or who have other diseases that may cause a false-positive RF. In fact, the prevalence of false-positive RFs in patients older than 75 years is between 2% and 25%. Although there may be an increased likelihood of developing RA in a RF-positive asymptomatic individual, the use of RF as a screening test performs poorly because of the high frequency of false-positive test results. RFs are most common in patients with RA, but they are also present in normal sera as well as in sera of patients with acquired immunodeficiency syndrome, hepatitis, various parasitic diseases, chronic bacterial infections such as tuberculosis and subacute bacterial endocarditis (SBE), tumors, chronic lymphocytic leukemia, and other hyper-globulinemic states such as cryoglobulinemia, primary Sjögren syndrome, chronic liver disease including chronic hepatitis C, sarcoidosis, and some chronic pulmonary diseases. For example, when RF is found in a patient with fever, arthralgia, and a heart murmur, SBE may be a more likely cause of a positive RF than RA. When found in patients with RA, RFs are usually specific for human IgG, are of high affinity, and include not only IgM RFs but also IgG, IgA, and IgE variants.

High levels of RF have been associated with a worse prognosis; there tend to be more involved joints when first seen by a physician, more erosions, and greater liga-mentous instability. However, RF titer does not correlate with disease activity and thus cannot be used to assess disease activity. A high level of RF is considered a risk factor for RA vasculitis. Other laboratory findings that are common in RA include leukocytosis (usually with a normal differential), thrombocytosis, anemia (normochromic, normocytic), normal uric acid (if the patient is not taking salicylates, which can raise uric acid levels), a negative ANA and anti-DNA antibody, and normal or elevated serum complement.

Anti-Cyclic Citrullinated Peptide Antibodies

Anti-cyclic citrullinated peptide (CCP) antibodies are autoantibodies directed against the acids formed by post-translational modification of arginine. During inflammation, the amino acid arginine can be enzymatically converted into citrulline, in proteins such as vimentin, in a process called citrullination. If their shapes are significantly altered, the proteins may be seen as antigens by the immune system, thereby generating an immune response. IgG anti-CCP antibodies are measured by ELISA using synthetic citrul-linated peptides. The 2010 American College of Rheuma-tology (ACR)/EULAR Rheumatoid Arthritis Classification Criteria now include anti-CCP testing. Anti-CCPs have the same sensitivity as RF, but the advantage is that they are more specific. Also anti-CCPs can be detected in early RA

and are better predictors of erosive disease than RF. There are patients who are both RF and CCP negative but have clinical signs of RA. They are labeled seronegative RA. As with RF, CCP levels cannot be used to monitor disease activity. However, RF and CCP combined can help in the diagnosis of RA. A false-positive CCP can sometimes be seen in diseases like tuberculosis, chronic lung diseases, and other connective tissue diseases. The newer genera-tion assays, anti-CCP antibody assays (anti-CCP2), have improved sensitivity and specificity compared with the original anti-CCP assays.

There have been several other antibodies described for diagnosing RA: 14-3-3η autoantibodies, alone and in com-bination with the 14-3-3η protein, RF, and/or anti-CCP identified most patients with early and established RA.[1] A number of other autoantibodies have been the subject of investigation in RA—anti – mutated citrullinated vimentin, Ig-binding protein, glucose-6-phosphate isomerase, type 2 collagen, mannose-binding lectin, ferritin, anti-RA33, anti-p68, anti-alpha enolase, antibodies to the enzyme peptidylarginine deiminase 4, etc. All of these require further studies for them to be widely used.

Antinuclear Antibodies

Lupus is another autoimmune disease which may have major joint manifestations. It usually causes a nonerosive, nondeforming symmetric arthropathy. Multiple joints are typically involved. The ankle and foot are less commonly involved than with RA. In addition, systemic features are more common. These include rash, fever, central nervous system involvement, renal disease, and serositis. Unlike RA, many types of autoantibodies are typically found in SLE and related syndromes. ANAs are a hallmark of SLE. These are antibodies directed against the cell nucleus. The ANA is positive in 95% to 99% of patients with lupus. The indirect immunofluorescence ANA is the method most commonly used. It is performed by diluting test sera and incubating with substrate cells. Traditionally, thin sections of frozen rat kidney or liver are used. However, cytocentrifuged preparations of cells from tissue culture such as Hep-2 can give optimal sensitivity and pattern discrimination. Any bound ANAs are then detected by fluorescein-tagged antihuman Ig. The sub-strate cell is then viewed under a fluorescence microscope. ANAs are reported by either intensity of fluorescence (i.e., 1+ to 4+) or by maximal dilution of serum giving a positive result. Values of 2+ or greater or titers of greater than 1:40 are considered abnormal. The pattern of the ANA is also re-ported (e.g., speckled, diffuse, rim, centromere). ANAs have different targets, and the pattern of immunofluorescence can provide differential diagnostic information.

Homogeneous patterns are least specific, and can be seen in up to 5% of normal patients, especially women and the elderly. In this setting, they are usually present in low titers. The rim pattern is characteristic of SLE. Nucleolar and speckled patterns are also seen and are associated with scleroderma, CREST (**C**alcinosis cutis, **R**aynaud phenomenon, **E**sophageal dysmotility, **S**clerodactyly, and **T**elangiectasia), mixed connective tissue disease (MCTD), and other diseases. Once a patient has been documented to have a positive ANA, it is usually not necessary to repeat the test unless a major change in therapy or status is detected. The ACR recommends testing for ANA only when there is a suspicion of a connective tissue disease like lupus. Positive tests must always be interpreted in context with the history, physical exam, and other laboratory tests. It should be noted that steroids and other immunosuppressant agents may lower ANA titers. Extractable nuclear antigens (ENAs) sometimes help sort the diagnosis.

Many diseases can produce anti–single-stranded DNA antibodies. These include liver diseases and drug-induced lupus. However, for the most part, only SLE (and MCTD) is associated with high-titer anti-dsDNA antibodies. These occur in nearly all SLE patients. In contradistinction to the ANA, levels of dsDNA antibodies are frequently used in monitoring disease activity, so it is often repeated in frequent intervals. Many other laboratory tests may be abnormal in SLE, and can be used in conjunction with the more specific tests for assessing disease activity. These include a low WBC (usually with neutropenia and lymphopenia), anemia (sometimes an autoimmune hemolytic anemia with positive Coombs), and thrombocytopenia. As suggested by the variety of ANA immunofluorescent patterns, ANAs may be directed against a number of different cellular constituents. Immunodiffusion and counterimmunoelectrophoresis can be performed using soluble components of cells (i.e., ENAs). The ENAs include anti-Ro, anti-La, anti-Smith and anti-ribonuclear protein (RNP). Anti-RNP is often accompanied by a speckled ANA and is seen in patients with SLE, or an overlap disease that is known as MCTD. Anti-Ro (SSA) and anti-La (SSB) are associated with Sjögren syndrome. In addition to nucleic acids, other protein antigens from both nuclei and cytoplasm have been shown to be targets of ANAs. The antinuclear specificities that are most common with SLE are anti–double-stranded DNA and anti-Smith. Anti-histone antibody and single-stranded DNA antibodies may be found in drug-induced lupus.

Antiphospholipid Syndrome

Many patients with lupus may have concomitant antiphospholipid syndrome (APLS). However, APLS may exist in patients without lupus too. Patients with APLS often present with ischemic toes, arterial and venous clots, or even emboli, resulting in strokes. It is characterized by elevated partial thromboplastin time (PTT), false-positive Venereal Disease Research Laboratories test, and antiphospholipid antibodies.

A factor has been known to exist in the serum of some SLE patients that prolongs the PTT. This inhibitor was frequently associated with false-positive serologic tests for syphilis. The factor could be absorbed from plasma by phospholipids. This factor became known as the lupus anticoagulant, even though approximately half of the patients with this serologic abnormality do not have SLE. In addition, although the inhibitor acts as an anticoagulant in vitro, patients with the lupus anticoagulant were not prone to excess bleeding. In fact, the opposite was found: they were prone to both arterial and venous thromboses as well as thrombocytopenia and fetal loss or miscarriage.

Standard antiphospholipid panels include the lupus anticoagulant, anti-cardiolipin antibodies, and β-2 glycoprotein. Anti-cardiolipin and anti-β-2-glycoprotein antibodies are usually ordered in IgG, IgM, and IgA forms. And generally, IgG antibodies have a higher predictive value than IgM and IgA; also the higher the elevation, the greater the positive predictive value of an association with APLS. Recently, a few centers started to measure anti-phosphatidylserine and other negatively charged phospholipids. However, they are not routinely used in clinical practice as there is not enough evidence in the literature to show its utility in diagnosis. Because these patients demonstrate a procoagulant state, treatment with anticoagulation is usually indicated.

Complement

The complement cascade contains at least 18 distinct plasma proteins. It is one of the major effector arms of the humoral immune system. Complement activation is thought to occur primarily by two mechanisms: the classic and the alternative. In the classic activation pathway, antigen–antibody complexes act on C1 and C2 to cause cleavage of C3. In the alternative pathway, complex polysaccharides act on properdin factors d and b to cause cleavage of C3. Once C3 is cleaved, the terminal components (C5–C9), which are common to both pathways, are activated. This leads to the lysis of the target cell and cellular membrane injury. Subsequently, many mediators are generated that trigger inflammation and anaphylaxis. C3 and C4 are measured by ELISA assays. CH50 is a measure of the total hemolytic complement and thus more a reflection of the classical pathway. Serum is diluted and added to sheep antibody-coated RBCs. The value reported is the reciprocal of the highest dilution able to lyse 50% of the RBCs. When immune complexes are formed and cleared from the body, the complement level is decreased. Serial measurements of C3, C4, or CH50 are useful in monitoring disease activity (particularly renal disease) in SLE. A decrease in complement level may precede the disease flare in lupus and related disorders. Decreased complement may also be seen in poststreptococcal glomerulonephritis or SBE. Genetic absence of complement proteins is rarely seen. C4 levels that are disproportionately lower than C3 may indicate cryoglobulinemia. CB-CAPs can be used in the diagnosis of lupus; however, its validity needs to be determined by further studies.

SERONEGATIVE SPONDYLOARTHROPATHIES

Another major group of rheumatic diseases that have frequent manifestations in the ankle and foot are the seronegative spondyloarthropathies. These include psoriatic arthritis, Reiter syndrome, ankylosing spondylitis, and the enteropathic arthritides. As with most forms of rheumatic disease, the diagnosis is made clinically.

Psoriatic arthritis has a number of different clinical presentations. These include spondylitis, RA-like asymmetric distal arthritis, dactylitis that causes sausage digits, and arthritis mutilans. Nail changes are common. There are no diagnostic lab findings, although an elevated ESR and slight elevation of uric acid are common. Psoriatic arthritis occurs more commonly in patients with tissue type human leukocyte antigens (HLA)-Cw6 and HLA-B27.

Reiter syndrome is associated with pauciarticular arthritis, frequently of the knees, ankles, metatarsals, and toes. Conjunctivitis, urethritis, prostatitis, sacroiliitis, and a skin rash (keratoderma blennorrhagicum—which preferentially affects the feet) are frequent clinical findings. Here too, an elevated ESR can be seen. Pyuria may also be a manifestation of Reiter syndrome when associated with prostatitis or urethritis (which may be asymptomatic). *Chlamydia* is one of the organisms thought to induce Reiter syndrome, and an effort should be made in the lab to identify this pathogen. Cultures are not reliable. The diagnostic test of choice for chlamydial infection of the genitourinary tract is nucleic acid amplification testing of vaginal swabs for women or first-catch urine for men. When appropriate, urethral, cervical, and rectal cultures should be performed. A variety of enteric pathogens such as *Salmonella*, *Shigella*, *Yersinia*, and *Campylobacter* can also induce Reiter syndrome. These may be confirmed by stool culture. Patients infected with *Chlamydia* are often also infected with gonorrhea, both sexually transmitted diseases. Probably the most important lab test when evaluating a patient with a mono- or pauciarticular arthritis, with urethritis, rash, and enteritis, is to rule out an infectious cause. Joint aspiration and culture can be performed and in gonorrhea infection is the best way to establish diagnosis.

Arthritis associated with Crohn disease and with ulcerative colitis will have negative stool and synovial fluid cultures. Intestinal histopathology should be helpful in confirming clinical suspicions of an inflammatory bowel disease. Anti–*Saccharomyces cerevisiae* antibodies may be positive in ulcerative and microscopic colitis. Pyoderma gangrenosum is an associated skin condition with ulcerative colitis and Crohn mainly involving the lower extremity.

Human immunodeficiency virus (HIV) infection has also been associated with a Reiter syndrome–like arthritis. Screening ELISA and confirmation with Western blot should be considered after appropriate history and physical examination and counseling.

It is well known that there is a relationship between HLA-B27 and ankylosing spondylitis. HLAs are present on the surface of nucleated cells and play a role in determining the genetic predisposition to a variety of immune-mediated processes, including autoimmune diseases. The sensitivity of this test is approximately 95% in ankylosing spondylitis, 80% in Reiter syndrome, and 50% in spondylitis associated

with inflammatory bowel disease. The background prevalence of this marker (6% to 10% in Whites) and the fact that only a small minority of HLA-B27-positive individuals will ever experience an arthropathy make the test of limited use. According to some authors, people with inflammatory low back pain have a 40% pretest probability of a positive HLA-B27.[2] When the test is ordered for patients with back pain that is not clinically suggestive of sacroiliitis, the test may yield more false-positive than true-positive results. Thus, a positive HLA-B27 may be of some value, but, as noted previously, it may result in the misclassification of diseases if it is relied on too heavily.

URIC ACID AND GOUT

Gout is one of the more common rheumatic diseases that affect the foot and ankle. When the metatarsal–phalangeal joint at the base of the big toe is affected, it is known as podagra. Approximately 50% of cases present with involvement of the big toe. However, other differential diagnoses must be kept in mind when diagnosing gout on the basis of podagra. A careful assessment is thus necessary **(Table 16-1)**. In its classic, acute presentation, it is not likely to be confused with RA or SLE. However, in its chronic tophaceous form, there are many features that can mimic RA, including polyarthritis, symmetry of joint involvement, nodules, fusiform swelling, and erosions. Sometimes, gout and RA may coexist. High uric acid may be seen in patients with RA for reasons unrelated to the type of arthritis present. Common causes of an increase in uric acid are: obesity, renal insufficiency, hypertension, alcohol intake, psoriasis, and genetic factors. In addition, patients with psoriasis have a higher than normal uric acid, attributed to rapid cell turnover in the skin. The use of such common drugs as salicylates, in low doses, immunosuppressive medications like tacrolimus, and diuretics can also precipitate gout. It should be stressed that an elevation of serum uric acid is not sufficient for the diagnosis of gout. In fact, hyperuricemia without joint/other manifestations has been described in more than 15% of certain populations. Current recommendations suggest that asymptomatic hyperuricemia should not be treated. However, if treatment with allopurinol

Table 16-1. Podagra Mimics
Septic arthritis/osteomyelitis
Rheumatoid arthritis
CPPD
BCP crystal disease/hydroxyapatite crystals
Calcium oxalate crystal deposition disease
Reactive arthritis
Trauma

BCP, basic calcium phosphate; CPPD, calcium pyrophosphate deposition disease.

is being considered, then obtaining an HLA-B58 should considered, particularly in Asian subpopulations (notably in Korean, Han Chinese, or Thai descent patients) because this HLA type is highly correlated with drug reactions. Further complicating the use of a serum uric acid in the diagnosis of gout is the fact that serum uric acid is frequently normal during an acute attack. The diagnosis is best established by joint aspiration and evaluation with compensated polarized light microscopy. The identification of needle-shaped, negatively birefringent crystals within neutrophils is diagnostic. A word of caution is necessary because it has been established that a variety of materials, including lipids, particulate matter from previous joint replacements, malignant cells, or other crystals such as previously injected intra-articular steroids, can be confused with those of uric acid.

CALCIUM PYROPHOSPHATE DEPOSITION DISEASE

Another crystal disease that can affect the foot and ankle must be distinguished from gout. That condition is calcium pyrophosphate deposition disease (CPPD). This is the arthritis associated with calcium pyrophosphate. Acute arthritis (or pseudogout) rarely affects the first metatarsophalangeal (MTP) joint the way gout does. More often, it affects the knees and wrists, but it may also involve the ankle and on occasion the first MTP. Although most often associated with a familial predisposition or with aging, a number of other diseases have been associated with CPPD. Many of these have characteristic laboratory features, including CPPD associated with diabetes, hemochromatosis (elevated iron, iron saturation, and ferritin), hyperparathyroidism (high parathyroid hormone [PTH], hypercalcemia, hyperchloremic acidosis), hypomagnesemia, hypophosphatasia, or hemosiderosis. As with gout, the diagnosis of CPPD is confirmed by joint aspiration and crystal search. CPPD crystals are positively birefringent when seen under compensated polarized light microscopy.

DIABETES

Diabetes has been associated with CPPD, although this is thought more likely to be the chance occurrence of two common diseases. Diabetes, however, does have major manifestations in diseases of the foot. These include peripheral neuropathy, Charcot joints, and diabetic ulcers with and without underlying osteomyelitis. The laboratory diagnosis of diabetes is, therefore, germane. Screening may be performed with a fasting blood glucose. Stress testing can include 2-hour postprandial sugars or a full glucose tolerance test. Hemoglobin (Hb)A1C or glycosylated hemoglobin may be useful in monitoring diabetic control in an individual patient. A HbA1C above 6.5% is considered indicative of diabetes. Usually by the time the foot complications of diabetes occur, the diagnosis is well established.

PERIPHERAL NEUROPATHY

There are many causes of peripheral neuropathy, other than diabetes, and vasculitis, including metabolic causes (e.g., thyroid—measure thyroid-stimulating hormone), lead and other heavy metal poisoning, toxic—both drug and alcohol related, various vitamin deficiencies, pernicious anemia, in which B_{12} levels can be used in the diagnosis, infections—Lyme, HIV, etc., deposition diseases—sarcoidosis, amyloidosis, etc.

SYNOVIAL FLUID ANALYSIS

Synovial fluid analysis is one of the most useful lab tests that can be performed in the evaluation of arthritis. It should be performed as part of the workup in every patient with a joint effusion. It is particularly important in the evaluation of septic arthritis.

Even in patients with an established diagnosis, it may provide evidence about the activity of disease. Alternatively, it may demonstrate the coexistence of another disease. For example, a patient with an underlying inflammatory arthritis such as RA may also have a superimposed infection. Similarly, a patient with RA or osteoarthritis may also have gout or pseudogout. Joint fluid has often been classified into five groups as mentioned in **Table 16-2**.

Although it is possible to measure antibodies in synovial fluid such as Lyme and RF, they are rarely performed any more due to lack of specificity and sensitivity.

Evaluation of the specimen under compensated polarized light microscopy is of critical importance. This is the only reliable method of diagnosing an acute attack of gout or pseudogout. Monosodium urate crystals are intensely negatively birefringent and form needles and rods. When found intracellularly, they are virtually diagnostic of gout. Calcium pyrophosphate dihydrate is weakly birefringent and often rhomboid in shape. Many other crystals have been described and include those composed of hydroxyapatite clumps, calcium oxalate, cholesterol, myeloma cell aggregates, depot steroids (from prior joint injections), particulate matter (from prior joint replacement), lipids, Charcot–Leyden crystals, and Igs. These crystals are found in a variety of clinical settings and may be useful in the diagnosis of many diseases.

METABOLIC BONE DISEASE

Stress fractures of the foot are common causes of foot pain. They may occur in patients with normal bone; however, osteoporosis may often contribute. There are many causes and risk factors for osteoporosis. Some of them are associated with laboratory abnormalities. Examples include steroid use (associated with hypokalemia), estrogen and testosterone deficiency states (measurement of specific hormone levels), renal disease (blood urea nitrogen, creatinine clearance), gastrointestinal and liver disease (liver function tests, tests

Table 16-2. Synovial fluid analysis

Joint Fluid	Amount	Appearance	WBCs	Characteristics
Normal	Less than 1 mL	Transparent, colorless, or straw colored	Less than 200 WBCs and less than 25% of them PMNs	Negative culture
Noninflammatory	Greater than 1 mL	Transparent with high viscosity, color may be more yellow	50 to 1,000 WBCs with less than 25% PMNs	Negative culture. Typically osteoarthritis
Inflammatory	Greater than 1 mL	Low viscosity, translucent but not transparent, yellowish colored	1,000 to 75,000 WBCs, PMNs typically greater than 50%	Negative culture. RA, psoriatic arthritis, Reiter syndrome, bowel-related SLE, scleroderma, Wegener granulomatosis, Sjögren syndrome, sarcoidosis, crystal-induced, etc.
Septic	Greater than 1 mL	Opaque fluid colored yellow to green	WBC counts often higher than 100,000 and greater than 85% are PMNs	Culture is typically positive for the respective organism
Hemarthrosis	Variable	Grossly and diffusely bloody fluid	Variable likely same as in peripheral blood	Negative culture. Trauma, PVNS, coagulation defects, and tumors

WBC, white blood cell, PVNS, pigmented villonodular synovitis, PMNs, olymorphonuclear leucocytes (neutrophils).

for particular types of diseases that cause hepatitis, or malabsorption), abnormalities of vitamin D, phosphate, and calcium metabolism (Ca^{2+}, PO_4^{2-}, 25-OH vitamin D, 24-hour urine for calcium), hyperthyroidism and hyperparathyroidism (TSH, thyroxine [T4], T4 uptake, triiodothyronine, T7 index, PTH, electrolyte abnormalities, calcium levels, urinary calcium), marrow replacement, such as with myeloma (serum immunoelectrophoresis, urine immunoelectrophoresis, ESR, CBC) or leukemia (CBC).

Autoimmune diseases: Like RA and SLE, not only may these illnesses cause an inflammatory arthritis that can involve the foot, but most are associated with osteoporosis.

Paget disease is another metabolic disease of bone that should be suspected as a cause of foot pain if there is an elevated alkaline phosphatase and high urinary hydroxyproline levels. Although it most often occurs in the spine, pelvis, skull, femur, and tibia, it may also occur in the small bones of the foot. Similarly, osteomalacia may also affect the lower extremity, and characteristic laboratory findings may be sought (e.g., calcium level, phosphorus, vitamin D, alkaline phosphate).

INFECTION

It is critical to diagnose infections of the foot promptly. Infection may involve the foot in a number of ways. These include direct puncture (with or without foreign body); trauma (e.g., motor vehicle accident) in the setting of ulcers (diabetic, vasculitic) as well as via hematogeneous spread. It is imperative to obtain appropriate cultures to identify the pathogen. They may involve the soft tissue, the joint, or deeper structures including the bone. Joint aspiration may be required to rule out septic arthritis. If there is evidence of

osteomyelitis, bone biopsy may be needed for both diagnosis and culture and sensitivity. Culturing an open ulcer may not be very helpful, because the organisms present may simply be contaminants, and not causative.

Many organisms can infect the foot. These include the following:

Bacterial: Typical staphylococcal and streptococcal infections affect the foot; however, in diabetics, *Pseudomonas* and even some anaerobic infections can be seen. Culture results will guide therapy in these. Lyme disease is a tick-borne illness caused by the bacteria *Borrelia burgdorferi*. It typically affects the knee, but may also affect the ankle and foot. In addition to history, ELISA is performed as a screening test, and a Western immunoblot is required for confirmation. IgG Lyme titers usually stay elevated long after Lyme disease is treated. Thus, a positive IgG titer only indicates past exposure and not necessarily an active infection. Mycobacterium infections in the joints are mainly seen in immunocompromised individuals. *Mycobacterium marinum* typically causes clusters of superficial nodules or papules in extremities after contaminated aquatic exposure. *Mycobacterium tuberculosis* may present as monoarticular joint swelling—acid fast bacilli (AFB) smear and culture should be ordered when there is a suspicion.

Fungal or parasitic: In an immunocompromised host, fungal or even parasitic joint infections may occur and relevant studies must be sent from joint fluid/serum per clinical suspicion. SBE will sometimes cause an immune-related arthritis, unrelated to direct infection. In the proper clinical setting (fever, heart murmur, embolic events), blood cultures are indicated.

Viral: Many viruses can cause arthritis, including the joints of the foot. These include viral infections like hepatitis C, B; mosquito-borne viral illnesses like dengue, chikungunya, etc. Dengue fever is diagnosed with IgM immunoassay ELISA. Chikungunya may have arthritis and arthralgia symptoms mainly in the back and lower extremity for weeks or sometimes years. Laboratory criteria include a decreased lymphocyte count consistent with viremia. However, a definitive laboratory diagnosis can be accomplished through viral isolation, reverse transcription polymerase chain reaction, or serologic diagnosis.

LÖFGREN SYNDROME

Löfgren syndrome is an acute form of sarcoidosis characterized by erythema nodosum (tender red nodules), bilateral hilar lymphadenopathy, and polyarthralgia or polyarthritis. The arthritis is often acute and involves the lower extremities, especially ankle joints. Besides the physical exam findings of inflammatory arthritis and imaging with lymphadenopathy, serum angiotensin-converting enzyme, vitamin D (1,25)-OH, and calcium levels are often increased; however, none of these abnormalities are specific.

VASCULITIS–VASCULOPATHIES

A variety of vasculitic syndromes may present with manifestations in the feet. One major mode of presentation is vascular insufficiency. This may initially cause claudication, and may later progress to pallor, cyanosis, ulceration, and eventually gangrene of the toes or feet. Often, small-vessel vasculitis will present as a rash or palpable purpura. Hydrostatic forces are thought to play a role in their preferential appearance in the lower extremities. Finally, neuropathy resulting from infarction of the vasa nervorum may have major manifestations in the foot, and sometimes, the first presentation of it may be a foot drop. This is a medical emergency. Immunologic causes of vasculitis often have characteristic laboratory findings. For example, active generalized granulomatosis with polyangiitis (GPA), formerly referred to as Wegener granulomatosis, is highly associated with antineutrophil cytoplasmic antibodies (ANCA).

These antibodies cause a characteristic pattern of cytoplasmic granular staining with immunofluorescence. The antibodies appear to be directed against proteinase 3 (PR3), a serine protease found in the primary granules of neutrophils. C-ANCA is found in 90% of cases of GPA and is usually not present in other types of vasculitis. The titers of C-ANCA parallel disease activity of GPA. They are not as commonly found in the limited forms of GPA. Antibodies directed against myeloperoxidase (MPO) produce a perinuclear pattern of staining referred to as P-ANCA. P-ANCAs are characteristic markers of systemic necrotizing vasculitis, and are seen in microscopic polyarteritis, idiopathic glomerulonephritis, and Churg–Strauss syndrome.

ANCA titers sometimes normalize posttreatment. Patients with concomitant C- and P-ANCA may have levamisole exposure, which is found in adulterated cocaine. The most common drugs that produce this include propylthiouracil, hydralazine, or minocycline.

Atypical ANCAs directed against targets other than MPO and PR3 are found in a wide variety of conditions. These include inflammatory bowel disease, liver disease, chronic infections, RA, HIV, and others. Mounting evidence directly implicates ANCAs in the pathogenesis of vasculitis.

HENOCH–SCHÖNLEIN PURPURA

Henoch–Schönlein purpura (HSP) is a disease of the skin and other organs like kidney. It causes palpable purpura (small hemorrhages), often with joint and abdominal pain. HSP is a systemic vasculitis (inflammation of blood vessels) and is characterized by deposition of immune complexes containing the antibody IgA mainly in skin and kidneys. Along with increased inflammatory markers, blood urea nitrogen, and creatinine, there is raised serum levels of IgA. The platelet count may be raised, and distinguishes it from diseases where low platelets are the cause of the purpura. On biopsy, immunofluorescence demonstrates IgA and C3 blood vessel wall.

CRYOGLOBULINEMIA

Cryoglobulins are usually immune complexes (rarely they include other serum constituents) that precipitate at low temperatures.

1. Type I cryoglobulinemia is associated with monoclonal Igs such as those occurring in Waldenström disease, lymphoma, or multiple myeloma. These are mostly of the IgM subtype.
2. Type II cryoglobulinemia is composed of a mix of polyclonal IgGs and monoclonal IgM-RF bound to autologous IgG.
3. Type III cryoglobulinemia is the most common type and contains polyclonal IgGs and polyclonal IgM-RF bound to polygonal IgG.

Many patients with type II or III cryoglobulins have hepatitis C infection. Thus, evaluation for hepatitis C with appropriate antibody tests is usually warranted. Hepatitis C infection may cause small-vessel vasculitis, often affecting the lower extremities. Hepatitis B, endocarditis, and many other infections may be associated with cryoglobulins. The typical presentation includes a palpable purpura on the lower extremities in nearly all patients. Ischemic toes may also develop. Patients with type II and type III cryoglobulinemia will have a false-positive RF.

Diagnosis requires the identification of a cryoprecipitate in the serum. Blood should be kept at body temperature (37°C) until the serum is separated. The serum is then kept at 4°C for 48 hours and examined for a precipitate. The precipitate is expressed as a percentage of the serum volume, and may be further characterized by electrophoresis and immunofix-ation. Complement activation may frequently be present on lab evaluation. In addition, evidence of glomerulonephritis and nephrosis may be present (e.g., active urine sediment, proteinuria, and abnormal renal function tests).

DERMATOMYOSITIS/POLYMYOSITIS

Dermatomyositis and polymyositis are characterized by inflammation of the muscles, which causes both pain and weakness. Dermatomyositis is also characterized by inflammation of the skin. Increased muscle enzymes are a hallmark, and muscle markers like creatine kinase, aldolase, myoglobin, and lactate dehydrogenase are elevated. Sometimes, aspartate transaminase and alanine transaminase are also increased as a result. Dermatomyositis is associated with autoantibodies, especially anti-Mi-2 antibodies, and to a lesser extent anti-Jo-1 antibodies, which are more commonly seen in polymyositis. Myositis-associated and myositis-specific antibodies including anti-Jo-1 and other anti-synthetase antibodies may be elevated.

SCLERODERMA

Scleroderma, also known as systemic sclerosis (SSc), is a chronic systemic autoimmune disease characterized by hardening (sclero) of the skin (derma) with widespread vascular dysfunction and progressive fibrosis of not only the skin but also internal organs. Limited cutaneous SSc may have features of CREST syndrome and only distal extremity involvement. Anti-DNA topoisomerase I (Scl-70) antibodies are generally associated with diffuse cutaneous SSc (dcSSc). Anticentromere antibody is usually associated with limited cutaneous SSc. Antibodies to RNA polymerase III are found in patients with dcSSc and are at increased risk for scleroderma renal crisis. All patients with newly diagnosed scleroderma should be appropriately cancer screened.

AUTOINFLAMMATORY DISEASES

Autoinflammatory diseases are a group of genetically diverse but clinically similar disorders characterized by recurrent fever associated with rash, serositis, lymphadenopathy, and musculoskeletal involvement. These fevers occur in the absence of any infections or malignancy. These include familial Mediterranean fever (FMF), tumor necrosis factor receptor-1 associated periodic syndrome, etc. Some people consider Still disease an autoinflammatory disease even though it has some features of that of RA. It is characterized by quotidian (daily) fevers, arthritis, and an evanescent rash.

Inflammatory markers, such as CRP and ESR, are elevated during disease flares and may sometimes be abnormal between episodes in these diseases. Genetic tests for various autoinflammatory diseases like FMF are available. Commonly, ferritin and IL-18 are substantially elevated in these diseases.

HYPERCOAGULABLE STATES

A number of hypercoagulable states may present in much the same way as the vasculitides. These include disorders of coagulation related to deficiency of factor C, factor S, and antithrombin III. Factor 5 Leiden mutation may also lead to a hypercoagulable state, especially in the homozygous form. Specific coagulation assays should be performed when these conditions are suspected, particularly if there is a family history of coagulopathy.

GENOME-WIDE ASSOCIATION STUDY

A genome-wide association study (GWAS) is an examination of many common genetic variants in different individuals to see if any variant is associated with a trait. GWAS typically focuses on associations between single-nucleotide polymorphisms and traits like major diseases by comparing patients with disease to that of normals, thus providing insights into associated molecular mechanisms. RA, SLE, ankylosing spondylitis, and some other autoimmune rheumatic diseases are complex genetic disease, where there is evidence of familial clustering, but not of Mendelian inheritance. Disease-associated loci identified to date reveals greater sharing of risk loci among the groups of seropositive (diseases in which specific autoantibodies are often present) or seronegative diseases than between these two groups. The nature of the shared and discordant loci suggests important differences and similarities among these diseases, and helps identify new therapeutic targets. This would help diagnose diseases in the at-risk population and also to develop targeted therapies in the future.[3]

NODULES

In addition to gout and RA, hyperlipidemia may cause skin nodules. Type II hyperlipoproteinemia may present with Achilles tendinitis and tenosynovitis. Asymmetric oligoarticular synovitis has been described in type IV hyperlipoproteinemia. Cholesterol and triglyceride profiles are useful in the evaluation of these disorders.

From this discussion, it is clear that laboratory testing is an invaluable part of the diagnostic process. However, it is best used only in a directed fashion and only as part of a complete evaluation that includes a history and physical examination.

REFERENCES

1. Maksymowych WP, Boire G, van Schaardenburg D, et al. 14-3-3η autoantibodies: diagnostic use in early rheumatoid arthritis. *J Rheumatol*. 2015;42(9):1587–1594.
2. Navarro-Compán V, de Miguel E, van der Heijde D, et al. Sponyloarthritis features forecasting the presence of HLA-B27 or sacroiliitis on magnetic resonance imaging in patients with suspected axial spondyloarthritis: results from a cross-sectional study in the ESPeranza Cohort. *Arthritis Res Ther*. 2015;17:265.

3. Kirino Y, Remmers EF. Genetic architectures of seropositive and seronegative rheumatic diseases. *Nat Rev Rheumatol.* 2015;11(7):401–414.

SELECTED BIBLIOGRAPHY

ARA Glossary Committee. *Dictionary of the Rheumatic Diseases: Vol II: Diagnostic Testing.* New York, NY: Contact Associates; 1985.

Kelley WN, Harris ED, Ruddy S, et al, eds. *Text Book of Rheumatology.* Philadelphia, PA: W. B. Saunders; 1997.

Khan MA, Kellner H. Immunogenetics of spondyloarthropathies. *Rheum Dis Clin North Am.* 1992;18:837.

McCarty GA. Autoantibodies and their relation to rheumatic diseases. *Med Clin North Am.* 1986;70:237–261.

Nolle B, Specks U, Ludermann J, et al. Anticytoplasmic autoantibodies: their immunodiagnostic value in Wegener granulomatosis. *Ann Intern Med.* 1989;111:28–40.

Paget S, Pellicci P, Beary JF, eds. *Manual of Rheumatology and Outpatient Orthopedic Disorders.* Boston: Little, Brown; 1993.

Sammaritano LR, Gharavi AE, Lockshin MD. Antiphospholipid antibody syndrome: immunologic and clinical aspects. *Semin Arthritis Rheum.* 1990;20:81.

Schumacher HR, ed. *Primer on the Rheumatic Diseases.* Atlanta: Arthritis Foundation; 1993.

Schumacher HR, Reginato AJ. *Atlas of Synovial Fluid Analysis and Crystal Identification.* Philadelphia: Lea & Febiger; 1991.

Sox HC Jr, Liang MH. The erythrocyte sedimentation rate: guidelines for rational use. *Ann Intern Med.* 1986;104:515–523.

CHAPTER 17

Metabolic Bone Disease Manifestations in the Foot

PANAGIOTA ANDREOPOULOU

This chapter focuses on skeletal dysplasias and metabolic bone diseases with manifestations in the feet. Although a strong association between osteoporosis and fractures has not yet been established, the contribution of this condition (which is quite common in postmenopausal women) to recurrent fractures and their healing process should not be overlooked. In addition, other rare or possibly under recognized metabolic bone diseases such as hypophosphatasia (HPP) and Paget disease may include foot lesions. Often the astute clinician may recognize the presence of a skeletal dysplasia in a patient with an already known or even not know diagnosis and then appropriately refer this patient for further evaluation and management.

SKELETAL DYSPLASIAS

Several syndromes associated with skeletal dysplasias may manifest with abnormalities of the feet. Often these are hereditary, and identification of a proband patient may have significant implications for the whole family. A careful clinical inspection and examination as well as evaluation of radiographic abnormalities may lead to the identification of a broader syndrome that may require a multidisciplinary management approach.

Genetic disorders of the skeleton are a clinically and genetically heterogeneous group of disorders of bone and/or cartilage characterized by abnormalities in growth, development, and/or homeostasis of the human skeleton.[1] They include the osteochondrodysplasias (primarily affecting bone and/or cartilage), the dysostoses (affecting a single bone or group of bones), the brachydactylies (primarily involving the hands and feet), and the lysosomal storage diseases. Although relatively rare individually, the skeletal dysplasias have an estimated birth prevalence of nearly 1/5,000.[2] It is now apparent that there are over 450 distinct genetic disorders of the skeleton that must be distinguished for specific genetic counseling, prognosis, and treatment. Of these conditions, 316 are associated with one or more of 226 different genes.

Osteopoikilosis

Osteopoikilosis ("spotted bones") is an autosomal dominant condition with an interesting radiographic appearance that may commonly affect the tarsal bones. If associated with connective tissue nevi and dermatofibrosis lenticularis disseminata, the disorder is the Buschke–Ollendorff syndrome.[3] Deactivating mutations in the *LEMD3* gene were identified.[4]

Osteopoikilosis (OMIM #166700) is usually an incidental finding. The bone lesions are asymptomatic, but if not understood can initiate a costly investigation for metastatic disease.[5] Family members at risk should be screened with a radiograph of a wrist and knee in early adult life. Joint contractions and limb length inequality may occur, especially in individuals with accompanying changes of melorheostosis (discussed below). The nevi usually involve the lower trunk or extremities and are small asymptomatic papules or yellow or white discs or plaques, deep nodules, or streaks.[3]

There are numerous, small, usually round or oval, foci of osteosclerosis. Commonly affected sites are the ends of the short tubular bones, metaepiphyses of long bones, and tarsal, carpal, and pelvic bones. Lesions remain stable for decades. Bone scan is normal.[5]

Dermatofibrosis lenticularis disseminata consists of unusually broad, markedly branched, interlacing elastin fibers in the dermis; however, the epidermis is normal.[3] Foci of osteosclerosis are thickened trabeculae that merge with surrounding normal bone or are islands of cortical bone that include haversian systems. Mature lesions appear to be remodeling slowly.

Osteopathia Striata

Osteopathia striata (OMIM #166500, autosomal dominant) features linear striations at the end of long bones and the ileum. Like osteopoikilosis, it is usually a radiographic diagnosis. Gracile linear striations are found in cancellous bone, particularly within metaepiphyses of major long bones and the periphery of the iliac bones. Carpal, tarsal, and tubular bones of the hands and feet are less often and more subtly affected. The striations appear stable for years. Bone scan is also normal.[5]

Melorheostosis

Melorheostosis (OMIM #155950), from the Greek words for limb, flow, and bone, refers to "flowing hyperostosis." The radiographic appearance resembles wax that has dripped down a candle. About 200 cases have been published[6] since the first description in 1922.[7] Melorheostosis occurs sporadically and may accompany osteopoikilosis.

Melorheostosis typically presents during childhood, usually with monomelic involvement; bilateral disease is characteristically asymmetrical. Cutaneous changes may overlie the skeletal lesions and include linear scleroderma-like patches and hypertrichosis. Fibromas, fibrolipomas, capillary hemangiomas, lymphangiectasia, and arterial aneurysms can also occur.[8] Soft tissue abnormalities are often noted before the hyperostosis. Pain and stiffness are the major symptoms. Affected joints may develop contractures, and leg length discrepancy can follow premature fusion of epiphyses. Bone lesions seem to advance most rapidly during childhood. In adult life, melorheostosis may not always progress.[9] Nevertheless, pain is more frequent when there is continuing subperiosteal bone formation.

Dense, irregular, and eccentric hyperostosis of both periosteal and endosteal surfaces of a single bone, or several adjacent bones, is the hallmark of melorheostosis.[6] Any bone may be affected, but the lower extremities are most commonly involved. Bone can also develop in soft tissues near skeletal lesions, particularly near joints. Melorheostotic bone is hyperemic and "hot" during bone scanning. Serum calcium, inorganic phosphate (Pi), and alkaline phosphatase levels are normal.

Melorheostosis features endosteal thickening during growth and periosteal new bone formation during adult life.[6] Affected bones are sclerotic with thickened, irregular lamellae. Marrow fibrosis may be present.[6] In the skin, unlike in true scleroderma, the collagen of the scleroderma-like lesions appears normal and has therefore been called linear melorheostotic scleroderma.[10]

Pachydermoperiostosis

Pachydermoperiostosis (hypertrophic osteoarthropathy: primary or idiopathic; OMIM #167100) causes clubbing of the digits, hyperhidrosis and thickening of the skin especially on the face and forehead (cutis verticis gyrata), and periosteal new bone formation, particularly in the distal extremities. Autosomal dominant and recessive inheritance with variable expression is established.[11] In 2008, autosomal recessive pachydermoperiostosis was elucidated by a loss-of-function mutation within the gene that encodes 15-hydroxyprostaglandin dehydrogenase.[12]

Men seem to be more severely affected than women and blacks more commonly than whites. Age at presentation is variable, but usually it is during adolescence. All principal features (clubbing, periostitis, and pachydermia) trouble some patients; others have just one or two. Clinical manifestations emerge over a decade and can then abate.[12] Progressive enlargement of the hands and feet may cause a paw-like appearance, and there may be excessive perspiration. Acro-osteolysis can occur. Fatigue and arthralgias of the elbows, wrists, knees, and ankles are common. Stiffness and limited mobility of both the appendicular and the axial skeleton may develop. Compression of cranial or spinal nerves has been described.

Cutaneous changes include coarsening, thickening, furrowing, pitting, and oiliness of the skin, especially the scalp and face. Myelophthisic anemia with extramedullary hematopoiesis may occur. Life expectancy is not compromised.

Severe periostitis thickens tubular bones distally: typically the radius, ulna, tibia, and fibula, and sometimes the metacarpals, tarsals/metatarsals, clavicles, pelvis, skull base, and phalanges. Clubbing is obvious, and acro-osteolysis can occur. The spine is rarely involved. Ankylosis of joints, especially in the hands and feet, may trouble older patients. The major challenge in differential diagnosis is secondary hypertrophic osteoarthropathy (pulmonary or otherwise). Here, however, the radiographic features are somewhat different, featuring periosteal reaction that is typically smooth and undulating.[13] In pachydermoperiostosis, periosteal proliferation is exuberant, irregular, and often involves epiphyses. Bone scanning in either condition reveals symmetrical, diffuse, regular uptake along the cortical margins of long bones, especially in the legs, causing a "double stripe" sign.

Nascent periosteal bone roughens cortical bone surfaces and undergoes cancellous compaction so that centrally it can be difficult to distinguish histopathologically from the original cortex. There may also be osteopenia of trabecular bone from quiescent formation. Mild cellular hyperplasia and thickening of blood vessels is found near synovial membranes, but synovial fluid is unremarkable.[14]

FIBROUS DYSPLASIA

Fibrous dysplasia of bone (FD) (OMIM #174800) is an uncommon skeletal disorder with a broad spectrum of clinical presentation. On one end of the spectrum, patients may present in later life with an incidentally discovered, asymptomatic radiographic finding that is of no clinical consequence. On the other end of the spectrum, patients may present early in life with a disabling disease. The disease may involve one bone (monostotic FD), multiple bones (polyostotic FD), or the entire skeleton (panostotic FD).[15–17] FD may be associated with extraskeletal manifestations, the most common of which is areas of cutaneous hyperpigmentation commonly referred to as café au lait macules. These lesions vary widely in size but have characteristic features that include jagged, "coast of Maine" borders, some relationship with the midline, and sometimes follow the developmental lines of Blaschko. FD can also be associated with hyperfunctioning endocrinopathies, including precocious puberty, hyperthyroidism, growth hormone (GH) excess, and Cushing syndrome. FD in combination with one or more of the extraskeletal manifestations is known as McCune–Albright syndrome (MAS).[18–21] A renal tubulopathy, which includes renal phosphate wasting, is one of the most common extraskeletal dysfunctions associated with polyostotic disease.[22] More rarely, FD may be associated with myxomas of skeletal muscle (Mazabraud syndrome)[23] or dysfunction of the heart, liver, pancreas, or other organs within the context of the MAS.[24]

FD is caused by missense mutations of the GNAS complex locus on chromosome 20q13.3.[25–27] GNAS encodes the alpha subunit of the stimulatory G protein ($G_s\alpha$) involved in the cyclic adenosine monophosphate (cAMP)-dependent signaling pathway. The mutation impairs the intrinsic GTPase activity of $G_s\alpha$, leading to persistent stimulation of adenylyl cyclase and aberrant production of cAMP (gain-of-function mutations).[28] Mutations of GNAS associated with FD and related disorders are never inherited and could theoretically occur at any time during postzygotic development. However, there is involvement of a pluripotent cell as the initial target of the disease, thus explaining how the mutation can be transmitted to derivatives of all three germ layers and be broadly distributed in patients with severe forms of the disease. At the same time, differences in the size and viability of the clone arising from the original mutated pluripotent cell could account for the variability of the clinical phenotype observed in the majority of FD patients.[29]

The pathology of FD is characterized by the development of fibro-osseous lesions that replace normal skeletal structures and impair normal skeletal functions.

The sites of skeletal involvement (the "map" of affected tissues) are established early in patients with FD. Ninety percent of the craniofacial lesions are established before the age of 5, and 75% of all sites of FD are evident by the age of 15; the implication is that essentially all clinically significant disease is present very early in life, probably by the age of 5.[17] Pathologic effects of $G_s\alpha$ mutations in osteogenic cells are most pronounced and evident during the phase of rapid bone growth, and account for the fact that childhood and adolescence are the periods during which the disease most commonly presents, is the most symptomatic, and is the period of peak rate of fractures.[30,31] The most common presenting features are a limp, pain, or a fracture. Any bone can be affected including the feet, although most commonly the ribs, long bones, and craniofacial bones are affected, whereas lesions in the spine and pelvis are typically less painful.[32] Pathologic fractures of weight-bearing limb bones are a major cause of morbidity. Deformity of limb bones, which is a common finding, is caused by expansion and abnormal compliance of lesional FD, fracture treatment failure, and occasionally local complications such as cyst formation.[29] Malignancy in FD is rare (less than 1%).[33] Rapid lesion expansion and disruption of the cortex on radiographs should alert the clinician to the possibility of sarcomatous change. Osteogenic sarcoma is the most common, but is not the only type of bone tumor that may complicate FD.

Diagnosis of FD must be established based on expert assessment of clinical, radiographic, and histopathologic features. Markers of bone turnover are usually elevated.[22] The extent of the skeletal disease is best determined with total body bone scintigraphy, which can be used to assess the skeletal disease burden and predict functional outcome.[34] Patients should be referred to an endocrinologist for screening and treatment of the metabolic derangements associated with FD, especially hypophosphatemia and GH excess.

Mutation analysis may be helpful in distinguishing FD from unrelated fibro-osseous lesions of the skeleton, which may mimic FD both clinically and radiographically (osteofibrous dysplasia, ossifying fibromas).[29] Multiple nonossifying fibromas, skeletal angiomatosis, and Ollier disease may sometimes enter the differential diagnosis. Distinction from these entities relies on histology and mutation analysis.

Acromelic and Acromicric Dysplasias

Acromelic dysplasia and acromicric dysplasia (AD) are because of inherited mutations in the gene for fibrillin-1 (FBN1). Fibrillin is a fibril-forming extracellular matrix protein with important roles in the development, growth, and maintenance of skeletal elements.[35]

The most well-known of these syndromes is Marfan syndrome, which is associated with handoff values with forefoot abduction and lowering of the midget (pes planus). Individuals with Marfan syndrome (OMIM #154700, autosomal dominant inheritance, 1 in 5,000) display major disease features in the skeleton: tall stature and arachnodactyly, scoliosis and chest deformities, joint hypermobility and muscle wasting, pes planus, and craniofacial abnormalities, including a highly arched palate. Multiple features in other organs (cardiovascular, ocular, skin, lung, and central nervous system) are also present. Prevalence of skeletal features changes with aging. In children, pes planus prevalence decreased from 73% to 65% between ages 0 and 6 years.[36]

The acromelic dysplasia group includes three rare disorders: Weill–Marchesani syndrome (WMS), geleophysic dysplasia (GD), and AD, all characterized by short stature, short and stubby hands and feet that are shorter than expected for their height, stiff joints, delayed bone age, cone-shaped epiphyses, thick skin, and heart disease. WMS is transmitted either by an autosomal dominant or an autosomal recessive, GD by an autosomal recessive, and AD by an autosomal dominant mode of inheritance.[37]

The skeletal features of WMS are the opposite of those found in Marfan syndrome. Patients (OMIM #608328) display short stature, brachydactyly (short and stubby hands and feet), hypermuscularity, and joint stiffness. However, ectopia lentis is typical of both syndromes.[38,39]

Syndromes of PTH Resistance: Pseudohypoparathyroidism

Brachydactyly of feet and ectopic subcutaneous ossifications are well-described features of pseudohypoparathyroidism (PHP).

In patients with PHP, failure of target tissues to respond appropriately to the biologic actions of parathyroid hormone (PTH), which is elevated, leads to functional hypoparathyroidism.

The signs and symptoms are principally manifestations of a reduced concentration of ionized extracellular calcium. Hypocalcemia causes tetany, which is increased neuromuscular irritability manifested as paresthesias in the distal extremities and face, muscle cramps, and, if severe, laryngospasm, seizures, or reversible heart failure. Other clinical features of chronic hypocalcemia include increased intracranial pressure, dry and rough skin, spondyloarthropathy, cataracts, and calcification of the basal ganglia that may rarely cause extrapyramidal neurologic dysfunction. Hypocalcemia can cause QT prolongation on an EKG. Patients can adapt to chronic hypocalcemia, and occasionally asymptomatic patients will be diagnosed only after a low serum calcium is detected after routine blood screening.[40]

Pseudohypoparathyroidism Type 1

The blunted nephrogenous cAMP response to PTH in subjects with PHP type 1 is caused by a deficiency of $G_s\alpha$, the signaling protein that couples PTH1R to stimulation of adenylyl cyclase. There are two forms of PHP type 1: generalized deficiency of $G_s\alpha$, because of mutations of the GNAS gene, are classified as PHP type 1a (PHP 1a; OMIM #103580), whereas more restricted deficiency of $G_s\alpha$, because of mutations that affect imprinting of GNAS, are classified as PHP type 1b (PHP 1b; OMIM #603233). PHP type 1c is likely a variant of PHP 1a.

Pseudohypoparathyroidism 1a

PHP 1a is the most common variant and readily recognized due to a constellation of clinical features termed Albright hereditary osteodystrophy (AHO) that includes short stature, round facies, brachydactyly of hands and/or feet, and/or mental retardation, ectopic subcutaneous ossifications, and obesity.[41,42]

PHP 1a results from heterozygous mutations on the maternal allele of the imprinted GNAS gene that reduce expression or function of the $G_s\alpha$ protein. These patients also have resistance to other hormones (e.g., thyroid-stimulating hormone [TSH], gonadotropins, calcitonin, and GH-releasing hormone). Primary hypothyroidism without goiter and GH deficiency are common.[43–46]

Patients with paternally inherited GNAS mutations have phenotypic features of AHO without hormonal resistance, a condition termed pseudopseudohypoparathyroidism (PPHP).[47]

Pseudohypoparathyroidism 1b

Patients with PHP 1b lack typical features of AHO but may still have mild brachydactyly. PTH resistance is the principal manifestation but some patients have mild TSH resistance.[48,49]

HYPOPARATHYROIDISM-RETARDATION-DYSMORPHISM SYNDROME

The hypoparathyroidism-retardation-dysmorphism syndrome (HRD, MIM #241410), also known as the Sanjad–Sakati syndrome, is a rare form of autosomal recessive hypoparathyroidism due to mutations in the TBCE gene encoding a protein required for the folding of tubulin. In addition to parathyroid dysgenesis, affected patients have severe growth and mental retardation, microcephaly, microphthalmia, small hands and feet, and abnormal teeth. This disorder is found almost exclusively in individuals of Arab descent.

PHP or PPHP may be suspected in patients who present with somatic features of AHO. However, several aspects of AHO, such as obesity, round face, brachydactyly, and mental retardation, also occur in other congenital disorders (e.g., Prader–Willi syndrome, acrodysostosis, Ullrich–Turner syndrome).

HYPERPHOSPHATEMIA/TUMORAL CALCINOSIS

Soft tissue calcifications may also be a consequences of chronic hyperphosphatemia. In the setting of chronic kidney disease (CKD), hyperphosphatemia promotes mineral deposition in soft tissues because it stimulates vascular cells to undergo osteogenic differentiation. Medial calcification of peripheral arteries associated with hyperphosphatemia may lead to calciphylaxis, a disorder with high mortality and morbidity.

Hyperphosphatemic Familial Tumoral Calcinosis

Hyperphosphatemic familial tumoral calcinosis (MIM #211900) is a rare autosomal recessive metabolic disorder notable for progressive deposition of calcium phosphate crystals in periarticular spaces and soft tissues. The biochemical hallmark of this condition is hyperphosphatemia due to increased renal tubular reabsorption of phosphate; however, there are normophosphatemic forms (MIM #610455). Mutations are found in GALNT3, FGF23, and KLOTHO. The mutations lead to loss of function, resulting in inadequate FGF23 protein levels or FGF23 action.[50–52] The majority of patients have those manifestations present by age 20.

Patients with familial tumoral calcinosis have heterotopic calcifications that are typically painless and slow growing, but may reach the size of an orange; however, the masses can become painful if they infiltrate into adjacent structures. Large calcified tophus-like nodules may be noted around the joints of the toes and the malleolus. However, the most frequently affected joints are hips, elbows, shoulders, and scapulae.[53]

The clinical complications are related to the infiltration of skin, marrow, teeth, blood vessels, and nerves. Range of motion is generally not affected unless the masses become large. A variably present feature of the disease is an abnormality in dentition. Biochemically, there is also increased 1,25(OH)2D3 with normal calcium and alkaline phosphatase levels. Urinary phosphate excretion is frequently low. Radiographs show large aggregates of irregularly dense calcified lobules located in regions known to be occupied by bursae.

More frequently, heterotypic calcification is associated with CKD–mineral bone disorder (MBD). The pandemic of CKD and end-stage renal disease and the role of the CKD–MBD in the associated mortality make the syndrome a major public health issue. The skeletal remodeling disorders caused by CKD contribute directly to the heterotopic mineralization, especially vascular calcification, and the disordered mineral metabolism that accompany CKD.[54,55]

Most soft tissue calcifications are attributed to the increased calcium phosphate product due to renal osteodystrophy and excess bone resorption. The syndrome of calciphylaxis is characterized by vascular calcifications in the tunica media of peripheral arteries that induce painful violaceous skin lesions, which progress to ischemic necrosis. This syndrome is associated with serious complications and high mortality.

Tumoral calcinosis is a form of soft tissue calcification that involves the periarticular tissues. Calcium deposits may grow to enormous size and interfere with the function of adjacent joints and organs.

Other common skeletal symptoms these patients report is slowly progressive bone pain that may be diffuse or localized with tenderness to local pressure and is aggravated by weight-bearing. Occasionally, it may mimic arthritis.

FIBRODYSPLASIA OSSIFICANS PROGRESSIVA

Fibrodysplasia ossificans progressiva (FOP: MIM #135100) is a rare heritable disorder of connective tissue characterized by congenital malformations of the great toes and progressive heterotopic endochondral ossification (HEO) in characteristic anatomic patterns.[56,57]

FOP, first described in 1692, has more than 800 cases reported and is among the rarest of human afflictions, with an estimated incidence of 1 per 2,000,000 individuals. All races are affected. Autosomal dominant transmission with variable expression and complete penetrance is established[58]; however, reproductive fitness is low and most cases are sporadic. Gonadal mosaicism has also been described.[59]

Malformations of the great toes are present at birth in all classically affected individuals. Typically, episodes of soft tissue swelling (flare-ups) leading to HEO begin during the first decade of life.[60,61] These patients become immobilized by the third decade of their life.

PAGET DISEASE OF THE BONE

The second most common bone disease after osteoporosis is Paget disease of the bone where the feet are only rarely affected; however, ankle arthritis may develop adjacent to paretic bone. This is a localized disorder of bone remodeling due to increased osteoclast-mediated bone resorption and subsequent compensatory increased born formation, resulting in a disorganized mosaic of woven and lamellar bone at affected skeletal sites. The affected bone is expanded in size, vascular and susceptible to deformity and fractures.[62] Although most patients are asymptomatic, some experience bone pain, arthritis, deformities, and fractures.

The pathophysiology is not fully elucidated but appears to be because of a combination of genetic and environmental factors. Paget disease occurs commonly in families and can be transmitted vertically in an autosomal dominant pattern. Fifteen percent to 30% of Paget disease patients have positive family histories of the disorder,[63–65] and the risk of a first-degree relative developing the condition is seven times greater than for someone without an affected relative.[66] Multiple genetic loci have been linked to familial Paget disease, and three genes have been identified. Mutations in SQSTM1 occur in 30% of patients with familial disease.[67]

There is a restricted geographic distribution for the occurrence of Paget disease: It is most common in Europe, North America, Australia, and New Zealand in persons of Anglo-Saxon descent and is extremely uncommon in Asia, Africa, and Scandinavia. Both genders are affected, with a slight male predominance, and presents after age 40 and most commonly after age 50.

Patients have elevated serum total alkaline phosphatase as well as other bone turnover markers (serum C-terminal telopeptide of collagen [CTX], urine N-terminal telopeptide of collagen [NTX], serum procollagen type 1 N-terminal propeptide [P1NP], serum bone-specific alkaline phosphatase).[68]

Paget disease may be monostotic or polyostotic and often asymmetric. The hands and feet are rarely affected. The most common sites of involvement include the pelvis, femur, spine, skull, and tibia and less commonly the humerus, clavicle, scapula, ribs, and facial bones. Most patients are asymptomatic, and the diagnosis often follows an incidentally noted elevated serum alkaline phosphatase (SAP) or when a radiograph taken for an unrelated problem reveals typical skeletal changes. Symptoms include bone pain from a site of pagetic involvement, either at rest or with motion, an unpleasant sensation of warmth, a bowing deformity of the femur or tibia with gait abnormalities that can lead to abnormal mechanical stresses, and severe secondary arthritis at joints adjacent to pagetic bone (e.g., the hip, knee, or ankle). Patients may also complain of back pain from enlarged pagetic vertebrae, vertebral compression fractures or spinal stenosis, and kyphosis. Skull-related manifestations include increase in head size with or without frontal bossing or deformity, headache, hearing loss, facial deformity, and dental problems. Fractures and malignant transformation may occur; however, they are not a feature of the foot lesions.

Bone scans are the most sensitive means of identifying possible pagetic sites, but are nonspecific, and also can be positive in nonpagetic areas that have degenerative changes or, more ominously, metastatic disease. Plain radiographs of bones noted to be positive on the bone scan provide the most specific information, because radiographic findings are usually characteristic to the point of being pathognomonic. Enlargement or expansion of bone, cortical thickening, coarsening of trabecular markings, and typical lytic and sclerotic changes may be found. Radiographs also show the condition of the joints adjacent to involved sites, identify fissure fractures, indicate the degree to which lytic or sclerotic lesions predominate, and demonstrate the presence or absence of deformity or fracture.

HYPOPHOSPHATASIA

HPP is the rare heritable rickets or osteomalacia (OMIM #146300, #241500, #241510)[69] characterized biochemically by subnormal activity of the tissue-nonspecific isoenzyme of alkaline phosphatase (TNSALP).[70,71] Although TNSALP is normally present in all tissues, HPP disturbs predominantly the skeleton and teeth. Muscle weakness is often an important finding. Approximately 350 cases have been reported, showing a remarkable range of severity with four overlapping clinical forms described according to patient age when skeletal disease is discovered: perinatal, infantile, childhood, and adult. Odonto-HPP features dental manifestations only. Generally, the earlier the skeletal problems, the more severe the clinical course. Perinatal and infantile HPP are very severe forms with high mortality if they remain untreated.

Interestingly, the adult form of HPP may present with recurrent foot fractures. Adult HPP usually presents during middle age, often with poorly healing, recurrent, metatarsal stress fractures.[72] Fractures can mend spontaneously, but healing may be delayed, including after osteotomy. Patients may recall rickets and/or premature loss of deciduous teeth during childhood. Chondrocalcinosis, pseudogout, and pyrophosphate arthropathy from calcium pyrophosphate dihydrate crystal deposition may occur.[70] Radiographs can show osteopenia, metatarsal stress fractures, chondrocalcinosis, and subtrochanteric femoral pseudofractures.

HPP rickets/osteomalacia is remarkable because serum levels of calcium and Pi are not reduced, and ALP activity is low, not high.[71] In childhood and adult HPP, approximately 50% of patients are hyperphosphatemic because of enhanced renal reclamation of Pi (increased TmP/GFR [the ratio of the maximum rate of tubular phosphate reabsorption to the glomerular filtration rate]).[70,71]

Three phosphocompounds accumulate endogenously in HPP: phosphoethanolamine, inorganic pyrophosphate (PPi), and pyridoxal 5′-phosphate (PLP). PPi assay is a research technique. If vitamin B_6 is not supplemented, elevated plasma PLP is an especially good marker for HPP. The worse the hypophosphatasemia (low serum ALP activity), the greater the plasma PLP, and the more severe the clinical manifestations.[70,71]

Mutation analysis of TNSALP is available commercially. Approximately 280 mutations (approximately 80% missense) have been identified.[73]

FOOT FRACTURES IN WOMEN WITH OSTEOPOROSIS

Osteoporosis is a skeletal disease characterized by low bone mass and microarchitectural deterioration of bone tissue with a consequent increase in bone fragility and susceptibility to fracture.[74] Clinically, osteoporosis has been difficult to define: A focus on bone mineral density (BMD) may not encompass all the risk factors for fracture, whereas a fracture-based definition will not enable identification of at-risk populations. In 1994, the World Health Organization (WHO)[75] convened to resolve this issue, defining osteoporosis in terms of BMD and previous fracture. Thus, the WHO definition does not take into account microarchitectural changes that may weaken bone independently of any effect on BMD. More recently, there has been a move toward assessment of individualized risk,[76] with the development of the FRAX algorithm,[77] a Web-based tool that uses clinical risk factors and/or BMD to calculate an individual's absolute risk of major osteoporotic or hip fracture over the next 10 years. This has the advantage of incorporating risk factors that are partly independent of BMD, such as age and previous fracture, and thus allows decisions regarding commencement of therapy to be made more readily. Osteoporosis-related fractures have a huge impact economically, in addition to their effect on health: The cost to the U.S. economy is around $17.9 billion per annum, with the burden in the U.K. being £1.7 billion[78] mostly because of hip fractures that contribute most to these figures. Thus, early diagnosis based on reasonable suspicion leading to diagnostic testing is paramount.

The 2004 report from the U.S. Surgeon General highlighted the enormous burden of osteoporosis-related fractures.[79] An estimated 10 million Americans over 50 years old have osteoporosis, and there are about 1.5 million fragility fractures each year. Another 34 million Americans are at risk of the disease. A study of British fracture occurrence indicates that population risk is similar in the UK.[80] Thus, one in two women aged 50 years will have an osteoporosis-related fracture in their remaining lifetime; the figure for men is one in five.

Osteoporosis is a common disease especially among postmenopausal women and aging men. After the occurrence of the first fracture, osteoporosis is no longer a "silent" disease, and the patient's risk for future fracture is increased severalfold.

However, there are conflicting data concerning whether foot fractures such as metatarsal fractures are associated with low BMD and thus might be sentinel fracture events.

The Multiple Outcomes of Raloxifene Evaluation (MORE) trial was a fracture outcomes study of postmenopausal women with osteoporosis. The location of first fractures among women with osteoporosis and no previous fractures at baseline was assessed after 3 years of follow-up in the placebo group. Patients were at least 2 years postmenopausal and up to 80 years of age (95% Caucasian), without severe or long-term disabling conditions, and had osteoporosis defined as femoral neck or lumbar spine BMD T-score below −2.5 based on the densitometer manufacturer's databases. The assessment included fractures of the ankle, calcaneus, tarsus, and metatarsus. Apart from the common and expected sites of fragility fractures such as vertebral and radius fractures, a small number of women experienced foot fractures as initial fractures, including ankle (0.6%) and metatarsal (0.6%) fractures. Fractures of the ankle and metatarsal each accounted for 4% to 6% of all fractures. No fractures of the calcaneus or tarsus were reported.[81]

Some studies have shown that patients with metatarsal fracture are at increased risk of osteoporosis at the spine,[82,83] whereas others have concluded that foot fractures are largely independent of spine BMD.[84]

Retrospectively analyzed data on 68 postmenopausal women concluded that low trauma metatarsal fracture is not a risk factor for low calcaneal (peripheral) BMD.[85] This was in agreement with a large longitudinal study,[84] which did not show that foot fractures had a statistically significant association with lumbar spine or calcaneal BMD, and had only a weak association with distal radius BMD.

A smaller cross-sectional study[82] showed that the prevalence of spinal osteoporosis in patients suffering from metatarsal fractures was similar to that in patients who had suffered wrist fractures and greater than that of their control group. These differences may be explained by differences in patient population (e.g., age, BMI), site of bone density assessment (axial as opposed to peripheral measurement), or study design (longitudinal vs. cross-sectional).

Tomczak et al. examined 21 patients (15 women and 6 men) who presented with unexplained metatarsal fractures. Twenty of the 21 had bone densities significantly below the mean for corresponding age, gender, and race. The average bone density for the 21 patients was 2.1 standard deviations (T −2.1) below the expected mean for the corresponding 30-year-old reference population and 1.7 standard deviations (z −1.7) below the mean for an age-, gender-, weight-, and ethnicity-matched population. The authors conclude that there is a previously unreported correlation between metatarsal insufficiency fractures and low bone mass in both genders, confirmed by the abnormal BMD testing.

FOOT STRESS FRACTURES

Overuse injuries in athletes have a prevalence of 76%.[86] The lower limb accounts for 80% to 95% of stress fractures.[87] There is increasing participation in endurance sports and marathon running, and the incidence of stress fractures in runners is 21% and higher in army recruits at 31%.[88–91]

Therefore, identifying stress fractures that are prone to delayed union or nonunion, such as when they are associated with reduced BMD, is essential.[83,92]

Postmenopausal women are particularly at risk of stress fractures. Also a worldwide estimate suggests that 1 billion people are vitamin D deficient, which may be a risk factor for stress fracture occurrence.[93] Therefore, it is essential to appropriately differentiate stress fractures that result from reduced BMD or vitamin D deficiency and those that are prone to nonunion due to the anatomical site.[94]

This will guide avoid over- or undertreating this condition.

With an aging population and an increase in exercising participants who are aged >50 years,[88,89] there will be an increased prevalence of osteoporotic stress fractures in the foot.[83]

The assessment of BMD in females is essential to avoid missing underlying causative pathology. In a patient cohort,[83] remarkably 95% of patients had underlying osteopenia or osteoporosis. Both prospective and retrospective studies have shown that gender is not a risk factor in musculoskeletal injuries, except for stress fractures, where female sex is a risk factor.[95,96]

The increase in stress fractures in females is multifactorial. The presence of the female athlete triad or any of its components increases the athletes' risk of stress fracture. Research has found that BMD, menstrual irregularity or absence of menses, and inadequate nutrition and thus deficits of energy intake, known together as the female triad, all increase stress fracture risk. In addition, low body mass index and increasing age all raise a women's risk of suffering a stress fracture.

In a cohort-controlled study spanning premenopausal ages ranging from 18 to 45 years matched for age, sport, and weekly training volume, the stress fracture group had significantly less trabecular BMD and cortical area.[97] Several other studies have not found a link between BMD and stress fractures in premenopausal women.[98–101] Postmenopausal women may be more prone to stress fractures as a result of reduced BMD.[102]

Tenforde et al.[103] found late menarche in 748 high school runners (age > 15 years) to be an independent risk factor for stress fractures. Menstrual history should be obtained in all women, and hormonal and structural abnormalities that may cause secondary amenorrhea (absence of menses for >6 months) should be further investigated.

Inadequate intake of calcium and vitamin D, or inadequate caloric intake, is associated with reduced bone mass.[104] Decreased bone mass increases the strain on the remaining bone, increasing the fatigue fracture risk.

Duckham et al.[105] found that nutritional psychopathology is associated with an increased risk of stress fractures in endurance athletes, which may be associated with menstrual dysfunction and compulsive exercise.

Vitamin D is produced by sunlight in the skin and is then converted to the active form (1,25-dihydroxycholecalciferol) in the liver and the kidney. Vitamin D increases calcium absorption in the gastrointestinal tract. A deficiency of vitamin D may lead to secondary hyperparathyroidism, which increases bone loss and possible stress fracture risk. Vitamin D deficiency is not uncommon in the general population.[106]

Sonneville et al.[107] compared dietary intake of calcium and vitamin D against the risk of stress fractures, and found that high vitamin D intake (rather than a high calcium intake) was protective against the development of stress fractures. The authors found a 50% reduction in the incidence of stress fractures in girls taking vitamin D who participated in a high-impact activity.

Currently, the Institute of Medicine guidelines suggest that 600 to 800 International Units of vitamin D is necessary for adequate bone health in most adults. Recently, McCabe et al.[108] recommend dosages up to 2,000 International Units, because vitamin D is safe and has a high therapeutic index and improves training efficiency. Vitamin D status should be routinely assessed so that athletes can be coached to maintain serum 25(OH) vitamin D concentration of >30 ng per mL.

PERIPHERAL DXA USE IN CLINICAL PRACTICE

A variety of peripheral dual-energy X-ray absorptiometry (DXA [pDXA]) devices are available for measuring the forearm, heel, or hand. In principle, these are attractive because they offer a quick, inexpensive, and convenient method of investigating skeletal status. In practice, however, these alternative types of measurement correlate poorly with central DXA, with correlation coefficients in the range $r = 0.5$ to 0.65.[109] The lack of agreement with central DXA has proved a barrier to reaching a consensus on how to interpret results from pDXA devices[110]; thus, these are not recommended for use in the clinical setting.

However, not all types of fractures are equally well predicted by the standard axial BMD measurements (spine and hip), which are best at predicting fractures at sites such as the hip, spine, forearm, humerus, and pelvis, and are relatively ineffective for fractures of the face, ankles, feet, and toes.[111]

OSTEONECROSIS

Regional interruption of blood flow to the skeleton can cause ischemic (aseptic or avascular) necrosis. Ischemia, if sufficiently severe and prolonged, will kill osteoblasts and chondrocytes. Clinical problems will arise if subsequent resorption of necrotic tissue during skeletal repair compromises the bone strength sufficiently to cause fracture, with subsequent deformity of bone and secondary damage to cartilage. It is estimated that there are approximately 15,000 new cases per year in the United States. The disease appears to occur more frequently in males than in females, with the overall male to female ratio being 8:1. The age of onset is variable, although in the majority of cases, the patient is less than 50 years of age. Female cases are on average 10 years older than male cases.

Osteonecrosis is often seen in association with a number of different conditions. Trauma with fracture, glucocorticoids, and alcoholism predispose to osteonecrosis. Accordingly, disorders that increase the size and/or number of adipocytes within critical areas of medullary space (e.g., alcohol abuse, Cushing syndrome) may ultimately compress sinusoids, thereby leading to infarction of bone. Other factors potentially involved in the pathogenesis of osteonecrosis include fat embolization, hemorrhage, and abnormalities in the quality of susceptible bone tissue. The factor V Leiden mutation (G1691A, Arg506Gln) is a common risk factor for thrombophilia.

The femoral head is the most common location for the development of osteonecrosis, although it may also occur at other sites including distal femur, humeral head, wrist, and foot. Patients may develop pain that can persist for weeks to months before radiographs show any change, although patients can be asymptomatic.

REFERENCES

1. Spranger J, Brill P, Poznanski A. *Bone Dysplasias. An Atlas of Genetic Disorders of Skeletal Development.* 2nd ed. Oxford: Oxford University Press; 2002.
2. Orioli IM, Castilla EE, Barbosa-Neto JG. The birth prevalence rates for skeletal dysplasias. *J Med Genet.* 1986;23:328–332.
3. Uitto J, Santa Cruz DJ, Starcher BC, et al. Biochemical and ultrastructural demonstration of elastin accumulation in the skin of the Buschke–Ollendorff syndrome. *J Invest Dermatol.* 1981;76:284–287.
4. Mumm S, Wenkert D, Zhang X, et al. Deactivating germline mutations in LEMD3 cause osteopoikilosis and Buschke-Ollendorff syndrome, but not sporadic melorheostosis. *J Bone Miner Res.* 2007;22:243–250.
5. Whyte MP, Murphy WA, Seigel BA. 99m Tc-pyrophosphate bone imaging in osteopoikilosis, osteopathia striata, and melorheostosis. *Radiology.* 1978;127:439–443.
6. Campbell CJ, Papademetriou T, Bonfiglio M. Melorheostosis: a report of the clinical, roentgenographic, and pathological findings in fourteen cases. *J Bone Joint Surg Am.* 1968;50:1281–1304.
7. Leri A, Joanny J. Une affection non decrite des os. Hyperostose "en coulee" sur toute la longueur d'un membre ou "melorheostose." *Bull Mem Soc Med Hop Paris.* 1922;46:1141–1145.
8. Applebaum RE, Caniano DA, Sun CC, et al. Synchronous left subclavian and axillary artery aneurysms associated with melorheostosis. *Surgery.* 1986;99:249–253.
9. Colavita N, Nicolais S, Orazi C, et al. Melorheostosis: presentation of a case followed up for 24 years. *Arch Orthop Trauma Surg.* 1987;106:123–125.
10. Wagers LT, Young AW Jr, Ryan SF. Linear melorheostotic scleroderma. *Br J Dermatol.* 1972;86:297–301.
11. Rimoin DL. Pachydermoperiostosis (idiopathic clubbing and periostosis). Genetic and physiologic considerations. *N Engl J Med.* 1965;272:923–931.
12. Uppal S, Diggle CP, Carr IM, et al. Mutations in 15-hydroxyprostaglandin dehydrogenase cause primary hypertrophic osteoarthropathy. *Nat Genet.* 2008;40:789–793.
13. Ali A, Tetalman MR, Fordham EW, et al. Distribution of hypertrophic pulmonary osteoarthropathy. *Am J Roentgenol.* 1980;134:771–780.
14. Lauter SA, Vasey FB, Hüttner I, et al. Pachydermoperiostosis: studies on the synovium. *J Rheumatol.* 1978;5:85–95.
15. Lichtenstein L, Jaffe HL. Fibrous dysplasia of bone: a condition affecting one, several or many bones, the graver cases of which may present abnormal pigmentation of skin, premature sexual development, hyperthyroidism or still other extraskeletal abnormalities. *Arch Pathol.* 1942;33:777–816.
16. Collins MT. Spectrum and natural history of fibrous dysplasia of bone. *J Bone Miner Res.* 2006;21(suppl 2):P99–P104.
17. Hart ES, Kelly MH, Brillante B, et al. Onset, progression, and plateau of skeletal lesions in fibrous dysplasia, and the relationship to functional outcome. *J Bone Miner Res.* 2007;22(9):1468–1474.
18. McCune DJ. Osteitis fibrosa cystica; the case of a nine year old girl who also exhibits precocious puberty, multiple pigmentation of the skin and hyperthyroidism. *Am J Dis Child.* 1936;52:743–744.
19. Albright F, Butler AM, Hampton AO, et al. Syndrome characterized by osteitis fibrosa disseminata, areas of pigmentation and endocrine dysfunction, with precocious puberty in females, report of five cases. *N Engl J Med.* 1937;216:727–746.
20. Danon M, Crawford JD. The McCune–Albright syndrome. *Ergeb Inn Med Kinderheilkd.* 1987;55:81–115.
21. Dumitrescu CE, Collins MT. McCune–Albright syndrome. *Orphanet J Rare Dis.* 2008;3:12.
22. Collins MT, Chebli C, Jones J, et al. Renal phosphate wasting in fibrous dysplasia of bone is part of a generalized renal tubular dysfunction similar to that seen in tumor-induced osteomalacia. *J Bone Miner Res.* 2001;16(5):806–813.

23. Cabral CE, Guedes P, Fonseca T, et al. Polyostotic fibrous dysplasia associated with intramuscular myxomas: Mazabraud's syndrome. *Skeletal Radiol.* 1998;27(5):278–282.

24. Shenker A, Weinstein LS, Moran A, et al. Severe endocrine and non endocrine manifestations of the McCune–Albright syndrome associated with activating mutations of stimulatory G protein GS. *J Pediatr.* 1993;123(4):509–518.

25. Weinstein LS, Shenker A, Gejman PV, et al. Activating mutations of the stimulatory G protein in the McCune-Albright syndrome. *N Engl J Med.* 1991;325(24):1688–1695.

26. Shenker A, Weinstein LS, Sweet DE, et al. An activating Gs alpha mutation is present in fibrous dysplasia of bone in the McCune-Albright syndrome. *J Clin Endocrinol Metab.* 1994;79(3):750–755.

27. Bianco P, Riminucci M, Majolagbe A, et al. Mutations of the GNAS1 gene, stromal cell dysfunction, and osteomalacic changes in non-McCune-Albright fibrous dysplasia of bone. *J Bone Miner Res.* 2000;15(1):120–128.

28. Landis CA, Masters SB, Spada A, et al. GTPase inhibiting mutations activate the alpha chain of Gs and stimulate adenylyl cyclase in human pituitary tumors. *Nature.* 1989;340(6236):692–696.

29. Bianco P, Gehron Robey P, Wientroub S. Fibrous dysplasia. In: Glorieux F, Pettifor JM, Juppner H, eds. *Pediatric Bone: Biology and Disease.* New York, NY: Academic Press/Elsevier; 2003:509–539.

30. Harris WH, Dudley HR, Barry RJ. The natural history of fibrous dysplasia. An orthopedic, pathological, and roentgenographic study. *J Bone Joint Surg Am.* 1962;44-A:207–233.

31. Leet AI, Chebli C, Kushner H, et al. Fracture incidence in polyostotic fibrous dysplasia and the McCune-Albright Syndrome. *J Bone Miner Res.* 2004;19(4):571–577.

32. Kelly MH, Brillante B, Collins MT. Pain in fibrous dysplasia of bone: age-related changes and the anatomical distribution of skeletal lesions. *Osteoporos Int.* 2007;19(1):57–63.

33. Ruggieri P, Sim FH, Bond JR, et al. Malignancies in fibrous dysplasia. *Cancer.* 1994;73(5):1411–1424.

34. Collins MT, Kushner H, Reynolds JC, et al. An instrument to measure skeletal burden and predict functional outcome in fibrous dysplasia of bone. *J Bone Miner Res.* 2005;20(2):219–226.

35. Sakai LY, Keene DR, Engvall E. Fibrillin, a new 350kD glycoprotein, is a component of extracellular microfibrils. *J Cell Biol.* 1986;103:2499–2509.

36. Stheneur C, Tubach F, Jouneaux M, et al. Study of phenotype evolution during childhood in Marfan syndrome to improve clinical recognition. *Genet Med.* 2014;16:246–250.

37. LeGoff C, Mahaut C, Wang LW, et al. Mutations in the TGFβ binding-protein-like domain 5 of FBN1 are responsible for acromicric and geleophysic dysplasias. *Am J Hum Genet.* 2011;89:7–14.

38. Faivre L, Gorlin RJ, Wirtz MK, et al. In frame fibrillin-1 gene deletion in autosomal dominant Weill-Marchesani syndrome. *J Med Genet.* 2003;40:34–36.

39. Sengle G, Tsutsui K, Keene DR, et al. Microenvironmental regulation by fibrillin-1. *Plos Genet.* 2012;8(1):e1002425.

40. Mantovani G. Pseudohypoparathyroidism: diagnosis and treatment. *J Clin Endocrinol Metab.* 2011;96:3020–3030.

41. Albright F, Burnett CH, Smith PH, et al. Pseudohypoparathyroidism—an example of "Seabright-Bantam syndrome." *Endocrinology.* 1942;30:922–932.

42. Chase LR, Melson GL, Aurbach GD. Pseudohypoparathyroidism: defective excretion of 3′,5′-AMP in response to parathyroid hormone. *J Clin Invest.* 1969;48:1832–1844.

43. Weinstein LS, Yu S, Warner DR, et al. Endocrine manifestations of stimulatory g protein alpha-subunit mutations and the role of genomic imprinting. *Endocr Rev.* 2001;22:675–705.

44. Mantovani G, Maghnie M, Weber G, et al. Growth hormone-releasing hormone resistance in pseudohypoparathyroidism type ia: new evidence for imprinting of the Gs alpha gene. *J Clin Endocrinol Metab.* 2003;88:4070–4074.

45. Germain-Lee EL, Groman J, Crane JL, et al. Growth hormone deficiency in pseudohypoparathyroidism type 1a: another manifestation of multihormone resistance. *J Clin Endocrinol Metab.* 2003;88:4059–4069.

46. Vlaeminck-Guillem V, D'Herbomez M, Pigny P, et al. Pseudohypoparathyroidism Ia and hypercalcitoninemia. *J Clin Endocrinol Metab.* 2001;86:3091–3096.

47. Albright F, Forbes AP, Henneman PH. Pseudo-pseudohypoparathyroidism. *Trans Assoc Am Physicians.* 1952;65:337–350.

48. Drezner M, Neelon FA, Lebovitz HE. Pseudohypoparathyroidism type II: a possible defect in the reception of the cyclic AMP signal. *N Engl J Med.* 1973;289:1056–1060.

49. Farfel Z. Pseudohypohyperparathyroidism-pseudohypoparathyroidism type Ib. *J Bone Miner Res.* 1999;14:1016.

50. Ichikawa S, Guigonis V, Imel EA, et al. Novel GALNT3 mutations causing hyperostosis-hyperphosphatemia syndrome result in low intact fibroblast growth factor 23 concentrations. *J Clin Endocrinol Metab.* 2007;92:1943–1947.

51. Ichikawa S, Lyles KW, Econs MJ. A novel GALNT3 mutation in a pseudoautosomal dominant form of tumoral calcinosis: evidence that the disorder is autosomal recessive. *J Clin Endocrinol Metab.* 2005;90:2420–2423.

52. Ichikawa S, Imel EA, Kreiter ML, et al. A homozygous missense mutation in human KLOTHO causes severe tumoral calcinosis. *J Clin Invest.* 2007;117(9):2684–2691.

53. Slavin RE, Wen J, Kumar D, et al. Familial tumoral calcinosis: a clinical, histopathologic, and ultrastructural study with an analysis of its calcifying process and pathogenesis. *Am J Surg Path.* 1993;17:788–802.

54. Mathew S, Lund R, Strebeck F, et al. Reversal of the adynamic bone disorder and decreased vascular calcification in chronic kidney disease by sevelamer carbonate therapy. *J Am Soc Nephrol.* 2007;18(1):122–130.

55. Davies MR, Lund RJ, Mathew S, et al. Low turnover osteodystrophy and vascular calcification are amenable to skeletal anabolism in an animal model of chronic kidney disease and the metabolic syndrome. *J Am Soc Nephrol.* 2005;16(4):917–928.

56. Connor JM, Evans DAP. Fibrodysplasia ossificans progressiva: the clinical features and natural history of 34 patients. *J Bone Joint Surg Br.* 1982;64:76–83.

57. Kaplan FS, Glaser DL, Shore EM, et al. The phenotype of fibrodysplasia ossificans progressiva. *Clin Rev Bone Miner Metab.* 2005;3:183–188.

58. Shore EM, Feldman GJ, Xu M, et al. The genetics of fibrodysplasia ossificans progressiva. *Clin Rev Bone Miner Metab.* 2005;3:201–204.

59. Janoff HB, Muenke M, Johnson LO, et al. Fibrodysplasia ossificans progressiva in two half-sisters. Evidence for maternal mosaicism. *Am J Med Genet.* 1996;61:320–324.

60. Rocke DM, Zasloff M, Peeper J, et al. Age and joint-specific risk of initial heterotopic ossification in patients who have fibrodysplasia ossificans progressiva. *Clin Orthop.* 1994;301:243–248.

61. Cohen RB, Hahn GV, Tabas JA, et al. The natural history of heterotopic ossification in patients who have fibrodysplasia ossificans progressiva. A study of 44 patients. *J Bone Joint Surg Am.* 1993;75:215–219.

62. Kanis JA. *Pathophysiology and Treatment of Paget's Disease of the Bone.* 2nd ed. London: Martin Dunitz; 1998.

63. Siris ES, Canfield RE, Jacobs TP. Paget's disease of bone. *Bull NY Acad Med.* 1980;56:285–304.

64. Morales-Piga AA, Rey-Rey JS, Corres-Gonzalez J, et al. Frequency and characteristics of familial aggregation of Paget's disease of bone. *J Bone Miner Res.* 1995;10:663–670.

65. McKusick VA. *Heritable Disorders of Connective Tissue.* 5th ed. St. Louis, MO: CV Mosby; 1972:718–723.

66. Siris ES, Ottman R, Flaster E, et al. Familial aggregation of Paget's disease of bone. *J Bone Miner Res.* 1991;6:495–500.

67. Hocking LJ, Herbert CA, Nicholls RK, et al. Genomewide search in familial Paget disease of bone shows evidence of genetic heterogeneity with candidate loci on chromosomes 2q36, 10p13, and 5q35. *Am J Hum Genet.* 2001;69:1055–1061.

68. Shankar S, Hosking DJ. Biochemical assessment of Paget's disease of bone. *J Bone Miner Res.* 2006;21(suppl 2):P22–P27.

69. McKusick-Nathans Institute of Genetic Medicine, Johns Hopkins University. 2008. Online Mendelian Inheritance in Man. https://www.ncbi.nlm. nih.gov/omim/. Accessed November 24, 2011.

70. Whyte MP. Hypophosphatasia: Nature's window on alkaline phosphatase function in humans. In: Bilezikian JP, Raisz LG, Martin TJ, eds. *Principles of Bone Biology.* 3rd ed. San Diego: Academic Press; 2008:1573–1598.

71. Whyte, MP. Hypophosphatasia. In: Thakker RV, Whyte MP, Eisman J, et al, eds. *Genetics of Bone Biology and Skeletal Disease.* San Diego, CA: Elsevier (Academic Press); 2013:337–360.

72. Khandwala HM, Mumm S, Whyte MP. Low serum alkaline phosphatase activity with pathologic fracture: case report and brief review of adult hypophosphatasia. *Endocr Pract.* 2006;12:676–681.

73. Mornet E. Tissue nonspecific alkaline phosphatase gene mutations database. Available online at http://www.sesep.uvsq.fr/Database.html. 2005. Accessed November 24, 2011.

74. Consensus development conference: diagnosis, prophylaxis and treatment of osteoporosis. *Am J Med.* 1993;941:646–650.

75. World Health Organization Study Group. Assessment of fracture risk and its application to screening for postmenopausal osteoporosis. *World Health Organ Tech Rep Ser.* 1994;843:1–129.

76. Kanis JA, Johnell O, Oden A, et al. Ten-year probabilities of osteoporotic fractures according to BMD and diagnostic thresholds. *Osteoporos Int.* 2001;12:989–995.

77. Kanis JA, McCloskey EV, Johansson H, et al. Case finding for the management of osteoporosis with FRAX—assessment and intervention thresholds for the UK. *Osteoporos Int.* 2008;19:1395–1408.

78. Ström O, Borgström F, Kanis JA, et al. Osteoporosis: burden, health care provision and opportunities in the EU: a report prepared in collaboration with the International Osteoporosis Foundation (IOF) and the European Federation of Pharmaceutical Industry Associations (EFPIA). *Arch Osteoporos.* 2011;6(1–2):59–155.

79. 79. *Bone Health and Osteoporosis: A Report of the Surgeon General.* Rockville, MD: U.S. Department of Health and Human Services; 2004

80. van Staa TP, Dennison EM, Leufkens HG, et al. Epidemiology of fractures in England and Wales. *Bone.* 2001;29:517–522.

81. Sontag A, Krege JH. First fractures among postmenopausal women with osteoporosis. *J Bone Miner Metab.* 2010;28(4):485–488. doi:10.1007/s00774-009-0144-9.

82. Varenna M, Binelli L, Zucchi F, et al. Is the metatarsal fracture in postmenopausal women an osteoporotic fracture? A cross-sectional study on 113 cases. *Osteoporos Int.* 1997;7:558–563.

83. Tomczak RL, VanCourt R. Metatarsal insufficiency fractures in previously undiagnosed osteoporosis patients. *J Foot Ankle Surg.* 2000;39(3):174–183.

84. Seeley DG, Kelsey J, Jergas M, et al. Predictors of ankle and foot fractures in older women. The Study of Osteoporotic Fractures Research Group. *J Bone Miner Res.* 1996;11:1347–1355.

85. Bridges MJ, Ruddick S. Are metatarsal fractures indicative of osteoporosis in postmenopausal women? *Foot Ankle Spec.* 2011;4(5):271–273.

86. Bennell KL, Crossley K. Musculoskeletal injuries in track and field: incidence, distribution and risk factors. *Aust J Sci Med Sport.* 1996;28(3):69–75.

87. Edwards PH Jr, Wright ML, Hartman JF. A practical approach for the differential diagnosis of chronic leg pain in the athlete. *Am J Sports Med.* 2005;33(8):1241–1249.

88. Pegrum J, Crisp T, Padhiar N, et al. The pathophysiology, diagnosis, and management of stress fractures in postmenopausal women. *Phys Sportsmed.* 2012;40(3):32–42.

89. Pegrum J, Crisp T, Padhiar N. Diagnosis and management of bone stress injuries of the lower limb in athletes. *BMJ.* 2012;344:e2511.

90. Lassus J, Tulikoura I, Konttinen YT, et al. Bone stress injuries of the lower extremity: a review. *Acta Orthop Scand.* 2002;73(3):359–368.

91. Milgrom C, Giladi M, Stein M, et al. Stress fractures in military recruits. A prospective study showing an unusually high incidence. *J Bone Joint Surg Br.* 1985;67(5):732–735.

92. Wolf JH. Julis Wolff and his "law of bone remodeling" [in German]. *Orthopade.* 1995;24(5):378–386.

93. Angeline ME, Gee AO, Shindle M, et al. The effects of vitamin D deficiency in athletes. *Am J Sports Med.* 2013;41(2):461–464.

94. Nattiv A, Kennedy G, Barrack MT, et al. Correlation of MRI grading of bone stress injuries with clinical risk factors and return to play: a 5-year prospective study in collegiate track and field athletes. *Am J Sports Med.* 2013;41(8):1930–1941.

95. Brunet ME, Cook SD, Brinker MR, et al. A survey of running injuries in 1505 competitive and recreational runners. *J Sports Med Phys Fitness.* 1990;30(3):307–315.

96. Shaffer RA, Rauh MJ, Brodine SK, et al. Predictors of stress fracture susceptibility in young female recruits. *Am J Sports Med.* 2006;34(1):108–115.

97. Schnackenburg KE, Macdonald HM, Ferber R, et al. Bone quality and muscle strength in female athletes with lower limb stress fractures. *Med Sci Sports Exerc.* 2011;43(11):2110–2119.

98. Giladi M, Milgrom C, Simkin A, et al. Stress fractures. Identifiable risk factors. *Am J Sports Med.* 1991;19(6):647–652.

99. Frusztajer NT, Dhuper S, Warren MP, et al. Nutrition and the incidence of stress fractures in ballet dancers. *Am J Clin Nutr.* 1990;51(5):779–783.

100. Cline AD, Jansen GR, Melby CL. Stress fractures in female army recruits: implications of bone density, calcium intake, and exercise. *J Am Coll Nutr.* 1998;17(2):128–135.

101. Lauder TD, Dixit S, Pezzin LE, et al. The relation between stress fractures and bone mineral density: evidence from active-duty Army women. *Arch Phys Med Rehabil.* 2000;81(1):73–79.

102. Myburgh KH, Hutchins J, Fataar AB, et al. Low bone density is an etiologic factor for stress fractures in athletes. *Ann Intern Med.* 1990;113(10):754–759.

103. Tenforde AS, Sayres LC, McCurdy ML, et al. Identifying sex-specific risk factors for stress fractures in adolescent runners. *Med Sci Sports Exerc.* 2013;45(10):1843–1851.

104. Ihle R, Loucks AB. Dose-response relationships between energy availability and bone turnover in young exercising women. *J Bone Miner Res.* 2004;19(8):1231–1240.

105. Duckham RL, Peirce N, Meyer C, et al. Risk factors for stress fracture in female endurance athletes: a cross-sectional study. *BMJ Open.* 2012;2(6).

106. Macdonald HM, Mavroeidi A, Fraser WD, et al. Sunlight and dietary contributions to the seasonal vitamin D status of cohorts of healthy postmenopausal women living at northerly latitudes: a major cause for concern? *Osteoporos Int.* 2011;22(9):2461–2472.

107. Sonneville KR, Gordon CM, Kocher MS, et al. Vitamin D, calcium, and dairy intakes and stress fractures among female adolescents. *Arch Pediatr Adolesc Med.* 2012;166(7):595–600.

108. McCabe MP, Smyth MP, Richardson DR. Current concept review: vitamin D and stress fractures. *Foot Ankle Int.* 2012;33(6):526–533.

109. Lu Y, Genant HK, Shepherd J, et al. Classification of osteoporosis based on bone mineral densities. *J Bone Miner Res.* 2001;16(5):901–910.

110. Blake GM, Chinn DJ, Steel SA, et al. A list of device specific thresholds for the clinical interpretation of peripheral x-ray absorptiometry examinations. *Osteoporos Int.* 2005;16(12):2149–2156.

111. Stone KL, Seeley DG, Lui LY, et al. BMD at multiple sites and risk of fracture of multiple types: long-term results from the Study of Osteoporotic Fractures. *J Bone Miner Res.* 2003;18(11):1947–1954.

CHAPTER 18

Gastrointestinal/Hepatic Disease Manifestations in the Lower Extremity

BRIAN P. BOSWORTH • YECHESKEL SCHNEIDER

Although the gastrointestinal (GI) system and the lower extremities would seem anatomically separate and distinct, it is not uncommon to encounter lower extremity manifestations of primary GI diseases. For example, disorders of malabsorption may present with vitamin deficiencies that lead to neuropathies or cutaneous findings. In addition, primary dermatologic findings on the lower extremities may be first presentations of inflammatory bowel diseases (IBDs). For these reasons, it is important for physicians to be aware of the link between the GI system and the lower extremities. This chapter focuses on primary GI disorders and their lower extremity manifestations, specifically neurologic, dermatologic, and rheumatologic findings because these will be most encountered by clinicians.

NEUROLOGIC ASSOCIATIONS

Disorders of the GI system, including luminal diseases of the stomach and bowel, as well as pancreatic and hepatic disorders, can lead to neurologic complications affecting the central nervous system (CNS) and the peripheral nervous system, both of which can present with lower extremity findings.

IBD is a chronic inflammatory GI disease comprised of Crohn disease (CD) and ulcerative colitis (UC), which can affect the entire GI tract, particularly the small and large intestines. The course for each individual patient can be highly variable, and many with the disease have relapsing and remitting disease. The underlying driving force of the disease is not entirely understood, but one's environment, genetics, and immune system (T_1 helper cells in CD and T_2 helper cells in UC) all play an important role. Most patients present between the ages of 15 and 40. CD may present with abdominal pain, diarrhea, GI tract obstruction, perianal fistulas or abscesses, and weight loss. UC often presents with bloody diarrhea, urgency, tenesmus, and pain with defecation.[1] Aside from GI-specific manifestations, IBD can be associated with extraintestinal manifestations that can affect multiple other organ systems including the nervous, dermatologic, vascular, orthopedic, and rheumatologic systems.[2] Neurologic involvement in IBD is one aspect of extraintestinal manifestation that can be seen in patients

with IBD. Peripheral neuropathy is a common neurologic manifestation, and may be related to medications including metronidazole and anti–tumor necrosis factor (TNF) agents, vitamin deficiencies, and immune-mediated changes.[3]

The reported incidence of neurologic manifestations in patients with IBD is thought to be approximately 3%,[4] of which the prevalence of peripheral neuropathy in particular has been reported to be as high as 13.4%,[5] with relatively comparable incidence in patients with UC and CD. These peripheral neuropathies may be sensory, motor, mixed, or autonomic. They may be acute or chronic, axonal or demyelinating, and may have various distributions.[6] Patients may also experience primary muscle involvement that may be confused with neuropathies; these can include inflammatory myopathies, dermatomyositis, polymyositis, rimmed vacuole myopathy, and granulomatous myositis.[3]

Peripheral neuropathies in IBD are not typically related to disease activity, and do not respond to treatment of the underlying IBD.[3] The underlying pathology of peripheral neuropathies may be immune-mediated, secondary manifestations of vitamin deficiencies (such as low vitamin B_{12} or vitamin B_6), or medication side effects (from metronidazole or anti-TNF agents). Patients may experience malabsorption secondary to surgical changes (e.g., vitamin B_{12} deficiency after ileal resections) or disease activity (ileal inflammation leading to decreased vitamin B_{12} deficiency).[7] Anti-TNF agents have been associated with peripheral and central demyelination, both new cases and aggravation of old cases. Natalizumab, which is an anti-integrin also approved for use in patients with IBD, has been associated with progressive multifocal leukoencephalopathy (PML) in patients with John Cunningham (JC) virus.[8]

Another notable neurologic condition associated with IBD is multiple sclerosis (MS). MS has been more frequently associated with UC than CD. The prevalence of MS is increased in patients with concomitant IBD.[9] Furthermore, patients with IBD are also more likely to have asymptomatic white matter lesions, although the clinical significance of these findings remains unclear.[10] The pathophysiology of this relationship is unclear, but likely is related to the underlying inflammatory and immunologic pathology that drives both

MS and IBD. Notably, anti-TNF agents are contraindicated in patients with MS, as they have been associated with new onset of demyelination and aggravation of preexisting disease.[11]

There have also been rare reports of fistulization from the rectum to the epidural and subdural spaces, leading to abscess formation and subsequent nerve compression with development of lower extremity weakness, pain, and other neurologic complications.[12,13] Although rare and uncommon, sudden onset of focal neurologic findings in the lower extremities should trigger an extensive workup, examining for peripheral neurologic conditions as well as brain and spinal cord pathology.

Hepatitis C virus (HCV) infection is one of the leading causes of cirrhosis, with significant morbidity and mortality globally.[14] It is often asymptomatic initially, but can become a chronic liver infection in over 80% of those infected with the virus.[15] HCV can independently be associated with peripheral neuropathy.[16] It is thought that HCV can trigger an immunologic response including production of antiganglioside antibodies (1 and 2), which may be related to the development of neuropathy.[17] Individuals infected with hepatitis C may also develop cryoglobulinemia, which is characterized by significant cryoglobulins (proteins that become insoluble complexes at cold temperatures) in the blood. Cryoglobulinemia can lead to deposition of immune complexes in small and medium-sized vessels with vascular inflammation, as well as mononeuropathy or mononeuropathy multiplex in 17% to 60% of patients.[3] Other hepatitides may also be associated with neurologic manifestations. Hepatitis A virus (HAV) is an acute, often self-limited hepatitis characterized by jaundice, abdominal pain, fever, nausea, vomiting, and diarrhea. HAV infection can rarely precede Guillain–Barré syndrome (which most commonly presents with ascending paralysis of the lower extremities).[18] Hepatitis B virus (HBV) is responsible for both acute and chronic hepatitis infections and may present with jaundice, abdominal pain, nausea, and vomiting. HBV infection can rarely be associated with Guillain–Barré syndrome,[19] as well as mononeuropathy multiplex and acute symmetrical vasculitic polyneuropathy (which presents as nonpalpable purpura, and acute-onset distal symmetric sensorimotor polyneuropathy).[20,21]

In terms of the CNS, multiple GI disorders (including IBD, HCV infection, and cirrhosis) have been associated with increased risk of stroke. This may present with focal neurologic deficits (isolated motor or sensory, or mixed) in the lower extremities. For example, patients may present with unilateral lower extremity weakness, numbness, or gait instability. Clinicians should have a low threshold to rule out a cerebral vascular accident in individuals who suffer from one of the aforementioned GI disorders and who present with focal neurologic findings. Cirrhotics often have an imbalance of prothrombotic and antithrombotic factors that are synthesized by the liver, which can make these individuals prone to hemorrhage or increased clot formation.[22] In those with IBD, the underlying mechanism driving an increased risk of stroke may be secondary to a systemic inflammatory state, leading to increased levels of factor V and VIII, fibrinogen, decreased levels of protein S and antithrombin, leading to a prothrombotic state. Other possible theories that have been proposed to explain why patients with IBD have an increased risk of clot formation include platelet dysfunction, increased von Willebrand factor, and increased levels of homocysteine.[3] Those with IBD have an increased risk of both arterial and venous thrombi.[6,23] Autopsy records estimate a prevalence as high as 30% for those with UC, and the incidence of thrombotic complications ranges from 0.5% to approximately 7% per year.[24] They are not related to the duration or the severity of IBD, but cerebrovascular events are more frequent during bouts of inflammation. There have also been case reports of ischemic strokes thought to be complications of anti-TNFα therapy. There have also been reports of thrombosis of the dural sinus and cerebral veins, and this, perhaps, is more common in the pediatric population.[25,26]

Acute liver failure (ALF, also known as fulminant hepatic failure) and cirrhosis may both be associated with encephalopathy, which can involve lower extremity findings. Encephalopathy seen in ALF is secondary to astrocyte swelling and progression to cerebral edema, with or without herniation.[27] In cirrhosis, encephalopathy is often thought to be driven by accumulation of toxins not cleared by the liver, which can be triggered by infections, GI bleeding, and constipation; in the case of cirrhosis, encephalopathy is known as portosystemic encephalopathy (PSE) or hepatic encephalopathy (HE).[28] Encephalopathy secondary to ALF or cirrhosis can manifest with subtle findings such as myoclonus or stark changes such as frank coma with posturing.[29] Although it would be rare to see isolated lower extremity manifestations in these conditions, one should still be aware of even subtle changes in the lower extremities as these help one recognize and grade the degree of HE. With resolution of liver disease, one would expect resolution of the neurologic manifestations. Although rare, after several episodes of PSE, cirrhotic patients can develop hepatic myelopathy, or a complex movement disorder known as acquired hepatocerebral degeneration. Hepatic myelopathy is caused by demyelination of the lateral corticospinal tracts and eventual axonal loss. It is characterized by a subacute progressive bilateral lower extremity weakness and spasticity, with minimal to no sensory abnormalities.[30,31] Acquired hepatocerebral degeneration presents with parkinsonism of predominantly lower body involvement, postural instability, and cranial dyskinesia; there may also be tremors, limb dystonia, and chorea.[32,33] In making these diagnoses, one must be careful to rule out metabolic etiologies (including hypoglycemia, hyponatremia), thiamine deficiency, as well as alcohol or recreational drug use. Patients should also undergo a CT of the head/brain to evaluate for evidence of intracranial bleed, and an MRI to rule out an ischemic event. An MRI can also be helpful in making the diagnosis, as it may reveal T1 bilateral high-signal abnormalities in the pallidum and substantia nigra, related to deposition of manganese.[34]

Medications

Promotility agents (such as metoclopramide), which may be utilized for patients with gastroparesis, has been shown to lead to the development of extrapyramidal side effects, acute dyskinesia, akathisia, tremor, parkinsonism, and tardive dyskinesia.[35] Anti-TNF agents (which include infliximab, adalimumab, certolizumab, and golimumab), as described earlier, can rarely cause or aggravate an underlying peripheral or central demyelinating disorder (including peripheral neuropathies and MS). They can be associated with dysesthesia, paresthesias, and ataxia; these symptoms may improve after discontinuation of the offending agent. Natalizumab, an anti-integrin agent, has been shown to cause PML via activation of the JC virus in those who are infected; this usually presents with dementia or confusion, but may also be associated with motor weakness. Metronidazole, when used for prolonged courses (such as for *Clostridium difficile* infection or intra-abdominal abscess), can cause ataxia, tremors, and peripheral neuropathy; these often resolve after discontinuation of the medication. Patients with IBD or autoimmune hepatitis may also be treated with steroids at some point during the course of their disease, sometimes for prolonged periods of time; this may lead to a steroid-related myelopathy and can occur with either acute or chronic use. One may also see proximal muscle wasting on physical examination with long-term steroid use. Cyclosporine, which may be used for severe IBD refractory to other medications, can also cause tremors and seizures.[6]

DERMATOLOGIC ASSOCIATIONS

GI manifestations in the lower extremities often involve both specific and nonspecific cutaneous findings. IBDs may present with cutaneous manifestations as their presenting symptom. Several hereditary polyposis syndromes (and familial colorectal cancer syndromes) are associated with cutaneous manifestations that one must be familiar with, as polyposis syndromes may confer an increased risk of colorectal malignancy. Certain GI-related malignancies may also be associated with skin conditions.

As mentioned earlier, those with IBD may develop extraintestinal manifestations, including dermatologic conditions. Most commonly, these include erythema nodosum (EN) and pyoderma gangrenosum (PG). The prevalence of cutaneous manifestations for patients with CD or UC is fairly similar (up to 23% of patients with CD and 19% of patients with UC).[36]

EN is a septal panniculitis, typically affecting the extensor surfaces of the lower extremities. It is the most common cutaneous manifestation of IBD, occurring in approximately 4% of all patients with IBD. Commonly seen in young women with IBD, EN is thought to reflect the underlying disease activity within the gut. Treatment is geared toward treatment of the underlying GI IBD symptoms.[37]

PG is another dermatologic condition that is often associated with IBD; 0.6% to 2% of patients with IBD may

develop PG,[37] whereas 20% of PG cases are associated with IBD.[38] It typically occurs at sites of previous trauma (referred to as pathergy). Unlike EN, PG does not necessarily reflect disease activity in the gut. Treatment ranges from localized to systemic therapies, and can include topical or intralesional corticosteroids, topical tacrolimus, anti-TNF agents such as infliximab or adalimumab, or systemic corticosteroids.[38,39]

Cutaneous polyarteritis nodosa (CPN) is another cutaneous manifestation of IBD, although much less frequently encountered than either EN or PG. It is a chronic vasculitis affecting small and medium-sized arteries. It often presents as a tender nodule on the lower extremities. It can be distinguished from EN and PG by excisional biopsy, which should show panarteritis and localized perivascular inflammation. CPN activity is not necessarily reflective of underlying active IBD. Treatment involves nonsteroidal anti-inflammatory drugs and low-dose corticosteroids.[40] Necrotizing vasculitis may also be seen in association with IBD, again less commonly than EN or PG. It can present with palpable purpura, or in advanced cases, even ulcerations and gangrene. It typically occurs on the lower extremities. Biopsy reveals a neutrophilic infiltrate and endothelial enlargement of postcapillary venules.[41,42]

It is important to be mindful that anti-TNF agents, which are used for many patients with IBD, can also be associated with the development of skin lesions. These can include palmoplantar pustulosis, eczema, xerosis cutis, and psoriasiform lesions.[43] Patients with IBD may also be at increased risk for the development of skin cancers; anti-TNF agents may increase the risk of melanoma, whereas immunomodulators (such as azathioprine and methotrexate) may increase the risk of nonmelanoma skin cancers.[44] Individuals taking these medications should undergo routine skin examinations with a dermatologist to examine for any concerning lesions.

Patients with IBD are at increased risk for the development of deep venous thrombosis (DVT) and thromboembolic disease.[45] Patients with DVTs may present with unilateral or bilateral lower extremity swelling and pain. It is important to ensure that all hospitalized patients with IBD be given some form of prophylaxis against DVTs. It is important to recognize that these patients are at an increased risk for the development of macrovesicular and microvesicular thrombosis to help prevent and ensure early recognition of these complications.[46]

Dermatitis herpetiformis is a cutaneous manifestation of Celiac disease, an immunologic disorder driven by antibodies that target gluten, specifically antigliadin and antitissue transglutaminase antibodies. It leads to changes in the duodenal mucosa, and endoscopy classically reveals villous atrophy of the duodenal mucosa with increased intraepithelial lymphocytes on biopsy (although some cases may present without these findings). It is almost always associated with human leukocyte antigen DQ2 and DQ8. The produced antibodies can deposit in the papillary dermis, which leads to recruitment of neutrophils and neutrophilic dermal microabscesses. These lesions typically start off as small herpetiform vesicles on an erythematous base and they are often pruritic. It is typically symmetric and can be seen on the knees, elbows, and shoulders. They are not responsive to topical therapies, but respond best to elimination of all gluten in one's diet.[47–49]

The four main familial colorectal cancer syndromes include Lynch syndrome, familial adenomatous polyposis (FAP) syndrome, juvenile polyposis syndrome, and Peutz–Jeghers syndrome (PJS). These can each be associated with skin findings that a physician should be able to recognize so as to help diagnose an underlying polyposis syndrome.[50] Lynch syndrome is a hereditary nonpolyposis colon cancer, and is the most common hereditary cancer. It is caused by inheritable mutations in the mismatch repair genes, MLH1, MSH2, MSH6, and PMS2. In addition to colon cancer, it is also responsible for hepatobiliary, small bowel, gynecologic (endometrial, ovarian), urologic, and brain malignancies.[51,52] Most of the skin manifestations seen in Lynch syndrome are associated with a specific variant referred to as Muir–Torre syndrome. Some of the dermatologic findings that can be seen include sebaceous adenomas, epitheliomas, carcinomas, and multiple keratoacanthomas.[53] These patients require surveillance colonoscopies as well as annual dermatologic follow-up and skin examinations.[54]

FAP is characterized by innumerable adenomatous polyps found in the colon, and carries an increased risk of colon cancer. It is caused by a mutation in the APC gene located on chromosome 5.[55] Gardner syndrome is a variant of FAP, and is associated with cutaneous manifestations, including lipomas, desmoid tumors, and epidermoid cysts. Epidermoid cysts are usually multiple, typically manifesting on the extremities or face, and can predate the appearance of intestinal polyps. Desmoid tumors may occur abdominally or extra-abdominally, especially in the inguinal region; these will appear as firm, well-circumscribed, nontender tumors. Similar to LS, FAP confers an increased risk for the development of colorectal cancer as well as noncolonic malignancies, and these include duodenal, liver, adrenal, thyroid, and brain malignancies.[56]

PJS is caused by a germline mutation in the STK11 gene on chromosome 19. It is characterized by hamartomatous polyposis, and PJS is associated with colorectal, small bowel, pancreatic, and gastric malignancies, as well as breast, uterine, and testicular cancer.[57,58] Cutaneous manifestations can be seen in 95% of patients with PJS and include mucocutaneous hyperpigmentation, small (1 to 5 mm) melanocytic macules. These lesions may be found on the mouth, nostrils, as well as dorsal and volar aspects of the hands and feet. They often precede the development of GI malignancy.

Cowden syndrome, known as multiple hamartoma syndrome, is caused by an abnormality in the phosphatase and tensin homolog (PTEN) tumor suppressor gene located on chromosome 10.[59] It is characterized by multiple hamartomas (in multiple organs), dermatologic findings, and an increased risk of colon, breast, and thyroid cancers.[60] The cutaneous findings include acral keratoses, facial papules, and oral papillomatosis. It has a female predominance. In the GI tract, it typically affects the colon, stomach, and esophagus. Mucocutaneous findings can be seen in almost all patients. Acral keratoses and keratosis punctata (on the palms and soles) are some of the more common findings in the lower extremities, but multiple other skin findings can be encountered.[61] Juvenile polyposis syndrome is another genetic hamartomatous polyposis syndrome, related to mutations in SMAD4 and BMPR1A genes. It can present with multiple juvenile polyps as well as hereditary hemorrhagic telangiectasias and digital clubbing.[57] Cronkhite–Canada syndrome is also characterized by GI polyposis and commonly involves nail dystrophy in up to 98% of all patients. Nail findings can include onycholysis, onychomadesis, and thinning and splitting of the nail bed. In addition, it can cause diffuse hyperpigmentation, especially in the soles, palms, and face. Additional symptoms include nausea, vomiting, diarrhea, and weight loss. It is typically seen in individuals in their fifties and affects those with Asian and European descent.[62,63]

Paraneoplastic Syndromes and GI Malignancies

GI malignancies may be associated with paraneoplastic-related skin manifestations that are important to recognize, as they may be the first presenting sign of a malignancy.[50] Gastric adenocarcinoma has been associated with palmoplantar keratoderma that is characterized by epidermal thickening leading to broad ridges and deep sulci in the palms and soles.[64] The sign of Leser–Trélat is the acute onset of multiple, eruptive seborrheic keratoses and may be secondary to an underlying GI malignancy (colon and stomach most commonly) in up to one-third of cases. This presents initially on the trunk and can spread to the extremities.[65] Bazex syndrome, also referred to as acrokeratosis paraneoplastica, is a rare acral psoriasiform dermatosis that may be associated with a GI malignancy (including squamous cell carcinoma of the esophagus and gastric cancer). It can present as erythematous plaques with scaling, hyperpigmentation, palmoplantar keratoderma, paronychia, and onycholysis. One may also see bulbous enlargement of distal phalanges with nail dystrophy.[66] Tylosis is also associated with palmoplantar hyperkeratosis and typically involves more than 50% of the acral surfaces, and has been associated with esophageal carcinoma.[67]

Glucagonomas, a glucagon-secreting pancreatic tumor, has a well-known association with necrolytic migratory erythema (NME). NME is characterized by painful and pruritic erythematous lesions, with central blisters and erosions, as well as hyperpigmentation. It can also be associated with brittle nails. NME in the absence of a glucagonoma can be seen in IBD, pancreatitis, nonpancreatic malignancies, cirrhosis, and intestinal malabsorption syndrome.

NUTRITIONAL DEFICIENCIES

The GI system is the main site for the absorption of essential micro- and macronutrients. Deficiencies of these nutrients may be secondary to malabsorption (secondary to CD, UC, prior surgeries including gastric bypass, pancreatic insufficiency) or poor intake (which may be secondary to anorexia, alcoholism, diets). Malabsorption might also result in poor absorption of vitamins, even when ingested in what should be adequate amounts. Vitamin A deficiency can result in phrynoderma—keratotic follicular papules on the anterolateral thighs. Vitamin A toxicity can also result in perifollicular hemorrhages. Chronic vitamin D deficiency can lead to osteomalacia and osteoporosis. A deficiency in vitamin B_3 (Niacin) can lead to pellagra; the classic tetrad of pellagra includes dermatitis, dementia, diarrhea, and death. The dermatitis can present as a bilateral, symmetric eruption that may be pruritic. Over time, the lesions may develop vesicles that coalesce into bullae, eventually becoming sharply marginated, keratotic, hyperpigmented plaques. Zinc deficiency can lead to acrodermatitis enteropathica, which is the clinical triad of diarrhea, alopecia, and periorificial and acral cutaneous eruption. One may see symmetric eczematous plaques that can progress into pustular and erosive plaques. In mild deficiency, one may see psoriasiform dermatitis.[68] Vitamin C deficiency, which is responsible for scurvy, can lead to splinter hemorrhages in the nail, perifollicular hemorrhages, and fractured, coiled hair.[69] Vitamin K deficiency may present with ecchymosis of the lower extremities, as a result of inability of the liver to synthesize vitamin K–dependent clotting factors.[70] Individuals with low albumin may present with lower extremity edema; this can be seen in patients with IBD (secondary to protein-losing enteropathy) or patient with cirrhosis (secondary to malnutrition and decreased liver synthesis of albumin). Low albumin can also impair wound healing.[71]

Vitamin deficiencies and malnutrition can also be responsible for the development of neurologic disease. Acute and chronic pancreatitis, as well as pancreatic adenocarcinoma, can lead to malabsorption of essential vitamins and minerals, which can lead to peripheral neuropathy secondary to vitamin deficiency. Active ileal CD or prior surgical resection of the ileum (in a patient with CD) can also lead to a deficiency of cobalamine (vitamin B_{12}). Vitamin B_{12} is absorbed in the ileum, and if the ileum is inflamed or has been removed, vitamin B_{12} deficiency can develop. When this happens, affected individuals can develop subacute combined posterior degeneration, a late-term myelopathy that leads to a loss of sensory and proprioceptive nerves. Other vitamin deficiencies with lower extremity neurologic manifestations include thiamine (vitamin B_1) and pyridoxine (vitamin B_6), both of which can lead to a polyneuropathy.[3,7]

RHEUMATOLOGIC ASSOCIATIONS

Rheumatologic manifestations of GI disorders can be encountered fairly commonly in clinical practice. The following will be a brief overview on some of the lower extremity rheumatologic findings one might see in individuals with primary GI disorders. There can also be GI symptoms in patients with primarily rheumatologic disorders, but that will not be covered in this chapter.

Spondyloarthropathies can occur in approximately 20% of patients with IBD, and this often includes peripheral arthritis of the lower extremities. Peripheral arthropathies may present in two ways. Type 1 is acute, self-limited, and typically affects fewer than five joints. Type 2 is chronic, symmetric, bilateral, and it often affects five or more joints (often small joints). Pauciarticular arthritis often parallels the underlying gut disease activity, whereas polyarticular arthritis does not.[72] Whipple disease, which is caused by *Tropheryma whippelii*, is a multisystem disorder that can present with polyarthritis (often symmetric and seronegative), lymphadenopathy, fever, and abdominal pain. One may see a positive periodic acid–Schiff stain on a duodenal biopsy (with intracytoplasmic inclusions); one may even see *T. whippelii* DNA on duodenal biopsy.[73] In reactive arthritis, affected individuals may have experienced a preceding GI infection, often *Yersinia* or *Salmonella*.[74] Hereditary hemochromatosis, an autosomal recessive disorder most commonly caused by a genetic defect of the HFE gene, leads to increased iron absorption and storage in the body. These patients develop arthritis secondary to iron deposition in the joints. They may also develop bronze discoloration of the skin, heart failure, diabetes, and cirrhosis, among other complications of iron deposition.

Furthermore, hepatitis B and C can also present with a polyarthritis. Hepatitis B may present with small joint polyarthritis, thought to be caused by immune complexes. Hepatitis C, as mentioned earlier, can be associated with cryoglobulinemia, which may present with the clinical triad of arthralgias, purpura, and weakness. It is important to think about underlying and concurrent GI disorders when performing a diagnostic workup for patients with arthritis and arthralgias.[75]

CONCLUSION

Primary GI disease can manifest with lower extremity symptoms. Recognition of these findings is important, as some may be presenting symptoms and signs of the primary disorder (such as in IBD or a familial polyposis syndrome), whereas others may reflect worsening of the GI disorder (including side effects from malnutrition). Close collaboration among health care providers is essential when taking care of patients with these disorders.

REFERENCES

1. Thoreson R, Cullen J. Pathophysiology of inflammatory bowel disease: an overview. *Surg Clin North Am.* 2007;87(3):575–585.
2. Ardizzone S, Puttini P, Cassinotti A, et al. Extraintestinal manifestations of inflammatory bowel disease. *Dig Liver Dis.* 2008;40:S253–S259.
3. Ferro J, Oliveira S. Neurologic manifestations of gastrointestinal and liver diseases. *Curr Neurol Neurosci Rep.* 2014;14(10):487.
4. Lossos A, River Y, Eliakim A, et al. Neurologic aspects of inflammatory bowel disease. *Neurology.* 1995;45(3):416–421.
5. Oliveira G, Teles B, Brasil É, et al. Peripheral neuropathy and neurological disorders in an unselected Brazilian population-based cohort of IBD patients. *Inflamm Bowel Dis.* 2008;14(3):389–395.

6. Cassella G, Tontini GE, Bassotti G, et al. Neurological disorders and inflammatory bowel diseases. *World J Gasteroenterol.* 2014;20(27):8764–8782.

7. Hwang C, Ross V, Mahadevan U. Micronutrient deficiencies in inflammatory bowel disease: from A to zinc. *Inflamm Bowel Dis.* 2012;18(10):1961–1981.

8. Singh S, Kumar N, Loftus E, et al. Neurologic complications in patients with inflammatory bowel disease. *Inflamm Bowel Dis.* 2013;19(4):864–872.

9. Gupta G, Gelfand J, Lewis J. Increased risk for demyelinating diseases in patients with inflammatory bowel disease. *Gastroenterology.* 2005;129(3):819–826.

10. Morís G. Inflammatory bowel disease: an increased risk factor for neurologic complications. *World J Gastroenterol.* 2014;20(5):1228–1237.

11. Thomas C, Weinshenker B, Sandborn W. Demyelination during anti-tumor necrosis factor α therapy with infliximab for Crohn's disease. *Inflamm Bowel Dis.* 2004;10(1):28–31.

12. Sacher M, Gopfrich H, Hochberger O. Crohn's disease penetrating into the spinal canal. *Acta Paediatr Scand.* 1989;78(4):647–649.

13. Hershkowitz S, Link R, Ravden M, et al. Spinal empyema in Crohn's disease. *J Clin Gastroenterol.* 1990;12(1):67–69.

14. Thomas D. Global control of hepatitis C: where challenge meets opportunity. *Nat Med.* 2013;19(7):850–858.

15. Grebely J, Page K, Sacks-Davis R, et al. The effects of female sex, viral genotype, and IL28B genotype on spontaneous clearance of acute hepatitis C virus infection. *Hepatology.* 2013;59(1):109–120.

16. Stübgen J. Neuromuscular diseases associated with chronic hepatitis C virus infection. *J Clin Neuromuscul Dis.* 2011;13(1):14–25.

17. Himoto T, Masaki T. Extrahepatic manifestations and autoantibodies in patients with hepatitis C virus infection. *Clin Dev Immunol.* 2012;2012:1–11.

18. Kadanali A, Kızılkaya M, Tan H, et al. An unusual presentation of hepatitis A virus infection: Guillain–Barré syndrome. *Trop Doct.* 2006;36(4):248–248.

19. Berger J. Guillain-Barré syndrome complicating acute hepatitis B. A case with detailed electrophysiological and immunological studies. *Arch Neurol.* 1981;38(6):366–368.

20. Mehndiratta M, Pandey S, Nayak R, et al. Acute onset distal symmetrical vasculitic polyneuropathy associated with acute hepatitis B. *J Clin Neurosci.* 2013;20(2):331–332.

21. Stübgen J. Neuromuscular disorders associated with hepatitis B virus infection. *J Clin Neuromuscul Dis.* 2011;13(1):26–37.

22. Sureka B, Bansal K, Patidar Y, et al. Neurologic manifestations of chronic liver disease and liver cirrhosis. *Curr Probl Diagn Radiol.* 2015;44(5):449–461.

23. Kappelman M, Horvath-Puho E, Sandler R, et al. Thromboembolic risk among Danish children and adults with inflammatory bowel diseases: a population-based nationwide study. *Gut.* 2011;60(7):937–943.

24. Zezos P, Kouklakis G, Saibil F. Inflammatory bowel disease and thromboembolism. *World J Gastroenterol.* 2014;20(38):13863–13878.

25. Barclay A, Keightley J, Horrocks I, et al. Cerebral thromboembolic events in pediatric patients with inflammatory bowel disease. *Inflamm Bowel Dis.* 2010;16(4):677–683.

26. DeFilippis EM, Barfield E, Leifer D, et al. Cerebral venous thrombosis in inflammatory bowel disease. *J Dig Dis.* 2015;16(2):104–108.

27. Scott T, Kronsten VT, Hughes RD, et al. Pathophysiology of cerebral oedema in acute liver failure. *World J Gastroenterol.* 2013;19(48):9240–9255.

28. White H. Neurologic manifestations of acute and chronic liver disease. *Continuum (Minneap Minn).* 2014;20:670–680.

29. Shawcross D, Wendon J. The neurological manifestations of acute liver failure. *Neurochem Int.* 2012;60(7):662–671.

30. Premkumar M, Bagchi A, Kapoor N, et al. Hepatic myelopathy in a patient with decompensated alcoholic cirrhosis and portal colopathy. *Case Reports Hepatol.* 2012;2012:735906.

31. Koo J, Lim Y, Myung S, et al. Hepatic myelopathy as a presenting neurological complication in patients with cirrhosis and spontaneous splenorenal shunt. *Korean J Hepatol.* 2008;14(1):89–96.

32. Fernández-Rodriguez R, Contreras A, De Villoria J, et al. Acquired hepatocerebral degeneration: clinical characteristics and MRI findings. *Eur J Neurol.* 2010;17(12):1463–1470.

33. Meissner W, Tison F. Acquired hepatocerebral degeneration. *Handb Clin Neurol.* 2011;100:193–197.

34. Maffeo E, Montuschi A, Stura G, et al. Chronic acquired hepatocerebral degeneration, pallidal T1 MRI hyperintensity and manganese in a series of cirrhotic patients. *Neurol Sci.* 2013;35(4):523–530.

35. Aggarwal A, Bhatt M. Chapter 43 – commonly used gastrointestinal drugs. In: Biller J, Ferro JM, eds, *Handbook of Clinical Neurology.* Vol 120. Elsevier; 2014:633–643.

36. Thrash B, Patel M, Shah K, et al. Cutaneous manifestations of gastrointestinal disease. *J Am Acad Dermatol.* 2013;68(2):211.e1–211.e33.

37. Farhi D, Cosnes J, Zizi N, et al. Significance of erythema nodosum and pyoderma gangrenosum in inflammatory bowel diseases. *Medicine.* 2008;87(5):281–293.

38. Callen J. Pyoderma gangrenosum. *The Lancet.* 1998;351(9102):581–585.

39. Reichrath J, Bens G, Bonowitz A, et al. Treatment recommendations for pyoderma gangrenosum: an evidence-based review of the literature based on more than 350 patients. *J Am Acad Dermatol.* 2005;53(2):273–283.

40. Pellicer Z, Santiago JM, Rodriguez A, et al. Management of cutaneous disorders related to inflammatory bowel disease. *Ann Gastroenterol.* 2012;25(1):21–26.

41. Iannone F, Scioscia C, Musio A, et al. Leucocytoclastic vasculitis as onset symptom of ulcerative colitis. *Ann Rheum Dis.* 2003;62(8):785–786.

42. Zlatanic J, Fleisher M, Sasson M, et al. Crohn's disease and acute leukocytoclastic vasculitis of skin. *Am J Gastroenterol.* 1996;91:2410–2413.

43. Cleynen I, Moerkercke W, Billiet T, et al. Characteristics of skin lesions associated with anti–tumor necrosis factor therapy in patients with inflammatory bowel disease. *Ann Intern Med.* 2015:10.

44. Long M, Martin C, Pipkin C, et al. Risk of melanoma and non-melanoma skin cancer among patients with inflammatory bowel disease. *Gastroenterology.* 2012;143(2):390.e1–399.e1.

45. Solem CA, Loftus EV, Tremaine WJ, et al. Venous thromboembolism in inflammatory bowel disease. *Am J Gastroenterol.* 2004;99:97–101.

46. Zitomersky N, Verhave M, Trenor C. Thrombosis and inflammatory bowel disease: a call for improved awareness and prevention. *Inflamm Bowel Dis.* 2011;17(1):458–470.

47. Collin P, Reunala T. Recognition and management of the cutaneous manifestations of celiac disease. *Am J Clin Dermatol.* 2003;4(1):13–20.

48. Marietta E, Black K, Camilleri M, et al. A new model for dermatitis herpetiformis that uses HLA-DQ8 transgenic NOD mice. *J Clin Invest.* 2004;114(8):1090–1097.

49. Caproni M, Antiga E, Melani L, et al. Guidelines for the diagnosis and treatment of dermatitis herpetiformis. *J Eur Acad Dermatol Venereol.* 2009;23(6):633–638.

50. Shah K, Boland C, Patel M, et al. Cutaneous manifestations of gastrointestinal disease. *J Am Acad Dermatol.* 2013;68(2):189.e1–189.e21.

51. Vasen H, Blanco I, Aktan-Collan K, et al. Revised guidelines for the clinical management of Lynch syndrome (HNPCC): recommendations by a group of European experts. *Gut.* 2013;62(6):812–823.

52. Lynch H, Lynch P, Lanspa S, et al. Review of the Lynch syndrome: history, molecular genetics, screening, differential diagnosis, and medicolegal ramifications. *Clin Genet.* 2009;76(1):1–18.

53. Ponti G, Ponz de Leon M. Muir-Torre syndrome. *Lancet Oncol.* 2005;6:980–987.

54. Cohen P, Kohn R, Kurzrock R. Association of sebaceous gland tumors and internal malignancy: the muir-torre syndrome. *Am J Med*. 1991;90(5):606–613.

55. Doxey B, Kuwada S, Burt R. Inherited polyposis syndromes: molecular mechanisms, clinicopathology, and genetic testing. *Clin Gastroenterol Hepatol*. 2005;3(7):633–641.

56. Jasperson K, Tuohy T, Neklason D, et al. Hereditary and familial colon cancer. *Gastroenterology*. 2010;138(6):2044–2058.

57. Schreibman I, Baker M, Amos C, et al. The hamartomatous polyposis syndromes: a clinical and molecular review. *Am J Gastroenterol*. 2005;100(2):476–490.

58. Beggs A, Latchford A, Vasen H, et al. Peutz-Jeghers syndrome: a systematic review and recommendations for management. *Gut*. 2010;59(7):975–986.

59. Jung I, Gurzu S, Turdean GS. Current status of familial gastrointestinal polyposis syndromes. *World J Gastrointest Oncol*. 2015;7(11):347–355.

60. Blumenthal G, Dennis P. PTEN hamartoma tumor syndromes. *Eur J Hum Genet*. 2008;16(11):1289–1300.

61. Farooq A, Walker LJ, Bowling J, et al. Cowden syndrome. *Cancer Treat Rev*. 2010;36:577–583.

62. Cronkhite L, Canada W. Generalized gastrointestinal polyposis. *New Engl J Med*. 1955;252(24):1011–1015.

63. Ward E, Wolfsen H. The non-inherited gastrointestinal polyposis syndromes. *Aliment Pharmacol Therapeut*. 2002;16(3):333–342.

64. Breathnach S, Wells G. Acanthosis palmaris: tripe palms. A distinctive pattern of palmar keratoderma frequently associated with internal malignancy. *Clin Exp Dermatol*. 1980;5(2):181–189.

65. Ponti G, Luppi G, Losi L, et al. Leser-Trélat syndrome in patients affected by six multiple metachronous primitive cancers. *J Hematol Oncol*. 2010;3(1):2.

66. Pecora AL, Landsman L, Imgrund SP, et al. Acrokeratosis paraneoplastica (Bazex' syndrome). Report of a case and review of the literature. *Arch Dematol*. 1983;119:820–826.

67. Varela A, Blanco Rodríguez M, Boullosa P, et al. Tylosis A with squamous cell carcinoma of the oesophagus ina Spanish family. *Eur J Gastroenterol Hepatol*. 2011;23(3):286–288.

68. Heath M, Sidbury R. Cutaneous manifestations of nutritional deficiency. *Curr Opin Pediatr*. 2006;18(4):417–422.

69. Nguyen R, Cowley D, Muir J. Scurvy: a cutaneous clinical diagnosis. *Australas J Dermatol*. 2003;44(1):48–51.

70. Barthelemy H, Chouvet B, Cambazard F. Skin and mucosal manifestations in vitamin deficiency. *J Am Acad Dermatol*. 1986;15(6):1263–1274.

71. Doweiko J, Nompleggi D. Role of albumin in human physiology and pathophysiology. *JPEN J Parenter Enteral Nutr*. 1991;15(2):207–211.

72. Brown S, Coviello L. Extraintestinal manifestations associated with inflammatory bowel disease. *Surg Clin North Am*. 2015;95(6):1245–1259.

73. Meunier M, Puechal X, Hoppe E, et al. Rheumatic and musculoskeletal features of whipple disease: a report of 29 cases. *J Rheumatol*. 2013;40(12):2061–2066.

74. Trabulo D, Mangualde J, Cremers I, et al. Reactive arthritis mimicking inflammatory bowel disease arthritis: a challenging diagnosis. *Acta Reumatol Port*. 2014;39(2):188–192.

75. Braun J, Sieper J. Rheumatologic manifestations of gastrointestinal disorders. *Curr Opin Rheumatol*. 1999;11:68–74.

CHAPTER 19

Acute Emergencies Related to Systemic Disease and How They Present in the Lower Extremity

EDWARD AMORES • RAHUL SHARMA

Several acute conditions occurring secondary to systemic disease processes may manifest in the lower extremities. Many patients who present to an Emergency Department, Urgent Care Center, or other acute care setting with a chief complaint of gait instability, leg weakness, ankle pain, foot paresthesias, or other symptoms may, in actuality, be suffering from a systemic illness. Although some findings are pathognomonic for specific diseases, others may be found in association with a multitude of processes. Further, pathology evident in the lower extremities may represent the entire symptomatology of a particular disease, or may encompass only a small portion of the findings evident on the complete physical exam of a patient with a given systemic illness.

In this chapter, we explore several different acute lower extremity findings, in the context of the systemic diseases they tend to occur in association with. Recognition of such lower extremity signs, symptoms, or findings as manifestations of specific systemic diseases may allow the astute clinician an opportunity to make diagnoses that might otherwise remain undetected or underdetected, and may also allow for treatment approaches that address the entire underlying disease state.

ACUTE LOWER EXTREMITY ARTERIAL OCCLUSION AS A MANIFESTATION OF ATHEROSCLEROTIC DISEASE

Atherosclerosis is a systemic disease process, where plaque formation leads to progressive narrowing of blood vessels and decreased tissue perfusion, and where the ever-present risk of sudden plaque rupture can cause sudden acute occlusion of arteries or veins, resulting in clinical emergencies such as cerebrovascular accidents, acute myocardial infarctions, abdominal aortic aneurysms, and limb ischemia.

Sudden occlusion of one or more arteries supplying the lower extremities can occur through several different extrinsic mechanisms, including embolic phenomena, external compression, tourniquetting, or compartment syndrome; the primary intrinsic mechanism whereby lower extremity arterial flow is compromised occurs with acute thrombosis of plaques within these arteries. Acute lower extremity arterial occlusion is often a pathognomonic sign of atherosclerotic disease.

Presentation

Patients will typically present acutely with complaints of pain and coolness to touch, and possibly mottling. Chief complaints registered in triage often include the terms "cool foot," or the more concerning "cold foot."

Signs and Symptoms

The six Ps classically associated with acute limb ischemia include pain, pallor, pulselessness, poikilothermia, paralysis, and paresthesias. However, it should be noted that patients presenting with acute limb ischemia may exhibit any combination of these signs and symptoms, or none at all. During the late stages of presentation, the clinician may note a mottled appearance to the affected leg, difficulty or inability to palpate a dorsalis pedis or posterior tibial pulse, and decreased tactile temperature. Swelling is commonly seen with venous occlusion, but can be seen with arterial occlusion as well.

Tests

Blood flow studies are useful when evaluating suspected arterial occlusions, but should not delay expert vascular consultation and expedited restoration of flow. Doppler ultrasound is used to visualize arterial flow or the lack thereof, whereas plethysmography is used to compare blood pressures in the ankles to blood pressures in the arms. Dividing the former by the latter gives a ratio known as the ankle-brachial index, which should be 0.9 or higher to be considered normal.[1] Lab studies, including a blood type and screen, and coagulation assays should also be sent.

Treatments and Therapies

Although progressive narrowing of arterial lumina in atherosclerotic disease is typically associated with worsening symptomatic claudication, sudden complete obstruction of lower extremity arterial vasculature represents a surgical emergency, and consultation with a vascular surgeon should be immediately obtained. Vessel bypass grafting, luminal stenting, and peripheral artery thrombolysis are methods used to restore blood flow, and to potentially to save a gravely threatened limb. Heparin administration should also be considered in order to limit the propagation of the thrombus and to protect collateral circulation. Atherectomy is a less commonly used technique for restoration of blood flow to compromised lower extremities.

Vessel bypass grafting involves restoration of blood flow by connecting a portion of the vessel proximal to an occlusion to a portion of the vessel distal to an occlusion. Synthetic vessel materials are often used to bridge across the occluded portion of the vessel.

Vessel stenting involves inserting a tube-like scaffold structure percutaneously into a vessel to ensure adequate flow through the vessel lumen. Stenting is often coupled with balloon angioplasty, to dilate the occluded vessel simultaneously as the stent is deployed.

Peripheral artery thrombolysis involves administration of a fibrinolytic agent near, or directly into, an arterial thrombus. Studies have demonstrated greater efficacy when the agent is delivered into the thrombus, and decreased risk of hemorrhage with intra-arterial over intravenous infusion.[2]

Atherectomy involves removal of atherosclerotic plaque from blood vessels, typically using catheter devices that cleave the plaque from the endoluminal walls. This technique differs from balloon angioplasty in that the plaque is cut away from the vessel rather than pressed into its walls.

A prior Cochrane systematic review comparing surgery to thrombolysis for the initial management of acute limb ischemia showed neither approach was superior in preventing limb amputation or death within 1 year; however, thrombolysis was associated with a higher risk of ongoing ischemia and of hemorrhagic complications.[3]

ACUTE LOWER EXTREMITY JOINT PAIN SECONDARY TO RHEUMATOID ARTHRITIS

Rheumatoid arthritis (RA) is an autoimmune disease, with both intra-articular and extra-articular manifestations. Intra-articular manifestations represent sequelae of inappropriate immune system activation against synovial tissue, with progressive destruction of joint articular surface linings and painful swelling that often limits joint range of motion.

Genetic predisposition appears to play a role in approximately half of all RA cases,[4] and many potential environmental RA triggers are thought to exist, including cigarette smoking.

Although a definitive cause of RA is not known, evolving appreciation for the interplay between genetic and environmental factors holds future promise for disease prevention.[5]

In the extremities, the synovial destruction of RA can manifest with decreased range of motion, painful joint swelling, and eventual deformation of joint angles. In advanced lower extremity disease, altered stance, abnormal gait, and asymmetric posture are often seen, and can place serious limitations on exercise tolerance and activities of daily living.

Presentation

Patients will typically present acutely with complaints of joint pain and swelling, although constitutional symptoms such as fever and malaise may precede focal joint symptoms. Patients who are aware of a diagnosis of RA may repeatedly present for care related to inadequately controlled pain. Episodic flares can prove particularly troublesome for some patients.

Signs and Symptoms

RA is characterized by both specific and nonspecific signs and symptoms; examples of the former include symmetric synovial inflammation affecting upper and lower extremity joints, progressive joint destruction, and extra-articular manifestations such as rheumatoid nodules on the skin. Examples of nonspecific signs and symptoms are numerous, and may be difficult to attribute directly to the presence of RA, because many of these same signs and symptoms are vague and identical to those found in many other disease states. Fever, malaise, weakness, and fatigue are examples of nonspecific RA symptoms.

Tests

Genetic testing can potentially reveal genes associated with RA. Higher incidence of human leukocyte antigen subsets has been found in RA patients compared to controls.[6] Autoantibodies such as rheumatoid factor, antinuclear antibodies, and the more specific anti-citrullinated protein antibodies (ACPAs) are also used to detect RA disease, although it is recognized that ACPA negative patients that develop RA may belong to a different RA patient subset. Several newer biomarkers of RA disease are currently being explored.

Radiography is the mainstay of serial surveillance in RA[7] and is used primarily to assess narrowing of joint spaces, alterations in joint alignment, development of articular surface erosions, and also to reveal fractures and dislocations (**Fig. 19-1**).

Magnetic resonance imaging allows for greater detail in evaluating joint pathology and earlier detection of disease, but is more time-consuming and costly. Ultrasonography is increasingly used to assess joint effusions, tendons, synovial surfaces, and other structures,[8] but is limited in that the quality of the images obtained are typically very operator dependent.

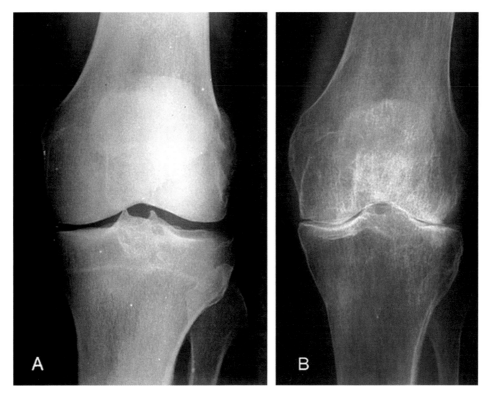

FIGURE 19-1. Knee joint space narrowing secondary to arthritis. (From Yochum TR, Rowe LJ. *Yochum and Rowe's Essentials of Skeletal Radiology.* 3rd ed. Philadelphia, PA: Lippincott Williams & Wilkins; 2004, with permission.)

Joint aspiration to obtain synovial fluid allows for laboratory assessment to help exclude joint sepsis, as well as crystalline arthritides as the precipitant cause of joint pain and swelling. Often, the white blood cell count level is useful to help distinguish inflammation from infection; a leukocyte count numbering below 50,000 per mL is expected in the former, whereas a cell count greater than 50,000 per mL is expected in the latter. Additionally, Gram stain or synovial fluid culture can further elucidate the infectious source in a suspected septic joint.[9]

Aspiration of joint fluid can also prove therapeutic, as patients will often note symptomatic relief with joint capsule decompression. Strict adherence to aseptic technique must be taken to avoid introducing infection into joint spaces.

Treatments and Therapies

Modern approaches to treatment of RA are focused on both symptomatic control and slowing of disease progression. Nonpharmacologic approaches include dietary control, regular exercise, physical therapy, and surgery. A recent Cochrane review examining the effects of dietary manipulation on symptom relief in patients with RA concluded that due primarily to study size limitations, the effects are still uncertain.[10] Pharmacologic therapies include nonsteroidal anti-inflammatory drugs (NSAIDs), oral and injected corticosteroids, disease-modifying antirheumatologic drugs (DMARDs), and immunosuppressive agents. Although the

American College of Rheumatology released its updated recommendations for the pharmacologic approach to treating RA,[11] most patients would benefit from a treatment regimen that incorporates several pharmacologic and nonpharmacologic approaches.

ACUTE LOWER EXTREMITY PATHOLOGIC FRACTURES SECONDARY TO METASTATIC MALIGNANT DISEASE

Malignant diseases include both "solid" tumors arising in tissue parenchyma and "liquid" tumors arising in the bloodstream. Spread of cancerous metastases to bone is common with primary lung, prostate, kidney, thyroid, and breast malignancies[12]; bony involvement is also common in multiple myeloma, and can be seen in association with lymphoma and leukemia. Although benign bone lesions can also compromise the structural integrity of bones comprising the appendicular skeleton, metastatic malignant disease must always be considered with sudden transverse femoral or tibial fractures precipitated by application of minimal force.

Malignancies metastatic to bone may weaken its architecture, often by stimulating osteoclasts that break down healthy bone tissue and release calcium into the blood. Metastases can also stimulate osteoblastic activity, causing abnormal bone growth. Diseased bone may have focal points of weakness, where minimal rather than substantial force may prove sufficient to fracture long bones.

Presentation

Patients will typically present complaining of long bone deformity and severe pain, sudden in onset after exposure to minimal force. Patients may report occurrence during an otherwise normal preceding activity, such as jogging, walking, or cutting to change direction while running. Patients with pathologic lower extremity fractures may report suddenly falling down, with subsequent inability to ambulate. Some patients will be unaware of an underlying cancer diagnosis at the time of presentation; therefore, the clinician's index of suspicion must remain high when caring for patients with long bone fractures who give a history of minimal preceding trauma.

Signs and Symptoms

Before presenting acutely with long bone fractures, patients with malignancies metastatic to bone may present with constitutional symptoms common to many cancers, or with symptomatology specific to the given primary cancer. Patients with malignancies metastatic to the long bones of the lower extremities may also note thigh pain, foreleg pain, or pain in one or more joints. Additionally, some patients may exhibit signs and symptoms of hypercalcemia secondary to osteoclast activity.

Tests

Radiologic tests can often reveal irregularities consistent with metastatic disease in patients who suffer pathologic fractures, typically demonstrating a fracture line through the abnormal bone. Often noted is cortical thinning, endosteal reabsorption, and cystic-appearing lytic lesions. Plain films will often suffice to reveal the pathologic fracture, whereas advanced imaging, such as computed tomography (CT) or magnetic resonance imaging (MRI), can serve to provide additional details useful in planning fracture fixation (**Fig. 19-2**).

Radiographic imaging may also suggest to the examiner which or what type of primary malignancy may underlie a pathologic fracture, although a definitive diagnosis requires examination of the affected tissue under a microscope. Assessing for the primary malignancy in patients with pathologic bone fractures often involves laboratory testing aimed at measuring the biomarkers of specific malignant diseases, and other screening tests.

Several primary cancers are commonly associated with bony metastases, with cancers of the breast, prostate, and lung comprising over 80% of the malignancies metastatic to bone.[13] Abnormal screening tests for any of these cancers in patients who have suffered pathologic long bone fractures can lead to a presumptive cancer diagnosis. Examples of such tests include prostate-specific antigen levels to screen for prostate cancer, mammography or ultrasound to screen for breast cancer, low-dose CT scanning to screen for lung cancer, and urine cytology to screen for kidney cancer.

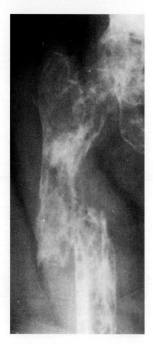

FIGURE 19-2. A pathologic femur fracture in a patient with lung cancer metastatic to bone. (Eisenberg RL. *An Atlas of Differential Diagnosis.* 4th ed. Philadelphia, PA: Lippincott Williams & Wilkins; 2003, with permission.)

Treatments and Therapies

Initially, the patient should be assessed for neurovascular compromise, and orthopedic consultation should be obtained immediately. Pain control and reduction and splinting of the affected extremity should be performed in a timely fashion. The definitive treatment of pathologic lower extremity long bone fractures is primarily orthopedic, focused on open reduction and internal fracture fixation using orthopedic hardware.

The general treatment of bony metastases may include radiation therapy and/or radioactive injection therapy to destroy cancer cells, bisphosphonate therapy to decrease the rate of bone reabsorption, and tumor ablative therapies.[14]

Treatment of the primary malignancy is often considered on a case-by-case basis, as pathologic fractures occurring secondary to malignant disease that has metastasized to bone are, by definition, associated with a tumor that has spread beyond its site of origin. Removal of a primary tumor that has already metastasized does not rid the body of cancer, and is often undertaken only for palliative reasons. The approach to treatment of the primary cancer in patients with pathologic fractures is therefore practically identical to the treatment of metastatic disease without fracture.

ACUTE LOWER EXTREMITY JOINT PAIN AND SWELLING AS A MANIFESTATION OF LYME DISEASE

Lyme disease, also known as borreliosis, is caused by bloodstream infection with *Borrelia burgdorferi*, a bacterium that infects mice and other mammals, and is often carried in the salivary glands of black-legged ticks of the *Ixodes* genus.[15] In the United States, *I. scapularis* and *I. pacificus* species serve as a vector of transmission to humans. Ticks acquire the infection while feeding on infected animals, and then transmit the infection to humans and other animals during subsequent feedings.

Patients who find a tick attached may take steps to remove the tick, and may also take a prophylactic antibiotic dose to prevent Lyme disease. Those who never notice the attached tick may be unaware of the possible exposure to *B. burgdorferi*, and may therefore never present to initiate early treatment. Should patients miss or fail to recognize early symptoms, such as the hallmark erythema migrans rash or the less specific influenza-like illness, they may instead present later with complaints related to disseminated infection, including pain in one or more joints.

Lyme arthritis is typically characterized as an intermittent oligoarticular arthritis primarily affecting large joints. The knees are the most commonly involved joints; painful swelling and decreased range of motion is often seen. Although initial arthritis symptoms may be due to active bacterial infection, chronic arthritis symptoms may be the sequelae of an inflammatory reaction to the causative bacteria in Lyme disease, causing damage to the cartilage lining joint articular surfaces; repeated cycles of inflammation might trigger progressive irreversible joint destruction that remains beyond the eradication of the bacterial infection.[16]

Presentation

Patients may present in the early stages of Lyme disease infection with vague complaints; only some will note the classic erythema migrans rash, described as a ring of erythema with central clearing. Patients may present in later stages of Lyme disease with diffuse myalgias, symptoms of Bell palsy, meningitis, atrioventricular conduction disturbance, and joint pains. A multitude of other symptoms may be seen in patients with Lyme disease, many of which are nonspecific and found in association with other illnesses. Often, making the diagnosis of Lyme disease requires a fairly high index of suspicion.

Signs and Symptoms

Clinicians may recognize the classic erythema migrans rash, or may elicit a history of potential tick exposure in patients with constitutional symptoms presenting in the early stages of Lyme disease infection. Practitioners in endemic areas may consider potential Lyme disease in nearly all patients with vague symptoms, whereas caregivers in areas where disease prevalence is low may fail to consider the possibility of Lyme disease early enough. Signs and symptoms of early Lyme disease may overlap those of viral syndromes, and can be easily missed or overlooked.

Nearly two-thirds of untreated patients will develop arthralgias, signaling progression from the first stage of Lyme disease to the second or third stage. Patients with early disseminated borreliosis may develop intermittent polyarticular arthritis affecting several large joints, typically progressing to monoarticular joint pain, most commonly affecting the knee joints.[17]

Tests

The Centers for Disease Control and Prevention (CDC) recommends a two-step approach to testing for the presence of Lyme disease, based on the idea that immunocompetent patients exposed to *B. burgdorferi* will subsequently develop antibodies to counter the infection, whereas patients not previously exposed will not carry these specific antibodies[18] (see Fig. 19-1). Enzyme-linked immunosorbent assay (ELISA) tests are considered reliable in excluding disease exposure when negative, but require confirmation when positive. Positive ELISA tests are followed by Western blot analysis, to ensure that the antibodies found through ELISA are truly directed against *B. burgdorferi* bacteria.

Polymerase chain reaction (PCR) can also be used to detect infection with *B. burgdorferi*, by replicating and amplifying bacterial DNA present in synovial and cerebrospinal fluid. However, PCR is error prone, and considered less reliable than serology for the detection of *B. burgdorferi* bacteria. PCR is not recommended by the CDC or cleared by the Food and Drug Administration[19] for the routine testing of potential Lyme disease patients.

Treatments and Therapies

Antibiotics are the mainstay of prophylaxis against and treatment of Lyme disease. Prophylaxis against Lyme disease seroconversion in adult patients, and in children aged 8 years or older weighing over 50 kg, who report removal of attached ticks within the past 72 hours, can be accomplished through the administration of a single 200 mg dose of doxycycline. Guidelines published by the Infectious Diseases Society of America also provide treatment regimens for both early and later stage Lyme disease.[20]

Symptomatic treatment of patients with negative PCR analysis of synovial fluid after appropriate antibiotic therapy noting persistent arthritis symptoms includes NSAIDs, intra-articular corticosteroid injections, and DMARDs. In refractory cases that fail to improve with the above measures, surgical synovectomy for amelioration of symptoms may be necessary (**Fig. 19-3**).[21]

ACUTE CALF PAIN AND SWELLING SECONDARY TO DEEP VENOUS THROMBOSIS AS A MANIFESTATION OF HYPERCOAGULABLE DISEASE STATES

Hypercoagulability describes an increased propensity to form clots within the circulatory system. Also known as thrombophilia, several genetic conditions are associated

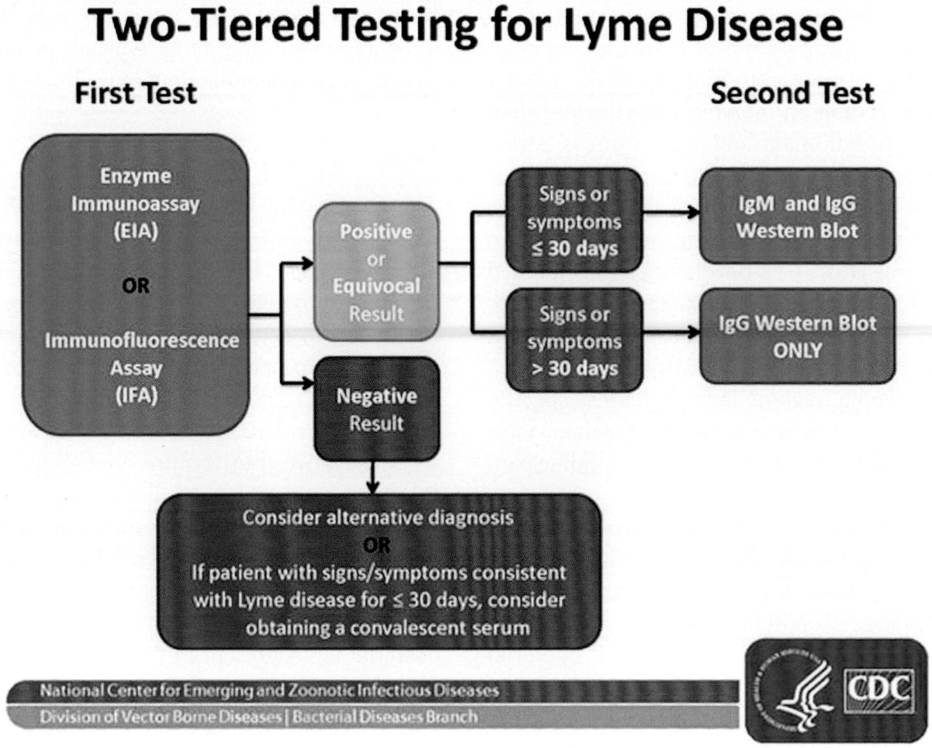

Two-Tiered Testing for Lyme Disease

First Test

Second Test

Enzyme Immunoassay (EIA)

OR

Immunofluorescence Assay (IFA)

→ Positive or Equivocal Result

→ Negative Result

Signs or symptoms ≤ 30 days → IgM and IgG Western Blot

Signs or symptoms > 30 days → IgG Western Blot ONLY

Consider alternative diagnosis

OR

If patient with signs/symptoms consistent with Lyme disease for ≤ 30 days, consider obtaining a convalescent serum

National Center for Emerging and Zoonotic Infectious Diseases
Division of Vector Borne Diseases | Bacterial Diseases Branch

CDC

FIGURE 19-3. CDC recommended approach to testing for suspected Lyme disease. (Obtained from http://www.cdc.gov/lyme/resources/twotieredtesting.pdf. Accessed January 17, 2017.)

with the prothrombotic state that defines hypercoagulability; numerous acquired risk factors for developing clots in the bloodstream have also been identified. Whether congenital or acquired, many hypercoagulable patients remain unaware of an increased risk of clot formation until after receiving an unexpected related diagnosis.

Although hypercoagulable disease states can increase the risk of thrombosis in both the arterial and venous circulatory subsystems, presenting symptoms may differ sufficiently to allow the clinician to surmise whether an arterial or venous thrombosis is the more likely cause of a patient's presentation. Patients with lower extremity deep venous thrombosis (DVT) will typically present with unilateral calf pain and swelling,[22] although symptoms may be minimal or absent. Patients may also note localized erythema and warmth that may appear clinically similar to cellulitis of the foreleg.

Patients with DVT of the lower extremity are at risk for embolization of the clot into the lungs.[23] More specifically, the thrombus may mobilize from the deep veins of the leg, traveling with deoxygenated blood through the right side of the heart into the pulmonary arteries. A very large pulmonary embolus (PE) that straddles the right and left pulmonary arteries is termed a saddle embolus, and may prove rapidly fatal if it completely impedes blood flow from the venous collecting system into the lungs, eliminating oxygen transfer and flow of oxygenated blood to the tissues.

DVT should be considered in patients presenting with complaints of calf pain and swelling, particularly if the patient

is known to have a disease associated with hypercoagulability or to have one or more prothrombotic risk factors. A high index of suspicion when evaluating patients with these symptoms may decrease the risk of missing the diagnosis.

Presentation

Patients with lower extremity DVT may present with any combination of calf pain, foreleg swelling, lower extremity erythema, and warmth, and the appearance of the affected lower extremity may closely resemble cellulitis (**Fig. 19-4**).

Patients with these complaints are at increased risk of pulmonary embolism, and may report additional symptomatology such as chest pain, dyspnea, or hemoptysis. Although patients with PE may report these or several other symptoms, it is important to note that some patients may remain asymptomatic, and clinicians must always consider the risk of silent embolization.

Signs and Symptoms

Patients may note any combination of calf pain, lower extremity swelling, localized erythema, and warmth, or may lack symptoms altogether. The physical exam alone is usually insufficient for either confirming or excluding a diagnosis of DVT, although clinicians may note calf pain on dorsiflexion of the foot, known as a positive Homan sign, in patients ultimately found to have a DVT. Nevertheless, although

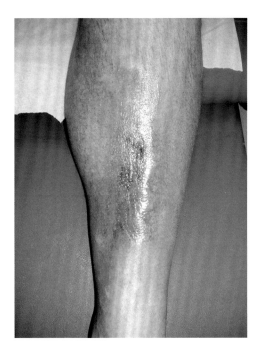

FIGURE 19-4. Postthrombotic leg ulcer. This photograph from a 50-year-old man with a history of DVT 2 years before demonstrates brownish hyperpigmentation of a large region of skin along the left calf. There is a small round ulcer within a central area of erythema and inflammation. The ankle region, and especially its medial aspect, is the most common site of venous leg ulcers, but they can also occur in the middle and lower calf, as depicted in the image. (From Geschwind J, Dake M. *Abrams' Angiography*. Philadelphia, PA: Wolters Kluwer; 2014, with permission.)

Table 19-1. Wells Score Criteria for Predicting the Probability of DVT		
Wells Score Estimates Probability of DVT		
The elements of the Wells score should be ascertained in the usual evaluation of a patient with suspected DVT.		
1 Point Each For: Active cancer Paralysis, paresis, recent plaster immobilization of lower limb Recently bedridden for >3 d or major surgery in past 4 wk Localized tenderness along distribution of deep venous system Entire leg swollen Calf swelling >3 cm compared to asymptomatic leg Pitting edema Collateral superficial veins		
−2 Points For: Alternative diagnosis as likely or more likely than that of DVT		
Probability:		
High	>3 points	
Intermediate	1 or 2 points	
Low	<0 points	

Obtained from http://www.ncbi.nlm.nih.gov/pmc/articles/PMC3183832/. Accessed January 17, 2017.

many potential causes of lower extremity pain and swelling are known to exist, DVT should always be considered in patients presenting with calf pain and swelling.

Tests

Ultrasonography is useful for detecting lower extremity DVT, and relies on identifying noncompressible portions of the venous anatomy. Ultrasound is limited in that it is operator dependent and is subject to error. A venogram also allows visualization of the venous circulation of the lower extremity, using radiographic imaging to detect flow of dye injected into the bloodstream.

Some clinicians use D-dimer assays that detect fibrin degradation products produced when clots are formed. Used in combination with a clinical decision tool known as The Wells score, these assays may serve to identify those patients who can safely forego Doppler imaging to reliably exclude DVT.

Lower sensitivity qualitative assays can safely exclude clot formation in patients deemed low risk by Wells score criteria, whereas higher sensitivity quantitative assays, with 98% sensitivity and a high negative predictive value, can exclude DVT in both low and moderate risk patients.[24] Both qualitative and quantitative D-dimer assays are considered unreliable in excluding clot formation in patients who are

considered to be at high risk of DVT, and should not be used in place of imaging studies in these patients (Table 19-1).

Treatments and Therapies

The treatment of lower extremity DVT is directed against extension and embolization of the clot. The mainstay of therapy is treatment with anticoagulants, designed to shift the balance between clot formation and clot dissolution from the former to the latter. Medications that shift this balance also increase the risk of unintended bleeding, which must be weighed on a case-by-case basis in patients with considerable bleeding risk, such as those who fall and injure themselves frequently.

In patients who cannot be adequately anticoagulated, because of fall risk or other reason, filters may be placed in the inferior vena cava to decrease the embolization risk. These filters are designed to trap larger clots that form in the lower extremities, serving as a physical barrier. Smaller clots may slip past the spokes of the filter however, and serve as a nidus for larger clot formation. In some cases, inferior vena cava filters are used in combination with anticoagulation to further decrease embolism risk.

Patients with newly diagnosed unexplained DVT will require a complete evaluation for hypercoagulable disorders, including testing for Protein C and Protein S deficiencies, the presence of Factor V Leiden, elevated homocysteine or fibrinogen levels, a mutation of the prothrombin gene, or one of several other congenitally acquired hypercoagulability disorders. Expeditious follow-up with the primary physician and prompt referral to a hematologist are recommended.

ACUTE ANKLE AND FOOT DEFORMITIES SECONDARY TO CHARCOT ARTHROPATHY AS A MANIFESTATION OF DIABETIC NEUROPATHY

Diabetes mellitus is a complex systemic disease process, with a multitude of potential manifestations and long-term sequelae, including diabetic neuropathies. Grouped broadly into autonomic, proximal, focal, and peripheral neuropathies,[25] diabetic neuropathies can cause a range of inappropriate symptoms, including autonomic dysfunction, muscle weakness, and paresthesias.

Diabetic patients who develop peripheral neuropathies may note paresthesias affecting the extremities, with the lower extremities typically affected before the upper extremities. These paresthesias may be characterized by pain, tingling, hypersensitivity to light touch, burning discomfort, and possibly decreased or altogether absent sensation to external stimuli. When patients lose the ability to appropriately sense painful or noxious stimuli, they may suffer injuries, yet remain unaware. The injuries suffered may be acute, such as immersion burn injuries, or indolent, such as progressive cellulitis secondary to skin abrasion or puncture injuries. Patients may fail to recognize these injuries until secondary symptoms are noted, as pain is either unappreciated or underappreciated.

Charcot arthropathy is a disease process whereby joint structures are progressively destroyed through repetitive injury occurring in the face of compromised sensation, such as those occurring in relation to the sensorimotor compromise noted with diabetic peripheral neuropathy. In the lower extremities, the term "Charcot foot" describes destruction of the joints of the ankle and foot, where fractures, dislocations, and loss of structural integrity can be seen in patients who lack the ability to feel pain, and who thus fail to modify or eliminate their exposure to the repetitive injuries, allowing damage to progress or accumulate. Although many disease processes are associated with peripheral neuropathies, and thus may be considered to be potential precipitants of a Charcot arthropathy, diabetes is widely considered to be one of the more common causes of peripheral neuropathy and the most common etiology of Charcot arthropathy.[26]

Presentation

Diabetic patients with Charcot arthropathy affecting the lower extremities may present with complaints of atraumatic ankle or foot pain, or instead with painless swelling, redness, and warmth, mimicking an infectious process. Patients may also note limited ability to bear weight, because of bony destruction leading to joint deformities and structural instability. Joint destruction may progress with continued attempted ambulation,

as the patient fails to recognize additional microtrauma or microfractures, further compromising joint stability.

Signs and Symptoms

During the initial destructive phase of Charcot neuropathic joint destruction, patients may note painful or painless swelling, redness, warmth, or trouble ambulating. During the subsequent convalescent phase, patients with Charcot arthropathy may actually note decreased swelling and warmth, although damage that has already occurred does not reverse itself, and can progress with continued weight-bearing activities. In the third reconstructive phase, healing begins, with fractured bones and deformed joints becoming somewhat more stable. Residual instability may persist, however, and deformities of the foot that developed in the earlier phases may increase the likelihood of developing ulcerative plantar lesions.[27]

Tests

Radiography is useful for assessing the bony destruction and potential joint compromise seen with Charcot arthropathy. Plain films can also be used to stage disease and to monitor progression (**Fig. 19-5**).

Bone scans may help differentiate neuropathic joint arthropathy from osteomyelitis; MRI imaging can provide greater anatomic detail and may also help differentiate Charcot arthropathy from osteomyelitis.

Laboratory tests have limited utility in evaluating Charcot arthropathy, although nonspecific markers of inflammation such as a complete blood count with differential, an erythrocyte sedimentation rate, or a C-reactive protein may indicate that infection is more likely than pure inflammation when elevated. Several other tests may help confirm or exclude the presence of diabetes, including glucose levels and glycosylated hemoglobin, as many other causes of neuropathic joint disease are known. In most cases, diabetics who develop Charcot arthropathy have had peripheral neuropathy for 10 to 15 years.[28]

Treatments and Therapies

The early treatment of Charcot arthropathy affecting the lower extremities is aimed at arresting progression of bony destruction and deformity. Serial contact casting using heavily padded plaster or other casting materials may control swelling, and limit progressive damage. Custom-made walking boots may serve a similar purpose. Limited weight-bearing may also play a role in restricting damage. Bisphosphonate therapy and calcitonin are currently debated as potentially useful adjuncts in the medical treatment of Charcot arthropathy.[29]

Surgical treatment may be required to stabilize unstable joints or to repair fractured bones. Amputation may be considered in cases where the feet are too damaged to allow weight-bearing, in which case prosthetic devices may be utilized. Patients should also be educated on how to protect

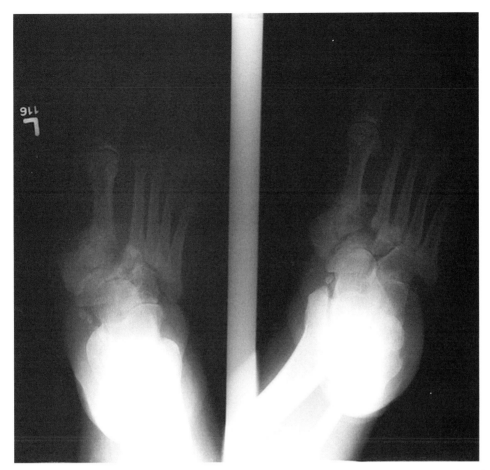

FIGURE 19-5. Radiographs of classic Charcot arthropathy showing bony projections, fractures, dislocations, bone disintegration, new bone formation, increased diastasis between metatarsal bases, and gross alteration in skeletal anatomy. (From Thordarson D. *Orthopaedic Surgery Essentials: Foot and Ankle.* Philadelphia, PA: Wolters Kluwer; 2012, with permission.)

the unaffected or lesser affected foot as it is more heavily loaded when the affected foot is made nonweight-bearing.

Specialized footwear and customized orthotics are often utilized in the long-term management of Charcot arthropathy. Patients should be closely followed to monitor for recurrent or worsening arthropathy symptoms, and to ensure that orthotics continue to fit well. Lastly, diabetic patients must also be followed closely by their primary physician and endocrinologist to optimize long-term glycemic control and diabetic disease management.

SUMMARY

Several systemic diseases may manifest wholly, or in part, with lower extremity findings. Recognition of the signs and symptoms involving the lower extremities that portend systemic illnesses often requires a high index of suspicion. Treating the primary disease processes that underlie the manifestations affecting the lower extremities is often necessary in order to adequately address the symptomatology that prompted a given patient to seek care. In those cases where patients are unaware of a yet undiagnosed systemic illness, education is necessary to ensure that the patient appreciates

how management of the primary disease can improve the overall outcome. Providing appropriate care beyond the initial presentation for acute symptomatology typically involves a concerted effort on the part of many providers, as well as collaboration from the patient receiving care, to maximize the overall outcome.

REFERENCES

1. Feringa HH, Bax JJ, van Waning VH, et al. The long-term prognostic value of the resting and postexercise ankle-brachial index. *Arch Intern Med.* 2006;166(5):529–535.
2. Kessel DO, Berridge DC, Robertson I. Infusion techniques for peripheral arterial thrombolysis. *Cochrane Database Syst Rev.* 2004;(1):CD000985.
3. Berridge DC, Kessel D, Robertson I. Surgery versus thrombolysis for acute limb ischaemia: initial management. *Cochrane Database Syst Rev.* 2013;(6):CD002784.
4. Barton A, Worthington J. Genetic susceptibility to rheumatoid arthritis: an emerging picture. *Arthritis Rheum.* 2009;61(10): 1441–1446.
5. Scott IC, Steer s, Lewis CM, et al. Precipitating and perpetuating factors of rheumatoid arthritis immunopathology—linking the triad of genetic predisposition, environmental risk factors and autoimmunity to disease pathogenesis. *Clin Rheum.* 2011;25(4):447–468.

6. Kapitany A, Zilahi E, Szanto S, et al. Association of rheumatoid arthritis with HLA-DR1 and HLA-DR4 in Hungary. *Ann N Y Acad Sci.* 2005;1051:263–270.

7. Van der Hejde DM. Radiographic imaging: the 'gold standard' for assessment of disease progression in rheumatoid arthritis. *Rheumatology.* 2000;39(1):9–16.

8. Wells AF, Haddad RH. Emerging role of ultrasonography in rheumatoid arthritis: optimizing diagnosis, measuring disease activity and identifying prognostic factors. *Ultrasound Med Biol.* 2011;37(8):1173–1184.

9. Faraj AA, Omonbude OD, Godwin P. Gram staining in the diagnosis of acute septic arthritis. *Acta Orthop Belg.* 2002;68(4):388–391.

10. Hagen KB, Byfuglien MG, Falzon L, et al. Dietary interventions for rheumatoid arthritis. *Cochrane Database Syst Rev.* 2009;(1):CD006400.

11. Singh JA, Furst DE, Bharat A, et al. 2012 update of the 2008 American College of Rheumatology recommendations for the use of disease-modifying antirheumatic drugs and biologic agents in the treatment of rheumatoid arthritis. *Arthritis Care Res.* 2012;64(5):625–639.

12. Feller L, Kramer B, Lemmer J. A short account of metastatic bone disease. *Cancer Cell Int.* 2011;11:24.

13. Maccauro G, Spinelli MS, Mauro S, et al. Physiopathology of spine metastasis. *Int J Surg Oncol.* 2011;2011:107969.

14. Coleman RE. Metastatic bone disease: clinical features, pathophysiology and treatment strategies. *Cancer Treat Rev.* 2001;27:165–176.

15. Burgdorfer W, Barbour AG, Hayes SF, et al. Lyme disease-a tick-borne spirochetosis? *Science.* 1982;216(4552):1317–1319.

16. Auwaerter PG. Point: antibiotic therapy is not the answer for patients with persisting symptoms attributable to lyme disease. *Clin Infect Dis.* 2007;45(2):143–148.

17. Girschick HJ, Morbach H, Tappe D. Treatment of lyme borreliosis. *Arthritis Res Ther.* 2009;11:258.

18. Lyme Disease. http://www.cdc.gov/lyme/. Updated August 2015. Accessed October 22, 2015.

19. Nelson C, Hojvat S, Johnson B, et al. Concerns regarding a new culture method for *Borrelia burgdorferi* not approved for the diagnosis of lyme disease. *MMWR Morb Mortal Wkly Rep.* 2014;63(15):333. http://www.cdc.gov/mmwr/preview/mmwrhtml/mm6315a4.htm?s_cid=mm6315a4_w. Accessed January 17, 2017.

20. Wormser GP, Dattwyler RJ, Shapiro ED, et al. The clinical assessment, treatment, and prevention of lyme disease, human granulocytic anaplasmosis, and babesiosis: clinical practice guidelines by the Infectious Diseases Society of America. *Clin Infect Dis.* 2006;43(9):1089–1134.

21. Smith BG, Cruz AI, Milewski MD, et al. Lyme disease and the orthopaedic implications of lyme arthritis. *J Am Acad Orthop Surg.* 2011;19(2):91–100.

22. Hirsh J, Lee AY. How we diagnose and treat deep vein thrombosis. *Blood.* 2002;99(9):3102–3110.

23. Kearon C. Natural history of venous thromboembolism. *Circulation.* 2003;107(23 Suppl 1):I22–I30.

24. Fancher TL, White RH, Kravitz RL. Combined use of rapid D-dimer testing and estimation of clinical probability in the diagnosis of deep vein thrombosis: systematic review. *BMJ.* 2004;329:821–824.

25. Boulton AJ, Vinik AI, Arezzo JC, et al. Diabetic neuropathies: a statement by the American Diabetes Association. *Diabetes Care.* 2005;28(4):956–962.

26. Rogers LC, Frykberg RG, Armstrong DG, et al. The charcot foot in diabetes. *Diabetes Care.* 2011;34(9):2123–2129.

27. van der Ven A, Chapman CB, Bowker JH. Charcot neuroarthropathy of the foot and ankle. *J Am Acad Orthop Surg.* 2009;17(9):562–571.

28. Tan AL, Greenstein A, Jarret SJ, et al. Acute neuropathic joint disease: a medical emergency? *Diabetes Care.* 2005;28(12):2962–2964.

29. Güven MF, Karabiber A, Kaynak G, et al. Conservative and surgical treatment of the chronic Charcot foot and ankle. *Diabet Foot Ankle.* 2013;4:21177.

CHAPTER 20

Foot Ulcers Associated with Hematologic Disorders

LEONARD A. LEVY

BACKGROUND

An often overlooked cause of lower extremity ulcers is diseases of the hematopoietic system. Although ulcers due to hematologic diseases are not as common as those due to venous and arterial disorders, podiatric physicians still need to include such conditions in their differential diagnosis. Ulcers of the foot and ankle secondary to blood dyscrasias may become more common as a result of modern medicine's ability to keep patients alive long enough to become victims of chronic diseases. Also, many pharmaceutical agents have among their side effects the ability to produce hematologic complications. The physician should not overlook hematologic disorders as being among the etiologic agents responsible for foot and ankle ulcers. Some of the conditions in which foot ulcers may occur associated with hematologic disorders are discussed.

SEVERITY OF FOOT AND LEG ULCERS

Many severity indices for foot and leg ulcers are based on size, depth, and duration. Staging based on depth is as follows:

- **Stage 1:** Nonblanchable erythema of intact skin, the heralding lesion of skin ulceration. In individuals with darker skin, discoloration of the skin, warmth, edema, induration, or hardness may also be indicators.
- **Stage 2:** Partial-thickness skin loss involving epidermis, dermis, or both. The ulcer is superficial and presents clinically as an abrasion, blister, or shallow crater.
- **Stage 3:** Full-thickness skin loss involving damage to or necrosis of subcutaneous tissue that may extend down to, but not through, underlying fascia. The ulcer presents clinically as a deep crater with or without undermining of adjacent tissue.
- **Stage 4:** Full-thickness skin loss with extensive destruction, tissue necrosis, or damage to muscle, bone, or supporting structures (e.g., tendon, joint capsule). Undermining and sinus tracts also may be present.

SICKLE CELL ANEMIA

Sickle cell anemia is an example of a hematologic disease that may cause ulcers affecting the lower extremities. The U.S. Cooperative Study of Sickle Cell Disease (SCD) reported that about 25% of patients with the disease over age 10 years had a history of leg ulcers.[1] The disease affects 50,000 to 100,000 people in the United States.[2] Its geographical distribution is variable, affecting 75% of patients in Jamaica but only 8% to 10% of North American patients.[3–5] Ulcers due to sickle cell anemia are less common in patients with α-gene deletion, high total hemoglobin level, or high levels of hemoglobin F. The pathogenesis of chronic ulcers in SCD is complex. Mechanical obstruction by dense sickled red cells, venous incompetence, bacterial infections, abnormal autonomic control with excessive vasoconstriction when in the dependent position, in situ thrombosis, anemia with decrease in oxygen carrying capacity, and decreased nitric oxide (NO) bioavailability leading to impaired endothelial function have all been proposed as potential contributing factors.[6,7] Patients have a marked reduction of NO, which is an important regulator of vascular tone, cell adhesion, and blood flow. This results in the development of a vasculopathy skewing the normal balance between vasoconstriction and vasodilatation in favor of vasoconstriction. As a result, there is NO deficiency leading to tissue ischemia and ulcer formation.[8] Ulcers are painful and often disabling complications of SCD, may affect 5% to 10% of adult patients, and may necessitate opioids. Those that are acute usually heal within a month, but those that are chronic may take 6 months. The SCD ulcers are more common in males and increase with age. Ulcers in sickle cell anemia typically occur in areas with thin skin and less subcutaneous fat, typically at the medial and lateral malleoli. However, sometimes the dorsum of the foot is affected as is the region over the Achilles tendon. These ulcers appear round and punched-out with raised margins, deep bases and necrotic slough varying in size from a few millimeters to large circumferential areas covering the entire distal lower extremity. The lesion is usually precipitated by minor trauma and spreads in size gradually.[9,10] Sickle cell anemia ulcers frequently are colonized with *Staphylococcus aureus*, *Pseudomonas aeruginosa*, and group A Streptococci. Typically patients with these ulcers develop wound infections which may be localized super-infections or recurrent cellulitis that heal slowly with residual hyperpigmentation and chronic scarring.[1]

Healing of this difficult to treat condition is reported as being 20 times slower than in similar types of refractory vascular lesions and is often recurrent.[11] Prevention includes the reduction of trauma with properly fitted shoes and compression stockings supported by application of emollients along with proper hygiene. When the ulcers occur moist, supportive dressing are indicated, but when they drain, absorbent dressing could be used. Topical antibiotics such as neomycin, polymyxin B, or bacitracin can be used if superinfection occurs. When there is necrotic tissue, debridement is indicated. There are reports that oral zinc sulfate accelerates healing.[12,13] The only Food and Drug Administration–approved treatment of sickle cell anemia–caused ulcers in adults is hydroxyurea, a cytotoxic, cytostatic drug also used for the prevention of the ulcers. Treatment with hydroxyurea starts with an initial dose of 15 mg per kg (10 to 20 mg per kg) once a day.[14] The dose may be increased in 5 mg/kg/day increments every 12 weeks to a maximum dose of 35 mg/kg/day. However, others suggest that hydroxyurea does not cause, prevent, or speed healing in SCD. Surgical intervention for recalcitrant ulcers using split-thickness skin grafting and myocutaneous flaps to bring blood supply to the area of ulceration has been used, but results are inconsistent.

ACUTE LEUKEMIA

In leukemia, specific or nonspecific lesions of the skin may occur. Specific lesions (leukemia cutis) contain leukemia cells, which directly infiltrate the epidermis, dermis, or subcutaneous fat. Nonspecific lesions, which are more common, are considered a cutaneous reaction to the ongoing malignancy process.

There have been reports of foot ulcers developing in children with newly diagnosed acute mixed lineage leukemia during induction chemotherapy. These ulcers may have a clinical resemblance to pyoderma gangrenosum, but on histopathologic examination, herpes simplex virus infection may be diagnosed. Treatment with oral acyclovir is ineffective, but the ulcer healed with intravenous acyclovir followed by oral valacyclovir. Viral infection remains an unusual but important cause of isolated extragenital cutaneous ulceration in the immunocompromised child.[15]

SPECIFIC LESIONS IN LEUKEMIA CUTIS

Leukemia cutis includes granulocytic sarcoma, chloroma, and myeloblastoma, representing localized or disseminated skin infiltration by blast cells. Leukemia cutis is usually a sign of relapse or dissemination of medullary disease. It is uncommon but is mostly found in people older than 50 years. Most often, it is associated with acute monocytic leukemia and acute myelomonocytic leukemia. It can be observed in any acute or chronic leukemia, including the leukemic phase of non-Hodgkin lymphoma and hairy cell leukemia. Skin pain, tenderness, and pruritus are usually absent, and most commonly, lesions are discrete, firm, violaceous or red-brown papules, nodules, or plaques. On occasion, ulcerative lesions are observed.

The differential diagnoses include bacterial, viral, and fungal dermatoses; drug eruptions; leukocytoclastic vasculitides; Sweet syndrome; and pyoderma gangrenosum. Leukemia cutis may occur simultaneously with or before the medullary disease. Leukemia cutis typically develops late in the course of established acute leukemia. In contrast, when it develops in association with chronic myelogenous leukemia or other myeloproliferative disorders, it is usually a sign of impending blastic transformation. Early cutaneous involvement occurs more frequently in acute myelomonocytic leukemia and monocytic leukemia. In addition, it is strongly associated with extramedullary involvement of other sites, including the meninges.

Histopathologically, leukemia cutis includes a diffuse and infiltrative population of mononuclear cells accompanied by granulocytic cells at various stages of maturation typically including eosinophilic myelocytes. Criteria for diagnosing leukemia cutis on skin biopsy are: chloroacetate esterase activity and Leu-M1 positivity; and the presence of lysozyme, α_1-antitrypsin, and α_1-antichymotrypsin serve as supportive findings, with lysozyme being the most consistent positive marker.

The prognosis for leukemia cutis is related directly to the prognosis for the systemic disease.[16]

THALASSEMIA MAJOR AND MINOR

Foot ulcers due to thalassemia minor are rare, but there have been cases reported. A 31-year-old Greek woman with thalassemia minor developed multiple painful ulcers on the ankles, toes, and dorsa of both feet, which were well defined and measured 2 to 10 mm in diameter. Also observed were punctate petechial hemorrhages. An acute vasculitis of the capillaries and fibrinoid necrosis of the vessel walls were observed microscopically with petechial hemorrhages and a lymphocytic infiltration in the surrounding connective tissue. No abnormalities were seen with lymphangiography, phlebography, and arteriography of the lower limbs. Although also rare, thalassemia major (Cooley anemia) ulcers have been reported. Patients with thalassemia major usually have hemoglobin levels of 9 g or less, and ulcers that form are probably due to lack of oxygen as a result of low hemoglobin A. These ulcers, like thalassemia minor, are usually found around the ankles unilaterally or bilaterally. Also a possible cause of leg ulcers is thalassemia intermedia, which occurs in patients with poorly controlled or untreated disease. This may be due to poor oxygen delivery because of the high oxygen affinity of hemoglobin F that may be more than 50% of the patient's total hemoglobin.[17]

THROMBOCYTHEMIA AND THROMBOCYTOSIS

In thrombocythemia, blood clots may develop in the feet as well as the brain and hands, less commonly, in other parts of the body such as the heart and intestines. When they affect the feet, there may be tingling.

The signs and symptoms of a high platelet count are linked to bleeding and blood clots. Symptoms may also include ulcers affecting the toes. Blood clots in the small vessels of the feet result in numbness and redness. This may lead to intense burning and throbbing in the plantar aspect of the foot. Bleeding occurs when the platelet count is higher than 1 million platelets per microliter of blood.

CRYOGLOBULINEMIA

Initially described by Wintrobe and Buell in 1933, cryoglobulins (CGs) were found in a patient with multiple myeloma. Patients with CGs are classified into three types. Type I are monoclonal, composed of immunoglobulin (Ig)M, IgG, IgA, and Bence Jones proteins in decreasing order of frequency. The serum level of monoclonal CGs is typically high, and they precipitate easily at cold temperatures. Type II CGs are mixed CGs composed of complexes of polyclonal IgG and monoclonal IgM rheumatoid factor. Type III CGs are mixed polyclonal CGs, most commonly composed of IgM and IgG and are usually present at very low levels in the serum. Type I cryoglobulinemia is associated with multiple myeloma, other hematologic proliferative disorders, rheumatoid arthritis, and autoimmune hemolytic anemia. Type II and III cryoglobulinemias are associated with chronic lymphocytic leukemia or lymphoma. Autoimmune diseases, such as Sjögren syndrome and rheumatoid arthritis, are found in patients with type II cryoglobulinemia. Type III cryoglobulinemia is seen in patients with systemic lupus erythematosus (SLE), periarteritis nodosa, idiopathic thrombocytopenic purpura, and hematologic proliferative disorders. Infections, including hepatitis B, mononucleosis, cytomegalovirus, subacute bacterial endocarditis, and toxoplasmosis, can be found in patients with cryoglobulinemias. The term essential cryoglobulinemia describes cryoglobulinemia with no clinical signs of underlying disease. Cryoglobulinemia was initially noted to occur predominantly in patients with myeloma, but it is now being detected in a growing number of infectious, collagen-vascular, and lymphoproliferative disorders. The major cause of cryoglobulinemia is now considered to be hepatitis C virus (HCV). Cutaneous manifestations are the most typical clinical sign of cryoglobulinemic vasculitis. They range from palpable purpura of the lower limbs to chronic torpid cutaneous ulcers typically located in the supramalleolar regions. The cutaneous involvement is often complicated by the occurrence of chronic leg ulcers with little or no tendency to heal and which spontaneously cause pain and severe discomfort to the patient. A case of HCV-positive type I cryoglobulinemia with severe leg ulcers and not responsive to antiviral and immunosuppressive treatment is described. This was followed by double filtration plasmapheresis for 6 months, with no other associated treatment. Before and after each session, an assessment of immunoglobulins, complement, cryocrit, and fibrinogen was made. HCV RNA

levels were determined in serum cryoprecipitate, in the supernatant before and after each session, and in the collection bag. No differences in pre- and postapheresis values were observed in the serum concentrations and the supernatant. However, the postapheresis cryoprecipitate showed a significantly reduced viral load ($P < 0.02$) as compared with the preapheresis values. Improvement in the ulcers in the leg occurred during apheresis with complete regression by the end of the cycle. Skin biopsy specimens from patients with primary mixed IgM–IgG cryoglobulinemia were examined by immunofluorescence, light, and electron microscopy. The biopsies taken from the involved skin of one patient with leg ulcers revealed small blood vessel occlusions by CG aggregates. Because a similar finding was not observed in the biopsy material taken from the other five patients who had no ulcerative skin lesions, it seems that the CG aggregates play a role in the development of the skin ulcerations in primary mixed IgM–IgG cryoglobulinemia.[18–20]

MYELOPROLIFERATIVE DISORDERS

As a result of impairment of the cutaneous microcirculation, hemorrheology, or the effect of hydroxyurea, ulcerations of the leg may occur in myeloproliferative disorders. The use of hydroxyurea may have as a side effect the presentation of such leg ulcers. In fact, the use of hydroxyurea in leg ulcers may result in a wound size increase. If the leg ulcers are due to hydroxyurea and the drug is stopped, typically healing occurs. An option is to use another cytotoxic agent if one is available, but it too may result in a leg ulcer. The differential diagnosis of myeloproliferative disease is vasculitis, cryoglobulinemeia, and pyoderma gangrenosum.

ANTIPHOSPHOLIPID SYNDROME

Antiphospholipid syndrome (APS) is an acquired, multisystemic disorder characterized by recurrent thromboses in the arterial system, venous system, or both. APS is classified into two groups: primary and secondary.

Secondary APS is often associated with SLE and infrequently with other diseases, such as lymphoproliferative disorders, autoimmune diseases, infections (e.g., syphilis, HIV, HCV), and drugs (e.g., procainamide, quinidine, hydralazine, phenytoin, chlorpromazine). Serologic markers for APS are antiphospholipid antibodies (β_2 glycoprotein I or anticardiolipins) or lupus anticoagulant.

The primary diagnostic criteria include arterial thrombosis, venous thrombosis, recurrent fetal loss, and thrombocytopenia. One of the listed primary criteria is required for diagnosis, combined with a sustained elevated titer of IgG anticardiolipin or lupus anticoagulant, which can be detected based on the prolonged activated partial thromboplastin time, Kaolin clotting time, or dilute Russell Viper venom time.

A large retrospective study from the Mayo Clinic of patients with lupus anticoagulant included 41% who had skin lesions as the first sign of APS. Cutaneous manifestations include livedo reticularis, necrotizing vasculitis, livedo vasculitis, thrombophlebitis, cutaneous ulceration and necrosis, erythematous macules, purpura, ecchymosis, painful skin nodules, and subungual splinter hemorrhages.[21,22]

LIVEDO RETICULARIS

Occasionally, livedo reticularis will cause ulcers of the foot. The disease is a condition associated with reddish blue, mottled, reticular, or blotchy discoloration that resembles a fishnet. Ulcerations occur only rarely, starting primarily in the summer months. A case was reported in which ulcers were present and caused by IgA anticardiolipin antibodies. As a result of treatment with warfarin and chloroquine as well as giving up birth control pills and smoking, cardiolipin can be included in all cases of livedo reticularis because treatment may be more effective in the event of positive antibody detection.[23]

REFERENCES

1. Sehgal S, Arunkumar B. Microbila flora and its significance in pathology of sickle cell disease leg ulcers. *Infection*. 1992;20(2):86–88.
2. Brawley O, Cornelius L, Edwards L, et al. NIH Conference Annals of Internal Medicine National Institutes of Health Consensus Development Conference statement: hydroxyurea treatment for sickle cell disease. *Ann Intern Med*. 2008;148(12):932–938.
3. Herrick JB. Peculiar elongated and sickle-shaped red blood corpuscles in a case of severe anemia. *Yale J Biol Med*. 2001;74(3):179–184.
4. Cummer C, LaRocco C. Ulcers of the legs in sickle cell anemia. *Arch Dermatol*. 1940;52(6):1015–1039.
5. Nolan V, Adewoye A, Baldwin C, et al. Sickle cell ulcers: associated with haemolysis and SNPsss in Klotho, TEK and genes of the TGF-B/BMP pathway. *Br J Haematol*. 2006;133(5):570–578.
6. Trent J, Kirsner R. Leg ulcers in sickle cell disease. *Adv Skin Wound Care*. 2004;17(8):410–416.
7. Wolfort F, Krizek T. Skin ulceration in sickle cell anemia. *Plast Reconstr Surg*. 1969;43(1):71–77.
8. Chirico E, Pialoux V. Role of oxidative stress in the pathogenesis of sickle cell disease. *IUMB Life*. 2012;64(1):72–80.
9. Eckmen J. Leg ulcers in sickle cell disease. *Hematol Oncol Clin North Am*. 1996;106(6):1333–1344.
10. Robinson S, Tasker S. Chronic leg ulcers of sickle cell anemia. *Cal West J Med*. 1946;64(4):250–252.
11. McMahon L, Tamary H, Askin M, et al. A randomized phase II trial of arginine butyrate with standard local therapy in refractory sickle cell leg ulcers. *Br J Haematol*. 2010;15(5):516–524.
12. Serjeant G, Galloway R, Gueri M. Oral zinc sulphate in sickle-cell ulcers. *Lancet*. 1970;31(2):891–892.
13. Ware RE, Aygun B. Advances in the use of hydroxyurea. *Hematology Am Soc Hematol Educ Program*. 2009;(1):62–69.
14. Platt O. Hydroxyurea for the treatment of sickle cell anemia. *N Engl J Med*. 2008;358(13):1362–1369.
15. Lau H, Lee AC, Tang SK. Isolated foot ulcer complicating acute leukemia: an unusual manifestation of herpes simplex virus infection simulating pyoderma gangrenosum. *Pediatr Hematol Oncol*. 2003;20(6):477–480.
16. Aksu AE, Saracoglu ZN, Sabuncu I, et al. Necrotic ulcer: a manifestation of leukemia cutis. *Skinmed*. 2012;10(2):108–110.
17. Berge G, Brehmer-Andersson E, Rorsman H. Thalassemia minor and painful ulcers of lower extremities. *Acta Derm Venereol*. 1970;50(2):125–128.
18. Josifova D, Gatt G, Aquilina G, et al. Double-filtration plasmapheresis in the treatment of leg ulcers in cryoglobulinemia. *J Clin Apher*. 2008;23(3):118–122. doi:10.1002/jca.20166.
19. Placik OJ, Zukowski ML, Lewis VL Jr. Cryoglobulinemia: dilemma for the reconstructive surgeon. *Plast Reconstr Surg*. 1993;91(2):348–351.
20. Berliner S, Weinberger A, Ben-Bassat M, et al. Small skin blood vessel occlusions by cryoglobulin aggregates in ulcerative lesions in IgM-IgG cryoglobulinemia. *J Cutan Pathol*. 1982;9(2):96–103.
21. Ruiz-Irastorza G, Crowther M, Branch W, et al. Antiphospholipid syndrome. *Lancet*. 2010;376(9751):1498–1509.
22. Alegre VA, Gastineau DA, Winkelmann RK. Skin lesions associated with circulating lupus anticoagulant. *Br J Dermatol*. 1989;120(3):419–429.
23. Magro CA, Guidolin F, Neto FB, et al. Livedo reticularis with ulcers in patients with IgA anticardiolipin. *An Bras Dermatol*. 2005;80(5):538–539.

CHAPTER 21

Lower Extremity Manifestations of Spine Disease

SRAVISHT IYER • TODD J. ALBERT

Spine complaints are extremely common: symptomatic lumbar disk herniation, for example, has a 2% lifetime prevalence; up to 10% of patients older than 60 may meet the clinical and radiographic criteria for lumbar stenosis.[1] In both cases, leg pain can often be seen as a primary manifestation of the disease. Practitioners who see patients with lower extremity pain in practice (e.g., foot and ankle surgeons, hip and knee surgeons) are almost certain to encounter patients with spine pathology in their clinics. These cases can frequently be difficult to manage as spine pathology and lower extremity pathology may overlap (e.g., hip osteoarthritis and spinal stenosis), leaving considerable doubt about the principal cause of the patients' complaints.[2] Successfully identifying these patients and providing them appropriate care requires that providers consider spine problems in their differential diagnoses when evaluating patients. In order to facilitate this differential, it is important to have a basic understanding of spinal anatomy, pathoanatomy, and common spinal complaints that may cause patients to present to a lower extremity clinic.

This chapter reviews basic spinal anatomy and neuroanatomy as it applies to the lower extremity. This review of the anatomy is then applied to three common conditions (cervical myelopathy, lumbar stenosis, and lumbar radiculopathy) that might cause patients to present to a lower extremity clinic. The pathophysiology, diagnosis, and management of each disease process are briefly discussed.

SPINE ANATOMY

Vertebral Anatomy

The spine consists of a total of 33 vertebrae (7 cervical, 12 thoracic, 5 lumbar, 5 sacral, and 4 coccygeal) (**Fig. 21-1A**). Although vertebrae in the sacrum and coccyx are fused, vertebrae in the cervical, thoracic, and lumbar spine articulate through a series of diarthrodial (i.e., synovial) joints that are stabilized by several ligaments and muscular attachments. The vertebra serves as a "building block" for the spine, and the 24 presacral vertebrae consist of a series of functional spinal units consisting of two vertebral bodies, the facet joint that forms the articulation between the two vertebrae and the intervertebral disk. Most vertebrae in the spine share a similar anatomy. Every vertebra consists of a vertebral body, pedicles, articular processes, pars interarticularis, transverse processes, lamina, and spinous process (**Fig. 21-1B**).

The vertebral body is a cylindrical mass of trabecular, cancellous bone that is found in the anterior aspect of the vertebral body. Vertebral bodies vary in size, generally increasing in size when moving more caudal in the spine. In the thoracic spine, the vertebral bodies have articulations for the ribs. In the cervical spine, vertebral bodies articulate with each other through saddle-shaped joints referred to as the "joints of Luschka" or uncovertebral joints. The intervertebral disk lies between the vertebral bodies of two adjacent vertebrae.

Just posterior to the vertebral body is the dorsal arch. In contrast to the vertebral body, whose anatomy is relatively simple, the dorsal arch consists of a series of processes that enclose the spinal canal, allow for articulation with the neighboring vertebral bodies, and provide attachment sites for ligaments and muscles. The dorsal arch of the vertebra is connected to the vertebral body by a pair of two stout pillars referred to as the pedicles. The dorsal "arch" is composed of a pair of flat surfaces called the lamina. These form the roof of the spinal canal. Where the lamina meet in the midline, a large process projects dorsally. This is called the spinous process.

The remaining portions of the dorsal arch (transverse process, articular processes, and pars interarticularis) are found at the junction of the lamina and the pedicles. At this point, the transverse processes extend to either side of the vertebral arch. In the thoracic spine, these articulate with the rib. The articular process extends superiorly and inferiorly from the junction of the lamina and the pedicles to form the superior articular process and inferior articular process, respectively. The area between the articular processes at the confluence of these various processes is referred to as the pars interarticularis. The superior articular process of a given vertebra articulates with the complementary inferior articular process of the level above. These processes have cartilage and form a diarthrodial joint called the facet joint. A vertebra typically has four facet joints (two with the vertebrae above and two with the vertebrae below). Typically, the superior articulating process is directed dorsally, whereas the inferior

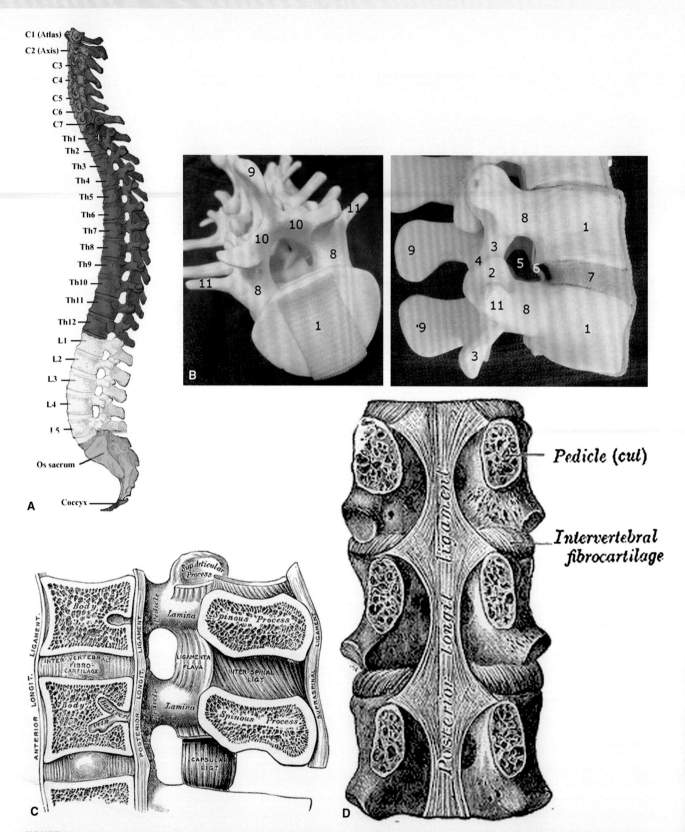

FIGURE 21-1. Important Anatomic Structures in the Spine. A: Image of the vertebral column depicting its segmental nature. **B:** Photographs of a spine model depicting various important anatomic landmarks: (1) vertebral body, (2) superior articular process, (3) inferior articular process, (4) facet joint; articulation between superior and inferior articular processes, (5) vertebral foramen, note the structures it is bounded by, (6) posterior longitudinal ligament, (7) intervertebral disk, (8) pedicles, (9) spinous process, (10) lamina, (11) transverse process. **C:** Profile of the spine illustrating the posterior longitudinal ligament along the dorsal surface of the vertebral body and the ligamentum flavum along the ventral surface of the lamina; hypertrophy or ossification of these soft tissue structures can reduce the space in the spinal canal. **D:** Posterior view of the posterior longitudinal ligament. Note that the ligament is thick centrally, but the lateral aspect of the disks is uncovered. (A: From Anatomical Chart Company, with permission. C and D: From Henry Vandyke Carter [Public domain], via Wikimedia Commons).

articular process is directed ventrally (toward the belly button). The specific orientation of the facet joints varies between the cervical, thoracic, and lumbar spine and is suited both to the types of loads and type of motion experienced by the specific spinal segments (e.g., rotation and lateral bending in the cervical spine and flexion/extension in the lumbar spine). The spinal nerve root exits the spinal cord from a space just anterior to the lateral aspect of the facet joint. This space, referred to as the intervertebral foramen, is bordered anteriorly by the intervertebral disk and posteriorly by the lateral aspect of the facet joint and ligamentum flavum, and the superior and inferior boundaries are formed by the pedicles of the levels above and below (**Fig. 21-1B**).

The discussion above highlights important structures that may contribute to compression of neural elements and lead to lower extremity symptoms. In addition to the bony structures mentioned earlier, soft tissue structures that might contribute to impingement include the posterior longitudinal ligament (PLL) and the ligamentum flavum (**Fig. 21-1C**). The PLL runs along the posterior surfaces of the vertebral bodies from the vertebral body of C2 to the sacrum and ventral to the spinal cord. The ligamentum flavum is an elastic structure that serves to help the vertebral column maintain a normal posture and runs dorsal to the spinal cord. The ligamentum flavum is actually a series of small ligaments that serve to connect adjacent vertebral lamina.

Neuroanatomy

Similar to the spine, the spinal cord is an anatomically segmented structure. There are 31 segments in the spinal cord: 8 cervical, 12 thoracic, 5 lumbar, 5 sacral, and 1 coccygeal. Each segment of the spinal cord innervates a single somite during development; this translates to each spinal nerve retaining its relationship with the characteristic areas of skin and muscles. The area of skin innervated by a single spinal segment is referred to as a dermatome. Although the relationship between spinal segment and dermatome in the trunk is quite simple and reflects the segmental nature of the spine, the relationship in the limbs is more complex because of the outgrowth of the limb buds during development.[3] These are illustrated in **Figure 21-2**.

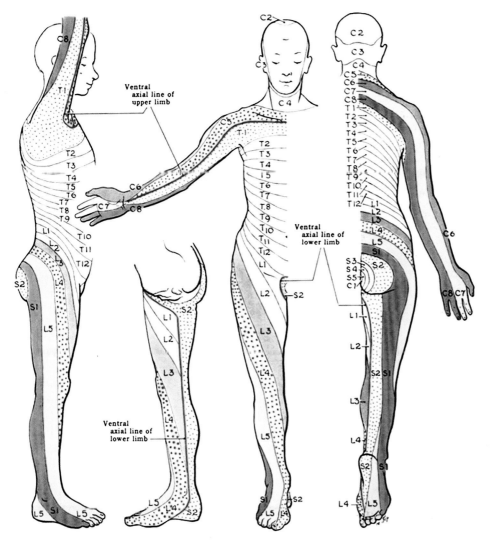

FIGURE 21-2. Depiction of a Dermatome Map. Note that each region is associated with a spinal level, for example, medial aspect of the foot is innervated by the L4 nerve root. Note that the distribution of the spine segments is relatively simple in the trunk but more complex in the extremities. (By Grant, John Charles Boileau. *An atlas of anatomy: by regions 1962*. Public domain, via Wikimedia Commons.)

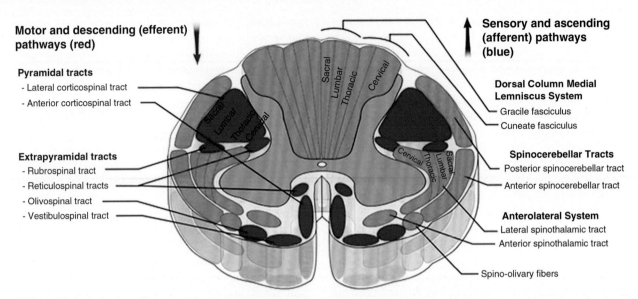

FIGURE 21-3. Cross-Sectional View of the Spine. Information in the spine is carried in characteristic areas. The red regions represent descending tracts. The pyramidal tracts (lateral) carry motor information from the motor cortex to the α motor neuron cells. The α motor neuron cells are located in the anterolateral region of the "H"-shaped central gray matter also seen in the image. The dorsal cord contains ascending afferent pathway and carries sensory input responsible for proprioception. (By Polarlys and Mikael Häggström [CC BY-SA 3.0, http://creativecommons.org/licenses/by-sa/3.0 or GFDL, http://www.gnu.org/copyleft/fdl .html], via Wikimedia Commons.)

Given the segmental nature of the cord, it is typically described in cross section. The cord consists of a roughly H-shaped area of gray matter that is surrounded by myelinated white matter. Each limb of the "H" shape of the gray matter can be divided into horns (posterior and anterior), whereas the white matter surrounding it is described as funiculi. Afferent fibers (i.e., sensory inputs from the limb) enter the cord via the dorsal roots and end on the ipsilateral side. Here, these inputs synapse on neurons in the ipsilateral gray matter in the posterolateral horn and feed into a complex system of sensory inputs. A portion of these inputs gives rise to the sensory pathways that ascend in the dorsal portion of the cord, whereas others feed into local reflex circuits. α motor neurons that innervate skeletal muscles can be found in the anterior horns. There are characteristic enlargements of the anterior horns in the cervical and lumbar regions (more α motor neurons) to account for motor innervation of the extremities. Anterior horn cells are arranged in cigar-shaped columns such that multiple levels may contribute to the function of a given muscle (i.e., the quadriceps is innervated by anterior horn cells corresponding to the L2 and L3 segments).[3] Output from the α motor neurons leaves the cord via the ventral roots. The remainder of the spinal cord has a fairly characteristic organization; fibers are generally organized by the type of information they carry. A complete understanding of this schema is beyond the scope of this chapter, but can be found in **Figure 21-3**.

The motor neuron cells in the anterior horn are modulated by a complex system of inputs from the corticospinal tracts that descend from the cerebral cortex as well as brain stem and diencephalic nuclei. The anterior horn cells are involved

in the reflex response. A reflex is defined as an involuntary response to a sensory input with circuitry that is contained entirely within the spinal cord. The deep tendon reflexes commonly tested in the clinical setting represent an example of a simple reflex loop (**Fig. 21-4**).[3] The reflex at the knee, for example, involves tapping the patellar tendon, which causes a small stretch of the quadriceps muscle. This stretch is detected by sensory neurons within the muscle and carried to the spine by the afferent pathway. These sensory neurons synapse onto the α motor neurons in the anterior horn of the spinal cord as well as an inhibitory interneuron. The α motor neuron receives a positive stimulus and acts to initiate quadriceps contraction, whereas the inhibitory interneuron suppresses the α motor neurons of the antagonist muscle group (hamstrings). These stimuli then exit the spinal cord via the ventral nerve roots, traveling via the femoral nerve to the quadriceps and via the tibial nerve to the hamstrings. Contraction of the quadriceps and relaxation of the hamstrings lead to knee extension, or the knee-jerk commonly seen on examination. From this example, it can be deduced that damage to the exiting nerve root (e.g., due to compression in the neural foramen) can diminish or eliminate the reflex response. Because of the segmental nature of the spine, reflexes are typically tied to a principal cord segment (in this case, L2). In this way, reflexes are important tools because they can be easily tested and can be used to localize lesions. The reflexes at the biceps, brachioradialis, triceps, and ankle (Achilles) are governed by a similar loop; the localization of these reflexes is shown in **Table 21-1**.

In truth, the monosynaptic reflex described above is a simplification.[3] The firing of the α motor neuron is modulated

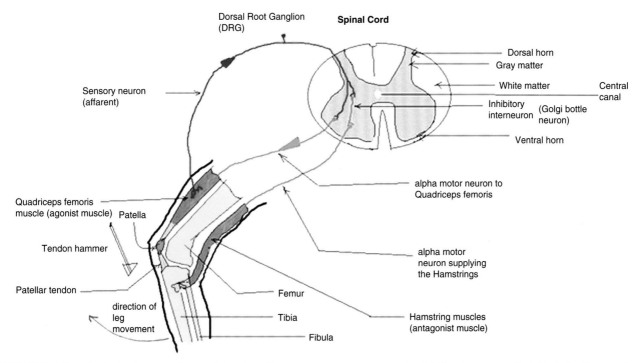

FIGURE 21-4. Example of a simple motor reflex consisting of an afferent neuron, α motor neuron, and an inhibitory interneuron. (By Amiya Sarkar [Own work] [CC BY-SA 4.0, http://creativecommons.org/licenses/by-sa/4.0], via Wikimedia Commons.)

by several inputs from the descending lateral cortical tracts. In general, the descending tracts serve to modulate the firing of the α motor neurons and allow volitional control of the upper and lower extremities. Injury to the lateral descending tracts, as can be seen in certain neurologic disorders or in compression of the cervical spine, can lead to increased muscle tone, hyperreflexia, and pathologic reflexes. It is important to understand the distinction between upper and lower motor neuron symptoms, and these are summarized in Table 21-2.

Finally, it is important to note that the human spinal cord reaches adult size faster than the vertebral column. As a result, it is typically shorter than the vertebral column, extending from the cervical spine to approximately the level of L1/L2.[3] Below this region, the spinal canal contains the spinal nerves for the lumbar vertebral levels, but these nerve roots are actually given off at higher levels and travel in the cord as a structure called the cauda equina (horse's tail) (**Fig. 21-5**).

SPINE PATHOLOGY WITH LOWER EXTREMITY FINDINGS

Cervical Spine

Cervical Myelopathy

Pathophysiology

The term myelopathy refers to compression of the spinal cord leading to upper motor neuron dysfunction. This compression encompasses a broad clinical spectrum and can involve radicular (nerve root, or lower motor neuron) symptoms in addition to central (spinal cord, or upper motor neuron) symptoms (**Table 21-2**).[4] In the radicular syndrome, compression of nerve root predominates. In this syndrome, patients typically complain of upper extremity symptoms, and lower extremity symptoms are rare. In the medial syndrome, patients complain of long tract signs (see diagnosis section), and lower extremity involvement is common. In the combined syndrome, patients present with both upper and lower extremity symptoms—this is the most common presentation of cervical spondylotic myelopathy (CSM). There are also vascular causes of myelopathy that can present with a mixed pattern of weakness and upper and lower extremity involvement.[4] CSM may also affect the anterior horn cells in the upper cervical spine leading to upper extremity weakness without lower extremity involvement.[4]

Table 21-1. Commonly Tested Reflexes with Associated Spinal Level	
Reflex	**Level**
Biceps reflex	C5, C6
Brachioradialis	C6
Triceps	C7, C8
Patellar tendon (knee-jerk)	L2, L3, L4
Achilles tendon (ankle-jerk)	S1, S2

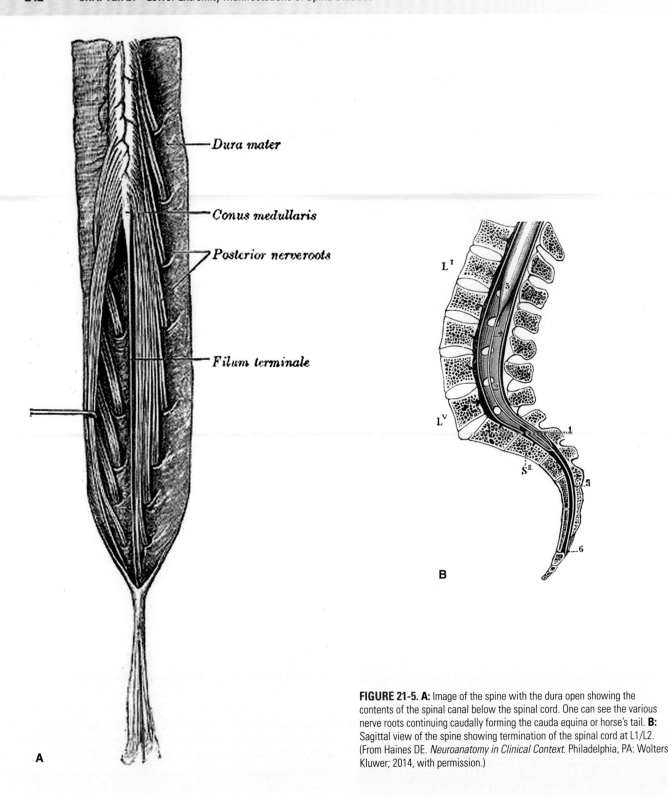

Dura mater

Conus medullaris

Posterior nerveroots

Filum terminale

A

L^I

L^V

S^{II}

B

FIGURE 21-5. A: Image of the spine with the dura open showing the contents of the spinal canal below the spinal cord. One can see the various nerve roots continuing caudally forming the cauda equina or horse's tail. **B:** Sagittal view of the spine showing termination of the spinal cord at L1/L2. (From Haines DE. *Neuroanatomy in Clinical Context.* Philadelphia, PA: Wolters Kluwer; 2014, with permission.)

Cervical spondylosis refers to degeneration of the cervical spine. This process begins with a loss of integrity of the intervertebral disk.[1] This process typically occurs with age, although a genetic predisposition toward disk degeneration may exist in some individuals. This process is typically asymptomatic. As the disk breaks down, it loses height and bulges outward into the spinal canal. This disk bulge may also occur laterally impinging on the spinal roots. Breakdown of the disk then leads to increased loads on the vertebral bodies and joints of Luschka (uncinate joints). In response, the uncinate joints and vertebra form more bone in order to better support the increased loads. Bone from the vertebral bodies can project into the canal and restrict the space available for the cord, whereas uncinate hypertrophy can cause lateral compression

Table 21-2.	Differences in the Clinical Presentation of Upper versus Lower Motor Neuron Disease	
Clinical Sign	**Upper Motor Neuron**	**Lower Motor Neuron**
Weakness	Yes	Yes
Atrophy	Mild atrophy possible	Yes
Fasciculations	Not present	Present
Reflexes	Increased	Decreased
Babinski/pathologic reflexes	Present	Absent
Tone	Increased	Decreased

congenitally narrow spinal canals and be at higher risk for developing myelopathy.[5]

Chronic compression of the spinal cord because of the static and dynamic factors described earlier leads to damage of the spinal cord through chronic distortion of the spinal cord microvasculature. Chronic compression of the cord leads to flattening, elongation, and stretching and eventual loss of the microvasculature. As compression proceeds, changes occur; the majority of changes are seen in the lateral funiculi and the corticospinal tracts.[5] More severe cases are associated with changes in the medial gray area and ventral aspect of the dorsal columns. The anterior columns appear to be relatively protected even in cases of severe compression.

Diagnosis and Lower Extremity Findings

Physical examination of patients with CSM demonstrates lower motor neuron signs at the level of the cervical lesions (i.e., in the upper extremity) and upper motor neuron signs at levels below the lesions (i.e., in the lower extremity). As most cases of CSM have combined compression of both the nerve root and the spinal cord, symptoms typically involve weakness, pain, and hyporeflexia in the upper extremity and spasticity and hyperreflexia in the lower extremities.[4]

Patients may present with subtle complaints related to gait instability and changes in gait and balance. Although there are certainly numerous causes for changes in gait patterns, difficulty with balance and difficulty with fine motor tasks

and nerve root impingement (**Fig. 21-6A**). Bulging of the disks and loss of disk height can also lead to infolding of the posterior soft tissues such as the ligamentum flavum and the PLL. These tissues can cause dynamic compression of the cord in flexion and extension (**Fig. 21-6 B**). Ossification of the PLL is most commonly seen in an Asian patient population and may lead to severe anterior cord compression (**Fig. 21-7**). Although the "normal" spinal canal has approximately 7 to 8 mm of space to accommodate intrusions from osteophyte formation and ossification, some patients may present with

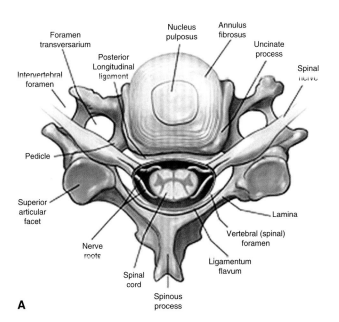

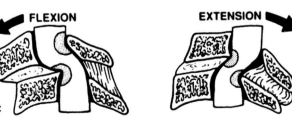

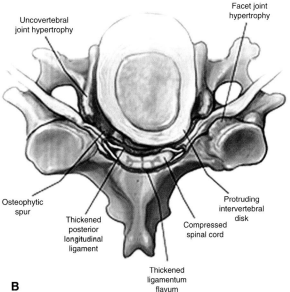

FIGURE 21-6. A: Normal cervical anatomy. **B:** Examples of degenerative changes in the cervical spine that can cause compression of the spinal cord. **C:** Example of dynamic compression of the spinal cord due to soft tissue impingement from the posterior longitudinal ligament or ligamentum flavum. (A and B: From Shen FH, Samartzis D, Fessler RG. *Text Book of the Surgical Spine*. Maryland Heights, Missouri: Elsevier; 2015. C: From Law MD Jr, Bernhardt M, White AA III. Cervical spondylotic myelopathy: a review of surgical indications and decision making. *Yale J Biol Med*. 1993;66(3):165–177.)

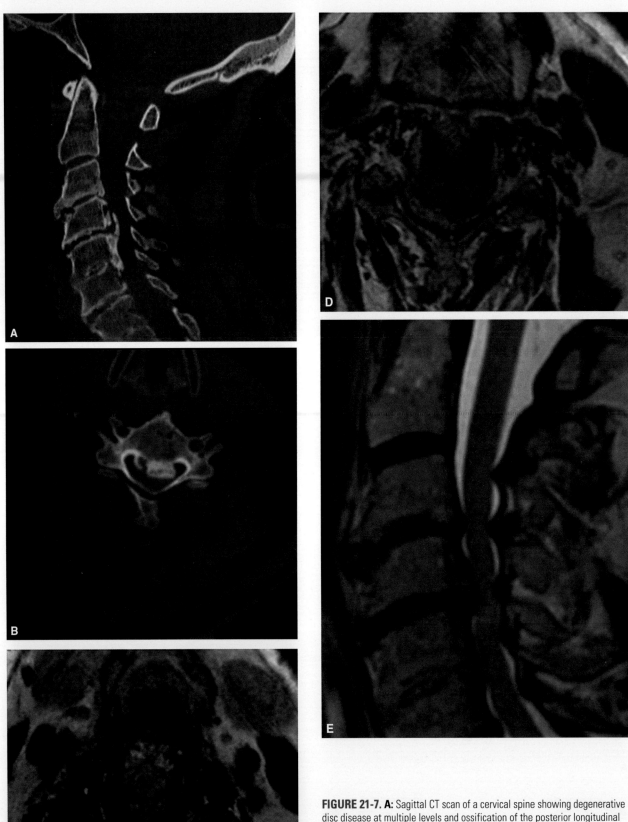

FIGURE 21-7. A: Sagittal CT scan of a cervical spine showing degenerative disc disease at multiple levels and ossification of the posterior longitudinal ligament. **B:** Axial image showing an ossified posterior longitudinal ligament narrowing the space available for the cord anteriorly. **C:** Axial MRI images showing a level without cord compression. **D:** Axial MRI through the same level seen on the CT scan in B. This image shows and example of severe cord compression. **E:** Sagittal MRI image showing compression of the spinal cord at multiple levels.

such as tandem walk should raise the examiner's suspicion for cervical pathology. In patients with these symptoms, it is important to also illicit a history of upper extremity function as they may complain of a loss of dexterity with fine motor tasks such as buttoning a shirt or handwriting.

On physical examination, patients with myelopathy present with a mix of upper and lower motor neuron findings in one or both upper extremities and primarily upper motor neuron symptoms in both lower extremities. Clinical signs typically include hyperreflexia, clonus, and other upper motor neuron signs such as a positive Babinski in the lower extremity.[6,7] The Babinski sign refers to dorsiflexion of the big toe when the sole of the foot is stroked by a sharp object (**Fig. 21-8A**). The clinical exam in patients who are suspected to have CSM should also include an exam of upper extremity reflexes; pathologic reflexes in the upper extremities include the Hoffman sign (**Fig. 21-8B**) and the inverted radial reflex (**Fig. 21-8C**).

Unfortunately, all physical exam maneuvers for CSM are limited by low sensitivity and specificity and these reflexes can sometimes be seen in healthy individuals.[8] However, gait imbalance, hyperreflexia, and Babinski's sign in patients presenting to a lower extremity clinic should raise suspicion and initiate a workup to rule out cervical compression as the cause of the patients' complaints.

Treatment

There is no predetermined course of CSM, and progression can vary between patients. However, it is generally agreed that once signs and symptoms of CSM are evident, there is no neurologic improvement without surgical intervention.[8,9] Deterioration, however, might follow a stepwise clinical course, with long periods of stability interrupted by periods of

marked decline. Conservative management has consisted of immobilization and cervical traction, but evidence for the role of conservative management in symptomatic CSM is limited.[8]

The decision between conservative and surgical management is more difficult in patients with mild symptoms or cervical stenosis without obvious clinical signs of myelopathy. These patients may be managed conservatively with periodic observation for signs of deterioration that might necessitate surgical intervention. Proponents of surgery, however, point to the progressive degenerative cascade of CSM and the risk of progressive (and potentially irreversible) neurologic injury as the rationale for early surgical intervention.[8,9] Changes on imaging that might encourage surgical change include: signal changes in the spinal cord in T2-weighted images and nerve root impingement found on magnetic resonance imaging.

Surgical intervention typically consists of decompression of the spine along with immobilization and fusion. More recent studies have suggested that hypermobility of the cervical spine might be a key factor in driving myelopathic changes. There are a variety of approaches and techniques available to decompress and stabilize the spine, but an in-depth discussion of these techniques is beyond the scope of this chapter.

Lumbar Spine

Lumbar Stenosis

Pathophysiology

Lumbar stenosis refers to the narrowing of the space available for the spine in the lumbar spine. Lumbar stenosis differs from cervical stenosis because it typically occurs below the level of the spinal cord. This fact is clinically relevant because compression of the cauda equina, unlike the spinal

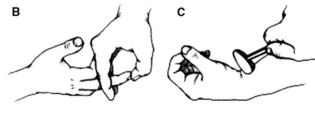

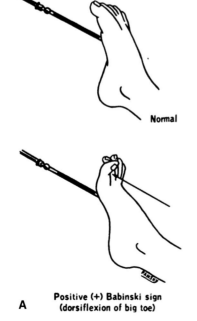

Normal

A **Positive (+) Babinski sign (dorsiflexion of big toe)**

FIGURE 21-8. A: Example of the Babinski sign; stroking a pen on the bottom of the foot should normally result in downgoing toes; upgoing toes is suggestive of upper motor neuron disease. **B:** Hoffman sign: the examiner flicking the middle finger as illustrated results in flexion of the other digits. **C:** Inverted radial reflex: Tapping the brachioradialis tendon leads to flexion of the digits (A: From House EL, Pansky B. *A Functional Approach to Neuroanatomy.* New York, NY: McGraw-Hill; 1960 [Public domain], via Wikimedia Commons. B and C: From Emerey SE. Cervical spondylotic myelopathy: diagnosis and treatment. *J Am Acad Orthop Surg.* 2001;9(6):376–388, with permission).

cord, does not affect the lateral descending and posterior ascending tracts. As a result, patients with lumbar stenosis, unlike patients with cervical stenosis, do not present with upper motor neuron complaints.

Like CSM, lumbar stenosis is a progressive, degenerative process that typically manifests clinically later in life (60s and 70s). Similar to the cervical spine, degeneration in the lumbar spine is thought to begin in the disk. As the structure of the disk changes with age, there is tearing of the disk contributing to disk degeneration, herniation, and loss of height. This again leads to abnormal spine biomechanics and abnormal loading of the spinal canal and degeneration of the facet joints.[1]

Lumbar facets are oriented approximately 90° in the sagittal plane. This orientation is optimal for flexion and extension in normal individuals. However, as the facet joints become inflamed, synovitis can lead to laxity and subluxation of the facet joints. This can cause instability of the vertebral column as one vertebra may "slip" forward, reducing the space available for the cord (**Fig. 21-9A**). This condition is referred to as degenerative spondylolisthesis (spondy = vertebral body and olithesis = slip in Greek) and contributes to lumbar stenosis.

In addition to laxity of the facet joints, degeneration and abnormal loading also lead to hypertrophy, osteophyte, and cyst formation. As noted in the anatomy section, the facet joints form the posterior border of the intervertebral foramen. Hypertrophy of these joints can lead to nerve root compression in the intervertebral foramen as well as compression of the thecal sac. Similarly, facet cysts can lead to nerve root impingement.

Degeneration of the disk also creates abnormal spaces across the vertebral bodies and vertebral endplates. This can lead to osteophyte formation and can contribute to compression of the thecal sac as well as the exiting nerve roots in the intervertebral foramen (**Fig. 21-9B**).

Causes of lumbar stenosis without degeneration include various congenital or developmental disorders such as congenital spondylolisthesis because of defect in the vertebral pars, achondroplasia, and other syndromes such as ankylosing spondylitis and Paget disease.[5]

Diagnosis and Lower Extremity Findings

Patients with lumbar stenosis most commonly present with lower extremity pain. Patients describe a feeling of leg numbness, fatigue, heaviness, cramping, burning, or weakness. Symptoms of stenosis are typically referred to as "neurogenic claudication" and typically worsen when patients are upright.[5,10] In an upright position, the lumbar spine assumes its most lordotic posture, which reduces the space available for the cord and contributes to compression. As a result, patients will typically complain of leg pain that is worst with standing or walking but relieved by sitting or bending forward.

Because of the exertional nature of the patients' complaints and the fact that lumbar stenosis typically affects an older population, it is important to differentiate neurogenic

claudication from vascular claudication. One important difference is that vascular claudication is typically relieved as soon as patients stop their exertional activities, whereas lumbar stenosis requires that patients change their posture in some way to reduce lumbar lordosis. For example, patients with vascular claudication might report an improvement in pain after they stop walking and stand for a few minutes, whereas lumbar stenosis patients will have the same pain even when standing because the spine remains extended. Sitting or leaning forward will result in relief of their symptoms. The "shopping cart sign" refers to the fact that many patients report an improvement in symptoms and mobility when leaning forward onto a shopping cart. Walking uphill is easier for patients with lumbar stenosis as the spine is relatively flexed during this activity while walking downhill is harder as the spine is extended. The opposite applies to patients with vascular claudication. Another common activity that might be elicited in the history is the stationary bike. Because this activity is performed in a seated position but still increases lower extremity oxygen demand, patients with vascular claudication will typically report increased pain after certain distances, whereas spinal stenosis patients are typically more comfortable with these activities.

Sometimes, patients with spinal stenosis may present with no leg pain but with low back pain radiating into the bilateral buttocks. In these cases, it can sometimes be difficult to differentiate pathology from the spine from pathology from the hip joint.[2] Although it is difficult to differentiate hip pathology from spine pathology on the history, the presence of a limp, limited hip internal rotation, and groin pain all suggest hip pathology instead of spine pathology.

Finally, patients with stenosis may also complain of radicular symptoms, that is, pain along a specified dermatome because of compression of a nerve in the lateral recess or intervertebral foramen. Low back pain is also a common complaint but in cases of isolated back pain, caution must be used to ensure that the patients' symptoms are consistent with stenosis (improves with sitting, flexing forward, etc.).

Examination of a patient with lumbar stenosis begins with a thorough history covering the points mentioned earlier. The history must also elicit any complaints of bowel or bladder dysfunction, progressive weight loss, fevers, chills, and history of cancer. Because lower extremity complaints may be the sign of a number of systemic diseases, a thorough medical history must also be obtained. The examination in the clinic begins with inspection and observation of postural changes (e.g., leaning forward when sitting). Examination of gait is important as patients with severe stenosis will walk or flex forward to reduce spine extension. The presence of a limp, however, should raise suspicion for a process localized to the lower extremity. A complete reflex exam should also be performed. It is not uncommon for patients with lumbar stenosis to have diminished reflexes, although this can be difficult to ascertain because reflexes tend to be diminished in older patients. Asymmetric reflexes should raise suspicion for spinal pathology. Complete strength testing of both lower

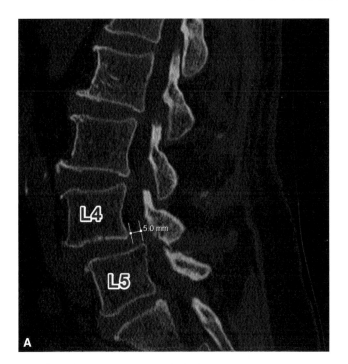

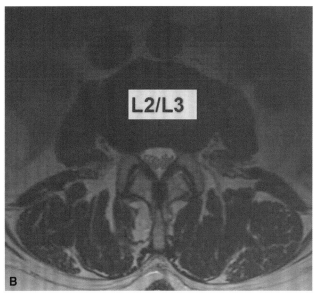

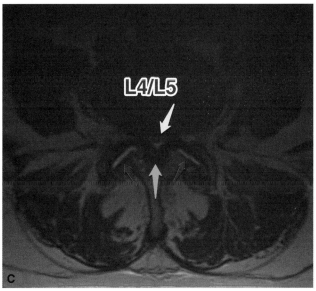

FIGURE 21-9. A: CT scan showing degenerative listhesis, that is, forward slippage of L4 on L5. **B:** Image of L2/L3 disk space showing no evidence of canal narrowing. **C:** In contrast, with axial image of L4/L5 showing fluid in the facet joints (*pink arrows*) that is likely responsible for the laxity and listhesis, a thickened ligamentum flavum (*green arrow*) leads the central stenosis (*yellow arrow*).

extremities should be performed. Although lower extremity weakness is not classically described in spinal stenosis, there may be some weakness found if there is a radicular component to the patients' disease. Special tests that may be performed include hyperextension of the spine to determine if this maneuver recreates the patients' pain. Upper motor neuron findings (such as hyperreflexia, clonus, Babinski, etc.) must be ruled out.

Diagnostic studies include plain radiographs, computed tomography, and magnetic resonance imaging.

Treatment

The North American Spine Society has released evidence-based guidelines for the diagnosis and treatment of lumbar stenosis.[11]

These guidelines recognize that the natural history of lumbar stenosis is largely unknown. Multiple prospective observational studies have shown that between 30% and 50% of lumbar stenosis patients have a favorable natural history with no significant progression of their symptoms and no limitations in activities of daily living. This seems to be the case regardless of the medical intervention used. Additionally, this group recognized that patients with stenosis do not suffer from rapid or catastrophic decline but, rather, a progressive worsening of symptoms. Conservative management may include analgesics, physical therapy, epidural steroid injections, and bracing. Nonsurgical treatment options can provide long-term relief, although there are only weak data to support this claim. Several studies have shown improved outcomes in patients with stenosis following surgical interventions; however, these are generally only recommended in cases with moderate or severe symptoms of stenosis. The Spine Patient Outcomes Research Trial (SPORT) indicated patients with lumbar stenosis for surgery if they met the following criteria: (1) history of neurogenic claudication or radicular symptoms for at least 12 weeks and (2) confirmatory cross-sectional imaging at one or more levels. This study demonstrated improved outcomes in the surgically treated cohort that have been shown to be maintained at up to 4-year follow-up,[12] although more recent investigation has shown a diminishing treatment effect at 8-year follow-up.[13]

Lumbar Radiculopathy

Pathophysiology

As noted in the anatomy section, the intervertebral disk sits between the adjacent vertebral bodies. It consists of three distinct parts: the vertebral endplates, the nucleus pulposus, and the annulus fibrosus (**Fig. 21-10**). The nucleus pulposus consists of aggrecan and other proteoglycans and type II collagen.[1] This environment is highly hydrophilic and retains water. Approximately 80% of the nucleus consists of water. As a result, the nucleus pulposus serves as something of a shock absorber for the intervertebral disk. The nucleus is surrounded by a lamellated layer of sheets called the annulus fibrosus. The annulus consists of type I collagen and serves to "contain" the nucleus; the structure of the annulus is best suited to resisting axial loads. Disk degeneration begins with loss of water in the nucleus pulposus; this is followed by biomechanical changes that lead to more forces being placed on the annulus. The annulus can then experience circumferential fissures that lead to disk herniation.[1]

In the lumbar spine, the lumbar disk is bounded posteriorly by the PLL in the midline. In effect, this renders the posterolateral part of the disk bare, making this the most likely location for disk herniation (**Fig. 21-1D**). Lumbar

disk herniations may be classified as central, posterolateral, foraminal, or extraforaminal. The location of the disk herniation is important as it guides localization of symptoms and allows for correlation with cross-sectional imaging. Ideally, the patients' symptoms should match the findings on imaging.

The herniated disk leads to nerve dysfunction through one of two mechanisms. First, compression on the nerve root causes mechanical dysfunction. Because spinal nerve roots lack the robust protective connective tissue sheaths that characterize peripheral nerves, they are thought to be especially susceptible to mechanical compression. Second, release of disk material in the vicinity of the nerve roots triggers an inflammatory cascade that also results in biologic nerve root dysfunction.[14]

Diagnosis and Lower Extremity Findings

Patients presenting with disk herniation may provide a long history of mild to moderate back pain or describe a specific incident that triggered the onset of their pain. The pain in cases of disk herniation is typically described as leg and back pain. The leg pain follows a dermatomal distribution (**Fig. 21-2**). Common sites of disk herniation include the L4-5 and L5-S1 levels. Examples of events that may trigger the onset of pain may include heavy lifting, bending, twisting, or a fall. Most patients presenting for this complaint typically have a complaint of pain, although numbness and weakness are also possible. The pain is typically described as a "radiating" pain extending to different parts of the lower extremity depending on the location of the herniation. For example, a herniation at L2 may present as pain in the medial thigh, whereas a herniation at L4–S1 will typically present as pain that radiates below the knee and into the foot. They must also elicit any complaints of bowel or bladder dysfunction, progressive weight loss, fevers, chills, and history of cancer. Particular attention must also be paid to peripheral causes of pain such as nerve (tumor, peripheral nerve compression, or diabetic neuropathy) or musculoskeletal causes of pain.

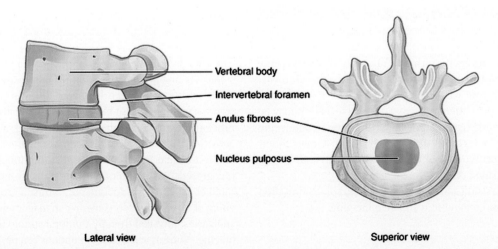

Vertebral body

Intervertebral foramen

Anulus fibrosus

Nucleus pulposus

Lateral view   **Superior view**

FIGURE 21-10. Superior and lateral views of the intervertebral disk showing the nucleus pulposus and annulus fibrosus. (From OpenStax College [CC BY 3.0, http://creativecommons.org/licenses/by/3.0], via Wikimedia Commons.)

The physical examination of patients with spinal stenosis begins with observation of gait. Patients with L5 herniations may exhibit a Trendelenburg gait because of weakness of the hip abductors. Patients may also lean away from the affected side as this maneuver is thought to release the mechanical pressure of the nerve root from the herniated disk. In advanced cases, patients may have a foot drop and exhibit a steppage-type gait pattern. A thorough neurovascular exam must be performed as well. Unlike lumbar stenosis, findings in disk herniation are typically unilateral. Asymmetric reflexes, weakness, or changes in sensation are all potential red flags for disk pathology.

Several clinical tests exist to confirm the diagnosis of disk herniation. In the presence of lumbar disk herniation (L3–S1), the affected nerve roots can be tensed during a straight leg raise maneuver. In this test, the leg is extended and passively raised (**Fig. 21-11**). In the arc of motion between approximately 30° and 70° of hip flexion, the nerve root is draped over the disk and tensed. The straight leg raise test is considered positive when this maneuver reproduces the patients' symptoms. The physician may also perform a straight leg raise on the contralateral extremity. If this reproduces symptoms in the affected limb, it is thought to increase the specificity of the finding[15]; however, estimates vary from 10% to 100%.[1,16] A variation of the straight leg raise, the slump test, can be performed with the patient in a seated position. The patient is asked to flex their neck and thoracic spine ("slump") and the foot is dorsiflexed and the knee extended. This maneuver causes the spinal cord to glide cephalad and increases the tension on the nerve roots; it has been shown to be more sensitive. Finally, in cases of upper lumbar disk herniation, the femoral nerve stretch test may be used. In this maneuver, the knee is flexed and the hip is extended with the patient in the prone or lateral decubitus position. Reproduction of the patients' pain (usually thigh pain) is indicative of upper lumbar root pathology (L1–L2 or L2–L3).

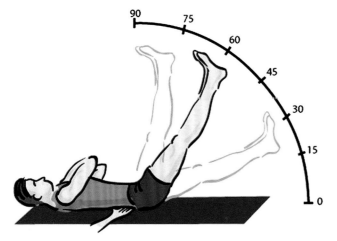

FIGURE 21-11. Picture of a straight leg raise; pain between 30° and 70° is suggestive of lumbar pathology. (By Davidjr74 [CC0], via Wikimedia Commons.)

Treatment

In patients presenting to the clinic with an acute disk herniation, the natural history has been documented in several studies with an observational arm. These studies show that between 50% and 60% of patients have improvement in their symptoms without surgery.[1] One widely cited retrospective trial found that 92% of patients return to work and 90% of patients have good to excellent outcomes after lumbar disk herniation.[17] However, critics of this study have raised the possibility of significant selection bias (the study investigators were nonoperative practitioners and only selected 58 of 347 patients referred to them for a second opinion) and point to a 10% dropout rate in the study cohort as evidence that the results may not be generalizable. The SPORT trial also followed a cohort of patients treated nonoperatively for lumbar disk herniation. In this group, 51% reported major improvement at 4-year follow-up.[18] This is similar to other more recent literature.[19,20]

Most trials designed to investigate the benefits of operative versus nonoperative intervention have suffered from significant crossover bias, and therefore limited conclusions can be drawn about the benefits of operative intervention. However, data from the SPORT trial (as-treated analysis) and Maine Lumbar Spine Study seem to suggest that operative intervention seems to produce improved outcomes compared to the nonsurgically treated group.[18,20] There is a 15% rate of reoperation following surgery for herniated disks.[21] Given this mixed data, there are few concrete operative indications for lumbar disk herniations except for progressive neurologic deficit.[1] Patients with a neurologic deficit in whom disk herniation is suspected should be referred to a spine surgeon expediently. Surgical intervention typically involves an open diskectomy or microdiskectomy, that is, entering the spinal canal after making an opening in the lamina and removing the offending disk material. Relative indications for surgery vary but, at the very least, require cross-sectional imaging findings that correlate with the patients' symptoms.

Nonsurgical treatment for disk herniation involves physical therapy and back school. Epidural steroid injections are commonly used in patients with lumbar disk herniation, especially if pain is too severe to initiate physical therapy.

REFERENCES

1. Cannada LK. *Orthopaedic Knowledge Update 11*. Rosemont, IL: American Academy of Orthopaedic Surgeons; 2014.
2. Fogel GR, Esses SI. Hip spine syndrome: management of coexisting radiculopathy and arthritis of the lower extremity. *Spine J*. 2003;3:238–241.
3. Nolte J. *The Human Brain: An Introduction to its Functional Anatomy*. Maryland Heights, MO: Mosby/Elsevier; 2009.
4. Bernhardt M, Hynes RA, Blume HW, et al. Cervical spondylotic myelopathy. *J Bone Joint Surg Am*. 1993;75:119–128.
5. Eismont FJ, Herkowitz HN, Garfin SR, et al. *Rothman-Simeone the Spine Online: Access to Continually Updated Online Reference*. Philadelphia, PA: Elsevier Science Health Science Division; 2006.
6. Harrop JS, Naroji S, Maltenfort M, et al. Cervical myelopathy: a clinical and radiographic evaluation and correlation to cervical spondylotic myelopathy. *Spine (Phila Pa 1976)*. 2010;35:620–624.

7. Rhee JM, Heflin JA, Hamasaki T, et al. Prevalence of physical signs in cervical myelopathy: a prospective, controlled study. *Spine (Phila Pa 1976)*. 2009;34:890–895.

8. Rhee JM, Shamji MF, Erwin WM, et al. Nonoperative management of cervical myelopathy: a systematic review. *Spine (Phila Pa 1976)*. 2013;38:S55–S67.

9. Karadimas SK, Erwin WM, Ely CG, et al. Pathophysiology and natural history of cervical spondylotic myelopathy. *Spine (Phila Pa 1976)*. 2013;38:S21–S36.

10. Issack PS, Cunningham ME, Pumberger M, et al. Degenerative lumbar spinal stenosis: evaluation and management. *J Am Acad Orthop Surg*. 2012;20:527–535.

11. Kreiner DS, Shaffer WO, Baisden JL, et al. An evidence-based clinical guideline for the diagnosis and treatment of degenerative lumbar spinal stenosis (update). *Spine J*. 2013;13:734–743.

12. Weinstein JN, Lurie JD, Tosteson TD, et al. Surgical compared with nonoperative treatment for lumbar degenerative spondylolisthesis. Four-year results in the spine patient outcomes research trial (SPORT) randomized and observational cohorts. *J Bone Joint Surg Am*. 2009;91:1295–1304.

13. Lurie JD, Tosteson TD, Tosteson AN, et al. Surgical versus nonoperative treatment for lumbar disc herniation: eight-year results for the spine patient outcomes research trial. *Spine (Phila Pa 1976)*. 2014;39:3–16.

14. Mulleman D, Mammou S, Griffoul I, et al. Pathophysiology of disk-related sciatica. I.—evidence supporting a chemical component. *Joint Bone Spine*. 2006;73:151–158.

15. Hudgins WR. The crossed straight leg raising test: a diagnostic sign of herniated disc. *J Occup Med*. 1979;21:407–408.

16. van der Windt DA, Simons E, Riphagen II, et al. Physical examination for lumbar radiculopathy due to disc herniation in patients with low-back pain. *Cochrane Database Syst Rev*. 2010;(2):CD007431. doi:10.1002/14651858.CD007431.pub2

17. Saal JA, Saal JS. Nonoperative treatment of herniated lumbar intervertebral disc with radiculopathy. An outcome study. *Spine (Phila Pa 1976)*. 1989;14:431–437.

18. Weinstein JN, Lurie JD, Tosteson TD, et al. Surgical versus nonoperative treatment for lumbar disc herniation: four-year results for the spine patient outcomes research trial (SPORT). *Spine (Phila Pa 1976)*. 2008;33:2789–2800.

19. Peul WC, van den Hout WB, Brand R, et al. Prolonged conservative care versus early surgery in patients with sciatica caused by lumbar disc herniation: two year results of a randomised controlled trial. *BMJ*. 2008;336:1355–1358.

20. Atlas SJ, Keller RB, Wu YA, et al. Long-term outcomes of surgical and nonsurgical management of sciatica secondary to a lumbar disc herniation: 10 year results from the maine lumbar spine study. *Spine (Phila Pa 1976)*. 2005;30:927–935.

21. Leven D, Passias PG, Errico TJ, et al. Risk factors for reoperation in patients treated surgically for intervertebral disc herniation: a subanalysis of eight-year SPORT data. *J Bone Joint Surg Am*. 2015;97:1316–1325.

CHAPTER 22

Lower Extremity Tendinopathy in the Setting of Systemic Disease

ANDREW J. ROSENBAUM • JASON P. TARTAGLIONE • MOSTAFA ABOUSAYED • MAXWELL C. ALLEY • JOSHUA S. DINES

Primary disorders of tendons are common musculoskeletal problems that represent diagnostic and treatment challenges for orthopedic surgeons, resulting in chronic and long-lasting morbidities. Recent studies have elucidated that tissue degeneration is the main pathophysiologic process responsible for tendon injuries and disorders, not inflammation.[1–6] Besides overuse, any process, intrinsic or extrinsic, that alters tendon morphology or disrupts the stepwise progression of tendon healing (inflammatory, proliferative, and maturation and remodeling phases), has the potential to cause tendon injury. This includes systemic diseases such as diabetes mellitus (DM), hypercholesterolemia, gout, rheumatoid arthritis, and genetic disorders that alter collagen form and function (i.e., Ehlers–Danlos syndrome, Marfan syndrome, and ochronosis).

Newer theories concerning the pathogenesis of tendinopathies suggest that both inflammatory and degenerative processes play roles in this complex disease entity[7] (Fig. 22-1). The most common tendons affected by tendinopathy in the foot and ankle include the Achilles, posterior tibial, peroneal,

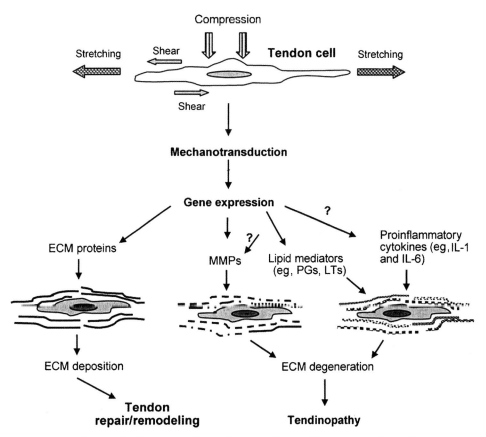

FIGURE 22-1. The biologic responses of tendon fibroblasts to repetitive mechanical loading conditions are shown. Depending on mechanical loading positions, the cellular mechanobiologic responses may lead to tendon physiologic remodeling or pathologic changes such as tendinopathy. ECM, extracellular matrix; MMP, matrix metalloproteinase; PG, prostaglandins; LT, leukotriene; IL, interleukin. (Reproduced from Wang JH, Iosifidis MI, Fu FH. Biomechanical basis for tendinopathy. *Clin Orthop Relat Res.* 2006;443:320–332.)

and flexor hallucis longus (FHL). It has been estimated that 11% of runners are afflicted by Achilles tendinopathy.[8] However, not all tendinopathies are associated with sporting activities, as it has been shown that approximately one-third of patients with Achilles tendinopathy do not participate in vigorous activities.[9] This is exemplified by the fact that the majority of people with radiographic evidence of tendinosis are asymptomatic.[7] Tendinopathies of the foot and ankle cause chronic pain and deformity and affect patients' overall quality of lives. Treatment options depend on the specific tendon involved, duration of symptoms, previous treatments, and patient factors including age, activity level, and medical comorbidities. Both nonsurgical and operative interventions can be used on a case-by-case basis. Unfortunately, there is a paucity in the literature of quality randomized controlled studies to help guide treatment.

In this chapter, we review the pathophysiology of tendinopathy and the risk factors predisposing patients to tendinopathy, particularly in the setting of systemic disorders, and review the evaluation and treatment of common foot and ankle tendinopathies.

DEFINITIONS

In the literature, the nomenclature used to describe tendon disorders has been confusing, and multiple terms are often used to describe the same disease process. Traditionally, the term *tendonitis* has been used to describe chronic pain or dysfunction of a tendon, with the implication that an inflammatory process is the primary underlying pathology. However, histologic review of surgical specimens from chronic tendinopathies of the Achilles, rotator cuff, patella, and extensor carpi radialis brevis has shown either absent or minimal inflammation.[1,2,4–6]

Throughout this chapter, the term "tendinopathy" will be used to describe a spectrum of tendon overuse disorders that include paratendinitis, tendonitis, and tendinosis. Paratendinitis is an acute inflammatory process affecting the paratenon and adjacent nontendinous tissues. In isolation, this pathologic process does not usually cause tendon rupture, is reversible, and can be treated with tenolysis in refractory cases.

Tendonitis is tendinopathy with the presence of a histologically proven inflammatory process. Studies have demonstrated that overloaded equine superficial digital flexor tendons undergo an acute phase of tendon injury that involves inflammatory cells early on in the injury process, which is followed by a degenerative process.[10,11] Tendinosis describes a degenerative process that lacks inflammation. These tendons have intrasubstance degeneration, which can be appreciated clinically by nodules within the tendon.

PATHOPHYSIOLOGY

Tendons are composed mainly of collagen fibrils, which are encased by an endotenon. Multiple collagen fibrils grouped together are surrounded by an epitenon that demarcates the actual tendon. In order to provide protection and lubrication and prevent friction, some tendons have a true enveloping synovial sheath (i.e., tibialis posterior and peroneal tendons), whereas other tendons are encased solely by a peritenon (i.e., Achilles). The extracellular matrix consists of collagen (65% to 80% of dry weight), most of which is Type I, which provides tendons with tensile strength. The mechanical behavior of tendons, which is viscoelastic in nature, is secondary to the cross-sectional area and length of the tendon. The larger a tendon's cross-sectional area, the greater the load to failure rate.[12] Tendons with longer fibers have decreased stiffness, equivalent load to failure rates, but increased elongation to failure rates.[13] The rest of the extracellular matrix is made up of 1% to 2% elastin and a ground substance that consists of 60% to 80% water, proteoglycans, and glycoproteins.[7] Tenoblasts and tenocytes form parallel rows between collagen fibers, making up 90% to 95% of tendons' cellular components.[7] Tendons carry their function through the musculotendinous junction, a richly innervated transitional area between the muscle and the tendon that experiences high mechanical forces, therefore making this region susceptible to injury. The enthesis, or osteotendinous junction, is an organized transition zone from tendon to bone allowing muscles to effectively transmit force to bone.

To date, the etiology and pathophysiology of tendinopathy are not well understood. As previously stated, tendinopathy was once believed to be the result of inflammation. However, through clinical practice, it has become recognized that anti-inflammatory medications do not relieve the pain associated with tendinopathy. In addition, using microdialysis, Alfredson et al.[14] demonstrated a lack of the inflammatory mediator prostaglandin E$_2$ in chronically affected Achilles tendons. However, clinical and basic science research often involves chronically affected tendons, making it possible that inflammation plays a role in the initial insult to chronically diseased tendons.

Histologically, chronic tendinopathy is characterized by degenerative changes, which include decreased cellularity and calcific, hypoxic, hyaline, mucoid, myxoid, fibrinoid, and fatty degenerations[2,4,15] (**Fig. 22-2**). Chronic tendinopathy is also characterized by an increase in Type III collagen, which has less cross-links than Type I collagen, conferring decreased tensile strength, as well as degeneration and loss of organization of collagen fibers mainly due to increased activity of matrix metalloproteinases.[16] Studies have shown that degenerative areas of tendons experience neovascularization.[17,18] Interestingly, using in vivo powered Doppler ultrasonography, various studies have demonstrated that neovascularization is often associated with patients who are symptomatic and experiencing pain.[17,19] Lastly, degenerative changes characterized by adhesions and increased number of fibroblasts and myofibroblasts are found in peritendinous tissues, most commonly occurring in tendons with synovial sheaths (posterior tibial and peroneal tendons).[20] Grossly, chronically diseased tendons have a disorganized appearance illustrated by a yellowish or brown color, palpable thickenings

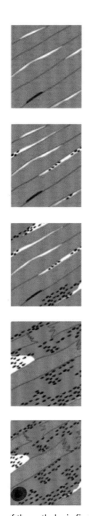

FIGURE 22-2. A summary of the pathologic findings associated with tendinopathy. (Reproduced from *UpToDate*, Wolters Kluwer Health.)

or nodules in the areas of chronic disease and degeneration that can be calcified.

There are currently three main theories describing the etiology of tendon degeneration that can progress to chronic tendinopathy and potential rupture: the mechanical, vascular, and neural theories.

The *mechanical theory* of tendinopathy describes how chronic repetitive damage to tendons over time could lead to a state of degeneration as opposed to inflammation. This theory states that repetitive loading of a tendon under physiologic loads progresses to degeneration and ultimate tendon failure. At rest, tendon collagen fibers are disorganized in a wave-like formation. As a tendon is loaded, these fibers begin to organize in a parallel manner. This occurs in the toe region of the stress–strain curve. Once the collagen fibers align and experience continued force, the tendon enters the elastic part of the stress–strain curve, which is characterized by a linear relationship between load and strain. It has been shown that normal physiologic loading of a tendon occurs between 4% and 8% strain.[21–26] At the higher end of the physiologic loading, tendons experience microscopic trauma, leading to degeneration and failure with repetitive stress. This repetitive

microtrauma can lead to the alteration of mechanical properties of tendons as well as a symptomatic tendon.[21,27–29] This theory fails to account for why specific areas of tendons have a predilection for injury and does not explain why some patients are symptomatic and others are not.

The *vascular theory* of tendinopathy is formed on the basis that tendons are metabolic structures with metabolic demands requiring an adequate vascular supply. The theory states that in the absence of an adequate blood supply, tendons undergo degeneration. Certain tendons, including the Achilles[30] and posterior tibial[31] tendons, have been shown to have areas of hypovascularity. For example, the watershed area of the Achilles tendon has been shown to occur in the midportion of the tendon as compared to areas closer to the proximal musculotendinous junction and distal enthesis.[32] However, using laser Doppler flowmetry, Astrom and Westlin[32] demonstrated that the Achilles tendon has uniform blood supply, except at the distal insertion.

The *neural theory* of tendinopathy is based on multiple observations from various studies trying to connect the role of tendon degeneration and neural-mediated causes. Tendons are highly innervated structures that have nerve endings closely associated with mast cells. It is theorized that tendon overuse causes overstimulation of nerves and subsequent degranulation of mast cells with the release of neuromodulators such as substance P, a nociceptive neurotransmitter and proinflammatory mediator,[33] and a calcitonin related peptide.[34] Increased levels of substance P have been found in rotator cuff tendinopathy,[35] and the neurotransmitter glutamate has been found in Achilles tendinopathy.[14] Lastly, Maffulli et al.[36] discovered a relationship between sciatica and Achilles tendinopathy, suggesting a connection between tendinopathy and a neural-mediated cause. Further research is needed to understand the full significance and role of relationship between nerve stimulation and tendinopathy.

It is likely that the combination of early inflammation and later degeneration plays a role in the pathogenesis of chronic tendon injury and tendinopathy. No one theory completely explains the etiology of tendinopathy; rather, it is likely a combination of the mechanical, vascular, and neural theories that best explains the pathogenesis. Further studies are needed to better understand the interconnectedness of these theories.

RISK FACTORS

The risk factors implicated in the development of tendinopathy can be stratified into two large categories: extrinsic and intrinsic (Table 22-1). Extrinsic risk factors, such as overuse, are those most commonly implicated. However, other extrinsic factors that must be recognized include training errors, fatigue, environmental conditions, footwear, equipment, and medications/nutritional supplementation. Intrinsic risk factors are innate to a given individual, and include one's genetic makeup, congenital disorders (e.g., alkaptonuria), limb malalignment, gender, aging, neurologic conditions, medical comorbidities (e.g., hypertension), and systemic diseases.

Table 22-1.	Risk Factors for the Development of Tendinopathy
Extrinsic	
Overuse	
Training errors	
Environmental conditions	
Poor equipment	
Poor ergonomics	
Medications/nutritional supplementation (e.g., fluoroquinolones)	
Intrinsic	
Increased age	
Increased body mass index	
Gender	
Biomechanical abnormalities	
Prior tendon lesions	
Limb malalignment	
Genetic makeup	
Medical comorbidities	
Systemic conditions	

The role of genetics in the development of tendinopathy is attributed to a sequence variation within the Type V collagen and Tenascin C genes.[37] Admittedly, the exact role of these genes in the pathophysiology of tendinopathy has yet to be defined. Aging has also been implicated because of its adverse effects on the mechanical properties of tendons, which may be due to reduced blood flow, local hypoxia, free radical production, impaired metabolism and nutrition, and advanced glycosylation end products (AGEs).[7]

The association between systemic disease and tendinopathy has been described in a multitude of studies, with diabetes, hypercholesterolemia, hyperuricemia, and obesity all implicated in the pathogenesis of tendon degeneration. Rheumatoid arthritis, in addition to many other autoimmune diseases, can also predispose patients to tendinopathy. In the setting of diabetes, tendon damage is caused by an excess of AGEs, which causes an oxidation-driven cross-linking of collagen. Unlike the enzymatically driven cross-linking of collagen, which has beneficial effects on tendon strength, AGE cross-linking compromises the biologic and mechanical integrity of tendons.[38] In both Type I and Type II DM, increased tendon thickness and structural abnormalities of the plantar fascia and Achilles tendon have been observed.

Tendon xanthoma is associated with heterozygous familial hypercholesterolemia (HeFH). This inherited disease involves a mutated low-density lipoprotein (LDL) receptor gene, leading to defective LDL catabolism.[39] The xanthoma, and subsequent tendon degeneration, occurs as cholesterol is deposited both extracellularly and inside histiocytes and other foam cells, triggering an inflammatory response and fibrous

reaction. The Achilles tendon is most commonly involved. Nonfamilial hypercholesterolemia may also contribute to tendinopathy. In one investigation, the concentration of serum lipids was found to be higher in subjects with an Achilles tendon rupture as compared to controls.[40] However, other works refute this, demonstrating tendon abnormalities only in subjects with familial hypercholesterolemia.[41]

Hyperuricemia can lead to monosodium urate (MSU) crystal deposition in tendon, in addition to other soft tissues and joints. These crystals, which are responsible for gout, can manifest in tendons as indolent nodules, which can be challenging to distinguish from other subcutaneous nodules, such as those seen in rheumatoid arthritis. In vitro studies have demonstrated that at serum uric acid levels of approximately 7 mg per dL, crystal precipitation begins to occur.[42] However, the in vivo development of MSU crystals is dependent on other factors as well; trauma, mechanical stress, decreased blood flow, and lower temperatures create an environment conducive to crystal deposition.[43]

There is a well-defined relationship between obesity and tendinopathy.[44] Although it was once thought that only load-bearing tendons were affected by obesity, the relationship between adiposity and tendinopathy is now recognized in non–load-bearing tendons as well.[45] This is due to an enhanced understanding of the systemic effects of adipose, specifically with regard to its role in the endocrine system. In other words, it is not simply the excess stress placed on tendons that leads to tendinopathy in the setting of obesity, but is also due to the bioactive peptides and hormones released by adipose tissue, such as chemerin, lipocalin 2, serum amyloid A3, leptin, and adiponectin.[46] These proteins stimulate a low-grade inflammatory response that disrupts the biologic milieu crucial for normal tendon homeostasis.[47] Further, obesity can lead to insulin resistance and the subsequent development of diabetes. As discussed previously, this disease is also implicated in tendinopathy.[48]

DIAGNOSIS

History and Physical Examination

A detailed history is imperative when concerned for tendinopathies of the foot and ankle, as patients' symptoms are often vague and present insidiously. A common complaint is pain in the region of the affected tendon that worsens with sustained activity or on weight bearing. Early on, pain is absent at rest, may decrease after a warm-up period, and is triggered by specific activities. With more advanced disease, patients describe continuous discomfort that is exacerbated by a broader spectrum of activities.

The clinician must identify any risk factors for tendinopathy, such as age, obesity, overuse, training errors, medication side effects, smoking, improper shoe wear, and systemic conditions.

Although patients may describe a specific injury, participation in a new sport or exercise, or an increase in the intensity of physical activity preceding the onset of symptoms, those with tendinopathy that is the manifestation of a systemic process may not. Therefore, clinicians must also inquire about concurrent musculoskeletal symptoms in other tendons or joints, which are most consistent with a systemic process.[49,50] Admittedly, the causes of tendinopathy do not solely occur independent of each other. Clinicians must therefore remember that one's presenting symptoms may be the cumulative result of several underlying processes.

The aforementioned relationship between tendinopathy and systemic disease elucidates the importance of obtaining thorough general health, medication, and past medical histories from patients in whom there is concern for a tendinopathy. Although some patients will present with a known diagnosis of one of those conditions, others may be unaware. This is commonly observed with DM, as approximately 25% of patients are unaware that they have the disease.[51]

Physical examination must include assessment of the entire body, as nonspecific findings such as body habitus may be of tremendous diagnostic utility. In a study investigating the relationship between fat distribution and tendinopathy, it was determined that Achilles tendon pathology is associated with central fat distribution in men and peripheral fat distribution in women.[48]

With regard to the foot and ankle examination, a comprehensive assessment is warranted. The examination should begin with visual inspection, which may reveal subtle differences as compared with the contralateral side. Such findings include swelling, muscle atrophy, skin breakdown, bruising, and deformity in the region of the affected tendon. With tendinopathy, discomfort is brought on by palpation along the affected tendon and during assessment of strength and function, which is usually diminished as well. A patient's alignment and neurovascular status must also be assessed during the examination.

In the foot and ankle, Achilles, posterior tibial, peroneal, tibialis anterior (TA), and FHL tendinopathies can result from underlying systemic processes. It is therefore important for clinicians to have a familiarity with the common examination findings associated with each of these. With Achilles tendinopathy, patients often present with pain and swelling in and around the tendon, and can also have palpable nodules, as seen in the setting of a xanthoma. Posterior tibial tendinopathy (PTT) is associated with the "too many toes" sign, which describes the increased number of toes evident on the lateral aspect of the involved foot when viewed from behind[52] (Fig. 22-3). In addition, when asked to stand on tiptoe, normal heel varus will not occur, and pain will ensue along the PTT. Tendinopathy of the peroneal tendons is frequently associated with lateral ankle pain, instability, and swelling. The pain can be reproduced with active dorsiflexion and eversion of the foot against resistance. In patients with TA, a bulbous enlargement of the tendon of the dorsal medial foot may be evident. If it is ruptured or severely attenuated, patients may have a foot drop. With FHL tendinopathy, posteromedial ankle pain may be present, and pain along the tendon will occur when the patient is asked to flex the hallux against resistance and with the foot in plantarflexion.

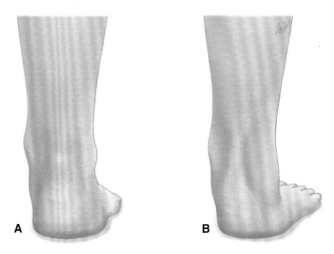

FIGURE 22-3. A: Normal posterior view of the foot. **B:** Evidence of arch collapse with "too many toes" sign. (Reproduced from *UpToDate*, Wolters Kluwer Health.)

Diagnostic Adjuncts

Plain radiographs should be the first imaging studies obtained, as they can exclude bony abnormalities and other pathologies as the cause of symptoms. Radiographs may also demonstrate osseous changes consistent with various systemic disorders, such as the erosive changes in the hallux consistent with gout (Fig. 22-4). Advanced imaging, such as ultrasound and magnetic resonance imaging (MRI), is warranted if the diagnosis remains unclear or if a patient fails to respond to conservative interventions.

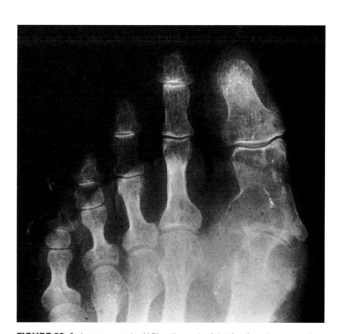

FIGURE 22-4. Anteroposterior (AP) radiograph of the forefoot demonstrating the destructive changes to the first metatarsophalangeal joint consistent with gout. (Reproduced from Rubin R, Strayer DS, Rubin E, eds. *Rubin's Pathology: Clinicopathologic Foundations of Medicine*. 6th ed. Philadelphia, PA: Lippincott Williams & Wilkins; 2012:1263.)

MRI is considered the standard for tendon imaging because of its excellent soft tissue contrast and visualization of intratendinous abnormalities.[53] It can also distinguish clinically similar entities, such as Achilles tendinosis and peritendinitis.[53] However, ultrasound has recently become a popular means of imaging tendons as it can be performed at a lower cost and has the advantage of dynamic real-time imaging.[54] Further, its high sensitivity, accuracy, and positive predictive value for tendon pathology of the foot and ankle are comparable to those of MRI.[54,55] When used in conjunction with Doppler techniques, ultrasound becomes even more advantageous, as it is able to delineate areas of neovascularization that are associated with tendinopathy.[18] In general, the ultrasound findings consistent with tendinopathy include increased cross-sectional and anterior–posterior tendon diameter, disruption of normal fibrillar patterns and irregular tendon structure, and hypoechoic areas within the tendon[56] (**Fig. 22-5**).

Laboratory studies are indicated if tendinopathy is thought to have resulted from a systemic condition. In addition to a complete blood count and metabolic panel, condition-specific labs must be obtained when the clinician is concerned for an underlying metabolic process as the cause of one's tendinopathy. Hemoglobin A1c (HbA1c) is beneficial in the workup for diabetes, and is representative of an individual's blood glucose control over the previous 2 to 3 months. An HbA1c >6.5% on two separate tests is consistent with the diagnosis of diabetes. The workup of rheumatoid arthritis and seronegative arthropathies, such as systemic lupus erythematosus, includes rheumatoid factor, antinuclear antibody, human leukocyte antigen B27, C-reactive protein, and an erythrocyte sedimentation rate.

When concerned that a tendinopathy is due to cholesterol metabolism, a lipid panel should be performed. In fact, Beeharry et al.[57] suggest that all young patients complaining of severe Achilles tendon pain for four or more days should have their serum cholesterol checked, as this is a common finding in patients with HeFH, as compared to control subjects. In another investigation, Gaida et al.[45] found that individuals with symptomatic Achilles tendinopathy had higher triglyceride

levels and lower high-density lipoprotein levels as compared with gender, age, and body mass index–matched controls.

A serum uric acid level must be obtained when the clinician's differential diagnosis includes MSU crystal deposition. In the work by Pineda et al.,[58] Achilles tendinopathy secondary to MSU deposition was more common in hyperuricemic as compared to normouricemic patients (15% vs. 1.9%, respectively).

TREATMENT

Available modalities for the treatment of foot and ankle tendinopathies range from conservative interventions to surgery. Although orthopedic surgeons and other musculoskeletal clinicians are typically able to manage such tendinopathies and the intrinsic and extrinsic risk factors most often responsible (e.g., overuse), those occurring in the setting of systemic disease often necessitate a multidisciplinary approach. Without treatment of the underlying condition, a patient's symptoms may fail to resolve, worsen, or recur following treatment. Further, systemic diseases such as obesity and diabetes predispose patients to inferior operative outcomes and complications.[59] In such instances, perioperative optimization is recommended with the assistance of a patient's endocrinologist, internist, or other specialist.

Most patients diagnosed with tendinopathy are initially treated with a 2- to 6-week period of rest with or without immobilization. However, there is no consensus on the exact period of rest needed, which is dependent on the extent of injury and the patient's level of activity. Medications such as nonsteroidal anti-inflammatory drugs (NSAIDs) and acetaminophen are also used at this time. Although NSAIDs provide short-term pain relief, they have not been shown to affect long-term outcomes. Further, there is no evidence to suggest that NSAIDs are more effective than acetaminophen for the treatment of tendinopathy.[60]

Following treatment with these modalities, a supervised physical therapy program can be initiated that is focused on stretching and strengthening (**Figs. 22-6** to **22-8**). Eccentric stretching and strengthening promotes the formation of new collagen and is associated with excellent results, particularly in the management of Achilles tendinopathy.[61] Ultrasound, laser, massage, and electrical stimulation have been used to supplement the rehabilitation process, but no conclusive evidence exists regarding the benefits of these modalities.[62–64] Other less traditional interventions, such as extracorporeal shock wave therapy (ESWT) and platelet-rich plasma (PRP), have begun to receive attention as novel techniques designed to improve tendon biology and mechanical integrity.

Repetitive low-energy ESWT is an alternative to surgery for both chronic tendinopathies that have failed other conservative interventions.[65–67] It works by introducing pressure waves at a diseased site which are converted into biochemical signals. These signals in turn stimulate the release of growth factors, increase vascularity, and enhance extracellular matrix production.[68] In a systematic review by Al-Abbad et al., benefits of

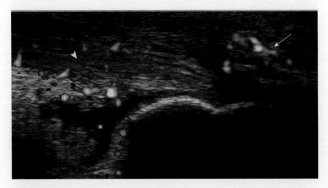

FIGURE 22-5. Ultrasound of the Achilles tendon demonstrating enthesitis (*arrow*), tendonitis (*arrowhead*), and retrocalcaneal bursitis (*). (Reproduced from *UpToDate*, Wolters Kluwer Health.)

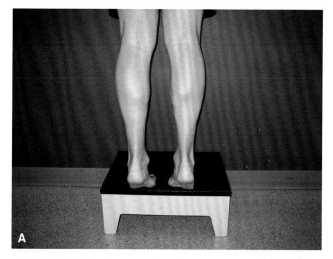

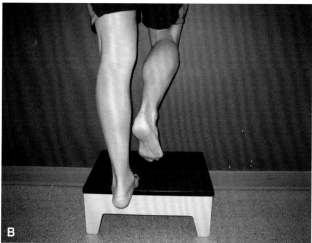

FIGURE 22-6. A: Eccentric Achilles strengthening exercise part 1: standing bilateral plantar flexion. **B:** Eccentric Achilles strengthening exercise part 2: standing unilateral controlled lowering. (Reproduced from Lotke PA, Abboud JA, Ende J. *Lippincott's Primary Care Orthopedics*. Philadelphia, PA: Wolters Kluwer; 2013. Figures 76-10, 76-11, with permission.)

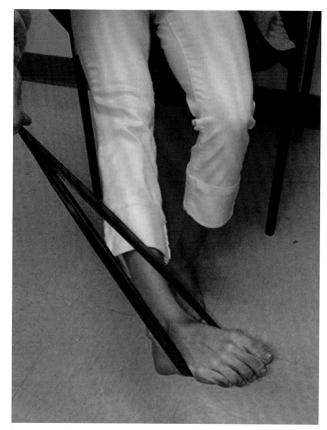

FIGURE 22-7. An example of a posterior tibial tendon strengthening exercise with a resistance band. (Reproduced from *UpToDate*, Wolters Kluwer Health.)

ESWT in the setting of chronic Achilles tendinopathy were consistently observed.[65] Rasmussen et al. found that patients with Achilles tendinopathy who were treated with ESWT improved their American Orthopaedic Foot and Ankle Society (AOFAS) scores to a significantly greater extent than those in a sham group at 3 months follow-up.[66] Further, ESWT may be of greater clinical utility when combined with an eccentric loading program, as described by Rompe et al.[67] Future research is needed regarding the optimal energy levels and the number of treatments necessary to achieve good results with ESWT. Studies with longer term follow-up would also be beneficial, as most literature has on the short-term benefits.[69]

Biologic therapies, such as PRP, attempt to facilitate the healing of degenerative tendons through the introduction of a high concentration of platelets and their respective growth factors to areas of diseased tendon.

The growth factors derived from these platelets include platelet-derived growth factor, transforming growth factor β, vascular endothelial growth factor, epidermal growth factor, insulin-like growth factors I and II, and fibroblast growth factor, which stimulate a healing response.[70] Specifically, they promote the formation of extracellular matrix and granulation tissue and stimulate cell growth, proliferation, angiogenesis, and cell migration. Platelets are found in extremely high concentrations in PRP as compared to normal plasma. Although the normal concentration of platelets is approximately 200,000 per μL, in PRP, it is approximately 2 million per μL.[71]

Monto[72] evaluated the role of PRP in treating chronic Achilles tendinopathy, and found it to be a beneficial intervention. At 6 months following treatment, abnormalities in MRI and ultrasound had resolved in 27 of 29 patients. At 24 months posttreatment, the average AOFAS score was 88; it was 34 pretreatment.[71] However, other investigations have not found PRP to be advantageous. In a randomized controlled trial by de Vos et al.,[73] eccentric exercises with a PRP injection did not result in greater improvement in pain and activity as compared to eccentric exercises with a saline placebo injection. As such, future research is required to enhance our understanding of PRP as a treatment for tendinopathy.

Surgical intervention is indicated if a patient has continued symptoms after 3 to 6 months of conservative treatments or if a tendon rupture has occurred. The general principles include debridement of abnormal tendon, the release of fibrous adhesions, and repair or tubularization of the remaining viable

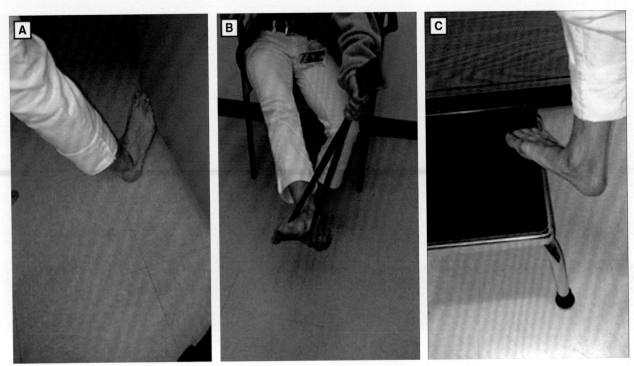

FIGURE 22-8. Exercises for the rehabilitation of peroneal tendinopathy. **A:** Isometric contraction against a wall with foot everted. **B:** Resistance band eccentric exercise. **C:** Heel drop and raise on step. (Reproduced from *UpToDate*, Wolters Kluwer Health; Courtesy of Timothy Draper, DO, AAFP, CAQ Sports Medicine.)

tendon. Tendon transfers and autograft- or allograft-based tendon reconstruction are used in severe cases of tendinopathy. Osseous procedures, such as the calcaneal osteotomies performed for PTT and pes planus, are designed to correct the underlying deformity and any malalignment.

CONCLUSION

Tendinopathies of the foot and ankle have traditionally been thought of as overuse injuries. Although this remains one of the most common causes of symptomatic lower extremity tendinopathy, the role of systemic disease must also always be considered, as metabolic derangements can adversely affect the mechanical and physiologic integrity of tendon. As the prevalence of metabolic disorders, such as DM and obesity, continues to rise in the United States, so too will the sequelae of these conditions.[73,74] Practitioners must therefore have a familiarity with the deleterious musculoskeletal effects of such diseases.

The evaluation of patients with a presumed tendinopathy of the lower extremity must begin with a complete history and physical examination. Admittedly, physical findings may fail to distinguish an overuse tendinopathy from that caused by a systemic process. However, patients may present with a previous diagnosis of a systemic disease. And in other patients, the history may aid practitioners in diagnosis, as complaints such as morning stiffness or involvement of multiple anatomic locations are often indicative of an underlying systemic process.

Although therapeutic interventions for lower extremity tendinopathies are most dependent on the tendon involved

and patients' prior treatments, those individuals with tendinopathy manifesting due to a systemic disease may benefit from additional treatments targeting the underlying process. These interventions, such as oral hypoglycemic medications for patients with diabetes, play a critical role not only in minimizing the musculoskeletal manifestations but also in controlling the sequelae of the disease process throughout the body. As such, we cannot overstate the pivotal role of musculoskeletal clinicians in the diagnosis and treatment of foot and ankle tendinopathies, particularly when due to systemic disease.

REFERENCES

1. Astrom M, Rausing A. Chronic Achilles tendinopathy: a survey of surgical and histopathologic findings. *Clin Orthop Relat Res.* 1995;316:151–164.
2. Hashimoto T, Nobuhara K, Hamada T. Pathologic evidence of degeneration as a primary cause of rotator cuff tear. *Clin Orthop Relat Res.* 2003;415:111–120.
3. Kannus P, Jozsa L. Histopathological changes preceding spontaneous rupture of a tendon. A controlled study of 891 patients. *J Bone Joint Surg Am.* 1991;73:1507–1525.
4. Khan KM, Maffulli N, Coleman BD, et al. Patella tendinopathy: some aspects of basic science and clinical management. *Br J Sports Med.* 1998;32:346–355.
5. Movin T, Gad A, Reinholt FP, et al. Tendon pathology in long-standing achillodynia. Biopsy findings in 40 patients. *Acta Orthop Scand.* 1997;68:170–175.
6. Potter HG, Hannafin JA, Morwessel RM, et al. Lateral epicondylitis: correlation of MR imaging, surgical, and histopathologic findings. *Radiology.* 1995;196(1):43–46.
7. Abate M, Silbernagel KG, Siljeholm C, et al. Pathogenesis of tendinopathies: inflammation or degeneration? *Arthritis Res Ther.* 2009;11:235.

8. James SL, Bates BT, Osternig LR. Injuries to runners. *Am J Sports Med.* 1978;6:40–50.

9. Rolf C, Movin T. Etiology, histopathology and outcome of surgery in achillodynia. *Foot Ankle Int.* 1997;18:565–569.

10. Marr CM, McMillan I, Boyd JS, et al. Ultrasonographic and histopathological findings in equine superficial digital flexor tendon injury. *Equine Vet J.* 1993;25:23–29.

11. Williams IF, McCullagh KG, Goodship AE, et al. Studies on the pathogenesis of equine tendonitis following collagenase injury. *Res Vet Sci.* 1984;36:326–338.

12. Williams LN, Elder SH, Bouvard JL, et al. The anisotropic compressive mechanical properties of the rabbit patellar tendon. *Biorheology.* 2008;45:577–586.

13. Yamamoto E, Hayashi K, Yamamoto N. Mechanical properties of collagen fascicles from the rabbit patellar tendon. *J Biomech Eng.* 1999;121:124–131.

14. Alfredson A, Thorsen K, Lorentzon R. *In situ* microdialysis in tendon tissue: high levels of glutamate, but not prostaglandin E2 in chronic Achilles tendon pain. *Knee Surg Sports Traumatol Arthrosc.* 1999;7:378–381.

15. Maffulli N, Wong J, Almekinders LC. Types and epidemiology of tendinopathy. *Clin Sports Med.* 2003;22:675–692.

16. Kader D, Saxena A, Movin T, et al. Achilles tendinopathy: some aspects of basic science and clinical management. *Br J Sports Med.* 2002;36:239–249.

17. Gissen K, Alfredson H. Neovascularization and pain in jumper's knee: a prospective clinical and sonographic study in elite junior volleyball players. *Br J Sports Med.* 2005;39:423–428.

18. Ohberg L, Lorentzon R, Alfredson H. Neovascularization in Achilles tendons with painful tendinosis but not in normal tendons: an ultrasonographic investigation. *Knee Surg Sports Traumatol Arthrosc.* 2001;9(4):233–238.

19. Knobloch K, Kraemer R, Lichtenberg A, et al. Achilles tendon and paratendon microcirculation in midportion and insertional tendinopathy in athletes. *Am J Sports Med.* 2006;34:92–97.

20. Jarvinen M, Jozsa L, Kannus P, et al. Histopathological findings in chronic tendon disorders. *Scand J Med Sci Sports.* 1997;7:86–95.

21. Curwin SL. The aetiology and treatment of tendinitis. In: Harries M, Williams C, Stanish WD, et al., eds. *Oxford Textbook of Sports Medicine.* 2nd ed. Oxford, UK: Oxford University Press; 1998: 610–632.

22. Krikendall DT, Garrett WE. Function and biomechanics of tendons. *Scand J Med Sci Sports.* 1997;7:62–66.

23. Magnusson SP, Hansen P, Aagaard P, et al. Differential strain patterns of the human gastrocnemius aponeurosis and free tendon, in vivo. *Acta Physiol Scnad.* 2003;177:185–195.

24. McGough RL, Debski RE, Taskiran E, et al. Mechanical properties of the long head of the biceps tendon. *Knee Surg Sports Traumatol Arthosc.* 1996;3:226–229.

25. Muramatsu T, Muraoka T, Takeshita D, et al. Mechanical properties of tendon and aponeurosis of human gastrocnemius muscle in vivo. *J Appl Physiol.* 2001;90:1671–1678.

26. Sheehan FT, Drace JE. Human patellar tendon strain. A non-invasive, in vivo study. *Clin Orthop Relat Res.* 2000;370:201–207.

27. Barnes GRG, Pinder DN. In vivo tendon tension and bone strain measurement and correlation. *J Biomech.* 1974;7:35–42.

28. Mosler E, Folkhard W, Knorzer E, et al. Stress-induced molecular re-arrangement in tendon collagen. *J Mol Biol.* 1985;182:589–596.

29. Wren TA, Lindsey DP, Beaupre GS, et al. Effects of creep and cyclic loading on the mechanical properties and failure of human Achilles tendons. *Ann Biomed Eng.* 2003;31:710–717.

30. Ahmed IM, Lagopoulos M, McConnell P, et al. Blood supply of the Achilles tendon. *J Orthop Res.* 1998;16:591–596.

31. Frey C, Shereff M, Greenidge N. Vascularity of the posterior tibial tendon. *J Bone Joint Surg Am.* 1990;72:884–888.

32. Astrom M, Westlin N. Blood flow in the human Achilles tendon assessed by laser Doppler flowmetry. *J Orthop Res.* 1994;12:246–252.

33. Garrett NE, Mapp PI, Cruwys SC, et al. Role of substance P in inflammatory arthritis. *Ann Rheum Dis.* 1992;51:1014–1018.

34. Hart DA, Frank CB, Bray RC. Inflammatory processes in repetitive motion and overuse syndromes; potential role of neurogenic mechanisms in tendons and ligaments. In: Gordon SL, Blair SJ, Fine LJ, eds. *Repetitive Motion Disorders of the Upper Extremity.* Rosemont, IL: American Academy of Orthopaedic Surgeons; 1995:247–262.

35. Gotoh M, Hamada K, Yamakawa H, et al. Increased substance P in subacromial bursa and shoulder pain in rotator cuff diseases. *J Orthop Res.* 1998;16:618–621.

36. Maffulli N, Irwin AS, Kenward MG, et al. Achilles tendon rupture and sciatica: a possible correlation. *Br J Sports Med.* 1998;32:174–177.

37. Magra M, Maffulli N. Genetic aspects of tendinopathy. *J Sci Med Sport.* 2008;11:243–247.

38. Abate M, Schiavone C, Pelotti P, et al. Limited joint mobility in diabetes and ageing: recent advances in pathogenesis and therapy. *Int J Immunopathol Pharmacol.* 2010;23:997–1003.

39. Beason DP, Abboud JA, Kuntz AF, et al. Cumulative effects of hypercholesterolemia on tendon biomechanics in a mouse model. *J Orthop Res.* 2011;29:380–383.

40. Ozgurtas T, Yildiz C, Serdar M, et al. Is high concentration of serum lipids a risk factor for Achilles tendon rupture? *Clin Chim Acta.* 2003;331:25–28.

41. Junyent M, Gilabert R, Zambón D, et al. The use of Achilles tendon sonography to distinguish familial hypercholesterolemia from other genetic dyslipidemias. *Arterioscler Thromb Vasc Biol.* 2005;25:2203–2208.

42. Choi HK, Mount DB, Reginato AM. Pathogenesis of gout. *Ann Intern Med.* 2005;143:499–516.

43. Schlesinger N, Thiele RG. The pathogenesis of bone erosions in gouty arthritis. *Ann Rheum Dis.* 2010;69:1907–1912.

44. Gaida JE, Cook JL, Bass SL. Adiposity and tendinopathy. *Disabil Rehabil.* 2008;30:1555–1562.

45. Gaida JE, Alfredson L, Kiss ZS, et al. Dyslipidemia in Achilles tendinopathy is characteristic of insulin resistance. *Med Sci Sports Exerc.* 2009;41:1194–1197.

46. Conde J, Gomez R, Bianco G, et al. Expanding the adipokine network in cartilage: identification and regulation of novel factors in human and murine chondrocytes. *Ann Rheum Dis.* 2011;70:551–559.

47. Cilli F, Khan M, Fu F, et al. Prostaglandin E2 affects proliferation and collagen synthesis by human patellar tendon fibroblasts. *Clin J Sport Med.* 2004;14:232–236.

48. Gaida JE, Alfredson H, Kiss ZS, et al. Asymptomatic Achilles tendon pathology is associated with a central fat distribution in men and a peripheral fat distribution in women: a cross sectional study of 298 individuals. *BMC Musculoskelet Disord.* 2010;11:41.

49. Batista F, Nery C, Pinzur M, et al. Achilles tendinopathy in diabetes mellitus. *Foot Ankle Int.* 2008;29(5):498–501.

50. Popelka S, Hromadka R, Vavrik P, et al. Isolated talonavicular arthrodesis in patients with rheumatoid arthritis of the foot and tibialis posterior tendon dysfunction. *BMC Musculoskelet Disord.* 2010;11:38.

51. American Diabetes Association. Diagnosis and classification of diabetes mellitus. *Diabetes Care.* 2012;35(Suppl 1):S64–S71.

52. Johnson KA. Tibialis posterior tendon rupture. *Clin Orthop Relat Res.* 1983;177:140–147.

53. Karjalainen PT, Soila K, Aronen HJ, et al. MR imaging of overuse injuries of the Achilles tendon. *Am J Roentgenol.* 2000;175(1):251–260.

54. Rockett MS, Waitches G, Sudakoff G, et al. Use of ultrasonography versus magnetic resonance imaging for tendon abnormalities around the ankle. *Foot Ankle Int.* 1998;19:604–612.

55. Grant TH, Kelikian AS, Jereb SE, et al. Ultrasound diagnosis of peroneal tendon tears. A surgical correlation. *J Bone Joint Surg Am.* 2005;87(8):1788–1794.

56. Leung JLY, Griffith JF. Sonography of chronic Achilles tendinopathy: a case-control study. *J Clin Ultrasound.* 2008;36(1):27–32.

57. Beeharry D, Coupe B, Benbow EW, et al. Familial hypercholes-terolaemia commonly presents with Achilles tenosynovitis. *Ann Rheum Dis.* 2006;65:312–315.

58. Pineda C, Amezcua-Guerra LM, Solano C, et al. Joint and tendon subclinical involvement suggestive of gouty arthritis in asymptom-atic hyperuricemia: an ultrasound controlled study. *Arthritis Res Ther.* 2011;13:R4.

59. Scott AT, Le IL, Easley ME. Surgical strategies: noninsertional Achilles tendinopathy. *Foot Ankle Int.* 2008;29(7):759–771.

60. Mafulli N, Longo UG, Petrillo S, et al. Management of tendinop-athies of the foot and ankle. *Orthop Trauma.* 2012;26(4):259–264.

61. Ohberg L, Lorentzon R, Alfredson H. Eccentric training in patients with chronic Achilles tendinosis: normalized tendon structure and decreased thickness at follow-up. *Br J Sports Med.* 2004;38(8):8–11.

62. Basford JR. Low intensity laser therapy: still not an established clinical tool. *Lasers Surg Med.* 1995;16:331–342.

63. Hamilton B, Purdam C. Patella tendinosis as an adaptive process: a new hypothesis. *Br J Sports Med.* 2004;38:758–761.

64. Robertson VJ, Baker KG. A review of therapeutic ultrasound; effectiveness studies. *Phys Ther.* 2001;81:1339–1350.

65. Al-Abbad H, Simon JV. The effectiveness of extracorporeal shock wave therapy on chronic Achilles tendinopathy: a systematic review. *Foot Ankle Int.* 2013;34(1):33–41.

66. Rasmussen S, Christensen M, Mathiesen I, et al. Shockwave ther-apy for chronic Achilles tendinopathy: a double-blind, randomized clinical trial of efficacy. *Acta Orthop.* 2008;79(2):249–256.

67. Rompe JD, Furia J, Maffulli N. Eccentric loading versus eccen-tric loading plus shock-wave treatment for midportion Achilles tendinopathy: a randomized controlled trial. *Am J Sports Med.* 2009;37(3):463–470.

68. Notarnicola A, Moretti B. The biological effects of extracorporeal shock wave therapy (eswt) on tendon tissue. *Muscles Ligaments Tendons J.* 2012;2(1):33–37.

69. Mani-Babu S, Morrissey D, Waugh C, et al. The effectiveness of extracorporeal shock wave therapy in lower limb tendinopathy: a systematic review. *Am J Sports Med.* 2015;43(3):752–761.

70. Eppley B, Woodell JE, Higgins J. Platelet quantification and growth factor analysis from platelet-rich plasma: implications for wound healing. *Plast Reconstr Surg.* 2004;114:1502–1508.

71. Woodell-May JE, Ridderman DN, Swift MJ, et al. Producing accurate platelet counts for platelet rich plasma: validation of a hematology analyzer and preparation techniques for counting. *J Craniofac Surg.* 2005;16(5):749–756.

72. Monto RR. Platelet rich plasma treatment for chronic Achilles tendinosis. *Foot Ankle Int.* 2012;33(5):379–385.

73. Licht H, Murray M, Vassaur J, et al. The relationship of obesity to increasing health-care burden in the setting of orthopaedic polytrauma. *J Bone Joint Surg Am.* 2015;97(18):e73.

74. Narayan KM, Boyle JP, Geiss LS, et al. Impact of recent increase in incidence on future diabetes burden: U.S., 2005–2050. *Diabetes Care.* 2006;29(9):2114–2116.

CHAPTER 23

Pedal and Lower Extremity Manifestations of HIV

KHURRAM H. KHAN • GEORGE S. ABDELMESSIEH • RIHAM M. WAHBA

Human immunodeficiency virus (HIV) has now spread to every country in the world, with a total of 33.3 million affected as per the 2009 UNAIDS global report; 189,165 cases of HIV and acquired immunodeficiency syndrome (AIDS) have been diagnosed and reported in New York City since the beginning of the epidemic. Tremendous research has been achieved on HIV over the past decade to improve health outcomes of people living with HIV. However, there has been very little written evaluating the prevalence of pedal complications of patients with HIV. The purpose of this study was to investigate pedal complications of HIV patients in an East Harlem foot clinic.

A retrospective chart review was performed for the treatment of pedal complication with the concurrence of the International Classification of Diseases, Ninth Revision (ICD-9) code 042.00; 153 HIV-infected adult patients' medical records fit the inclusion–exclusion criteria. There were 88 females and 65 males in the 40- to 74-year age group, the average age being 55.1 years. The most common pedal complaints were onychomycosis in 107 patients (70%), neuropathy in 101 patients (66%), tyloma in 62 patients (41%), tinea pedis in 60 patients (39%), xerosis in 59 patients (39%), and longitudinal melanonychia in 10 patients (7%). The most co-common morbidity was diabetes in 37 patients (24%). Of those with neuropathy, only 18% were diagnosed with diabetes, showing that neuropathy is a significant finding in HIV+ patients on its own.

Our retrospective review sheds some light on the pedal complications in this patient population, which has not been extensively studied in the past. Further research is warranted to examine the complications more closely in a larger pool, with specific comparisons to be made between HIV neuropathy and diabetic neuropathy.

This is a literature review of PubMed and Medline with the purpose of the study to look for some of the most common pedal complications and the prevalence of each in HIV-infected persons to establish the prevalence and compare them to the results of our study performed at Foot Clinic of New York. The data of their prevalence among such high-risk group are lacking, and there is no one study that discusses the problem collectively.

Very little has been written in regard to the pedal complication in the HIV population. A wide spectrum of pedal complications are associated with HIV infection, but it is important to remember that not all are related to the infection itself and the same complications could happen in normal immune-competent persons. HIV infection can alter the clinical presentation and course of any condition, and many conditions may be more severe in an HIV-infected person. Infection should always be considered in any presentation involving the feet.

Depending on the stage of a patient's disease, opportunistic infections (OIs) may be responsible for the pedal complications. If the CD4 count is >300 cells per μL, then an OI is less likely.

HISTORICAL PERSPECTIVE

AIDS was first described in the United States in 1981. It is caused by a lentivirus (subfamily of retroviruses), the Latin word "lentus" meaning slow, denoting the long latent phase between infection and clinical presentation. Retroviruses use the enzyme reverse transcriptase to generate proviral DNA from RNA (reverse of the usual direction of genetic transcription). The term HIV was accepted in 1986 and there are two types. HIV-1 is a rapidly mutating virus that is more virulent and rapidly progressive than HIV-2, which is predominantly found in West Africa. HIV-1 is divided into three groups of M (main group), which is further subdivided into at least 11 subtypes or clades, O (outlier group) and N (new group). HIV-2 is divided into groups A to G. The most common group worldwide is HIV-1 type M.[1]

A decade after the first description of AIDS, the epidemic has become a worldwide public health problem. Initially, HIV transmission occurred predominantly among homosexuals and intravenous drug users in developed countries, and among heterosexuals in developing countries.

Subsequently, HIV transmission among heterosexuals increased also in developed countries. Currently, HIV seroprevalence among heterosexuals varies from 0.1% to 1.4% in Europe and 0.3% to 0.6% in North America to as high as 39% in some regions of sub-Saharan Africa.[2] The majority of the 40 million people living with HIV/AIDS (of whom 70% are in sub-Saharan Africa) are young adults, but about 3 million are 50 years old or older. Since the introduction of highly active antiretroviral therapy (HAART) in the mid-1990s, HIV-infected patients live longer, and the proportion of deaths due to diseases of aging has increased.[3] Although

FIGURE 23-1. New HIV Diagnoses in the United States for the Most-Affected Subpopulations, 2015. (CDC. Diagnoses of HIV infection in the United States and dependent areas, 2015. *HIV Surveillance Report* 2016;27. Subpopulations representing 2% or less of HIV diagnoses are not reflected in this chart. Abbreviation: MSM, men who have sex with men.)

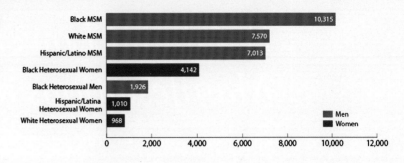

men who have sex with men remain the group at highest risk in the United States, there is an increasing burden of the disease among African-Americans, heterosexual men and women, and young people.[4]

At the end of 2013, an estimated 1.2 million persons aged 13 and older were living with HIV infection in the United States, including an estimated 161,200 (13%) persons whose infections had not been diagnosed.[5]

The Centers for Disease Control and Prevention (CDC) reports in 2015 that 39,513 people were diagnosed with HIV infection in the United States and estimates 265,330 new infections could occur in the next five years, if current testing, treatment, and pre-exposure prophylaxis (PrEP) trends remain the same (**Fig. 23-1**).

To remedy this situation, the CDC currently recommends voluntary "opt-out" HIV screening at health care centers, which means that HIV testing is performed unless the patient declines.[7]

ETIOLOGY AND PATHOGENESIS

HIV is an RNA virus (retrovirus) that binds to the CD4 antigen, mainly expressed on the surface of helper T lymphocytes and dendritic cells, including Langerhans cells. Coreceptors for HIV are the chemokine receptors CCR5 and CXCR4. Viral RNA undergoes reverse transcription to DNA, which is incorporated into the host DNA. Viral replication occurs by transcription of proviral DNA into viral mRNA, which is associated with a decline in the CD4 cell count and consequently impaired cellular immunity. After initial exposure, HIV replicates within dendritic cells of the skin and mucosa before spreading through lymphatic vessels and developing into a systemic infection. This leaves a window of opportunity for postexposure prophylaxis (PEP) using antiretroviral drugs to block replication of HIV.[8]

HIV is transmitted through blood, semen, vaginal secretions, and breast milk. The virus has also been isolated from saliva, tears, urine, amniotic fluid, and cerebrospinal fluid.[7,9] The routes of HIV transmission are sexual intercourse, sharing infected needles or syringes, transfusion of blood or blood products, from mother to baby during birth or breast-feeding, and occupational exposure of health care professionals. The approximate risks of infection are listed in **Table 23-1**.

In comparison to the risks shown in the table, the average transmission risk after percutaneous exposure of a health care professional is 6% to 30% for hepatitis B virus (HBV) and 2% for hepatitis C virus (HCV). To minimize the risk of blood-borne pathogen transmission from patients, all health care professionals should adhere to standard precautions, including hand washing, protective barriers, and care in the use and disposal of needles and sharp instruments.[10] Semen represents the main vector for HIV dissemination. HIV-1 replication may occur in macrophages in the testis and/or prostate, which may constitute pharmacologic sanctuaries protecting the virus against HAART. Persistence of virus release into the semen may occur despite an undetectable blood viral load (BVL).[11] Vertical transmission of HIV from mother to baby is increased with CD4 counts <500 cells per μL, intrapartum use of invasive procedures, rupture of membranes >6 hours, and labor >5 hours. HAART reduces the risk of mother to baby transmission from about 18% to less than 1%.[12] HIV infection is usually diagnosed by detecting antibodies in a serum sample. There is a delay (window period) between infection and a positive HIV antibody test, varying from 2 to 6 weeks and up to 3 months. During this time, the person is often very infectious with a high viral load, but antibody tests may be false-negative. Therefore, plasma should be tested for HIV p24 antigen and RNA by a technique such as polymerase chain reaction.[1]

Table 23-1. Approximate HIV Transmission Risk Following a Single Exposure to HIV Infection

	% Risk
Vaginal or anal insertive intercourse	0.03–0.09
Vaginal or anal receptive intercourse	0.1–3
Oral (fellatio)	0.04
Occupational:	
Mucous membrane contact	0.1
Needle-stick injury	0.3
Transfusion of 1 unit of blood	90–100

(Data from Pattman R, Snow M, Handy P, et al. *Oxford Handbook of Genitourinary Medicine, HIV, and AIDS.* Oxford, UK: Oxford University Press; 2008:345–548.)

When the CD4 counts are <200 cells per µL certain AIDS defining illnesses, such as OTs, can develop (Appendix 1) (see **Table 23-2**).

Apart from these OIs, other AIDS defining conditions include CD4 count <200 cells per mm^3, non-Hodgkin lymphoma (NHL), Kaposi sarcoma (KS), invasive cervical cancer, HIV encephalopathy, and wasting syndrome due to HIV. If untreated, the average time between HIV infection and AIDS is about 10 years. BVL predicts the likely rate of disease progression and indicates response to therapy. BVL <5,000 copies per mL generally suggests a low rate of progression in the next 5 years and >55,000 copies per mL is associated with increased progression. HIV-associated OIs can affect virtually any organ or system, and are caused by organisms those are rarely pathogenic if the cellular immune system is intact.

APPENDIX 1:

Organisms Causing Opportunistic Infections in HIV+ Patients

1. Bacteria: *Salmonella, Mycobacteria (M. tuberculosis, M. kansasii, M. avium-intracellulare* complex, *M. genavense, M. simiae, M. celatum), Bartonella henselae,* and *B. quintana*
2. Viruses: Herpes simplex, Cytomegalovirus, Varicella zoster virus, Human papillomavirus, Epstein–Barr virus, Hepatitis B, Hepatitis C, Polyoma virus, Pox virus, Parvovirus, Adenovirus, Erythrovirus B19
3. Fungi: *Candida, Pneumocystis jiroveci (carinii), Cryptococcus neoformans, Histoplasma capsulatum, Aspergillus* species, *Coccidioides immitis, Penicillium marneffei, Blastomyces*
4. Protozoa/Parasites: Cryptosporidiosis, Microsporidiosis, *Isospora belli, Strongyloides stercoralis, Toxoplasma gondii,* Leishmaniasis

Infection

Since the introduction of HAART in the mid-1990s, there has been a dramatic decrease in the incidence of OIs in HIV-infected subjects.[13] This decrease is due to restoration of cell-mediated immunity induced by HAART, whereas protease inhibitors used during HAART may have a direct effect against the proteases of parasites.[16] However, patients remain vulnerable to OIs for approximately 2 months after starting HAART. Sometimes OIs occur despite increased CD4 counts because of impaired functioning of CD4 effector memory T cells and deregulation of B cells that may persist despite changes in the CD4 count.[17]

Table 23-2. CD4$^+$ Count and Opportunistic Conditions in HIV Infection

CD4$^+$ Count (cells/mm^3)	Infectious Complications	Noninfectious Complications
>500	Acute retroviral syndrome Candidal vaginitis	Persistent generalized lymphadenopathy Guillain–Barré syndrome Myopathy Aseptic meningitis
200–500	Pneumococcal and other bacterial pneumonias Pulmonary tuberculosis Herpes zoster Oropharyngeal candidiasis Kaposi sarcoma Oral hairy leukoplakia	Cervical neoplasia and cancer B-cell lymphoma Anemia Mononeuropathy multiplex Idiopathic thrombocytopenic purpura Hodgkin lymphoma Lymphocytic interstitial pneumonia
<200	*Pneumocystis* pneumonia Disseminated histoplasmosis and coccidioidomycosis Miliary and extrapulmonary tuberculosis Progressive multifocal leukoencephalopathy	Wasting Peripheral neuropathy HIV-associated dementia Cardiomyopathy Vacuolar myelopathy Progressive polyradiculopathy Non-Hodgkin lymphoma
<100	Disseminated herpes simplex Toxoplasmosis Cryptococcosis Cryptosporidiosis, chronic Microsporidiosis Candidal esophagitis	
<50	Disseminated cytomegalovirus Disseminated *Mycobacterium avium* complex	

(Data from Refs. 8, 12–15.)

The resurgence of tuberculosis (TB) in the United States is largely linked to the HIV epidemic. Multidrug-resistant (MDR)-TB and extensive drug-resistant TB have emerged as threats to TB control. HIV infection may be associated with primary MDR-TB, possibly by causing malabsorption of anti-TB drugs and acquired rifamycin resistance. HIV-infected patients with MDR-TB have increased mortality.[18]

Prophylaxis against disseminated *Mycobacterium avium-intracellulare* complex infection with azithromycin or clarithromycin is recommended for all patients with CD4 counts <50 cells per μL.

Malignancy

HIV-1 may contribute to the development of malignancy through several mechanisms, including infection by oncogenic viruses, impaired immune surveillance, or imbalance between cellular proliferation and differentiation.[14]

The incidence of certain malignancies is increased with impaired cellular immunity. The AIDS defining cancers (ADCs) are KS, NHL, and cervical carcinoma, which are associated with DNA viruses, namely KS-associated herpes virus, Epstein–Barr virus, and human papillomavirus (HPV), respectively.[19]

In the pre-HAART era, approximately 10% of HIV-infected persons had cancer. HAART has dramatically reduced the incidence and mortality of KS and NHL, but has not significantly decreased the incidence of cervical or anal cancer. Although reduced, the incidence of KS and NHL remains higher in HIV-infected than noninfected patients.[12,19,20]

Since the introduction of HAART, rates of non-ADCs have increased and they currently comprise about 70% of cancers in HIV-infected people.[21] Non-ADCs include carcinoma of the anus, lung, breast, skin, conjunctiva, head and neck, liver, testis and prostate, Hodgkin lymphoma, plasma-cell neoplasia, multiple myeloma, leukemia, melanoma, and leiomyosarcoma.[22,23] The risk of HPV-associated cancers of the anus, cervix, oropharynx, penis, vagina, and vulva is increased among HIV-infected persons. The risk increases with advancing immunosuppression, reflecting gradual loss of control over HPV-infected keratinocytes. Infection with oncogenic HPV may facilitate HIV acquisition.[24,25]

Currently, malignancies are the most frequent cause of death (around a third) of HIV-infected patients. Non-ADC accounts for more morbidity and mortality than ADC in the HAART era. The reasons include the decreased occurrence of OIs and ADCs, longer survival of HIV-infected patients, and the possible oncogenic role of HIV itself. The use of HAART is associated with lower rates of non-ADCs.[26]

Treating cancer in HIV-infected patients remains a challenge because of late presentation, immunosuppression, drug interactions, compounded side effects, and the potential effect of chemotherapy on CD4 count[3] and HIV-1 viral load.[17] Nonetheless, HIV-infected patients with cancer should receive the same treatment as HIV-uninfected patients.[27]

CURRENT THERAPY

Since the approval of zidovudine as the first anti-HIV drug two decades ago, remarkable advances in the understanding of HIV/AIDS pathogenesis and drug development have led to the current availability of more than 30 drugs and fixed dose combinations to treat HIV infection (Appendices 2 and 3).

The median survival after AIDS diagnosis has increased significantly during the HAART era, which has transformed HIV from an almost uniformly fatal condition to a chronic disease. Other benefits of HAART include potential reduction of HIV transmission among adults and decrease of mother to child transmission.

However, in countries where early access to HAART is not readily available, death is still most often due to AIDS-related disorders such as OIs and advanced AIDS status.[28]

HIV drug resistance may be intrinsic or acquired as a result of mutations in viral proteins. The overall prevalence of baseline genotypic resistance is about 30%. Resistance is disseminated by transmission of resistant mutations selected during therapy. To minimize the development of drug resistance, a combination of at least three drugs from at least two different classes should be used (Appendices 4 and 5) (see **Table 23-3**).[7]

The benefits of beginning HAART at CD4 counts <200 cells per μL are well documented. Recent studies

---

APPENDIX 2:

Classification of Antiretroviral Drugs

1. Reverse transcriptase inhibitors: impair conversion of viral RNA to proviral DNA
   a. NRTIs
   b. NNRTIs
2. Protease inhibitors: prevent protease processing of viral subunits leading to assembly of infective virions
3. Fusion inhibitors: prevent binding of HIV to CD4 or chemokine receptors (CCR5 or CXCR4)

APPENDIX 3:

Antiretroviral Drugs[1]

NRTIs	NNRTIs	PIs	FIs
Abacavir	Delavirdine	Amprenavir	Enfuvirtide
Didanosine	Efavirenz	Atazanavir	Maraviroc
Emtricitabine	Etravirine	Fosamprenavir	Raltegravir
Lamivudine		Indinavir	
Stavudine		Lopinavir	
Tenofovir		Nelfinavir	
Zalcitabine		Ritonavir	
Zidovudine		Saquinavir	

APPENDIX 4:

Standard Regimens for HAART

1. 2 NRTIs plus 1 NNRTI tenofovir/emtricitabine or abacavir /lamivudine
2. 2 NRTIs plus 1 PI (usually boosted with low-dose ritonavir)
3. Triple nucleoside analog combinations

There is controversy about the guidelines for initiating HAART, especially the CD4 cell count at which HAART should be started (Appendix 5).

APPENDIX 5:

Current Guidelines for Initiating HAART[28]

1. All symptomatic HIV-infected patients
2. All asymptomatic HIV-infected persons with CD4 cell counts <350 cells/μL
3. In patients with higher CD4 cell counts, treatment indications include
   a. High viral load (>100,000 copies/mL)
   b. Rapid CD4 cell count decline (>100/μL/year)
   c. HBV or HCV coinfection
   d. HIVAN
   e. Risk factors for non-AIDS diseases, particularly cardiovascular diseases

Table 23-3. Recommendations for Initiation of HAART in Treatment-naïve, Non-pregnant Adults

Patient Status[a]	Recommendation
Symptomatic HIV disease	HAART recommended
CD4$^+$ T-cell count ≤200	HAART recommended
CD4$^+$ T-cell count <350 but >200	Consider HAART, individualize to patient
CD4$^+$ T-cell count ≥350 but ≤500	HAART generally not recommended (see text)
CD4$^+$ T-cell count >500	HAART generally not recommended

HAART, highly active antiretroviral therapy.
[a]CD4$^+$ T-cell counts in cells/mm^3. The closer the CD4$^+$ T-cell count is to 200, the stronger the recommendation, particularly if the plasma HIV RNA level is high (>100,000/mL) or the CD4$^+$ T-cell count is declining rapidly (>100 cells/mm^3/yr). (Data from Refs. 8, 12–15.)

have suggested that 350 cells per μL should be the minimum threshold for initiation of HAART.[28,29]

However, the costs and possible side effects of HAART are important considerations in the debate about the indications for initiating therapy (see **Tables 23-4** to **23-6**).

Table 23-4. Side Effects, Contraindications, and Interactions of Nucleoside and Nucleotide Reverse Transcriptase Inhibitors

Agent	Common Side Effects	Serious Side Effects	Contraindications	Interactions	Comments
Abacavir (ABC)	Hypersensitivity (5%–8%) with morbilliform rash; GI complaints; fever, dyspnea, cough, malaise, usually in first 6 weeks, may be confused with influenza or other intercurrent illnesses; nausea, vomiting; headache	Life-threatening systemic hypersensitivity reaction if rechallenged after developing hypersensitivity (usually within hours of restarting dose)	History of ABC hypersensitivity; avoid with end-stage liver disease	Overlapping resistance with ddI, insufficient data for recommendation	Hepatic metabolism
Didanosine (ddI)	Nausea	Pancreatitis, lactic acidosis, peripheral neuropathy	Use with ribavirin contraindicated because of increased toxicity	TDF increases ddI concentration, is antagonistic, and inhibits T-cell recovery; avoid combination or dose reduce ddI; D4T increases risk of pancreatitis and lactic, avoid coadministration	Renal elimination, do not take with food
Emtricitabine (FTC)	Minimal; occasional hyperpigmentation of palms and soles, especially in dark-skinned persons	None	None	3TC has similar action and resistance profile, avoid coadministration	Renal elimination

(continued)

Table 23-4. Side Effects, Contraindications, and Interactions of Nucleoside and Nucleotide Reverse Transcriptase Inhibitors (*continued*)

Agent	Common Side Effects	Serious Side Effects	Contraindications	Interactions	Comments
Lamivudine (3TC)	Minimal	None	None	FTC has similar action and resistance profile; avoid coadministration	Renal elimination
Stavudine (D4T)	Headache, nausea (uncommon)	Lactic acidosis and hepatic steatosis, pancreatitis, lipodystrophy, peripheral neuropathy	Avoid in patients with neuropathy, lipoatrophy, previous NRTI-associated lactic acidosis	Antagonism with AZT, increased pancreatitis and lactic acidosis with ddl, avoid coadministration	Renal elimination
Tenofovir (TDF)	Minimal	Nephrotoxicity, especially in patients with preexisting renal disease	None	ddl: avoid coadministration or use reduced dose of ddl; ATV must be boosted with ritonavir (300/100 qd); caution when used in patients with underlying renal disease	Renal elimination
Zidovudine (AZT, ZDV)	Headache, nausea, malaise, macrocytosis; within 4 wk after start of therapy, nearly all pts have MCV >100 µm³	Bone marrow suppression with anemia or neutropenia, lactic acidosis and hepatic steatosis, lipoatrophy, myopathy (leg pain, increased CPK)	Avoid in patients with anemia	D4T: antagonism avoid coadministration, Ribavirin: increased risk for anemia Methadone: increases AZT levels	Dose adjustment needed with renal impairment

CPK, creatine phosphokinase; MCV, mean corpuscular volume; NRTI, nucleoside reverse transcriptase inhibitors.
(Data from Refs. 8, 12–15.)

Table 23-5. Side Effects, Contraindications, and Interactions of Nonnucleoside Reverse Transcriptase Inhibitors

Agent	Serious Side Effects	Contraindications	Interactions[a]
Delavirdine (DLV)	Hepatotoxicity, Stevens–Johnson syndrome	Not recommended for use in pregnancy	Cytochrome P450 metabolites
Efavirenz (EFV)	Hepatotoxicity	Not recommended for use in pregnancy; can cause neural tube defects	Cytochrome P450 metabolites
Nevirapine (NVP)	Severe hepatotoxicity and/or rash, including Stevens–Johnson syndrome	Do not start in women with CD4 > 250 or men with CD4 > 400 because of risk of fulminant hepatic necrosis	Cytochrome P450 metabolites

[a]NNRTIs decrease PI concentrations; PI dose adjustment needed with many PIs (FPV, ATV, LPV); discontinuation of NNRTI-based regimens may lead to NNRTI resistance because of long half-life; consider step-wise discontinuation or substitution of PI.

HAART in individuals with an OI increases the risks of subtherapeutic antiretroviral exposure and the development of resistance, or supratherapeutic levels resulting in adverse effects. Recommendations advise starting HAART 2 to 4 weeks after initiating treatment of the OI.[30]

Monitoring

The effectiveness of therapy is monitored by CD4 cell counts and BVL. Effective therapy should result in at least a 10-fold decrease in HIV-1 RNA copies per mL in the first month and suppression to <50 copies per mL by 24 weeks.[28] Monitoring

Table 23-6. Side Effects, Contraindications, and Interactions of Protease Inhibitors

Agent	Common Side Effects	Serious Side Effects	Contraindications	Interactions	Comments
Atazanavir (ATV)	GI intolerance, indirect hyperbilirubinemia and/or jaundice/scleral icterus	Prolonged QTc; less metabolic toxicity (hyperlipidemia, insulin resistance) than with other PIs	Contraindicated with PPIs; dosing separation required with H2-inhibitor or antacids	Cytochrome P450 metabolites,[a] antacids, PPIs; RTV boosting required when combined with TDF, EFV, and probably NVP; avoid use with IDV because of increased risk for hyperbilirubinemia	
Darunavir (DRV)	GI intolerance	Hepatotoxicity, hyperlipidemia, insulin resistance and/or diabetes, fat accumulation		Cytochrome P450 metabolites[a]	Indicated for PI-experienced patients; RTV boosting required
Fosamprenavir (FPV), rash	GI intolerance	Hepatotoxicity, hyperlipidemia, insulin resistance and/or diabetes, fat accumulation	Use with caution in patients with sulfonamide allergy	Cytochrome P450 metabolites[a]	
Indinavir (IDV)	Asymptomatic indirect hyperbilirubinemia, nephrolithiasis, hyperlipidemia, insulin resistance, xerosis, alopecia, paronychia	Nephrolithiasis, indinavir nephropathy with azotemia, diabetes, hyperlipidemia, fat accumulation		Cytochrome P450 metabolites,[a] avoid use with ATV because of increased risk for hyperbilirubinemia	
Lopinavir/ ritonavir (LPV/RTV)	GI intolerance	Hepatotoxicity, hyperlipidemia, insulin resistance and/or diabetes, fat accumulation		Cytochrome P450 metabolites[a]	
Nelfinavir (NFV)	Diarrhea, altered taste	Hyperlipidemia, insulin resistance and/or diabetes, fat accumulation, hepatotoxicity		Cytochrome P450 metabolites[a]	The only PI that cannot be boosted; less effective than boosted PIs or EFV; administer with food to increase drug levels; fiber supplements decrease diarrhea
Ritonavir (RTV)	GI intolerance and diarrhea, improved when taken with food; perioral paresthesias	Hyperlipidemia, insulin resistance and/or diabetes, hepatotoxicity, fat accumulation		Cytochrome P450 metabolites[a]	Better tolerated and less toxic at boosting doses (100–400 mg/day)
Saquinavir (SQV)	GI intolerance, headache	Hyperlipidemia (possibly less than with other PIs except ATV), fat accumulation, insulin resistance and/or diabetes		Cytochrome P450 metabolites[a]	RTV boosting required
Tipranavir (TPV)	GI intolerance	Hepatotoxicity, hyperlipidemia, intracerebral hemorrhage	Not for HAART naïve; bleeding diathesis or recent neurosurgery	Cytochrome P450 metabolites,[a] vardenafil	Greater risk of hepatotoxicity and hyperlipidemia than other PIs; only for PI-experienced patients; RTV boosting required

[a]Cytochrome P450 metabolites: rifamycins, terfenadine, midazolam, voriconazole, methadone (reduces levels by 50%), simvastatin, lovastatin, clarithromycin.
GI, gastrointestinal; HAART, highly active antiretroviral therapy; PI, protease inhibitor; PPI, proton pump inhibitor.

for toxicity during HAART should include baseline and follow-up evaluation of renal, hepatic, and cardiovascular function, and serum lipid profile.

Antiviral drugs associated with

- **Potential Peripheral Neuropathy (PN) are didanosine, stavudine, and zalcitabine.** Stavudine is the most prevalent for PN.31
- **Myopathy and leg pain is zidavudine.**
- **Perioral paresthesia is ritonavir.**

HAART regimens are not able to eradicate HIV because of the persistence of virus in cellular reservoirs (predominantly long-lived memory CD4 T cells) and anatomical sanctuary sites (brain and possibly testis or prostate).

The enhanced immunity resulting from HAART converts a subclinical infection to a symptomatic infection because of the expansion of CD4 memory cells.[1]

PEP for health care professionals should be considered if contact with HIV occurred through percutaneous injury (needles, instruments, bone fragments, bites), exposure of broken skin, or exposure of mucous membranes (including the eye). There is no risk of HIV transmission if intact skin is exposed to HIV-infected body fluids (e.g., urine). Despite the lack of evidence from prospective randomized studies, it is recommended that PEP be commenced within 72 hours after exposure and continued for 4 weeks. PEP usually includes the three drugs zidovudine plus lamivudine plus nelfinavir. Alternatives are stavudine or tenofovir for zidovudine, and lopinavir and ritonavir for nelfinavir.[8]

THE PRIMARY STUDY

Methods

The primary study is a cohort of subjects who visited the Foot Center of New York located in East Harlem between April 2000 and April 2009. ICD-9 code 042.00 (HIV seropositive) was used to screen over 10,000 charts, and 250 unique HIV+ subjects were identified. After applying our inclusion–exclusion criteria 153 HIV+ subjects were selected for review. The documentation reviewed were the subject's medical records that included relevant medical history and progress notes for each visit to the Foot Clinic of New York. All HIV+ identified subjects were kept confidential and secure, and only identified data were recorded. No direct contact was performed.

Of a total of 153 subjects, 88 were females and 65 were males in the 40- to 74-year age group, the average age being 55.1 years. Using these documents, master data were created to investigate our study goal; age, gender, and pedal complication such as onychomycosis, tyloma, xerosis, tinea pedis, hallux abductovalgus and/or hammer toes, and neuropathy were recorded.

Inclusion criteria: Our study sample of 153 subjects with documented positive diagnosis of HIV. Exclusion Criteria: The subjects were excluded if they were younger than 18 years of age, or the subjects' medical record was not legible.

Results

There were 88 female subjects and 65 male subjects between the age of 40 and 74 years, with the average age being 55.1 years.

The most common pedal complications were onychomycosis seen 107 subjects (70%), neuropathy in 101 subjects (66%), tyloma in 62 subjects (41%), tinea pedis in 60 subjects (39%), xerosis in 59 subjects (39%), and longitudinal melanonychia in 10 subjects (7%) (**Fig. 23-2**).

Out of 153 HIV+ subjects, 107 subjects were diagnosed with neuropathy. Of those, only 28% were diagnosed with comorbidity of diabetes; 72% of HIV+ subjects had neuropathy without the comorbidity of diabetes, demonstrating that neuropathy is a significant finding in our HIV+ patients presenting for foot care (**Fig. 23-3**).

ONYCHOMYCOSIS AND TINEA PEDIS

Onychomycosis is a common podiatric condition that has become an increasing problem as the number of patients with HIV infection has grown. Although it is not among the most severe infections that affect HIV+ patients, it tends to be more extensive, is refractory to treatment, and has a

FIGURE 23-2. Pedal complications in HIV-seropositive patient at FCNY.

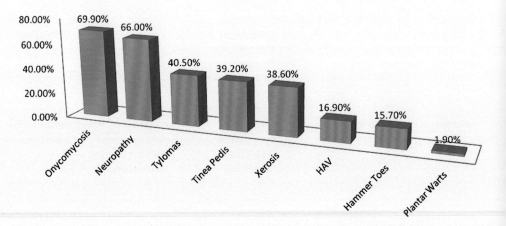

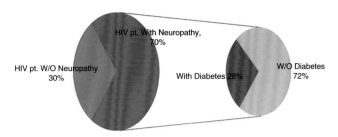

FIGURE 23-3. Neuropathy in HIV-seropositive patients with versus without diabetes mellitus.

unique clinical presentation in this patient population. It is important for the podiatric physician to be aware of the epidemiology, clinical presentation, diagnosis, and treatment of onychomycosis in HIV+ patients.

Onychomycosis occurs worldwide, and its incidence has been steadily increasing. Up to 50% of all nail disorders are caused by fungal infection, and approximately 30% of patients with cutaneous fungal infection also have fungal nail disease. But the overall prevalence does not present the whole story. Many host and environmental factors contribute to the growing incidence of fungal nail infections, including an aging population, a growing prevalence of diabetes, and an increasing number of people who have AIDS and HIV infection. In patients with HIV infection, onychomycosis is one of the earliest fungal infections to emerge, often appearing when the CD4-lymphocyte count drops to approximately 450 cells per mm^3 (normal range, 1,200 to 1,400). The condition becomes more common as the CD4-lymphocyte count falls lower. Onychomycosis has been reported to occur in 2.7% to 32%

of AIDS patients with relatively serious disease (symptomatic or CDC stage IV). Toenails are more frequently involved than fingernails. In contrast to the distal site of onset for onychomycosis in nonimmunocompromised patients, the infection often starts as proximal white subungual onychomycosis.[9]

Methods

There is lack of national data and studies regarding the prevalence of the pedal complications in HIV patients and AIDS patients.

Searching PubMed and Medline using "HIV + Onychomycosis" as a key word resulted in 77 results; 44 were reviewed, 23 studies indicated the prevalence of onychomycosis in HIV patients, with their distribution according to country being 1 Brazil, 1 Canada, 3 France, 2 India, 1 Mexico, 3 Spain, 11 USA. For the most relevant studies, see **Table 23-7** and **Figure 23-4**.

PLANTAR VERRUCA

One of the most common podiatric medical manifestations of HIV infection is plantar verrucae. Plantar verrucae, commonly known as plantar warts, are benign hyperkeratotic neoplasms caused by infection of epidermal keratinocytes in the stratum corneum and granulosum with HPV; HPV is a circular, double-stranded DNA virus enclosed in a nonenveloped protein capsid. Infection often follows trauma-induced exposure and inoculation of viral particles into the basal cell layer of the epithelium. Infection with HPV stimulates rapid proliferation

Table 23-7 Onychomycosis Prevalence and Causative Agents Compared by the Country of Origin

Country	Prevalence	Causative Organisms	Notes
Brazil[32]	32%	*Candida albicans, C. parapsilosis, C. tropicalis, C. guilliermondii, Trichophyton rubrum, T. mentagrophytes, Fusarium solani, Scytalidium hyalinum, S. japonicum, Aspergillus niger, Cylindrocarpon destructans,* and *Phialophora reptans*	
Canada[33]	500 subjects, 400 Canadian and 100 Brazilian, with the prevalence of onychomycosis of 23.2%. The prevalence of onychomycosis in the Canadian samples was 24.0% (96 of 400) and in the Brazilian samples was 20.0% (20 of 100)	Dermatophytes: *Candida* species: nondermatophyte, 73:2:2 (Canadian and Brazilian samples: dermatophytes 95.5% vs. 90.9%, Candida species 3.0% vs. 0%, and nondermatophyte molds 1.5% vs. 9.0%)	■ Onychomycosis (WSO), 3.6%; proximal subungual onychomycosis (PSO), 1.8% (Canadian and Brazilian samples: distal and lateral superficial onychomycosis [DLSO] 21.2% vs. 15.0%, WSO 3.3% vs. 5.0%, and PSO 1.5% vs. 3.0%) ■ Predisposing factors: CD4 count of approximately 370, a positive family history of onychomycosis, a history of tinea pedis, and walking barefoot around pools

(continued)

Table 23-7. Onychomycosis Prevalence and Causative Agents Compared by the Country of Origin (*continued*)

Country	Prevalence	Causative Organisms	Notes
France[34]	The prevalence of onychomycosis is 30.3% (47 out of 155) of HIV-seropositive patients versus 12.6% of controls ($P < .001$)	Total cultured: 27 *Dermatophyte* species (total): 12 *Trichophyton rubrum*: 10 *Trichophyton mentagrophytes*: 2 *Trichosporon cutaneum*: 1 *Candida* species (total): 9 *Candida albicans*: 2 *Candida parapsilosis*: 3 *Candida tropicalis*: 1 *Candida ciferrii*: 1 *Candida famata*: 1 *Candida guilliermondii*: 1 *Aspergillus* species (total): 5 *Aspergillus ustus*: 1 *Aspergillus candidus*: 1 *Aspergillus niger*: 1 *Aspergillus versicolor*: 2 *Scytalidium dimidiatum*: 1 *Rhodotorula* species: 4 *Penicillium* species: 5 *Cladosporium* species: 2 *Fusarium* species: 2 *Dotryotrichum piluliferum*: 1 Mold fungi: 2	■ Superficial onychomycosis in 2 patients, and proximal onychomycosis in 2 patients; 43 patients had total or distal-lateral onychomycosis. ■ Risk factors: Low CD4$^+$ count and advanced stages of the disease
India[35]	19.2% (48 out of 250 pt) with toenail involvement. 24% (60 out of 250 pt) with onychomycosis, toenail in 38 patients (63.33%), fingernail in 12 patients (20%), whereas 10 (16.66%) patients had involvement of both	■ 13 positive dermatophyte cultures: *Trichophyton rubrum* was isolated on 11 and *Trichophyton mentagrophytes* on 2 cultures. ■ 19 nondermatophytic cultures: *Aspergillus niger* was isolated on 3 and *Candida* spp. on 12 while *Cladosporium* spp, *Scytalidium hyalinum*, *Penicillium* spp., and *Gymnoascus dankaliensis* on 1 each	■ 21 pt (35%) respondents had DLSO, 5 (8.33%) had proximal subungual onychomycosis (PSO), 1 (1.66%) had superficial white onychomycosis (SWO), whereas 33 (55%) had total dystrophic onychomycosis (TDO) ■ 19 (31.66%) patients had associated tinea pedis
India[36]	5 pt out of 185 (2.7%) had toenail onychomycosis. 11 pt out of 185 (6%) had dermatophytosis of the nails. 6 pt had it in the finger nails, 4 in the toenails and 1 in both. Toenails were involved in 5 pt where 4 had toenail involvement only and in 1 fingernails and toenails were involved		■ Distal subungual onychomycosis (DLSO) in 3 cases and proximal white subungual onychomycosis (PWSO) in 3 cases, nail dystrophy in 4 cases, and superficial white in 1 case. ■ Tinea pedis in 7 pt out of 185 (3.7%). ■ Tinea pedis was associated with onychomycosis in 5 patients.

Table 23-7. Onychomycosis Prevalence and Causative Agents Compared by the Country of Origin (*continued*)

Country	Prevalence	Causative Organisms	Notes
Spain[37]	80 out of 303 HIV+ patients (26.4%) have onychomycosis. 61 out of 303 pt (20.1%) have nonungual mycosis		■ Association of the disease with CD4+ count: <200 cells/mm^3 ■ 14 pt out of 54 pt (25.9%) were diagnosed with onychomycosis, whereas in pt with >200 cells/mm^3 the prevalence was 26.4% (65 pt out of 246) ■ In terms of antiretroviral therapy: 55 pt out of 219 who received the therapy (25.1%) had onychomycosis compared to 25 pt out of 84 (29.8%) who did not receive the therapy and were diagnosed with onychomycosis
USA[38]	11%–67% of HIV+ pt Toenails more than fingernails. Proximal white subungual onychomycosis is the most frequent type in HIV+ population	*Trichophyton rubrum:* 58.1% *Candida albicans:* 11.3% *Trichophyton mentagrophytes:* 9.7% Molds: 8.1% *Epidermophyton floccosum:* 4.8% *Pityrosporum ovale:* 3.2% Not cultured: 4.8%	Risk Factors: Aging population CD4+ count below 450 cells/mm^3 Associated morbidities such as DM

USA[39]	Not discussed	Dermatophytes
		  Trichophyton rubrum: 36 (58%)
		  Trichophyton mentagrophytes (interdigital): 6 (10%)
		  Epidermophyton floccosum: 3 (5%)
		Yeasts
		  Candida albicans: 7 (11%)
		  Pityrosporum ovale (*Malassezia furfur*): 2 (3%)
		Molds
		  Scopulariopsis brevicaulis: 4 (7%)
		  Aspergillus fumigatus: 1 (2%)[40]
			Proximal white subungual onychomycosis is the rarest form of onychomycosis in the general population. This form has been associated with AIDS[41] and is considered an early clinical marker of HIV infection

	Clinical form	Prevalence	Common agents
Tinea pedis: clinical forms and common etiologic agents	Interdigital	Common	*Trichophyton rubrum* *Trichophyton mentagrophytes* *Epidermophyton floccosum*
	Vesicular	Occasional	*Trichophyton mentagrophytes*
	Moccasin	Frequent	*Trichophyton rubrum*

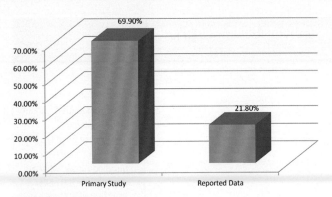

FIGURE 23-4. Onychomycosis prevalence.

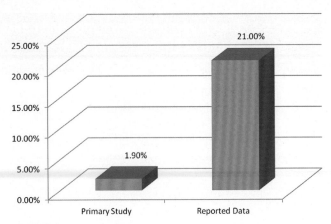

FIGURE 23-5. Plantar warts.

of the squamous epithelium, producing the visible clinical manifestation of a verruca, commonly known as a wart.

Although more than 100 different serotypes of HPV have been identified, three types have primarily been associated with plantar warts: HPV types 1, 2, and 4.[42] Whitaker et al and Davis et al demonstrated plantar verruca in HIV+ patients caused by HPV type 66 and type 69.[43,44]

Although environmental and physical factors such as infection location, amount of weight-bearing pressure on the lesion, and moisture each play a role in determining the exact clinical appearance of plantar verrucae, the type of HPV infecting the tissue has been linked to the general clinical manifestation of these warts. There are three main clinical types or morphologies of plantar verrucae. Verruca plantaris, generally associated with HPV-1 infection, manifests as a single nodule lying deep within a hyperplastic and hyperkeratotic epidermis. These warts are usually painful and are characterized by punctate bleeding because of a large number of blood vessels invading the lesion at an angle perpendicular to the plane of the skin. Mosaic warts, generally associated with HPV-2 infection, are superficial warts that are intimately connected, forming a mosaic pattern on the skin. The third clinical type is known as punctate or seed-corn verrucae and is generally associated with HPV-4 infection. Clinically, this type of wart presents as single lesions that are smaller and more superficial than verruca plantaris lesions. These lesions do not display the punctate bleeding of verruca plantaris.[45]

Methods

Searching PubMed and Medline using HIV, plantar verruca, warts, and verruca as key words yielded 13 results, and 7 were reviewed after the exclusion of the others, which were either case reports or do not include HIV+ patient population as the study group.

Unfortunately, there are not that many studies looking at the prevalence of the disease in the special population. According to Johnston et al., of the 504 participants surveyed in 2008, 63 were infected with HIV (12.5%). The prevalence of plantar verrucae in patients with HIV was 20.6% (13 of 63), whereas the prevalence of plantar verrucae in patients without HIV was 4.7% (21 of 441), with most of the verrucae

being observed among 36- to 45-year-olds and 46- to 55-year-olds (16 of 34 and 11 of 34, respectively). White participants demonstrated a 7.6% prevalence of plantar verrucae (23 of 304), and nonwhite participants had a prevalence of 5.5% (11 of 200). In this analysis, there was no association between race/ethnicity and the prevalence of plantar verrucae ($P = 0.49$). Men were significantly more likely than women/transgender/other to present with plantar warts (8.4% vs. 3.1%, P = 0.03).[42]

Blanes et al. found that the prevalence of viral warts is 21.4% in the HIV+ patient population (65 out of 303 patients). Most of the warts are observed among patients with CD4+ count below 200 cells per mm^3 (18 out of 54 patients, 33.3%) compared to patients with CD4+ count more than 200 cells per mm^3 (55 out of 246 patients, 22.4%) ($P = 0.08$). Patients receiving antiretroviral therapy (ART) had a prevalence of 26.9% (59 out of 219 patients), whereas patients who do not receive the therapy demonstrated a prevalence of 16.7% (14 out of 84 patients) ($P = 0.6$). In this study, there were no data regarding the prevalence in terms of age, sex, ethnicity, and comorbidities.[37]

Our study of 153 HIV-infected adult patients' medical records fit the inclusion–exclusion criteria. There were 88 females and 65 males in the 40-to 74-year age group, the average age being 55.1 years. A total of 3 of 153 patients were diagnosed with plantar verruca; all of them were male patients and their ages were 32, 50, and 66 years, with the average age being 49.3 years (**Fig. 23-5**).

HAV AND HAMMER TOES

Methods

Searching PubMed and Medline using HIV, AIDS, HAV, Hallux Valgus, Bunion, Hammertoes, Hammer toes, Pedal deformities, and foot deformities as key words, the results of the search show the following: NO studies had shown a correlation between HIV and Bunion or hammertoe deformities, the only combination of HIV and Pedal deformities resulted in 9 results and none of them correlate HIV and Bunion or Hammertoes.

Hence, there are no studies to compare with our study conducted at Foot Clinic of New York.

Results

Hallux abducto valgus and/or hammertoes, 19%
Hallux abducto valgus, 26 subjects (16.9%)
Hammer toe, 24 subjects (15.7%)

PERIPHERAL NEUROPATHY

PN is a common and often progressive condition frequently seen in primary care.[46]

PN is characterized as a generalized, relatively homogeneous process affecting many peripheral nerves and predominantly affecting distal nerves. The epidemiology of PN is limited because the disease presents with varying etiology, pathology, and severity. Toxic, inflammatory, hereditary, and infectious factors can cause damage to the peripheral nerves resulting in PN.[47]

HIV-associated distal neuropathic pain (DNP) remains one of the most prevalent and debilitating complications of HIV disease.[48]

DNP is associated with advanced HIV disease and may be a complication of ART or anti-TB drugs, specifically isoniazid (INH).[49]

The chronic pain associated with PN, or neuropathic pain[50] and numbness[51] are significantly the most common symptoms and can significantly diminish patients' quality of life (QoL) and be challenging to treat.[46]

Wadley et al. found pain was the primary symptom reported by participants with HIV-associated sensory neuropathy (HIV-SN; 76%, 172 of 226), followed by numbness (48%, 108 of 226), and pins and needles (46%, 105 of 226). About three-quarters of participants rated their symptoms as being of moderate to severe intensity. Symptoms were always present in the feet and only 23% experienced symptoms proximal to the feet.[50]

Biraguma and Rhoda studied a sample of 185 adults living with HIV/AIDS and attending the outpatient clinic. The subjective PN screen and the World Health Organization Quality of Life Scale Brief Version were used to collect the data. Data were analyzed to determine if significant differences existed between QoL scores in participants with and without PN symptoms. The results indicated that 40.5% of respondents experienced PN. QoL in participants with PN showed significantly lower scores in the physical ($P = 0.013$) and psychological ($P = 0.020$) domains when compared with those who did not have PN.[52]

In Cameroon, Luma et al. have noted that PN has a negative impact on the QoL of HIV/AIDS patients, which exists in different clinical patterns of which HIV-SN is the most common affecting up to two-thirds of patients with advanced disease in some settings. Out of 295 patients studied, 21% had HIV-SN. In HIV-SN patients the median duration of HIV infection was 79.8 months (IQR, 46–107.5) and their

median CD4 count was 153 cells per μL (IQR, 80–280). A total of 83.9% patients had neuropathic symptoms prior to HAART initiation and 16.1% after HAART initiation. This indicates that initiation of HAART will decrease the incidence and the prevalence of PN.[53]

However, despite the use of HAART as the main option for management of patients living with HIV is associated with decreased morbidity and mortality, which is due to its effectiveness in inhibiting viral replication, this effectiveness is not without adverse drug effects (ADRs). Cross-sectional clinical chart review of adult Cameroonian patients on HAART between 2003 and 2009 at the Douala General Hospital was done in search of reported HAART-associated ADRs. Sixty-six (19.5%) of the 339 patients on HAART reported ADRs. Among those who reported ADRs, 29.6% were on D4T-3TC-EFV, 29.3% on D4T-3TC-NVP, 16% on AZT-3TC-EFV, and 10.8% on AZT-3TC-NVP. PN was the most common ADR and represented 21.2% of all ADRs. Patients on D4T-containing regimens were more likely to develop ADR (odds ratio [OR] = 3.5; 95% confidence interval [CI], 1.5–9.8, $P < 0.01$) and 56.1% of all ADRs were associated with D4T (Stavudine).[54]

Similarly, Shurie et al. indicated that the overall prevalence of DSP among the study participants was 34.6% (110/318), of which 81 of 110 (73.6%) were symptomatic and 29 of 110 (26.4%) were asymptomatic. The prevalence of DSP among HAART-treated patients was 48% (98/204) and among untreated individuals 10.5% (12/114). The prevalence of DSP among 30 mg stavudine in combination with HAART regimen users was 43% (52/121) and 74% (40/54) among 40 mg stavudine in combination with HAART regimen users.

Among zidovudine in combination with HAART regimen–treated individuals, 20.7% (6/29) were found to have DSP. And among recent (<6 months) HAART and INH (as standard anti-TB)-exposed study participants, 12 (52%) had DSP and among HAART-untreated INH (as standard anti-TB)-exposed study participants, DSP was found in 2 (25%) of them. Among sociodemographic variables, older participants were 5.3 times more likely to develop DSP as compared with younger ones.

In conclusion, the prevalence of Distal sensory polyneuropathy was high with age and the combined use of 40 mg high-dose Stavudine with HAART were important risk factors for DSP.[55]

But Oshinaike et al. state a different opinion, wherein in their study of 323 patients with HIV, they found the prevalence of PN among those on HAART as 42.3% (60/142 patients) compared to 36.5% (66/181 patients) among HAART-naïve individuals, which is insignificant ($P = 0.29$). On the other hand, they found that the independent associations with PN were increasing age ($P = 0.03$) and current exposure to stavudine ($P = 0.00$), which is statistically significant.[56]

Yet another question that needs to be answered is, does race play a role in the prevalence of the disease and is race considered to be a potential risk factor? Anziska et al. tried to answer that question. Between April and October 2009, as part of the NIH Women's Interagency HIV Study, 1,414 women, 973 of whom were HIV infected, were clinically evaluated for PN. Utilizing available clinical, laboratory, and sociodemographic variables, they conducted a cross-sectional analysis of factors associated with HIV-distal sensory polyneuropathy (DSPN). A total of 36% of HIV-infected women met our definition of HIV-DSPN; 41.3% of African-Americans, 34.8% of Whites, and 24.7% of Hispanics had DSPN. Age, hepatitis C coinfection, and diabetes were each significantly associated with HIV-DSPN. After controlling for age, diabetes, hepatitis C coinfection, alcohol use, current dideoxynucleoside reverse transcriptase inhibitor use, current CD4 count, and plasma HIV viral load, HIV-DSPN was significantly associated with ethnicity; the OR was 1.67 ($P = 0.001$) in African-Americans compared to other racial groups. The study concludes that the likelihood of HIV-DSPN was higher in African-Americans compared to other racial groups. HIV-DSPN was more common in those coinfected with hepatitis C, older individuals, and diabetics. And further prospective studies are needed to explore the relationship between gender, race, and HIV-DSPN, and the mechanistic basis for racial differences.[57]

Shikuma et al. add to the risk factors the effect of CD4 count, age, body mass index (BMI), height, and peripheral blood mononuclear cell oxidative phosphorylation (PBMC OXPHOS) activity. In 132 subjects, the median (IQR) epidermal nerve fiber density (ENFD; fibers per mm) values were 21.0 (16.2–26.6) for the distal leg and 31.7 (26.2–40.0) for the proximal thigh. By linear regression, lower CD4 count ($P < 0.01$), older age ($P < 0.01$), increased BMI ($P = 0.04$), increased height ($P = 0.02$), and higher PBMC OXPHOS activity as measured by Complex IV (CIV) activity ($P = 0.02$) were associated with lower distal leg ENFD.[58]

Wadley et al.[50] state that increasing age and height were independently associated with the development of SN among patients who had used stavudine.

According to Mullin et al., of 326 evaluable participants, 81 (32 men, median age 38 years, median CD4 142 cells per μL) were enrolled in the ART/CD4 < 200 group, 78 (17 men, median age 37 years, median CD4 345 cells per μL) in ART/CD4 > 200, 81 (30 men, median age 37 years, median CD4 128 cells per μL) in no ART/CD4 < 200 and 86 (22 men, median age 33 years, median CD4 446 cells per μL) in no ART/CD4 > 200. Numbness was the most commonly reported symptom. DSP prevalence ranged from 43.2% in ART/CD4 < 200 to 20.9% in no ART/CD4 > 200. DSP was more common among men (adjusted odds ratio [aOR] 1.9; 95% CI, 1.2–3.3) and older participants (aOR 2.7; 95% CI, 1.1–6.2 for age 40+ vs. <30 years), and stavudine and didanosine expose HIV-infected patients to an additional avoidable risk of DSP.[51]

Evans et al.[59] conducted AIDS Clinical Trials Group Longitudinal Linked Randomized Trial; participants who initiated combined antiretroviral therapy (cART) in randomized trials for ART-naïve patients were annually screened for symptoms/signs of PN. PN was defined as at least mild loss of vibration sensation in both great toes or absent/hypoactive ankle reflexes bilaterally. Symptomatic peripheral neuropathy (SPN) was defined as PN and bilateral symptoms.

Results

A total of 2,141 participants were followed from January 2000 to June 2007. Rates of PN/SPN at 3 years were 32.1/8.6% despite 87.1% with HIV-1 RNA 400 copies per mL or less and 70.3% with CD4 greater than 350 cells per μL. Associations with higher odds of PN included older patient age and current neurotoxic antiretroviral therapy (nART) use. Associations with higher odds of SPN included older patient age, nART use, and history of diabetes mellitus. Associations with lower odds of recovery after nART discontinuation included older patient age. Associations with higher odds of PN while on nART included older patient age and current protease inhibitor use.

Concluding associations with higher odds of SPN while on nART included older patient age, history of diabetes, taller height, and protease inhibitor use.[60]

Multicenter prospective, cross-sectional analysis conducted in six US academic medical centers, with 1,539 patients enrolled, demonstrated HIV-SN in 881 participants (57.2%). Of these, 38.0% reported neuropathic pain. Neuropathic pain was significantly associated with disability in daily activities, unemployment, and reduced QoL. Risk factors for HIV-SN after adjustment were advancing age (OR 2.1 [95% CI, 1.8–2.5] per 10 years), lower CD4 nadir (1.2 [1.1–1.2] per 100 cell decrease), current cART use (1.6 [1.3–2.8]), and past "D-drug" use (specific dideoxynucleoside analog antiretrovirals) (2.0 [1.3–2.6]). Risk factors for neuropathic pain were past D-drug use and higher CD4 nadir.[61]

In another cross-sectional study, approximately half (49%) of the study population (598 HIV-infected patients) were diagnosed with DSP, and 30% of the study population were diagnosed with SDSP. In multivariate analyses, the OR (95% CI) of DSP was independently associated with ART use (OR 1.7, 1.0–2.9), age (per 10-year increment) (OR 1.7, 1.4–2.2), and prior TB (OR 2.0, 1.3–3.0). Pain or paresthesias were reported as moderate to severe by 70% of those with SDSP. Stavudine use was significantly associated with DSP. DSP is a clinically significant problem in urban HIV-infected Africans. Our findings raise the possibility that the incidence of DSP may be reduced with avoidance of stavudine-containing regimens in older subjects, especially with a history of prior TB infection.[62]

Cherry et al. conducted a multinational cross-sectional study and found the prevalence of neuropathy was 42% in Melbourne (n = 100), 19% in Kuala Lumpur (n = 98), and 34% in Jakarta (n = 96). In addition to treatment exposures, increasing age ($P = 0.002$) and height ($P = 0.001$) were independently associated with neuropathy. *Age ≥40 years and height cutoffs of ≥170 cm* predicted neuropathy. And the risk of neuropathy following stavudine was 20% in younger, shorter patients, compared with 66% in older, taller individuals.[63]

On the contrary, Oshinaike et al.[56] found that gender ($P = 0.99$), height ($P = 0.07$), use of HAART ($P = 0.50$), duration of HAART treatment ($P = 0.10$), and lower CD4 count ($P = 0.12$) were not associated with an increased PN risk.

Methods

Searching PubMed and Medline using Antiretroviral medications, Complications, Epidemiology, HIV, Neuropathy, Peripheral Neuropathy, Prevalence as key words resulted in 1,504 articles, and only 245 articles relate to the prevalence of PN in HIV patients and antiretroviral recipients.

Exclusion criteria are case reports, studies conducted in children, studies that do not include any data on the prevalence of the pathology, and articles published in languages other than English.

Results were classified by the region, Australia 2, Cameroon 2, Ethiopia 1, India 1, Malawi 2, Nigeria 1, Rwanda 1, South Africa 3, UK (Tanzania population) 1, USA 13 (1 done in Kenya), multinational 2, and systemic review 1.

Results

The prevalence of PN among HIV patients derived from 30 studies varied from 3.9% to 57.2%, with 32.4% being the average. Another systematic literature review study states the prevalence of PN among HIV patients derived from 25 studies varied from 1.2% to 69.4%.[64] All the results are compared in **Table 23-8**.

Table 23-8. Comparison of the Studies, Classified by the Country of Origin

Country	Prevalence	Risk Factors	Notes
Australia31 Multinational cross-sectional study	Prevalence of neuropathy was 42% in Melbourne (n = 100), 19% in Kuala Lumpur (n = 98), and 34% in Jakarta (n = 96).	Treatment exposures, increasing age (P = 0.002) and height (P = 0.001) were independently associated with neuropathy And the risk of neuropathy following stavudine was 20% in younger, shorter patients, compared with 66% in older, taller individuals	Age and height cutoffs of ≥170 cm or ≥40 years predicted neuropathy
Cameroon[53]	21%	83.9% had neuropathic symptoms prior to HAART initiation and 16.1% after HAART initiation	Median duration of HIV infection was 79.8 months (IQR, 46–107.5) and their median CD4 count 153 cells/μL (IQR, 80–280)
Cameroon[54]	21.2% developed PN as ADR of HAART	Patients on D4T-containing regimens were more likely to develop ADR (OR = 3.5; 95% CI, 1.5–9.8, P < 0.01) and 56.1% of all ADRs were associated with D4T	
Ethiopia[55]	34.6%	The prevalence of DSP among highly active antiretroviral HAART-treated individuals was 48% (98/204) and among untreated individuals it was 10.5% (12/114). The prevalence of DSP among 30 mg stavudine in combination with HAART regimen users was 43% (52/121) and 74% (40/54) among 40 mg stavudine in combination with HAART regimen users. Among zidovudine in combination with HAART regimen–treated individuals, 20.7% (6/29) were found to have DSP. Older participants were 5.3 times more likely to develop DSP as compared to young ones	81 of 110 (73.6%) were symptomatic and 29 of 110 (26.4%) were asymptomatic
India[65]		Stavudine is a major risk factor for peripheral neuropathy	Peripheral neuropathy and anemia were highly prevalent ADRs
Malawi[66]	Prevalence rates (95% confidence interval) of toxicities after 1 year on stavudine were: peripheral neuropathy 21.3% (16.5–26.9), incidence rates per 100 person-years (95% confidence interval) during the second year on stavudine were: peripheral neuropathy 19.8 (14.3–26.6)	Stavudine therapy	ADR of HAART reported: lipodystrophy 14.7% (2.4–8.1), high lactate syndromes 0.0% (0–1.4), diabetes mellitus 0.8% (0–2.8), Pancreatitis 0.0% (0–1.5). Stavudine-associated toxicities continued to accumulate during the second year of ART, especially peripheral neuropathy

(continued)

Table 23-8. Comparison of the Studies, Classified by the Country of Origin (*continued*)

Country	Prevalence	Risk Factors	Notes
Malawi[67]	428 out of 1173 (13%)	D4T 40 mg	Leg pain or numbness was reported in 1,173 patients (35%); 228 (7%) were prescribed amitriptyline and 200 (6%) were switched to AZT.
Nigeria[56]	39.0% of which 23% were symptomatic.	Risk factors: increasing age ($P = 0.03$) and current exposure to stavudine ($P = 0.00$)	Patients on HAART, 60/142 (42.3%) had SN compared to 66/181 (36.5%) HAART-naïve individuals ($P = 0.29$). Gender ($P = 0.99$), height ($P = 0.07$), use of HAART ($P = 0.50$), duration of HAART treatment ($P = 0.10$), and lower CD4 count ($P = 0.12$) were not associated with an increased SN risk
Rwanda[52]	40.5%		QoL in participants with PN showed significantly lower scores in the physical ($P = 0.013$) and psychological ($P = 0.020$) domains when compared with those who did not have PN
South Africa[49]	3.9%	>3 months of ART use increases the incidence of PN	
South Africa[50]	57%	Increasing age and height were independently associated with the development of SN among patients who had used stavudine.	Pain was the primary symptom reported by participants with HIV-SN (76%, 172 of 226), followed by numbness (48%, 108 of 226), and pins and needles (46%, 105 of 226). About three-quarters of participants rated their symptoms as being of moderate to severe intensity. Symptoms were always present in the feet and only 23% experienced symptoms proximal to the feet.
South Africa[62]	49% of the study population were diagnosed with distal SP, and 30% of the study population were diagnosed with symptomatic DSP.	In multivariate analyses, the odds ratio (OR) (95% confidence interval) of DSP were independently associated with ART use (OR 1.7, 1.0–2.9), age (per 10-year increment) (OR 1.7, 1.4–2.2), and prior TB (OR 2.0, 1.3–3.0). Stavudine use was significantly associated with DSP.	Pain or paresthesias were reported as moderately severe by 70% of those with SDSP
UK (Tanzania)[51]	The prevalence ranged from 43.2% in ART/CD4 < 200 to 20.9% in no ART/CD4 > 200	DSP was more common among *men* (adjusted odds ratio [aOR] 1.9; 95% confidence interval [CI], 1.2–3.3) and *older participants* (aOR 2.7; 95% CI, 1.1–6.2 for age 40 + vs. <30 years). Stavudine and didanosine expose HIV-infected patients to an additional avoidable risk of DSP.	Distal sensory polyneuropathy is common among those participants with no ART exposure and a CD4 count above 200 cells/μL Access to non-neurotoxic ART regimes as well as earlier HIV diagnosis and initiation of ART is needed.
USA (Kenya)[68]	PN per 100 person-years was 21.9 (n = 236) among D4T (stavudine) users and 6.9 (n = 7) among ZDV (zidovudine) users ($P = 0.0002$)	D4T (stavudine) was associated with 2.7 greater risk of PN than ZDV (zidovudine) (adjusted hazard ratio, 2.7, $P = 0.009$)	

Table 23-8. Comparison of the Studies, Classified by the Country of Origin (*continued*)

Country	Prevalence	Risk Factors	Notes
USA[57]	36% of the total subjects had PN. 41.3% of African-Americans, 34.8% of Whites, and 24.7% of Hispanics had PN.	Age, hepatitis C coinfection, and diabetes were each significantly associated with HIV-DSPN. After controlling for age, diabetes, hepatitis C coinfection, alcohol use, current dideoxynucleoside reverse transcriptase inhibitor use, current CD4 count, and plasma HIV viral load, HIV-DSPN was significantly associated with ethnicity; the odds ratio was 1.67 ($P = 0.001$) in African-Americans compared to other racial groups	
USA[64]	1.2%–69.4%		Systematic literature review
USA[69]	20%		Multinational study
USA[59]	Rates of peripheral neuropathy were 32.1% despite 87.1% with HIV-1 RNA 400 copies/mL or less and 70.3% with CD4 greater than 350 cells/μL	Associations with higher odds of peripheral neuropathy included older patient age, current nART use, and diabetes mellitus. Associations with lower odds of recovery after nART discontinuation included older patient age. Associations with higher odds of PN while on nART included older patient age, history of diabetes, taller height, and protease inhibitor use.	
USA[61]	57.2%	Risk factors for HIV-PN after adjustment were advancing age (odds ratio, 2.1 [95% confidence interval, 1.8–2.5] per 10 years), lower CD4 nadir (1.2 [1.1–1.2] per 100-cell decrease), current cART use (1.6 [1.3–2.8]), and past "D-drug" use (specific dideoxynucleoside analog antiretrovirals) (2.0 [1.3–2.0]). Risk factors for neuropathic pain were past D-drug use and higher CD4 nadir	Neuropathic pain was significantly associated with disability in daily activities, unemployment, and reduced quality of life

CONCLUSIONS

- Very little has been written on the pedal complications in a cohort of patients presenting to a specialty foot clinic
- Our results are surprising compared to published results on similarly studied topics
- Neuropathy has been shown to be a common complication of HIV.[70]
- Neuropathies associated with HIV are Guillain–Barré syndrome, chronic inflammatory demyelinating neuropathy, polyradiculoneuropathy, and distal symmetrical polyneuropathy.[37]
- Neuropathy although associated with the HIV infection itself is also associated with the antiretroviral drugs.[70]
- Nucleoside reverse transcriptase inhibitor–associated mitochondrial dysfunction, inflammation, and nutritional factors seem to be the most common link.[71]

- Adverse effects of antiretroviral drugs vary by drug, by ethnicity, by individual, and by interaction with other drugs.[72]
- Our study using a retrospective review sheds some light on the pedal complications in the HIV+ population, which has not been extensively studied in the past.
- Further research is warranted to examine the complications more closely in a larger pool with specific comparisons to be made between HIV neuropathy and diabetic neuropathy.
- Nail changes are seen in 68% of the HIV+ population compared to 34% in the noninfected group.
  - Onychomycosis was the most common finding at 30.3% versus 12.6% of controls.
  - Longitudinal melanonychia (14.8%) secondary to HIV medications.[71]
- Other findings in this study included clubbing (5.8%), transverse lines (7.1%) , onychoschizia (7.1%), and leukonychia (14.3%).[33]

- Gupta et al.[33] found 23% prevalence of onychomycosis in HIV+ population. The main predisposing factor was a CD4 count of ~370, positive family history of onychomycosis, a history of tinea pedis, walking barefoot around pools.

- Surprisingly, our study had only one patient with verruca plantaris. In a study recently published in *JAPMA*, controlling for age, race, and sex, patients with HIV were 4.5 times more likely to present with verrucae compared to patients without HIV ($P = 0.0002$).[15]

- Limitations of this study: This retrospective, observational study was based on the codes of diagnoses and procedures and also the sample comprised patients who visited the clinic in East Harlem, New York, and does not generalize to other populations.

REFERENCES

1. Pattman R, Snow M, Handy P, et al. *Oxford Handbook of Genitourinary Medicine, HIV, and AIDS.* Oxford, UK: Oxford University Press; 2008:345–548.
2. Hudson CP. AIDS in rural Africa: a paradigm for HIV-1 prevention. *Int J STD AIDS.* 1996;4:236.
3. Nguyen N, Holodniy M. HIV infection in the elderly. *Clin Interv Aging.* 2008;3:453.
4. Fenton KA. Changing epidemiology of HIV/AIDS in the United States: implications for enhancing and promoting HIV testing strategies. *Clin Infect Dis.* 2007;45(Suppl 4):S213–S220.
5. Centers for Disease Control and Prevention (CDC). Prevalence of Diagnosed and Undiagnosed HIV Infection—United States, 2008–2012. MMWR 2015; 64:657–662
6. CDC. Estimated HIV incidence among adults and adolescents in the United States, 2007–2010. HIV Supplemental Report 2012. https://www.cdc.gov/hiv/library/reports/hiv-surveillance.html.
7. Heyns CF, Fisher M. The urological management of the patient with acquired immunodeficiency syndrome. *BJU Int.* 2005;95:709.
8. Young TN, Arens FJ, Kennedy GE, et al. Antiretroviral post-exposure prophylaxis (PEP) for occupational HIV exposure. *Cochrane Database Syst Rev.* 2007;1:CD002835.
9. Heyns CF, Groeneveld AE, Sigarroa NB. Urologic complications of HIV and AIDS. *Nat Clin Pract Urol.* 2009;6:32.
10. Beltrami EM, Williams IT, Shapiro CN, et al. Risk and management of blood-borne infections in health care workers. *Clin Microbiol Rev.* 2000;13:385.
11. Le Tortorec A, Dejucq-Rainsford N. HIV infection of the male genital tract —consequences for sexual transmission and reproduction. *Int J Androl.* 2010;33:e98.
12. Garcia-Tejedor A, Maiques V, Perales A, et al. Influence of highly active antiretroviral treatment (HAART) on risk factors for vertical HIV transmission. *Acta Obstet Gynecol Scand.* 2009;88:882.
13. Ives NJ, Gazzard BG, Easterbrook PJ. The changing pattern of AIDS-defining illnesses with the introduction of highly active antiretroviral therapy (HAART) in a London clinic. *J Infect.* 2001;42:134.
14. Barbaro G, Barbarini G. HIV infection and cancer in the era of highly active antiretroviral therapy. *Oncol Rep.* 2007;17:1121.
15. Warnke D, Barreto J, Temesgen Z. Antiretroviral drugs. *J Clin Pharmacol.* 2007;47(12):1570–1579.
16. Pozio E, Morales MA. The impact of HIV-protease inhibitors on opportunistic parasites. *Trends Parasitol.* 2005;21:58.
17. French M, Keane N, McKinnon E, et al. Susceptibility to opportunistic infections in HIV-infected patients with increased CD4 T cell counts on antiretroviral therapy may be predicted by markers of dysfunctional effector memory CD4 T cells and B cells. *HIV Med.* 2007;8:148.
18. Suchindran S, Brouwer ES, Van Rie A. Is HIV infection a risk factor for multi-drug resistant tuberculosis? A systematic review. *PLoS One.* 2009;4:e5561.
19. Nutankalva L, Wutoh AK, McNeil J, et al. Malignancies in HIV: pre- and post-highly active antiretroviral therapy. *J Natl Med Assoc.* 2008;100:817.
20. Palefsky J. Human papillomavirus-related disease in people with HIV. *Curr Opin HIV AIDS.* 2009;4:52.
21. Crum-Cianflone N, Hullsiek KH, Marconi V, et al. Trends in the incidence of cancers among HIV-infected persons and the impact of antiretroviral therapy: a 20-year cohort study. *AIDS.* 2009; 23:41.
22. Bedimo RJ, McGinnis KA, Dunlap M, et al. Incidence of non-AIDS-defining malignancies in HIV-infected versus noninfected patients in the HAART era: impact of immunosuppression. *J Acquir Immune Defic Syndr.* 2009;52:203.
23. Engels EA, Biggar RJ, Hall HI, et al. Cancer risk in people infected with human immunodeficiency virus in the United States. *Int J Cancer.* 2008;123:187.
24. Silverberg MJ, Chao C, Leyden WA, et al. HIV infection and the risk of cancers with and without a known infectious cause. *AIDS.* 2009;23:2337.
25. Auvert B, Lissouba P, Cutler E, et al. Association of oncogenic and noncogenic human papillomavirus with HIV incidence. *J Acquir Immune Defic Syndr.* 2010;53:111.
26. Bonnet F, Chêne G. Evolving epidemiology of malignancies in HIV. *Curr Opin Oncol.* 2008;20:534.
27. Klibanov OM, Clark-Vetri R. Oncologic complications of human immunodeficiency virus infection: changing epidemiology, treatments, and special considerations in the era of highly active antiretroviral therapy. *Pharmacotherapy.* 2007;27:122.
28. Hammer SM, Eron JJ Jr, Reiss P, et al. Antiretroviral treatment of adult HIV infection: 2008 recommendations of the International AIDS Society-USA panel. *JAMA.* 2008;300:555.
29. When To Start Consortium, Sterne JA, May M, et al. Timing of initiation of antiretroviral therapy in AIDS-free HIV-1-infected patients: a collaborative analysis of 18 HIV cohort studies. *Lancet.* 2009;373:1314.
30. Manzardo C, Zaccarelli M, Agüero F, et al. Optimal timing and best antiretroviral regimen in treatment-naive HIV-infected individuals with advanced disease. *J Acquir Immune Defic Syndr.* 2007;46(Suppl 1):S9.
31. Anwikar SR, Bandekar MS, Smrati B, et al. HAART induced adverse drug reactions: a retrospective analysis at a tertiary referral health care center in India. *Int J Risk Saf Med.* 2011;23(3):163–169. doi:10.3233/JRS-2011-0532.
32. Cambuim II, Macêdo DP, Delgado M, et al. Clinical and mycological evaluation of onychomycosis among Brazilian HIV/AIDS patients. *Rev Soc Bras Med Trop.* 2011;44(1):40–42.
33. Gupta AK, Taborda P, Taborda V, et al. Epidemiology and prevalence of onychomycosis in HIV-positive individuals. *Int J Dermatol.* 2000;39(10):746–753.
34. Cribier B, Mena ML, Rey D, et al. Nail changes in patients infected with human immunodeficiency virus. A prospective controlled study. *Arch Dermatol.* 1998;134(10):1216–1220.
35. Surjushe A, Kamath R, Oberai C, et al. A clinical and mycological study of onychomycosis in HIV infection. *Indian J Dermatol Venereol Leprol.* 2007;73(6):397–401.
36. Kaviarasan PK, Jaisankar TJ, Thappa DM, et al. Clinical variations in dermatophytosis in HIV infected patients. *Indian J Dermatol Venereol Leprol.* 2002;68(4):213–216.
37. Blanes M, Belinchón I, Merino E, et al. [Current prevalence and characteristics of dermatoses associated with human immunodeficiency virus infection]. *Actas Dermosifiliogr.* 2010;101(8):702–709.
38. Levy LA. Epidemiology of onychomycosis in special-risk populations. *J Am Podiatr Med Assoc.* 1997;87(12):546–550.
39. Aly R, Berger T. Common superficial fungal infections in patients with AIDS. *Clin Infect Dis.* 1996;22(Suppl 2):S128–S132.

40. Dompmartin D, Dompmartin A, Deluol AM, et al. Onychomycosis in AIDS: clinical and laboratory findings in 62 patients. *Int J Dermatol.* 1990;29(5):337–339.

41. Weismann K, Knudsen EA, Pedersen C. White nails in AIDS/ARC due to *Trichophyton rubrum* infection. *Clin Exp Dermatol.* 1988;13:24–25.

42. Johnston J, King CM, Shanks S, et al. Prevalence of plantar verrucae in patients with human immunodeficiency virus infection during the post-highly active antiretroviral therapy era. *J Am Podiatr Med Assoc.* 2011;101(1):35–40.

43. Whitaker JM, Palefsky JM, Da Costa M, et al. Human papilloma virus type 69 identified in a clinically aggressive plantar verruca from an HIV-positive patient. *J Am Podiatr Med Assoc.* 2009;99(1):8–12.

44. Davis MD, Gostout BS, McGovern RM, et al. Large plantar wart caused by human papillomavirus-66 and resolution by topical cidofovir therapy. *J Am Acad Dermatol.* 2000;43(2 pt 2):340–343.

45. Whitaker JM, Gaggero GL, Loveland L, et al. Plantar verrucae in patients with human immunodeficiency virus. Clinical presentation and treatment response. *J Am Podiatr Med Assoc.* 2001;91(2):79–84.

46. Hammersla M, Kapustin JF. Peripheral neuropathy: evidence-based treatment of a complex disorder. *Nurse Pract.* 2012;37(5):32–39; quiz 39–40. doi:10.1097/01.NPR.0000413482.44379.ff.

47. Nguyen VH. POEMS syndrome diagnosed 10 years after disabling peripheral neuropathy. *Case Rep Med.* 2011;2011:126209. doi:10.1155/2011/126209.

48. Keltner JR, Vaida F, Ellis RJ, et al. Health-related quality of life 'well-being' in HIV distal neuropathic pain is more strongly associated with depression severity than with pain intensity. *Psychosomatics.* 2012;53(4):380–386. doi:10.1016/j.psym.2012.05.002.

49. Evans D, Takuva S, Rassool M, et al. Prevalence of peripheral neuropathy in antiretroviral therapy naïve HIV-positive patients and the impact on treatment outcomes—a retrospective study from a large urban cohort in Johannesburg, South Africa. *J Neurovirol.* 2012;18(3):162–171. doi:10.1007/s13365-012-0093-2.

50. Wadley AL, Cherry CL, Price P, et al. HIV neuropathy risk factors and symptom characterization in stavudine-exposed South Africans. *J Pain Symptom Manage.* 2011;41(4):700–706. doi:10.1016/j.jpainsymman.2010.07.006.

51. Mullin S, Temu A, Kalluvya S, et al. High prevalence of distal sensory polyneuropathy in antiretroviral-treated and untreated people with HIV in Tanzania. *Trop Med Int Health.* 2011;16(10):1291–1296. doi:10.1111/j.1365-3156.2011.02825.x.

52. Biraguma J, Rhoda A. Peripheral neuropathy and quality of life of adults living with HIV/AIDS in the Rulindo district of Rwanda. *SAHARA J.* 2012;9(2):88–94. doi:10.1080/17290376.2012.683582.

53. Luma HN, Tchaleu BC, Doualla MS, et al. HIV-associated sensory neuropathy in HIV-1 infected patients at the Douala General Hospital in Cameroon: a cross-sectional study. *AIDS Res Ther.* 2012;9(1):35. doi:10.1186/1742-6405-9-35.

54. Namme Luma H, Doualla MS, Choukem SP, et al. Adverse drug reactions of Highly Active Antiretroviral Therapy (HAART) in HIV infected patients at the General Hospital, Douala, Cameroon: a cross sectional study. *Pan Afr Med J.* 2012;12:87.

55. Shurie JS, Deribew A. Assessment of the prevalence of distal symmetrical polyneuropathy and its risk factors among HAART-treated and untreated HIV infected individuals. *Ethiop Med J.* 2010;48(2):85–93.

56. Oshinaike O, Akinbami A, Ojo O, et al. Influence of age and neurotoxic HAART use on frequency of HIV sensory neuropathy. *AIDS Res Treat.* 2012;2012:961510. doi:10.1155/2012/961510.

57. Anziska Y, Helzner EP, Crystal H, et al. The relationship between race and HIV-distal sensory polyneuropathy in a large cohort of US women. *J Neurol Sci.* 2012;315(1–2):129–132. doi:10.1016/j.jns.2011.11.009.

58. Shikuma C, Gerschenson M, Ananworanich J, et al. Determinants of epidermal nerve fibre density in antiretroviral-naïve HIV-infected individuals. *HIV Med.* 2012;13(10):602–608. doi:10.1111/j.1468-1293.2012.01024.x.

59. Evans SR, Ellis RJ, Chen H, et al. Peripheral neuropathy in HIV: prevalence and risk factors. *AIDS.* 2011;25(7):919–928. doi:10.1097/QAD.0b013e328345889d.

60. Ellis RJ, Rosario D, Clifford DB, et al. Continued high prevalence and adverse clinical impact of human immunodeficiency virus-associated sensory neuropathy in the era of combination antiretroviral therapy: the CHARTER Study. *Arch Neurol.* 2010;67(5):552–558. doi:10.1001/archneurol.2010.76.

61. Maritz J, Benatar M, Dave JA, et al. HIV neuropathy in South Africans: frequency, characteristics, and risk factors. *Muscle Nerve.* 2010;41(5):599–606. doi:10.1002/mus.21535.

62. Cherry CL, Affandi JS, Imran D, et al. Age and height predict neuropathy risk in patients with HIV prescribed stavudine. *Neurology.* 2009;73(4):315–320. doi:10.1212/WNL.0b013e3181af7a22.

63. Ghosh S, Chandran A, Jansen JP. Epidemiology of HIV-related neuropathy: a systematic literature review. *AIDS Res Hum Retroviruses.* 2012;28(1):36–48. doi:10.1089/AID.2011.0116.

64. Cherry CL, Affandi JS, Brew BJ, et al. Hepatitis C seropositivity is not a risk factor for sensory neuropathy among patients with HIV. *Neurology.* 2010;74(19):1538–1542. doi:10.1212/WNL.0b013e3181dd436d.

65. van Oosterhout JJ, Mallewa J, Kaunda S, et al. Stavudine toxicity in adult longer-term ART patients in Blantyre, Malawi. *PLoS One.* 2012;7(7):e42029. doi:10.1371/journal.pone.0042029.

66. Beadles WI, Jahn A, Weigel R, et al. Peripheral neuropathy in HIV-positive patients at an antiretroviral clinic in Lilongwe, Malawi. *Trop Doct.* 2009;39(2):78–80. doi:10.1258/td.2008.080213.

67. McGrath CJ, Njoroge J, John-Stewart GC, et al. Increased incidence of symptomatic peripheral neuropathy among adults receiving stavudine- versus zidovudine-based antiretroviral regimens in Kenya. *J Neurovirol.* 2012;18(3):200–204. doi:10.1007/s13365-012-0098-x.

68. Robertson K, Kumwenda J, Supparatpinyo K, et al. A *multinational study* of neurological performance in antiretroviral therapy-naïve HIV 1 infected persons in diverse resource constrained settings. *J Neurovirol.* 2011;17(5):438–447. doi:10.1007/s13365-011-0044-3.

69. Hahn K, Husstedt IW. HIV associated neuropathy. *Der Nervenarzt.* 2010;81(4):409–417.

70. Kallianpur AR, Hulgan T. Pharmacogenetics of nucleoside reverse transcriptase inhibitor associated peripheral neuropathy. *Pharmacogenomics.* 2009;10(4):623–637.

71. Wang X, Chai H, Lin PH, et al. Roles and mechanisms of HIV protease inhibitor Ritonavir and other anti-HIV drugs in endothelial dysfunction of porcine pulmonary arteries and human pulmonary artery endothelial cells. *Am J Pathol.* 2009;174:771–781.

72. Cribier B, Mena ML, Rey D, et al. Nail changes in patients infected with human immunodeficiency virus: a prospective controlled study. *Arch Dermatol.* 1998;134:1216–1220.

CHAPTER 24

Foot Complications of Obesity

LOUIS J. ARONNE • ANTHONY CASPER • REKHA KUMAR • LEON IGEL • ALPANA SHUKLA

Obesity is recognized as a chronic disease state that affects multiple organ systems, and is closely associated with type 2 diabetes, cardiovascular disease, sleep apnea, and osteoarthritis. The World Health Organization defines a person with a body mass index (BMI) of 30 or more as obese, and a person with a BMI between 25 and 30 as overweight. According to 2009 to 2010 data from the National Health and Nutrition Examination Survey published in 2012, US prevalence of obesity remains high, with greater than one-third of US adults and one-sixth of US children and adolescents affected. In 2008, the annual medical costs associated with obesity in the USA were estimated at $147 billion. Once thought to be a problem solely in affluent countries, overweight and obesity are now on the rise globally in many developing countries.

Increasing BMI has a negative impact on the foot in several areas, ranging from dermatologic complications to orthopedic, vascular, and neurologic conditions as well. Increasing BMI, specifically abdominal fat mass, is strongly associated with foot pain and disability stemming from metabolic complications such as inflammation, as well as mechanical consequences because of increases in pressure, gait alterations, and problems with balance. Although these issues are prevalent in the adult community, as evidenced by the approximate 51% of adults with obesity who reported their foot health as being in fair to poor condition according to the 2012 National Foot Health Assessment, it is now recognized that weight-related disorders of the foot affect the adolescent population as well.[1] A 2009 Dutch national survey of family practices concluded that children aged 2 to 17 years with overweight and obesity reported considerably more ankle and foot complications compared to those with normal weight. The results also revealed that there was no significant difference between the two groups with respect to reported upper extremity issues, which suggests that the increase in fat mass may be directly correlated to the lower extremity complications.[2]

The goal for patients with overweight or obesity is modest weight reduction, which is known to improve several medical complications of obesity. Producing any change in weight for an individual must begin with a difference in energy expenditure and energy intake. Therefore, to specifically attain weight loss, one must achieve a net negative energy balance where energy expenditure exceeds energy intake. The two major components of creating a negative energy balance are a calorie-restricted diet and physical activity. The activity level of an individual is not only a contributing factor for obesity and diabetes but has also proven to influence cardiovascular health, bone and joint diseases, as well as depression.[3] An obvious hindrance to physical activity is lower extremity pain or injury, which can lead to weight gain, thus creating a vicious cycle that leads to increased immobility and further weight gain. The opposite is also true, where primary weight gain from increased caloric intake and the development of an obesogenic environment leads to decreased activity and worsening of the primary complication. The overweight and obese populations are consequently at an increased risk of developing foot complications, leading to the lowering of one's quality of life.[1,4]

DERMATOLOGIC OBESITY COMPLICATIONS

Obesity is associated with a number of dermatologic conditions. Much of the pathophysiology of these dermatologic complications is unknown, but demonstrates strong correlation with elevated weight. Obesity can affect many pathways that disrupt the normal function of the integumentary system such as temperature control, skin barrier function, lymphatic drainage, and wound healing capabilities.[5] Obesity's effect on the lymphatic system is demonstrated by the direct relationship seen between the increased weight of a patient and the increased risk of that patient developing lymphedema[6] in the postoperative setting. In addition, patients with BMI > 50 kg/m^2 are at risk of developing primary lymphedema. Currently, the mechanism by which obesity increases the incidence of lymphedema is unclear; however, it is believed that the overgrowth of adipose tissue impedes the flow of lymphatic fluid.[6] The obstruction of flow results in the accumulation of fluid in the lower extremities, beginning with the feet and spreading proximally.[7] Eventually, this progresses into a chronic inflammatory state.[7] Weight reduction has exhibited some benefit in relieving the burden of lymphedema, further demonstrating the effect obesity and overall weight gain has on the lower limbs.[7]

Another common dermatologic issue frequently linked to obesity is the development of skin infections. Obesity's effect on the skin barrier function as well as the lymphatic system has been shown to increase the incidence of skin infections and cellulitis.[7,8] The presence or growth of erythematous plaque, which appears commonly in skin folds and other intertriginous areas, increases the development of abrasions and results in moisture retention, creating an optimal environment for bacterial and fungal growth.[7] Obesity is one of the most prevalent factors predisposing individuals to fungal infections of the feet and nails.[5] The Achilles Project, which was a large-scale assessment conducted across Europe in patients with normal, overweight, and obese BMI classifications, revealed that of patients who conveyed having fungal foot disease, 35.1% reported having at least some discomfort in walking and 17.6% reported experiencing limitations in activities of daily living.[9] These results demonstrate that fungal foot infections are debilitating to all patients, regardless of BMI. Fungal foot diseases in patients with obesity may be even more debilitating because of a potential impairment of the wound healing function of the integumentary system.[7,10] Impaired wound healing is a consequence of an excess accumulation of adipose tissue, which subsequently causes reduced perfusion at the injured site, limiting the delivery of oxygen and essential nutrients.[7,10]

Lower extremity pressure ulcers have also been observed more frequently in individuals with obesity because of difficulty with mobilization and decreased sensitivity to pressure.[5] Increased weight also has the ability to produce physical changes to foot shape. These musculoskeletal changes, coupled with decreased pressure sensation, increase exposure to unalleviated pressure.[5,10] Particularly damaging in feet, the unalleviated pressure leads to ischemia and tissue necrosis.[10] The main factors leading to the development of pressure ulcers are high amounts of force (typically over bony prominences within the soft tissue), high levels of friction, and prolonged contact, all of which would be amplified in patients with obesity.[10] According to a cross-sectional study on the association of pressure ulcers and BMI classification, participants who were classed as morbidly obese had twice as many pressure ulcer occurrences compared to those with BMIs below 40.[11]

ORTHOPEDIC COMPLICATIONS FROM OBESITY

The burden of extra stress on the foot as a result of obesity impacts the mechanics of activity, such as an individual's gait. Obesity affects gait in two predominant ways: changes in foot structure (increased thickness of the plantar fat pad) and changes in motor operations (compensatory movements due to lack of muscular strength and power).[12] Excess weight places additional pressure on the foot, which can lead to a variety of biomechanical concerns. A 2012 study showed that there is a correlation between obesity and foot pain, and that those with a higher fat mass were more likely to suffer from foot pain.[12] This correlation remained even after being adjusted for skeletal muscle mass.[12] A possible explanation for this association is that as a patient's weight increases, the strain placed on muscles and tendons of the foot to function at a basic capacity will also increase, giving patients with overweight and obesity a high likelihood of developing foot disorders like tendonitis. Tendonitis, a condition in which

a tendon becomes inflamed and irritated, is an anticipated disorder because of the altered gait patients with obesity experience. This was demonstrated by a separate 2012 study, which determined that patients with obesity are twice as likely to experience tendonitis of the foot compared to those with a normal BMI.[13] Tendonitis can severely limit function of the inflamed area, and, in this case, would decrease the mobility of the patient with obesity.

Plantar fasciitis, which is the inflammation of the plantar fascia, is the most common source of reported foot pain.[14] Plantar fasciitis is reported most in patients who work long hours on their feet and/or run for long durations. An array of factors may increase the risk of developing plantar fasciitis, such as age, foot structure, and weight.[14] Obesity drives an individual toward developing plantar fasciitis because of overuse of the fascia. Patients with obesity tend to have increased step widths causing greater dorsiflexion and less plantarflexion.[15] This increases the tension on the fascia, constantly creating microtears. The repetitive overstretching and continual formation of these microtears cause the fascia to become irritated and inflamed. The correlation between obesity and plantar fasciitis is reflected in the mechanical gait disturbance, regularly seen in patients with obesity, to compensate for larger thigh widths and greater weight stability.[15]

Osteoarthritis is the most prevalent form of arthritis, especially common in the overweight and obese populations.[16] Similar to plantar fasciitis, osteoarthritis is established as a *wear and tear* disease.[16] The additional trauma placed on the bones of the foot severely impacts the joint cartilage; the extra weight causes more stress on the cartilage per movement, leading to quicker deterioration.[16] When evaluating risk factors for heel pain, it was reported that patients with obesity are up to five times more likely than normal weight patients to present with heel-specific pain, a common indication of osteoarthritis in the foot.[16] Another study reviewed data on foot positioning and force in patients with obesity and revealed that patients with obesity have a more toe-out stance.[17] Most obese patients adapt this posture as a way for the body to support the added weight and maintain balance while conducting a movement, such as walking.[17] Additional data also presented in the study established that the obese population also typically has a larger midfoot weight-bearing area.[17] An increase of this area has proven to critically harm the plantar tendons of the arch, making osteoarthritis in the foot increasingly common in patients with obesity.[17]

VASCULAR/NEUROLOGIC OBESITY COMPLICATIONS

Obesity has a significant influence on cardiovascular diseases.[18] The pathophysiology of obesity as a risk factor for cardiovascular disease includes leptin resistance, increased total blood volume, increased cardiac output, and lower total peripheral resistance, among others.[18] One of the cardiovascular diseases that can be produced secondary to obesity is peripheral artery disease (PAD). PAD is an occlusive lower extremity disease that occurs when the arteries of the lower extremities lose their compliance as a result of increased peripheral and visceral fat, hypertension, elevated triglycerides, and dyslipidemia.[19] This disease has shown strong associations with decreased quality of life because of limited functionality of the lower extremities and possible amputation.[20] Claudication is the most common symptom of PAD, which is exacerbated in patients with overweight and obesity because of the confounding lower leg effects that have been previously discussed. A 2012 systematic review also identified obesity as an independent risk factor for major cardiovascular events in patients with established PAD, making obesity a compounding condition after the diagnosis of PAD.[21]

Obesity is also considered one of the contributing factors to the rise in incidence of venous ulceration.[22] A main cause of venous ulcers as a result of obesity is chronic venous insufficiency by way of mechanical obstruction from increased adiposity and valvular incompetence.[5] Valvular incompetence occurs in a patient who is overweight or obese because they experience increased intra-abdominal pressure.[10] This intra-abdominal pressure is then relayed to the lower extremities, increasing the distal venous pressure of the femoral veins, resulting in venous stasis.[10,23] The increased pressure also disrupts the commissures of the valves during dilation, leading to valvular dysfunction.[23] Venous stasis and eventual blood pooling cause damage to the capillaries of the lower extremities, initiating an inflammatory response and culminating in endothelial damage.[24] Venous stasis ulcers are said to account for 80% of all reported lower extremity ulcerations, and have been shown to be more common in those with obesity.[5,24]

Peripheral neuropathy and its association with obesity has long been discussed due to increased thickness of the subcutaneous tissue, which was presumed to act as an insulator to nerve pulses, reducing the magnitude of the response.[25] A 2005 study confirmed these reports, showing a correlation between BMI and a reduction in amplitude of motor and sensory nerve responses.[25] Another proposed pathway for obesity's influence on neuropathy development is the chronic exposure to abnormal insulin levels, manifesting as increased vascular resistance within the larger vasculature, causing damage to the vessel. The smaller vessels are comparably damaged, producing poor circulation in the lower extremities inducing peripheral neuropathy. In 2011, a study looked at the clustering of cardiometabolic disorders and their effect on peripheral vascular disease (PVD) and peripheral neuropathy; the results revealed that patients with obesity have twice the probability of experiencing both peripheral neuropathy and PVD.[19]

PREVENTIONS AND INTERVENTIONS

Obesity can be considered a "gateway" disease because of its prevalence of secondary complications, as evidenced by the array of foot disorders that can occur as a direct result of obesity. As noted by most studies listed earlier, a majority of

the foot complications have a significant impact on the quality of life of those burdened. There are few treatments for the prevention or rehabilitation of the disorders listed; however, the prevailing notion for all conditions is that weight reduction would improve outcomes. In the treatment of lymphedema, the main goal is reduction of limb girth, for which there are limited options.[7] Reducing the girth of the lower extremities can be accomplished with the use of elastic compression stockings or compressive bandaging.[7,10] The elastic mildly compresses the leg to increase blood flow to the area, serving to prevent swelling and pooling.[7,19] Compression stockings, because of their mechanism of enhancing blood flow, are also a main option for the management of PAD and the prevention of venous stasis ulcers.[22] The treatment of skin infections is increasingly important because of their potential severity and obesity's prevalence in causing such diseases.[5] Skin infection treatments are broken down into two strategies: preinfection (prevention) and postinfection (intervention). Preinfection intervention begins most importantly with increased awareness from the individual; heightened cognizance of dermatologic disorders can lead to better prevention along with earlier diagnosis and therapy, leading to improved outcomes.[9] Preinfection interventions would also include vigilant cleaning of the feet with a mild soap, carefully rinsing and drying all crevices of the feet, moisturizing the feet daily, and avoiding trauma to the area.[10] Postinfection intervention includes treating the area with an antibacterial or antifungal medication, as determined by the treating practitioner and contingent on the type of infection.[10] As for the orthopedic disorders, treatment commonly involves the use of orthotic devices. When it comes to plantar fasciitis, foot orthotics that provide support to the arch and the heel of the foot have been shown to lessen the stress on the plantar fascia.[26] Padded socks may also be used to supply additional support and may even help prevent the development of plantar fasciitis.[26] The intervention for tendonitis of the Achilles is centered around reducing the inflammation of the affected area.[27] Treatments include rest, icing the inflamed area, and anti-inflammatory medications if needed.[27] Conversely, the main treatment for osteoarthritis is physical activity along with a well-tolerated regime of anti-inflammatory medications.[17] Although many osteoarthritic patients will avoid activity as a result of the pain and decreased mobility often experienced, mild to moderate activity will help reduce discomfort and increase functionality.[17] For more severe cases, surgical interventions can be utilized.

CONCLUSION

As the incidence of obesity rises, the secondary complications that are highly correlated with excess weight gain and adiposity will also rise, including a wide array of foot disorders. Obesity causes complications of the foot through several different systems such as dermatologic, vascular, orthopedic, and neurologic. Although causation between obesity and foot disease needs to be further elucidated, there is clear correlation between these conditions. Developing a foot complication along with obesity presents a challenge for both patients and physicians because of the vicious cycle that is created from inactivity and additional weight gain. The development of a foot disorder may lead to further weight gain in a patient with overweight and obesity, and further weight gain may lead to additional foot problems. The ideal treatment plan for patients is modest weight reduction coupled with the designated noninvasive intervention, such as compression stockings, padded socks, orthotics, hygienic foot care, and patient awareness. The latter may be the most important to help prevent these complications from occurring and recognizing the optimal time to see a physician. All too commonly, minor foot problems go unnoticed or, even worse, are ignored by the patient, leading to worsening of the condition.

REFERENCES

1. Institute for Preventive Foot Health. National Foot Health Assessment 2012. http://www.ipfh.org/resources/surveys/national-foot-health-assessment-2012/. Accessed January 17, 2017.
2. Krul M, van der Wouden JC, Schellevis FG, et al. Musculoskeletal problems in overweight and obese children. *Ann Fam Med.* 2009;7(4):352–356. doi:10.1370/afm.1005.
3. Warburton DER, Nicol CW, Bredin SSD. Health benefits of physical activity: the evidence. *CMAJ.* 2006;174(6):801–809. doi:10.1503/cmaj.051351.
4. Jelinek HF, Fox D. Foot health and elevated body mass index. *Foot Ankle Online J.* 2009;2(8):10 13. doi:10.3827/faoj.2009.0208.0004.
5. Scheinfeld NS. Obesity and dermatology. *Clin Dermatol.* 2004;22(4):303–309. doi:10.1016/j.clindermatol.2004.01.001.
6. Mehrara BJ, Greene AK. Lymphedema and obesity: is there a link? *Plast Reconstr Surg.* 2014;134(1):154e–160e. doi:10.1097/PRS.0000000000000268.
7. Yosipovitch G, DeVore A, Dawn A. Obesity and the skin: skin physiology and skin manifestations of obesity. *J Am Acad Dermatol.* 2007;56(6):901 916. doi:10.1016/j.jaad.2006.12.004.
8. Huttunen R, Syrjänen J. Obesity and the risk and outcome of infection. *Int J Obes.* 2013;37(3):333–340. doi:10.1038/ijo.2012.62.
9. Katsambas A, Abeck D, Haneke E, et al. The effects of foot disease on quality of life: results of the Achilles Project. *J Eur Acad Dermatol Venereol.* 2005;19(2):191–195. doi:10.1111/j.1468-3083.2004.01136.x.
10. García Hidalgo L. Dermatological complications of obesity. *Am J Clin Dermatol.* 2002;3(7):497–506. doi:10.2165/00128071-200203070-00006.
11. Drake DJ, Swanson M, Baker G, et al. The association of BMI and Braden total score on the occurrence of pressure ulcers. *J Wound Ostomy Continence Nurs.* 2010;37(4):367–371. doi:10.1097/WON.0b013e3181e45774.
12. Tanamas SK, Wluka AnE, Berry P, et al. Relationship between obesity and foot pain and its association with fat mass, fat distribution, and muscle mass. *Arthritis Care Res.* 2012;64(2):262–268. doi:10.1002/acr.20663.
13. Butterworth PA, Landorf KB, Smith SE, et al. The association between body mass index and musculoskeletal foot disorders: a systematic review. *Obes Rev.* 2012;13(7):630–642. doi:10.1111/j.1467-789X.2012.00996.x.
14. Waclawski ER, Beach J, Milne A, et al. Systematic review: plantar fasciitis and prolonged weight bearing. *Occup Med (Lond).* 2015;65(2):97–106. doi:10.1093/occmed/kqu177.
15. Frey C, Zamora J. The effects of obesity on orthopaedic foot and ankle pathology. *Foot Ankle Int.* 2007;28(9):996–999. doi:10.3113/FAI.2007.0996.
16. Felson DT. Weight and osteoarthritis. *Am J Clin Nutr.* 1996;63(Suppl 3):430S–432S.
17. Messier SP. Obesity and osteoarthritis: disease genesis and nonpharmacologic weight management. *Med Clin North Am.* 2009;93(1):145–159. doi:10.1016/j.mcna.2008.09.011.
18. Lavie CJ, Milani RV, Ventura HO. Obesity and cardiovascular disease. risk factor, paradox, and impact of weight loss. *J Am Coll Cardiol.* 2009;53(21):1925–1932. doi:10.1016/j.jacc.2008.12.068.
19. Ylitalo KR, Sowers M, Heeringa S. Peripheral vascular disease and peripheral neuropathy in individuals with cardiometabolic clustering and obesity: National Health and Nutrition Examination Survey 2001–2004. *Diabetes Care.* 2011;34(7):1642–1647. doi:10.2337/dc10-2150.
20. Hirsch AT, Murphy TP, Lovell MB, et al. Gaps in public knowledge of peripheral arterial disease: the first national PAD public awareness survey. *Circulation.* 2007;116(18):2086–2094. doi:10.1161/CIRCULATIONAHA.107.725101.
21. Cronin O, Morris DR, Walker PJ, et al. The association of obesity with cardiovascular events in patients with peripheral artery disease. *Atherosclerosis.* 2013;228(2):316–323. doi:10.1016/j.atherosclerosis.2013.03.002.
22. Mekkes JR, Loots MAM, Van Der Wal AC, et al. Causes, investigation and treatment of leg ulceration. *Br J Dermatol.* 2003;148(3):388–401. doi:10.1046/j.1365-2133.2003.05222.x.
23. Willenberg T, Schumacher A, Amann-Vesti B, et al. Impact of obesity on venous hemodynamics of the lower limbs. *J Vasc Surg.* 2010;52(3):664–668. doi:10.1016/j.jvs.2010.04.023.
24. Collins L, Seraj S. Diagnosis and treatment of venous ulcers. *Am Fam Physician.* 2010;81(8):989–996. http://www.ncbi.nlm.nih.gov/pubmed/20387775. Accessed January 17, 2017.
25. Miscio G, Guastamacchia G, Brunani A, et al. Obesity and peripheral neuropathy risk: a dangerous liaison. *J Peripher Nerv Syst.* 2005;10(4):354–358. doi:10.1111/j.1085-9489.2005.00047.x.
26. Prevention and Treatment of Plantar Fasciitis, Institute for Preventive Foot Health (IPFH). http://www.ipfh.org/foot-conditions/foot-conditions-a-z/plantar-fasciitis/prevention-and-treatment-of-plantar-fasciitis/. Accessed February 18, 2016.
27. Prevention & Treatment of Achilles Tendinitis, Institute for Preventive Foot Health (IPFH). http://www.ipfh.org/foot-conditions/foot-conditions-a-z/achilles-tendinitis/prevention-treatment-of-achilles-tendinitis/. Accessed February 18, 2016.

CHAPTER 25

Lower Extremity Signs and Symptoms of Multiple Sclerosis

MARY ANN PICONE • HUNTER VINCENT • KAREN BLITZ-SHABBIR •
CLOVER YOUN WEST • JEMIMA AKINSANYA

Multiple sclerosis (MS) frequently presents with deficits of the lower extremities, particularly gait disorders, motor weakness, balance problems, and spasticity. The goal of this chapter is to discuss the most common lower extremity impairments associated with MS, including their signs and symptoms, prevalence, pathophysiology, diagnosis, assessment tools, and treatment.

MS is a chronic multifocal autoimmune inflammatory demyelinating disease of the central nervous system (CNS). The pathologic hallmarks of MS lesions include breakdown of the blood–brain barrier, perivascular infiltrates of mononuclear cells, multifocal inflammation, oligodendrocyte loss, gliosis, axonal damage, and neurodegeneration.[1]

It is predominantly a T cell–mediated inflammatory disorder with overproduction of proinflammatory cytokines. These cytokines weaken the blood–brain barrier, allowing T cells to enter the CNS and attack myelin. The resulting demyelination slows conduction of electrical impulses along nerve axons and decreases the speed at which information travels down them. Axonal damage occurs early on in the disease course and is considered the major cause of neurologic disability. MS clinical symptoms vary from person to person depending on the number and location of demyelinating lesions within the brain and spinal cord. Brain atrophy is the cumulative effect of demyelination and axonal loss.[2]

MS is the most common neurologic disorder of young adults in the United States, and is increasing in prevalence both in the United States and worldwide, with the median prevalence estimated at nearly 33 per 100,000 globally as of 2013.[3] Approximately 450,000 people are diagnosed in the United States and 2.5 million people worldwide. Most people are diagnosed between the ages of 20 and 45 years. Women outnumber men in a 3:1 ratio.[3]

The cause of MS is still unknown. However, the development of MS is thought to involve both a genetic predisposition and exposure to environmental and infectious triggers. Exposure to Epstein–Barr virus after early childhood, low vitamin D levels, cigarette smoking, high-salt diets, and obesity have all been shown to potentially trigger a proinflammatory state, leading to a predisposition for developing MS. High-salt diets have been shown to induce pathogenic Th17 cells.[3] Genetic factors seem to play a role as well. There tends to be a higher incidence of MS in Caucasians and people of Northern European descent, and genetically the strongest association maps to the HLA-DRB1 allele of the class II major histocompatibility complex region.[4]

MS CLASSIFICATION

MS disease course descriptions (phenotypes) are clinically important for interdisciplinary communication, treatment decision-making algorithms, clinical trial selection, and patient prognosis.

Clinically Isolated Syndrome

Clinically isolated syndrome (CIS) is characterized as the first episode of neurologic symptoms, lasting at least 24 hours, caused by an inflammatory or demyelinating lesion in the CNS, but not sufficient enough to satisfy the McDonald diagnostic criteria for MS.[5] The neurologic symptoms can be monofocal, affecting only a single neurologic region such as the optic nerve in optic neuritis, or multifocal, affecting multiple neurologic areas of the body.[6] The risk of CIS progressing to MS can vary depending on the presence of a CNS-occupying lesion.[6] When CIS is present with at least one demyelinating lesion in the CNS, the patient has a 60% to 80% risk of a second neurologic episode and being diagnosed with MS.[7] In CIS patients without a CNS lesion, the risk decreases to approximately 20%.[8] Preliminary clinical trials show that early treatment of patients with CIS can decrease the risk of a second neurologic episode and the conversion to "clinically definite MS."[9,10]

Relapsing Remitting MS

Relapsing remitting MS is the most common disease course, encompassing approximately 85% of initial MS diagnosis. This MS disease classification is defined by exacerbations of disease symptoms, also known as relapses, followed by periods of remission where no apparent clinical worsening or progression of the disease occurs. However, changes can still be seen on magnetic resonance imaging (MRI) examination. Neurologic symptoms often include changes in vision, numbness, fatigue, spasticity, muscle spasms, bowel/bladder problems, and cognitive difficulty.[11,12] However, the presentation of relapsing remitting MS is oftentimes extremely variable between patients and unique to each individual.

Patients may experience complete recovery of function and resolution of symptoms following a relapse, or only partial, leading to increased disability.

Primary Progressive MS

Primary progressive MS is a disease course characterized by worsening neurologic status from the onset of diagnosis, usually without relapses or remissions, affecting approximately 10% to 15% of MS patients.[13] Primary progressive MS usually affects men and women equally, and is often diagnosed later in life around the fourth or fifth decade.[14] In addition, primary progressive MS tends to present with an increased number of spinal cord lesions with less inflammatory cells, versus relapsing remitting MS, which usually presents with brain lesions ("plaques") containing a larger number of inflammatory cells.[15] It is common for patients with primary progressive MS to experience difficulty with walking and mobility, which can potentially limit their ability to continue working.[13,16]

Secondary Progressive MS

Secondary progressive MS generally presents initially as a relapsing remitting disease course, upward of 90% of cases,[17] but eventually transitions into a disease course defined by progressive disability that is independent of relapse activity. A majority of untreated patients with relapsing remitting MS usually transition to secondary progressive MS approximately 10 years after diagnosis.[18] Although research is mixed, between 15% and upward of 50% of patients with relapsing remitting disease will advance to secondary progressive MS.[14] The onset of secondary progressive MS is of large clinical significance, because it has been shown to be the most important determining factor for long-term prognosis with MS, and its prevention is a crucial primary target for treatment[5,17,19] (**Fig. 25-1**).

DIAGNOSTIC STUDIES

Despite recent advances and improvements in imaging techniques, the diagnosis of MS remains primarily a clinical diagnosis. Signs and symptoms referable to white matter lesions disseminated in time and space within the neuraxis should be seen, whereas other MS mimics have been ruled out. In 2010, the revised version of the McDonald diagnostic criteria for MS was developed utilizing MRI much more than in the past to help identify patients earlier in the disease course[20] (**Table 25-1**).

No one laboratory test is diagnostic, but several tests may help support the diagnosis. Examination of cerebrospinal fluid (CSF) from a lumbar puncture could confirm the diagnosis and rule out other disease conditions. CSF studies usually show an increase in immunoglobulin G (IgG) index and intrathecal IgG antibody production, as well as two or more oligoclonal bands. In addition, evoked potentials of the visual, somatosensory, and auditory systems may show delayed conduction latencies. Furthermore, blood work testing is done to rule out confounding diagnoses and mimics.

MRI has made a tremendous impact in the early diagnosis of MS lesions. It is the most sensitive test that is currently available to detect MS lesions. It can help estimate lesion load and extent of disease activity, and measure brain volume and atrophy. Clinicians rely on MRI to monitor disease progression, evaluate therapeutic response, and serve as prognostic indicator of disease worsening. Typical MS lesions on MRI are ovoid in shape and tend to be located in the periventricular white matter, as well as in the posterior fossa, spinal cord, corpus callosum, and subcortical regions. They are often situated perpendicular to the ventricles. When gadolinium dye is injected, lesions may enhance in areas of acute inflammation because of disruption of the blood–brain barrier. Higher strength (7 T) MRIs can also detect lesions in normal-appearing white matter and gray matter.

Spinal cord lesions are usually located peripherally, with the dorsolateral cord being the most common plaque location. Lesions are typically less than two vertebral segments long, occupying less than half of the cross-sectional area of the cord.[21] Lesions that occupy three or more vertebral segments in length or that are centrally located should raise suspicion for the diagnosis of neuromyelitis optica (**Fig. 25-2A to C**).

Functional Assessment

Mobility/Ambulation

Patients with MS can present with a wide variety of clinical symptoms depending on the number and location of MS lesions within the brain and spinal cord. Commonly, the presence and location of CNS lesions result in lower limb dysfunction, which manifests as difficulty with walking. Approximately 75% of MS patients experience significant difficulty with walking.[22] In addition, lower leg function has been shown to be the most important bodily function when compared to other areas of the body for patients with MS.[23] Studies have shown that impaired mobility and ambulation are directly correlated with reduction in patient quality of life, activities of daily living, and overall productivity.[24] Walking limitations have also contributed to increased unemployment for MS patients, often linked to decreased productivity in the workplace.[25]

In many cases, the source of lower limb dysfunction can be traced back to the spinal cord. It has been shown that lesions in the pyramidal tracts can contribute to weakness and spasticity, whereas dorsal column and cerebellar lesions can contribute to loss of coordination and proprioception.[26]

Many common symptoms of MS can result in an abnormal gait pattern, most frequently exhibited as unsteadiness or a slowed cadence. Such symptoms include ataxia, sensory ataxia, imbalance, foot drop, weakness, spasticity, tremor, vertigo, visual impairment, and cognitive deficits. When a normal gait pattern is altered, it ultimately causes an increased expenditure of energy while walking. A common gait dysfunction seen in MS is foot drop. Though foot drop in

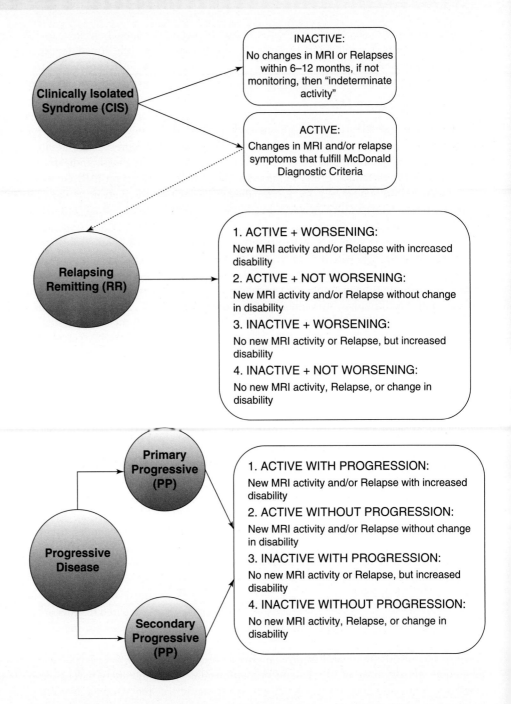

FIGURE 25-1. 2013 Multiple sclerosis phenotype classifications. (Images created by Dr. Hunter Vincent with information from The National MS Society.)

non-MS patients is typically caused by damage to the peroneal nerve, in MS patients, the foot drop is related to upper motor neuron dysfunction causing focal weakness in dorsiflexion, monoparesis, or hemiparesis. On examination, the forefoot drags and is unable to clear during the swing phase of gait.

Because of the heterogeneous presentation of MS, it is not uncommon for disability to fluctuate from day to day based on mood and environment, even without signs of disease progression.[27] The significance of walking and ambulation dysfunction in the course of MS disease progression should not be overlooked, and accurate assessment is needed to understand subtle changes in each patient's unique disease presentation.

Proper measurement of a patient's ambulation and balance is essential for assessing disease worsening, which are important indicators for disease progression. Identifying subtle changes in lower extremity dysfunction can ensure proper treatment and rehabilitation, as well as initiation of appropriate disease-modifying therapy.[28] There are many standardized assessments that aggregate multiple aspects of physical function to assess disease status. Some analyze ambulation or balance alone, whereas others test a hybrid of both. **Table 25-2** summarizes a literature search on functional assessments of the lower extremity. The most commonly used functional exams will be explained in further detail.

Table 25-1. 2010 Revised McDonald Diagnostic Criteria for Multiple Sclerosis[20]

Clinical (Attacks)	Lesions	Additional Criteria to Make Diagnosis (DX)
2 or more	Objective clinical evidence of 2 or more lesions or objective clinical evidence of 1 lesion with reasonable historical evidence of a prior attack	None. Clinical evidence alone will suffice; additional evidence desirable but must be consistent with MS
2 or more	Objective clinical evidence of 1 lesion	Dissemination in space, demonstrated by ■ 1 T2 lesion in at least two MS typical CNS regions (periventricular, juxtacortical, infratentorial, spinal cord); **OR** ■ Await further clinical attack implicating a different CNS site
1	Objective clinical evidence of 2 or more lesions	Dissemination in time, demonstrated by ■ Simultaneous asymptomatic contrast-enhancing and nonenhancing lesions at any time; **OR** ■ A new T2 and/or contrast-enhancing lesions(s) on follow-up MRI, irrespective of its timing; **OR** ■ Await a second clinical attack
1	Objective clinical evidence of 1 lesion	Dissemination in space, demonstrated by ■ 1 T2 lesion in at least two MS typical CNS regions (periventricular, juxtacortical, infratentorial, spinal cord); **OR** ■ Await further clinical attack implicating a different CNS site **AND** Dissemination in time, demonstrated by ■ Simultaneous asymptomatic contrast-enhancing and nonenhancing lesions at any time; **OR** ■ A new T2 and/or contrast-enhancing lesions(s) on follow-up MIR, irrespective of its timing; **OR** ■ Await a second clinical attack

(From Polman CH, Reingold SC, Banwell B, et al. Diagnostic criteria for multiple sclerosis: 2010 Revisions to the McDonald criteria. *Ann Neurol.* 2011;69(2):292–302. doi:10.1002/ana.22366, with permission.)

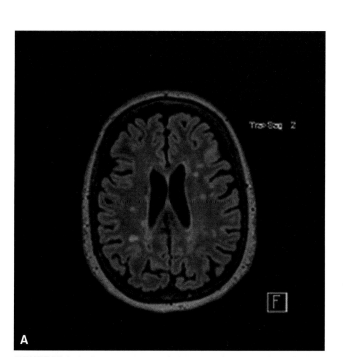
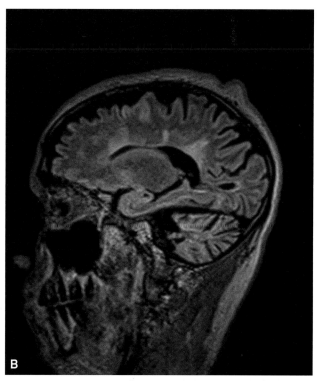

FIGURE 25-2. A: Ovoid, periventricular white matter lesions demonstrated on axial FLAIR image. **B:** Periventricular lesions characteristically seen as Dawson's fingers on sagittal FLAIR image. **C:** Sagittal T2-weighted image of cervical spine lesion. (Images courtesy of Dr. John Morgan, Holy Name Medical Center.)

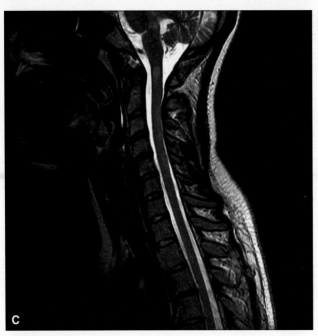

FIGURE 25-2. (*continued*)

Clinical Observation

Although direct observation and assessment of a patient's walking lacks the objective grading scale of more standardized tests, it is often the initial approach to identify changes in a patient's mobility. Regardless of whether a standardized assessment is performed, regular gait and mobility assessment should be a standard occurrence during patient visits.

Expanded Disability Status Scale

The Kurtzke Expanded Disability Status Scale (EDSS) is one of the most well-documented MS-specific functional scales. It is considered the gold standard for establishing objective disability status and monitoring disease progression. The EDSS applies a numerical value from 0 to 10 to a patient's disability, primarily associating disease progression with ambulatory difficulty. The lower numbers on the EDSS (1 to 4.5) evaluate disease impairments, but all patients within this range are fully ambulatory without aid. The middle numbers on the scale (4.5 to 7.5) assess difficulty with ambulation. A patient's numerical disability value is based on their ability to walk a maximum distance of 500 m and the presence and

Table 25-2. Functional Assessments Involving the Lower Extremity in Multiple Sclerosis

Type	Assessment Name	Data Measured	Limitations
Mobility/Ambulation			
Direct observation	Clinical examination	Physician's clinical interpretation of walking and mobility	
	Kurtzke Expanded Disability Severity Scale[29]	Evaluates impairment and disability detected, followed by assessment of maximum walking distance and aids required. Scored 0–10	The use of aids is dependent on psychosocial factors[26]
	Multiple Sclerosis Functional Composite (MSFC)[30]	Evaluates walking with a timed 25-foot walk, upper extremity function with nine-hole peg test, and cognitive function with paced auditory serial addition test	
	Dynamic Gait Index (DGI)[31]	8-part evaluation examining gait, balance, and fall risk; Functional Gait assessment (FGA) and 4-Item Dynamic Gait Index are variations	
	25-ft Timed Walk[25]	Gait speed	Only a measure of speed. Not effective for level of activity.[26] Poor test for patients with minimal disease severity[25]
	Six Spot Step Test (SSST)[32]	Ambulation, coordination, and balance. Patient walks from one end to the other of a delineated rectangular field, kicking cylindrical blocks out of their marked circles	Requires specific testing field with setup[25]
	2- or 6-min walk[33,34]	Distance traveled and walking stamina	Highly variable depending on pain, mood, motivation[26]
	Kinetic Gait Analysis	Computer-analyzed gait analysis	Costly, time consuming, not ideal for large groups[26]
	Video Gait Analysis	Video-based scoring system of gait[35,36]	

Table 25-2. Functional Assessments Involving the Lower Extremity in Multiple Sclerosis (*continued*)

Type	Assessment Name	Data Measured	Limitations
	Physiological Cost Index[26]	Ambulation/mobility given a score based on change between resting and active heart rate to measure energy consumption	Not good for patients with dysautonomia related to MS[37]
	Physiological Profile Approach (PPA)[38]	Clinical tests of vision, cutaneous sensation of the feet, leg muscle force, step reaction time, and postural sway. Scored 0–2 to assess risk of falls	Time to perform: 30 min, equipment is needed, imprecise measure of physiologic mechanisms, not measuring functional tasks or balance control systems[26]
Self-reported	Rivermead Mobility Index (RMI)[39]	Mobility-derived disability, ranging from ability to turn in bed to running, and an observation of standing without aid	Relies on a patient's subjective assessment[26]
	Hauser Ambulation Index[40] (Hauser)	Semiquantitative scale (0–10) based on time to walk 25 feet and use of aids	Relies on a patient's subjective assessment, and the use of aids is also dependent on psychosocial factors[26]
	Multiple Sclerosis Walking Scale (MSWS-12)[41]	12 questions with five responses regarding limitations of mobility	Relies on a patient's subjective assessment[26]
	EuroQol-5 dimension Index (EQ-5D)[42]	Five descriptive questions including mobility, self-care, usual activities, pain/discomfort, and anxiety/depression with three potential responses	
	UK Neurological Disability Scale (UKNDS)[43]	12 subsections including mobility, scored 0–5 based on use of aids	Relies on a patient's subjective assessment[26]
	Functional Independence Measures (FIM)[44]	Includes 18 items with four levels of response, with sections for mobility and locomotion	Relies on a patient's subjective assessment[26]
	Barthel Index[45]	Assesses activity including mobility, based on use of aids and ability to walk a distance or climb stairs	Relies on a patient's subjective assessment[26]
	Short Form 36 (SF-36)[46]	8-part questionnaire about overall quality of life, but includes physical functioning and ambulation	Relies on a patient's subjective assessment,[26] not specific to MS, floor and ceiling effects[47]
	Multiple Sclerosis Quality of Life Inventory (MSQLI)[30]	Health Status Questionnaire (SF-36), plus nine symptom-specific measures: fatigue, pain, bladder function, bowel function, emotional status, perceived cognitive function, visual function, sexual satisfaction, and social relationships	
	Multiple Sclerosis Quality of Life (MSQOL-54)[47]	12 subscales along with two summary scores, and two additional single-item measures, including physical function, role limitations—physical, role limitations—emotional, pain, emotional well-being, energy, health perceptions, social function, cognitive function, health distress, overall quality of life, and sexual function	Relies on a patient's subjective assessment[26]
	Multiple Sclerosis Impact Scale[48]	29 questions regarding limitations secondary to MS (each scored 1–5)	Relies on a patient's subjective assessment[26]
	Patient Determined Disease Steps (PDDS)[49]	Scored from 0 (normal) to 8 (bedridden), with scores between 3 and 7 specifically focused on patient-reported walking limitations	Relies on a patient's subjective assessment[26]

(*continued*)

Table 25-2. Functional Assessments Involving the Lower Extremity in Multiple Sclerosis (*continued*)

Type	Assessment Name	Data Measured	Limitations
	Functional Assessment of Multiple Sclerosis (FAMS)[50]	44 questions divided into six subscales: mobility, symptoms, emotional well-being (depression), general contentment, thinking/fatigue, and family/social well-being	Relies on a patient's subjective assessment
	Physical activity diary	Patient records daily activity or recalls daily activity after each week	Patient compliance can be poor, and time consuming for patients[26]
	Activities-specific Balance Confidence Scale (ABC)[51]	16-item questionnaire in which respondents rate their confidence that they can maintain their balance in the course of daily activities. Scored 0–10 and averaged	Subjective, does not identify type of balance problems, and not related to falls[52]
Activity trackers	Pedometer	Number of steps	Not effective for qualitative assessment[26]
	Accelerometer[25,26]	Steps, distance, energy expenditure	Not effective for qualitative assessment[26]
Balance			
Direct observation	Balance Evaluation Systems Test (BESTest)[48]	36 items, grouped into six systems: "Biomechanical Constraints," "Stability Limits/Verticality," "Anticipatory Postural Adjustments," "Postural Responses," "Sensory Orientation," and "Stability in Gait." Each item scored 0–4 and totaled	Time to perform: 30 min, no studies of fall risk, equipment is needed[52]
	Functional Reach[53]	Maximal distance a person can reach beyond the length of their arm while maintaining a fixed base of support in the standing position. A reach less than or equal to 6 inches predicts fall	Only one task evaluated, does not identify type of balance problem[26]
	Tinetti Gait and Balance[54]	14-item balance and 10-item gait test. Predicts the risk of having one fall in the next year	Poor specificity, ceiling effect, does not identify type of balance problem[52]
	Timed Up and Go (TUG)[55]	Time required for a person to rise from a chair, walk 3 m, turn around, walk back to the chair, and sit down	Ceiling effect, only one functional task, does not identify type of balance problem[52]
	Berg Functional Balance Scale[56]	14-item functional assessment including sitting, standing, and postural transitions. Items scored from 0 to 4 points	Poor sensitivity, does not identify the type of balance problem, ceiling effect, does not test dynamic balance[52]
	One-Leg Stance[57]	Eyes open and arms on the hips, patients stand unassisted on one leg. Participants unable to perform for at least 5 s are at increased risk for injurious fall	Only one task of static balance is evaluated, no identification of the type of balance problem, not continuously related to falls[52]
Spasticity			
	Ashworth Scale[58]	Muscle spasticity on a scale from 0 to 4 depending on tone, resistance, and range of motion	Does not differentiate lower levels effectively. Evaluator error
	Modified Ashworth Scale[59]	Muscle spasticity on a scale including 0, 1, 1+, 2, 3, 4 evaluating tone, resistance, spastic catch, and range of motion	Evaluator error
	Tardieu Scale[60]	Muscle reaction (0–5) at three different speeds (V1, V2, V3)	Evaluator error
	Modified Tardieu Scale[61]	Muscle reaction (0–5) at three different speeds (V1, V2, V3), and accounts for Joint angle	Evaluator error
	Multiple Sclerosis Spasticity Scale (MSSS-88)[62]	88 questions regarding the impact of spasticity on a patient's overall function	Based on the patient's subjective response

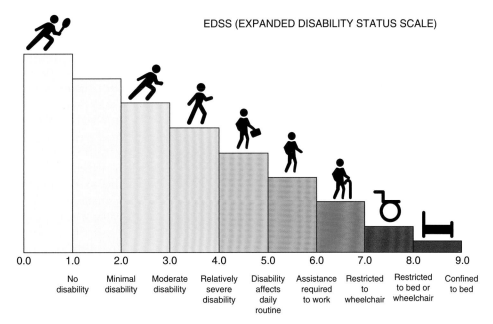

FIGURE 25-3. Expanded Disability Status Scale.

type of assistive device needed. EDSS progression is more heavily weighted toward dependence on assistive devices. For patients within this range on the EDSS, there is often wide variability in functional disability, because many patients requiring assistive devices have the ability to walk the same maximum distances as patients not requiring assistive devices. In addition, day-to-day variations in patient symptoms can have large effects on walking distance and have been shown to cause changes of approximately 1.5 points on the scale.[27] For scores greater than 7.5, all patients are bedbound or confined to a wheelchair, with very severe degrees of functional disability[30] (Fig. 25-3).

The EDSS has been criticized for its lack of psychometric input, leading to low sensitivity, poor reliability, and inability to correlate with disease changes.[63] The most pertinent flaw in the EDSS is that it is too heavily focused on ambulation, and not sensitive enough for overall disability. However, it remains a mainstay in clinical assessment of disability in MS and is routinely used for outcome measurements with clinical trials.

Timed Walking Tests

Although not specific to MS, timed walking tests are easy point of care functional exams that provide quantitative data in the assessment of ambulatory dysfunction. The three most common walking tests are the timed 25-foot walk (T25), 2-minute timed walk, and 6-minute timed walk. The T25 is commonly used as a measure of ambulation speed[26] and gait disturbances in MS. It is one of three functional measurements in the Multiple Sclerosis Functional Composite (MSFC),[30] which has shown moderate correlations with the EDSS.[64] Independently of its involvement in the MSFC, the T25 has been shown to correlate with EDSS across different disease severities and types,[65] as well as the Incapacity Status Scale, Rivermead Mobility Index, and frequency of falls.[66]

The patient is shown a well-demarcated 25-foot path, and instructed to start from a static standing position and walk as quickly as possible to the end, while remaining safe. The patient is timed twice for the exam, and all normal assistive devices are to be used for the exam. The test is limited by its inability to detect changes in patients with minimal disease severity or ambulatory dysfunction, and it is not a good measurement of a patient's walking stamina; however, it has shown to have high test–retest reliability and validity.[67]

The timed 2- and 6-minute walk are also commonly used timed walking tests; however, the longer duration is better suited for assessing patient stamina and endurance.[68] Each test measures the total distance walked in either 2 or 6 minutes. The 6-minute walking test has shown strong correlations with the T25, EDSS, MSFC, and Multiple Sclerosis Walking Scale in assessing patient disability.[34] In addition, the tests have been used to analyze changes in gait during times of fatigue. Both the 2- and 6-minute walking tests have been shown to be better than the T25 at detecting clinically significant improvement following rehabilitation programs.[69] The 6-minute walking test is oftentimes limited by space, as it is best to perform the test in a space requiring minimal turns. In addition, for patients with severe fatigue or loss of endurance, the 6 minute walk may require too much energy expenditure, and the 2-minute walking test would be more suitable in such cases. Research has shown the 2-minute walking test to be statistically similar to the 6-minute walking test.[70]

Multiple Sclerosis Walking Scale-12

The Multiple Sclerosis Walking Scale 12 (MSWS-12) is a 12-item questionnaire used to assess patient-reported impact of MS on walking.[41] Each question has a numerical answer between 1 and 5, and the total aggregate score creates a standardized level for how a patient feels their walking is affected by MS. The MSWS-12 has been extensively validated as a reliable and accurate clinical measure[71] in both community and hospital settings. The MSWS-12 has illustrated a very high correlation with the EDSS overall, but is predominately focused on correlation in the lower levels of disease impairment (EDSS 1 to 4.5). It has also shown strong correlations with oxygen cost of walking during 6-minute walking tests,[72] as well as the T25.[71] One of the strongest elements of the MSWS-12 is its responsiveness to change, making it a logical choice for clinical trial application.

Health Status Questionnaire

The Short Form 36 (SF-36) health status questionnaire is one of the most widely used patient-reported surveys for health-related quality of life. Studies have shown that this survey can differentiate not only between different diseases, but also between severity within a specific disease.[73] The SF-36 is a set of 36 questions that requires approximately 10 minutes for the patient to complete, with little to no intervention from a health care professional. It is comprised of eight categories: physical functioning, role limitations due to physical problems, bodily pain, general health perceptions, vitality, social functioning, role limitations due to emotional problems, and mental health.[74] From the eight sections, two aggregate scores are created, including one for physical functioning and the other for mental functioning. Although the SF-36 is not specifically focused toward MS sequelae, the physical functioning aggregate score is largely applicable for a functional assessment of the lower extremity. Studies have shown the physical functioning aggregate score and the role limitations due to physical functioning score were able to differentiate MS from other diseases.[47] In addition, the aggregate scores can be applied to other health assessments that are more specific to MS, including the Multiple Sclerosis Quality of Life Inventory (MSQLI) and the Multiple Sclerosis Quality of Life 54 (MSQOL-54). Within the MSQLI health assessment, the physical functioning portion from the SF-36 has illustrated correlations with the EDSS and Ambulation Index.[74]

Multiple Sclerosis Impact Scale

The Multiple Sclerosis Impact Scale is a set of 29 questions, 20 assessing physical functioning and 9 assessing psychological functioning that are specific to MS patients and seek to determine the impact of the disease on a specific patient. The scale determines a full range of impairment with MS, including physical functioning, and has exhibited correlations with the EDSS and the MSFC.[75] The survey is a self-reported survey that has exhibited good variability, minimal ceiling and floor effects, and high internal consistency.[48] The questionnaire takes approximately 5 to 10 minutes to complete, and has shown validity and reliability in multiple MS populations, including postal surveys[48,75] and hospital settings.[76] In addition, the survey illustrated good responsiveness to change when examined alone and when compared to other self-reported surveys, which could provide better longitudinal analysis of disease progression.[77]

Functional Assessment of Multiple Sclerosis

The Functional Assessment of Multiple Sclerosis (FAMS) is a 44-question patient-reported survey that encompasses six different areas of overall well-being in MS patients. The six subsections are: mobility, symptoms, emotional well-being (depression), general contentment, thinking/fatigue, and family/social well-being. When the patient is completing the survey, they are asked to answer the question based on the previous 7 days of their life. The FAMS takes approximately 20 minutes to complete, which can be a limitation if under time constraints, and a higher score represents higher quality of life.[78] The FAMS is a simple and easy survey that provides reliable and valid information about a patient's lower extremity function. Although not a specific patient survey on mobility such as the MSWS-12, the mobility section of the FAMS has been shown to illustrate strong correlations to the Kurtzke EDSS and Scripps Neurologic Rating Scale.[50]

Accelerometer

Of late, the use of accelerometers has become widespread with the everyday user through devices such as fitness trackers; however, their application has also expanded into clinical application. Accelerometers measure human movement in multiple planes, whereas a pedometer only tracks human steps. They have been used in many preliminary studies specifically focused on their application in MS.[60,79,80] Initial research has shown accelerometer to be a better quantitative measure of overall activity, versus qualitative measure of ambulation, and it has shown correlation with other standardized walking tests such as the 5-minute walk test.[81] In addition, when accelerometry has been used to measure patients' household and habitual ambulation, it has been predictive of outcomes in walking capacity assessments such as the 2-minute timed walk and the 6-minute timed walk.

Balance

Approximately 75% of patients with MS report issues with balance. Because of the integral role of balance in many aspects of physical functioning, its effect on disease state is quite significant. In general, balance is maintained by the interconnectedness of multiple sensory systems including the motor, somatosensory, and visual/vestibular systems. Because of the variable nature of CNS lesions in MS, none or all of these systems may be affected, leading to variable levels of balance dysfunction in multiple aspects of physical functioning from ambulation, turning, standing still, and spatial awareness. Increasing difficulty with balance in patients with lower levels of disease impairment (EDSS 0 to 4.5) can be difficult to detect and can present in many different forms from reductions in gait velocity and stride length,[82] to compensatory gait actions,[83] decreases in functional reach,[84] and even increased stride cadence at slow speeds.[85] Alterations in the somatosensory system can manifest as changes in peripheral sensory signals and proprioception that can further affect ambulation, as well as postural control, which can lead to increased energy expenditure because of compensatory adaptations.[86] Vestibular system manifestations can result in vertigo, unstable gaze with head movement, and gait ataxia.[87] Vertigo has been reported in up to 20% of all patients with MS.[88] Disturbances in vision can also have drastic effects on balance, and most commonly present as optic neuritis, visual field defects, and saccadic eye movements. The visual system is extremely important when patients have deficits in the somatosensory system, because patients often compensate with the visual system to adjust for postural instability and loss of proprioception.[87] The multifactorial etiology of balance impairment in MS makes reliable and accurate evaluation difficult, and multiple methods of assessment are encouraged to ensure thorough assessment of a patient's functional status.

Tinetti Gait and Balance

The Tinetti Gait and Balance test is a hybrid assessment of balance and gait, which is used to predict an individual's risk of having at least one fall in the next year. Although not specifically used for MS patients, it is the oldest clinical balance assessment tool and commonly used to assess the geriatric demographic. The maximum score is 40, and individuals scoring less than 36 are at greater risk for having a fall.[54] The test is an easy point-of-care assessment requiring approximately 20 minutes to perform, with little to no additional setup, that has been shown to have high interrater reliability and a sensitivity of 93% in regard to identifying patients that will fall.[89] However, the test is limited by its lack of specificity, in that only 11% of nonfallers were identified. In addition, the exam has been shown to have a ceiling effect, and does not adequately assess patients with mild impairments.[90]

Timed Get Up and Go Test

Previously known as the "Get Up and Go" test, the Timed Get Up and Go (TUG) test is a short, simple, and reliable clinical assessment of balance that has been used in multiple populations including geriatrics, Parkinson disease, and MS. It has illustrated correlations with fall risk in elderly[91] and is correlated with disease severity in Parkinson disease. The test requires a patient to sit in a chair, rise, walk out 3 m, turn around, walk back to the chair, and sit back down. It has proven to be one of the more reliable balance assessments because it is based on stopwatch time, rather than subjective scales. When compared to the timed 10 m walk and timed 30 m walk, the TUG test showed strong correlations.[92] The TUG test is limited by its inability to discern differences between gait and balance as individual deficits, but rather assesses them as a unified concept. In addition, the exam illustrates a ceiling effect, in that the exam is not as strong at identifying impairments in patients with mild disease symptoms.

Berg Balance Scale

The Berg Balance Scale (BBS) is another balance assessment that has been used in geriatrics, but shows validity for patients with MS.[56,93] The test is a 14-item functional assessment that evaluates sitting, standing, and postural transitions on a scale from 0 to 4, and requires approximately 15 minutes to complete. The BBS has been shown to have high interrater reliability when compared to the timed 6-minute walk.[94] Similar to many other balance assessments, the test is limited by its ceiling effect and its inability to identify the specific balance problem. The test also does not assess dynamic balance[52] and may not be the most effective at identifying clinically significant changes in disability.[95]

One-Leg Stance

First published by Fregly and Graybiel,[57] in 1968, the one-leg stance test is the oldest balance assessment tool, first used in tests for the military. This test is not specifically used for assessing MS, but has been used as a measure of postural stability for many neurologic disorders. The patient is instructed to balance on one foot unsupported with eyes open, without bracing the legs against each other. Then the patient closes their eyes and attempts to maintain balance for 30 seconds. The time is stopped if the patient's foot touches the floor, the foot touches the support leg, hopping occurs, or the patient's arms touch something.[96] Although the exam is performed with both eyes open and closed, the eyes closed progression is oftentimes too difficult for many patients with balance disorders because of the needed compensation from the visual system. Patients who are unable to perform the test for more than 5 seconds are at significantly increased risk for falls. Similar to the TUG test, the use of a stopwatch for timing creates reliable quantitative data.[52] The test is limited because it only assesses a single type of static balance, and does not address the type of balance issue.

Spasticity

Muscle spasticity is a very common symptom of MS, affecting approximately 80% of MS patients. In fact, about one-third of MS patients are thought to have spasticity that impacts their daily life.[97] The classic presentation of an upper motor neuron lesion, spasticity is defined by velocity-dependent increase in muscle tone caused by excitability of the muscle stretch reflex.[74] It is commonly represented by the clasp knife phenomenon, also known as the "spastic catch," which can be overcome with continued force. At lower speeds, the spastic catch is diminished.[98] The etiology of spasticity development is thought to be largely due to the loss of inhibitory control over spinal reflexes, leading to hyperexcitability of the spinal reflexes.[75] However, given the large variability of upper motor neuron lesions in MS and the array of neurologic adaptations, the exact mechanism is likely multifaceted. With MS, spasticity can be triggered by various stimuli, including position changes, cold and hot temperatures, urinary retention, urinary tract infections, constipation, pain, pressure ulcers, or infection.[5] Spasticity can present in a myriad of ways, both painful and painless, most commonly seen as muscle stiffness or spasms, decreased active or passive range of motion, impaired voluntary movements, or sensation of muscle tightening. Tendon reflexes are exaggerated, and clonus may be present at the ankle.[99] It is generally classified into two groups: flexor and extensor spasticity.[73] Flexor spasticity in the lower limb generally presents as involuntary bending of the hips and knees, commonly affecting the hamstring muscles, whereas extensor spasticity results in straightening of the leg, targeting the quadriceps and adductors, and extensor spasms of the extensor hallucis longus.[99] Patients with extensor hallucis longus spasms can show abrasion to the great toe because of irritation from rubbing against the inside of the shoe. Knee extension, inversion of the foot, and plantarflexion of the ankle can be seen either unilaterally or bilaterally. Untreated, spasticity can cause pain, muscle atrophy, and fixed contractions. Spasticity can also cause a scissoring gait pattern because of adduction at the hip joint.

Spasticity can significantly influence quality of life by affecting patients' ambulation, ability to sit, and ability to sit in a wheelchair, which could lead to pressure ulcers and permanent contractures.[76] Patients may often require the use of a cane to help with stability, in which case they should be instructed to use the cane on their stronger side. However, when patients have concomitant areas of weakness in the lower extremities, spasticity can sometimes be beneficial by increasing stability and providing just enough functional support to allow patients to transfer, stand, or walk.[5] Because of the large effects spasticity plays in patients' quality of life, proper assessment and monitoring of spasticity is important for monitoring disease progression and initiating applicable treatment options.

Modified Ashworth Scale

The Modified Ashworth Scale is the most popular clinical assessment scale for measuring spasticity in patients with MS. It is a revised version of the original Ashworth scale, and categorizes spasticity based on muscle tone, the presence of a spastic catch, and range of motion affected.[59] The original Ashworth scale was set on a scale from 0 to 4, but the Modified Ashworth added a 1+ characterization, to better characterize lower levels of spasticity (**Table 25-3**).

Table 25-3. Modified Ashworth Scale

Grade	Description
	Modified Ashworth Scale
0	No increased muscle tone
1	Slight increase in tone, spastic catch with release present or minimal resistance at end range of motion (ROM) during flexion and extension
1+	Slight increase in tone, spastic catch with minimal resistance throughout remainder of movement (less than half of ROM)
2	Further increased muscle tone throughout most ROM, but affected part easily moves
3	Considerable increase in muscle tone, passive movement difficult
4	Muscle rigid in flexion or extension

TREATMENT

Proper assessment of lower extremity dysfunction can lead to initiation of appropriate disease-modifying therapy to slow the underlying demyelinating process, as well as proper symptomatic treatment and rehabilitation.

Disease-Modifying Therapies

There are currently 14 disease-modifying therapies that are Food and Drug Administration (FDA) approved for relapsing forms of MS. They have been shown to slow disease progression and disability, while decreasing the number of relapses and MRI lesions. Research has shown that the earlier patients are diagnosed and treated, the better their chances are of delaying long-term disability and development of secondary progressive MS.

The first-line injectable therapies include glatiramer acetate and the interferon betas: interferon β-1b (subcutaneous), interferon β-1a (subcutaneous), interferon β-1a (intramuscular), peginterferon β-1a (subcutaneous). A more recently approved injectable therapy is daclizumab, which is a monoclonal antibody. The more recently developed oral medications include fingolimod, teriflunomide, and dimethyl fumarate. The currently approved monoclonal antibody intravenous infusion therapies include natalizumab and alemtuzumab. Additionally, ocrelizumab, a B cell–directed monoclonal antibody, is currently being evaluated by the FDA for possible future approval as an intravenous infusion therapy for both primary progressive and relapsing forms of MS.

Gait and Ambulation

Various approaches can be taken to treat gait disorders based on the specific gait dysfunction. Physical therapy is often the mainstay of treatment focusing on strengthening, therapeutic exercise, stretching, spasticity reduction, gait training, balance retraining, and generalized conditioning techniques. Neurorehabilitation focuses on regaining or improving function with the use of therapeutic exercise, compensatory mechanisms, appropriate assistive devices, or equipment that can compensate for lost functioning. Exercises can improve the postural changes that can occur related to CNS-induced weakness, scoliosis, pain, or poor postural practices. Improved posture can help facilitate gait and walking speed. Generalized conditioning programs have been shown to improve endurance and gait pattern. Such conditioning can also promote general cardiopulmonary health and cognitive functioning.[100]

Focused strategies can address specific functional deficits. For example, a foot drop due to inherent weakness in dorsiflexion can be controlled with an ankle-foot orthosis (AFO), which maintains the ankle at a 90° angle. This prevents foot drag in the swing phase of gait, helps normalize the gait pattern, and can decrease the patient's overall energy expenditure. There are various bracing options available, such as a custom solid

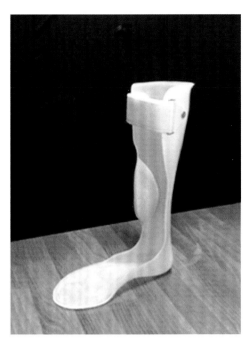

FIGURE 25-4. Ankle-foot orthosis.

lightweight plastic AFO, a plastic AFO with metal hinges that facilitates dorsiflexion or plantarflexion depending on dysfunction. A newer energy return AFO is available that utilizes natural flex built into the material of the AFO to provide dorsiflexion assist. Less expensive prefabricated braces are available with energy return design. These are well suited for patients who do not require custom fitting (**Fig. 25-4**).

There are two newer devices that incorporate electrical stimulation to assist with dorsiflexion. The WalkAide and Bioness L300 use functional electrical stimulation, which sends low-level electrical impulses to the peroneal nerve to signal dorsiflexion. The WalkAide uses a tilt sensor built into the stimulator that can track the angle and speed of the leg. The Bioness L300 utilizes a gait sensor that attaches to the shoe and communicates with the functional stimulation cuff around the leg via a wireless stimulator. These devices work well in patients with isolated dorsiflexion weakness. However, if other weakness-causing inversion or eversion at the ankle or recurvatum at the knee is present, custom AFOs may be a better option. Therefore, full evaluation by a physical therapist or physician is often required to determine which device may be most appropriate or best suited to compensate for the patient's specific deficit (**Figs. 25-5** and **25-6**).

There is one pharmacologic agent that is FDA approved to increase walking speed. Ampyra (dalfampridine) is an extended release preparation of 4-aminopyridine, which in a Phase III clinical trial that showed efficacy in MS.[25] About 35% to 40% of subjects were classified as responders in the Phase III clinical trial.[25] The use of this drug is limited to patients who have had no history of seizure, and the safety of the drug in patients with mild renal impairment is unknown.

Balance

Physical therapy can utilize various approaches to improve balance and coordination, from simple balance boards to more sophisticated functional training systems. The use of assistive devices may also improve balance by providing direct support in the form of a walker, rolling walker, or cane. Assistive devices may also assist balance in patients with proprioceptive deficits by allowing proprioceptive input that cannot be perceived normally via the lower extremity or spinal cord. Patients who use a cane to assist with lower extremity

FIGURE 25-5. WalkAide.

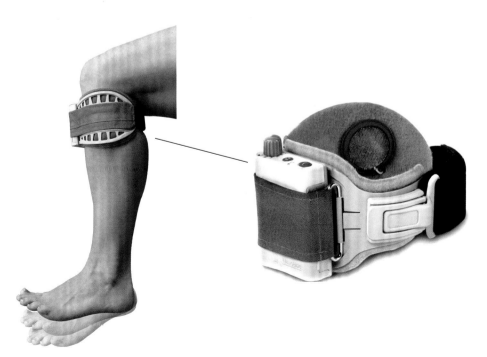

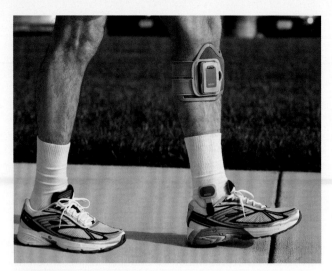

FIGURE 25-6. Bioness L300.

weakness or balance difficulties should be instructed to utilize the cane on their stronger side.

Spasticity

The treatment of spasticity depends on the severity of increased muscle tone, the muscles involved, and functional limitation produced in the patient. Treatment can include stretching, range of motion exercises, weight-bearing, physical therapy, occupational therapy (OT), positioning and splinting modalities, massage, ice/cold therapy, focal treatments, and medication. Commonly used oral medications for spasticity include baclofen, tizanidine, and benzodiazepines. Although these medications are effective in many cases, their side-effect profile, which includes sedation and excessive loss of tone, can limit their usefulness. The muscle relaxant dantrolene was used in the past as well, but due to its adverse effects of hepatotoxicity and muscle weakness, it is currently used less frequently.

Intrathecal baclofen may be considered when there has been insufficient control of spasticity with other treatment options, when there are unacceptable side effects to oral medications, or if a more precise dosing system is required.[101] The benefit of intrathecal baclofen is that the medication is introduced directly into the spinal cord where it acts, with no first-pass effect. The intrathecal baclofen pump is surgically implanted and programmable. The medication is instilled in the reservoir, and inert gases inside the pump create a pressure, pushing the medication into the tubing and into the spinal canal. A battery-powered microprocessor controls flow rate and can be reprogrammed with the use of an external computerized device. The baclofen pump requires refilling and needs to be replaced after 5 to 7 years of use depending on the size of the pump and the concentration used (**Fig. 25-7**).

Focal treatments such as botulinum toxin and chemodenervation with phenol nerve blockade can be considered in some instances, particularly when targeting specific small

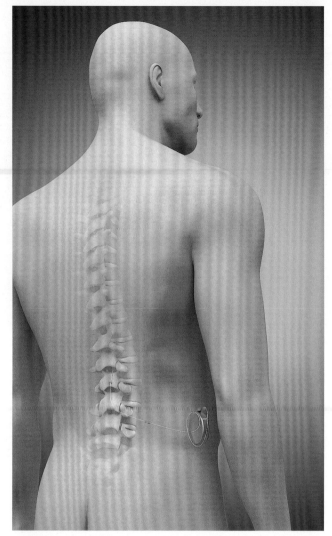

FIGURE 25-7. Intrathecal baclofen pump.

muscle groups.[101] Botulinum toxin is made from a neurotoxin produced by the bacterium *Clostridium botulinum*. The toxin decreases the release of acetylcholine through its high-affinity bonds to cholinergic nerve terminals, causing a neuromuscular blockade. It is often used to relieve increased tone in certain muscle groups. It takes full effect within 1 to 4 weeks after injection and has an effect lasting for 2 to 6 months. Botulinum toxin is often used for small muscle groups to relieve tone in the hands and feet, but this may not be an appropriate choice when treating large muscle groups as there is a dose limit. In certain situations, when noninvasive approaches prove to be unsuccessful, tenotomy (tendon release), which is the surgical cutting of a tendon, may be considered. Tenotomy can be used to lengthen contracted tendons related to severe spasticity. With comprehensive rehabilitation, it can be used in certain muscle groups such as triceps surae or hip adductors to enhance function or facilitate positioning.

Additionally, OT is another treatment modality that can be used to improve function and quality of life for patients. OT focuses on "occupation," which is defined as the daily tasks that take our time and energy and provide meaning to our lives. OT evaluates and offers interventions for self-care activity, productive activity, and leisure activity. OT identifies barriers to participation in activity and educates patients on energy conservation and compensatory strategies to achieve occupational goals.[102]

OTHER CONSIDERATIONS

It is also important to keep in mind other comorbidities or circumstances that may factor into the assessment of mobility in the MS patient. Patients who have bladder infections can have transient worsening of lower extremity weakness and spasticity. A distended bladder due to urinary retention can also act as a noxious stimulus and increase spasticity. Depression can decrease a patient's desire to move around and exercise, and cognitive deficits and fatigue can contribute to immobility. Sensory disturbances, visual impairment, muscle spasms, obesity, and dependent edema may all contribute to difficulty with ambulation. Furthermore, pain is a common symptom in MS patients. There is no evidence that pain is more common in patients with more versus less disability.[103] In many instances, symptoms such as pain can be debilitating and interfere with lower extremity functioning. Disorders originating from the foot such as plantar fasciitis or heel spurs can contribute to pain with ambulation. The most prevalent types of pain in MS patients include headache and dysesthetic limb pain.[103] Other types of pain include central or neuropathic pain, which can often be mediated with treatments such as antidepressants, antiepileptic medications, or benzodiazepines.[104]

Several of these considerations are illustrated in the following case:

A 40-year-old female was diagnosed with relapsing remitting MS 6 years ago. She initially presented with left optic neuritis, but now complains of gradual worsening of her gait over the past 6 months. She has experienced dragging of her right leg, especially after walking for longer than 10 minutes. She reported falling twice, particularly noting tripping due to the right foot drag. She also has noted increase in stiffness in her right leg and often circumducts it when she walks. She is very heat sensitive. She has been on Copaxone (glatiramer acetate) as a disease-modifying therapy. She has history of overactive bladder, and slowness in getting to the bathroom has resulted in occasional episodes of incontinence. Her T25 foot walk was 30 seconds. She has needed to use a cane to help her with stability.

Considerations for this patient include the following:

1. Consider a change in disease-modifying therapy because she has had worsening of her disease while on Copaxone.
2. Evaluate the weakness and spasticity contributing to her walking difficulties. Treatment with an antispasticity medication such as baclofen may be helpful. Physical therapy to help with gait assistance and core strengthening would be advisable. She should also be evaluated for a right ankle-foot orthotic or a functional stimulator such as a WalkAide that could assist with the right foot drop.
3. Consider treatment with dalfampridine (Ampyra), which is a potassium channel blocker that has the potential to improve walking speed.
4. Refer for urology evaluation. Evaluation and treatment of overactive bladder by a urologist can help improve bladder control.
5. Educate the patient on maintenance of proper temperature regulation by methods such as air-conditioning of the house and cooling devices such as a cooling vest to help with heat sensitivity.

When treating MS, comprehensive management plan evaluating and treating the underlying disease process as well as symptoms is the best approach. With these things in mind, cognitive, functional, and mobility assessments should be repeated periodically as the disease changes and progresses, with treatments adjusted accordingly.

CONCLUSION

MS is a common neurologic disorder affecting approximately 2.5 million people worldwide, with significant impact on lower extremity functioning in a large subset of patients. The lower extremity manifestations are classically a result of demyelinating lesions of upper motor neurons in the brain and spinal cord, resulting in pain, weakness, paresthesias, and spasticity. The combination of such symptoms most commonly presents as ambulatory and balance dysfunction. The variable presentation of physical impairment and complex clinical picture of MS makes accurate assessment and management of such lower extremity manifestations quite challenging.

Clinical assessment of lower extremity symptoms can be evaluated on a symptom-specific basis, such as the Modified Ashworth Scale for spasticity or physician evaluation of muscle strength or sensation. Conversely, lower extremity symptoms can also be assessed through more comprehensive functional evaluations such as the EDSS or SF-36, as well as patient-reported surveys such as the MSWS-12 and Multiple Sclerosis Impact Scale. Furthermore, quantitative measures such as the Tinetti Gait and Balance, TUG, and timed walking tests can provide more objective data for monitoring progression. Proper utilization and execution of such assessments are essential for identifying changes in lower extremity function, as well as initiating proper treatment.

Although there is no curative agent for MS as a whole, disease-modifying therapies continue to be developed, attempting to slow the progression of the disease or minimize the chances of relapse. However, multiple treatment modalities are available for treating individual lower extremity symptoms and can be used to improve patient quality of life and overall function.

When examining the many diseases or disorders that affect the lower extremity, it is important to include MS in the differential. Although there is much to learn about the underlying physiology and mechanism of MS, understanding the lower extremity manifestations and their impact on MS patients can lead to drastic improvements in patient care.

REFERENCES

1. Lassmann H, Brück W, Lucchinetti CF. The immunopathology of multiple sclerosis: an overview. *Brain Pathol.* 2007;17:210–218. doi:10.1111/j.1750-3639.2007.00064.x.

2. Milo R, Miller A. Revised diagnostic criteria of multiple sclerosis. *Autoimmun Rev.* 2014;13(4–5):518–524. doi:10.1016/j.autrev.2014.01.012.

3. Kleinewietfeld M, Manzel A, Titze J, et al. Sodium chloride drives autoimmune disease by the induction of pathogenic TH17 cells. *Nature.* 2013;496(7446):518–522. doi:10.1038/nature11868.

4. Ascherio A, Munger KL. Environmental risk factors for multiple sclerosis. Part I: the role of infection. *Ann Neurol.* 2007;61(4): 288–299. doi:10.1002/ana.21117.

5. MS Practice. Spasticity and Multiple Sclerosis. June 2009; 1–10. https://www.msaustralia.org.au/file/278/download?token=cK4rr3lc. Accessed June 14, 2016.

6. Marcus JF, Waubant EL. Updates on clinically isolated syndrome and diagnostic criteria for multiple sclerosis. *Neurohospitalist.* 2013;3(2):65–80. doi:10.1177/1941874412457183.

7. Newland PK, Fearing A, Riley M, et al. Symptom clusters in women with relapsing-remitting multiple sclerosis. *J Neurosci Nurs.* 2012;44(2):66–71. doi:10.1097/JNN.0b013e3182478cba.

8. Ziemssen T, Rauer S, Stadelmann C, et al. Evaluation of study and patient characteristics of clinical studies in primary progressive multiple sclerosis: a systematic review. *PLoS One.* 2015;10(9).e0138243. doi:10.1371/journal.pone.0138243.

9. Confavreux C, Vukusic S. Natural history of multiple sclerosis: a unifying concept. *Brain.* 2006;129(pt 3):606–616. doi:10.1093 /brain/awl007.

10. Sturm D, Gurevitz SL, Turner A. Multiple sclerosis: a review of the disease and treatment options. *Consult Pharm.* 2014;29(7):469–479. doi:10.4140/TCP.n.2014.469.

11. Hawker K. Progressive multiple sclerosis: characteristics and management. *Neurol Clin.* 2011;29(2):423–434. doi:10.1016/j .ncl.2011.01.002.

12. Bashir K, Whitaker JN. Clinical and laboratory features of primary progressive and secondary progressive MS. *Neurology.* 1999;53(4):765–771. doi:10.1212/WNL.53.4.765.

13. Society NM. Primary progressive MS (PPMS). http://www .nationalmssociety.org/What-is-MS/Types-of-MS/Primary-progressive-MS. Accessed January 1, 2016.

14. Koch M, Kingwell E, Rieckmann P, et al. The natural history of secondary progressive multiple sclerosis. *J Neurol Neurosurg Psychiatry.* 2010;81(9):1039–1043. doi:10.1136/jnnp.2010.208173.

15. Scalfari A, Neuhaus A, Daumer M, et al. Onset of secondary progressive phase and long-term evolution of multiple sclerosis. *J Neurol Neurosurg Psychiatry.* 2014;85(1):67–75. doi:10.1136 /jnnp-2012-304333.

16. Scalfari A, Neuhaus A, Daumer M, et al. Age and disability accumulation in multiple sclerosis. *Neurology.* 2011;77(13):1246–1252. doi:10.1212/WNL.0b013e318230a17d.

17. Trapp BD, Nave KA. Multiple sclerosis: an immune or neurodegenerative disorder? *Annu Rev Neurosci.* 2008;31:247–269. doi:10.1146/annurev.neuro.30.051606.094313.

18. Stadelmann C, Albert M, Wegner C, et al. Cortical pathology in multiple sclerosis. *Curr Opin Neurol.* 2008;21(3):229–234. doi:10.1097/01.wco.0000318863.65635.9a.

19. Tintoré M, Rovira A, Martínez MJ, et al. Isolated demyelinating syndromes: comparison of different MR imaging criteria to predict conversion to clinically definite multiple sclerosis. *Am J Neuroradiol.* 2000;21(4):702–706.

20. Polman CH, Reingold SC, Banwell B, et al. Diagnostic criteria for multiple sclerosis: 2010 revisions to the McDonald criteria. *Ann Neurol.* 2011;69(2):292–302. doi:10.1002/ana.22366.

21. Katz Sand IB, Lublin FD. Diagnosis and differential diagnosis of multiple sclerosis. *Continuum (Minneap Minn).* 2013;19(4 Multiple Sclerosis):922–943. doi:10.1212/01.CON.0000433290.15468.21.

22. Swingler RJ, Compston DA. The morbidity of multiple sclerosis. *Q J Med.* 1992;83(300):325–337.

23. Heesen C, Böhm J, Reich C, et al. Patient perception of bodily functions in multiple sclerosis: gait and visual function are the most valuable. *Mult Scler.* 2008;14(7):988–991. doi:10.1177/1352458508088916.

24. Sutliff MH. Contribution of impaired mobility to patient burden in multiple sclerosis. *Curr Med Res Opin.* 2010;26(1):109–119. doi:10.1185/03007990903433528.

25. Bethoux F. Gait disorders in multiple sclerosis. *Continuum (Minneap Minn).* 2013;19(4):1007–1022. doi:10.1212/01 .CON.0000433286.92596.d5.

26. Pearson OR, Busse ME, van Deursen RWM, et al. Quantification of walking mobility in neurological disorders. *QJM.* 2004;97(8):463–475. doi:10.1093/qjmed/hch084.

27. Albrecht H, Wötzel C, Erasmus LP, et al. Day-to-day variability of maximum walking distance in MS patients can mislead to relevant changes in the Expanded Disability Status Scale (EDSS): average walking speed is a more constant parameter. *Mult Scler.* 2001;7(2):105–109.

28. Association of British Neurologists. *Guidelines for the Use of Beta Interferons and Glatiramer Acetate in Multiple Sclerosis.* London, UK: ABN; 2001.

29. Kurtzke JF. Rating neurologic impairment in multiple sclerosis: an expanded disability status scale (EDSS). *Neurology.* 1983;33(11):1444–1452.

30. Fischer JS, Rudick RA, Cutter GR, et al. The Multiple Sclerosis Functional Composite Measure (MSFC): an integrated approach to MS clinical outcome assessment. National MS Society Clinical Outcomes Assessment Task Force. *Mult Scler.* 1999;5(4):244–250.

31. McConvey J, Bennett SE. Reliability of the Dynamic Gait Index in individuals with multiple sclerosis. *Arch Phys Med Rehabil.* 2005;86(1):130–133.

32. Nieuwenhuis MM, Van Tongeren H, Sørensen PS, et al. The six spot step test: a new measurement for walking ability in multiple sclerosis. *Mult Scler.* 2006;12(4):495–500.

33. Brooks D, Parsons J, Hunter JP, et al. The 2-minute walk test as a measure of functional improvement in persons with lower limb amputation. *Arch Phys Med Rehabil.* 2001;82(10):1478–1483. doi:10.1053/apmr.2001.25153.

34. Goldman MD, Marrie RA, Cohen JA. Evaluation of the six-minute walk in multiple sclerosis subjects and healthy controls. *Mult Scler.* 2008;14(3):383–390. doi:10.1177/1352458507082607.

35. Lord SE, Halligan PW, Wade DT. Visual gait analysis: the development of a clinical assessment and scale. *Clin Rehabil.* 1998;12(2):107–119.

36. Wiles CM, Newcombe RG, Fuller KJ, et al. Controlled randomised crossover trial of the effects of physiotherapy on mobility in chronic multiple sclerosis. *J Neurol Neurosurg Psychiatry.* 2001;70(2):174–179.

37. Merkelbach S, Haensch CA, Hemmer B, et al. Multiple sclerosis and the autonomic nervous system. *J Neurol.* 2006;253(Suppl 1):I21–I25. doi:10.1007/s00415-006-1105-z.

38. Lord SR, Clark RD. Simple physiological and clinical tests for the accurate prediction of falling in older people. *Gerontology.* 1996;42(4):199–203.

39. Collen FM, Wade DT, Robb GF, et al. The Rivermead Mobility Index: a further development of the Rivermead Motor Assessment. *Int Disabil Stud.* 1991;13(2):50–54.

40. Hauser SL, Dawson DM, Lehrich JR, et al. Intensive immunosuppression in progressive multiple sclerosis. A randomized, three-arm study of high-dose intravenous cyclophosphamide, plasma exchange, and ACTH. *N Engl J Med.* 1983;308(4):173–180. doi:10.1056 /NEJM198301273080401.

41. Hobart JC, Riazi A, Lamping DL, et al. Measuring the impact of MS on walking ability: the 12-Item MS Walking Scale (MSWS-12). *Neurology*. 2003;60(1):31–36.

42. Sidovar MF, Limone BL, Lee S, et al. Mapping the 12-item multiple sclerosis walking scale to the EuroQol 5-dimension index measure in North American multiple sclerosis patients. *BMJ Open*. 2013;3(5). doi:10.1136/bmjopen-2013-002798.

43. Sharrack B, Hughes RA. The Guy's neurological disability scale (GNDS): a new disability measure for multiple sclerosis. *Mult Scler*. 1999;5(4):223–233.

44. Keith RA, Granger CV, Hamilton BB, et al. The functional independence measure: a new tool for rehabilitation. *Adv Clin Rehabil*. 1987;1:6–18.

45. Mahoney FI, Barthel DW. Functional evaluation: the barthel index. *Md State Med J*. 1965;14:61–65.

46. Ware J, Snow KK, Kosinski M, et al. *SF-36 Health Survey Manual and Interpretation Guide*. Boston, MA: Nimrod Press; 1993.

47. Vickrey BG, Hays RD, Harooni R, et al. A health-related quality of life measure for multiple sclerosis. *Qual Life Res*. 1995;4(3):187–206.

48. Hobart J, Lamping D, Fitzpatrick R, et al. The Multiple Sclerosis Impact Scale (MSIS-29): a new patient-based outcome measure. *Brain*. 2001;124(pt 5):962–973.

49. Learmonth YC, Motl RW, Sandroff BM, et al. Validation of patient determined disease steps (PDDS) scale scores in persons with multiple sclerosis. *BMC Neurol*. 2013;13:37. doi:10.1186/1471-2377-13-37.

50. Cella DF, Dineen K, Arnason B, et al. Validation of the functional assessment of multiple sclerosis quality of life instrument. *Neurology*. 1996;47(1):129–139.

51. Powell LE, Myers AM. The Activities-specific Balance Confidence (ABC) Scale. *J Gerontol A Biol Sci Med Sci*. 1995;50A(1):M28–M34.

52. Mancini M, Horak FB. The relevance of clinical balance assessment tools to differentiate balance deficits. *Eur J Phys Rehabil Med*. 2010;46(2):239–248.

53. Duncan PW, Weiner DK, Chandler J, et al. Functional reach: a new clinical measure of balance. *J Gerontol*. 1990;45(6):M192–M197.

54. Tinetti ME. Performance-oriented assessment of mobility problems in elderly patients. *J Am Geriatr Soc*. 1986;34(2):119–126.

55. Podsiadlo D, Richardson S. The timed "Up & Go": a test of basic functional mobility for frail elderly persons. *J Am Geriatr Soc*. 1991;39(2):142–148.

56. Berg KO, Wood-Dauphinee SL, Williams JI, et al. Measuring balance in the elderly: validation of an instrument. *Can J Public Health*. 1992;83(Suppl 2):S7–S11.

57. Fregly AR, Graybiel A. An ataxia test battery not requiring rails. *Aerosp Med*. 1968;39(3):277–282.

58. Lee KC, Carson L, Kinnin E, et al. The Ashworth Scale: a reliable and reproducible method of measuring spasticity. *J Neuro Rehab*. 1989;3:205–209.

59. Bohannon RW, Smith MB. Interrater reliability of a modified Ashworth scale of muscle spasticity. *Phys Ther*. 1987;67(2):206–207.

60. Patrick E, Ada L. The Tardieu Scale differentiates contracture from spasticity whereas the Ashworth Scale is confounded by it. *Clin Rehabil*. 2006;20(2):173–182. doi:10.1191/0269215506cr922oa.

61. Mehrholz J, Wagner K, Meissner D, et al. Reliability of the Modified Tardieu Scale and the Modified Ashworth Scale in adult patients with severe brain injury: a comparison study. *Clin Rehabil*. 2005;19(7):751–759.

62. Hobart JC, Riazi A, Thompson AJ, et al. Getting the measure of spasticity in multiple sclerosis: the Multiple Sclerosis Spasticity Scale (MSSS-88). *Brain*. 2006;129(pt 1):224–234. doi:10.1093/brain/awh675.

63. Hobart J, Freeman J, Thompson A. Kurtzke scales revisited: the application of psychometric methods to clinical intuition. *Brain*. 2000;123(pt 5):1027–1040.

64. Rudick RA, Cutter G, Reingold S. The multiple sclerosis functional composite: a new clinical outcome measure for multiple sclerosis trials. *Mult Scler*. 2002;8(5):359–365.

65. Kalkers NF, de Groot V, Lazeron RH, et al. MS functional composite: relation to disease phenotype and disability strata. *Neurology*. 2000;54(6):1233–1239.

66. Bethoux FA, Palfy DM, Plow MA. Correlates of the timed 25 foot walk in a multiple sclerosis outpatient rehabilitation clinic. *Int J Rehabil Res*. 2016;39(2):134–139. doi:10.1097/MRR.0000000000000157.

67. National Multiple Sclerosis Society Clinically isolated syndrome (CIS). Timed 25-foot Walk. http://www.nationalmssociety.org/For-Professionals/Researchers/Resources-for-Researchers/Clinical-Study-Measures/Timed-25-Foot-Walk-(T25-FW)."http://www.nationalmssociety.org/For-Professionals/Researchers/Resources-for-Researchers/Clinical-Study-Measures/Timed-25-Foot-Walk-(T25-FW).

68. Bethoux F, Bennett S. Evaluating walking in patients with multiple sclerosis: which assessment tools are useful in clinical practice? *Int J MS Care*. 2011;13(1):4–14. doi:10.7224/1537-2073-13.1.4.

69. Baert I, Freeman J, Smedal T, et al. Responsiveness and clinically meaningful improvement, according to disability level, of five walking measures after rehabilitation in multiple sclerosis: a European multicenter study. *Neurorehabil Neural Repair*. 2014;28(7):621–631. doi:10.1177/1545968314521010.

70. Gijbels D, Eijnde BO, Feys P. Comparison of the 2- and 6-minute walk test in multiple sclerosis. *Mult Scler*. 2011;17(10):1269–1272. doi:10.1177/1352458511408475.

71. McGuigan C, Hutchinson M. Confirming the validity and responsiveness of the Multiple Sclerosis Walking Scale-12 (MSWS-12). *Neurology*. 2004;62(11):2103–2105. doi:10.1212/01.WNL.0000127604.84575.0D.

72. Motl RW, Dlugonski D, Suh Y, et al. Multiple Sclerosis Walking Scale-12 and oxygen cost of walking. *Gait Posture*. 2010;31(4):506–510. doi:10.1016/j.gaitpost.2010.02.011.

73. Riazi A. Using the SF-36 measure to compare the health impact of multiple sclerosis and Parkinson's disease with normal population health profiles. *J Neurol Neurosurg Psychiatry*. 2003;74(6):710–714. doi:10.1136/jnnp.74.6.710.

74. National Multiple Sclerosis Society. Health Status Questionnaire (SF-36). http://www.nationalmssociety.org/For-Professionals/Researchers/Resources-for-Researchers/Clinical-Study-Measures/Health-Status-Questionnaire-(SF-36).

75. McGuigan C, Hutchinson M. The multiple sclerosis impact scale (MSIS-29) is a reliable and sensitive measure. *J Neurol Neurosurg Psychiatry*. 2004;75(2):266–269. doi:10.1136/jnnp.2003.016899.

76. Riazi A. Multiple Sclerosis Impact Scale (MSIS-29): reliability and validity in hospital based samples. *J Neurol Neurosurg Psychiatry*. 2002;73(6):701–704. doi:10.1136/jnnp.73.6.701.

77. Hobart JC, Riazi A, Lamping DL, et al. How responsive is the Multiple Sclerosis Impact Scale (MSIS-29)? A comparison with some other self report scales. *J Neurol Neurosurg Psychiatry*. 2005;76(11):1539–1543. doi:10.1136/jnnp.2005.064584.

78. Yorke AM, Cohen ET. Functional assessment of multiple sclerosis. *J Physiother*. 2015;61(4):226.

79. Shammas L, Zentek T, von Haaren B, et al. Home-based system for physical activity monitoring in patients with multiple sclerosis (Pilot study). *Biomed Eng Online*. 2014;13:10. doi:10.1186/1475-925X-13-10.

80. Busse ME, Pearson OR, Van Deursen R, et al. Quantified measurement of activity provides insight into motor function and recovery in neurological disease. *J Neurol Neurosurg Psychiatry*. 2004;75(6):884–888.

81. Hale L, Williams K, Ashton C, et al. Reliability of RT3 accelerometer for measuring mobility in people with multiple sclerosis: pilot study. *J Rehabil Res Dev*. 2007;44(4):619–627.

82. Martin CL, Phillips BA, Kilpatrick TJ, et al. Gait and balance impairment in early multiple sclerosis in the absence of clinical disability. *Mult Scler*. 2006;12(5):620–628.

83. Thoumie P, Mevellec E. Relation between walking speed and muscle strength is affected by somatosensory loss in multiple sclerosis. *J Neurol Neurosurg Psychiatry*. 2002;73(3):313–315.

84. Frzovic D, Morris ME, Vowels L. Clinical tests of standing balance: performance of persons with multiple sclerosis. *Arch Phys Med Rehabil.* 2000;81(2):215–221.

85. Thoumie P, Lamotte D, Cantalloube S, et al. Motor determinants of gait in 100 ambulatory patients with multiple sclerosis. *Mult Scler.* 2005;11(4):485–491.

86. Rougier P, Faucher M, Cantalloube S, et al. How proprioceptive impairments affect quiet standing in patients with multiple sclerosis. *Somatosens Mot Res.* 2007;24(1–2):41–51. doi:10.1080/08990220701318148.

87. MS Australia. Balance for People with Multiple Sclerosis. MS Practice:1–10. https://www.msaustralia.org.au/file/274/download?token=kKMkvZHS.

88. Frohman EM, Frohman TC, Zee DS, et al. The neuro-ophthalmology of multiple sclerosis. *Lancet Neurol.* 2005;4(2):111–121. doi:10.1016/S1474-4422(05)00992-0.

89. Topper AK, Maki BE, Holliday PJ. Are activity-based assessments of balance and gait in the elderly predictive of risk of falling and/or type of fall? *J Am Geriatr Soc.* 1993;41(5):479–487.

90. Yelnik A, Bonan I. Clinical tools for assessing balance disorders. *Neurophysiol Clin.* 2008;38(6):439–445. doi:10.1016/j.neucli.2008.09.008.

91. Whitney JC, Lord SR, Close JCT. Streamlining assessment and intervention in a falls clinic using the Timed Up and Go Test and Physiological Profile Assessments. *Age Ageing.* 2005;34(6):567–571. doi:10.1093/ageing/afi178.

92. Nilsagard Y, Lundholm C, Gunnarsson LG, et al. Clinical relevance using timed walk tests and "timed up and go" testing in persons with multiple sclerosis. *Physiother Res Int.* 2007;12(2):105–114.

93. Cattaneo D, Regola A, Meotti M. Validity of six balance disorders scales in persons with multiple sclerosis. *Disabil Rehabil.* 2006;28(12):789–795. doi:10.1080/09638280500404289.

94. Toomey E, Coote S. Between-rater reliability of the 6-minute walk test, berg balance scale, and handheld dynamometry in people with multiple sclerosis. *Int J MS Care.* 2013;15(1):1–6. doi:10.7224/1537-2073.2011-036.

95. Downs S, Marquez J, Chiarelli P. The Berg Balance Scale has high intra- and inter-rater reliability but absolute reliability varies across the scale: a systematic review. *J Physiother.* 2013;59(2):93–99. doi:10.1016/S1836-9553(13)70161-9.

96. Lewis C, Shaw K. One Legged (single limb) Stance Test. *Phys Ther Rehab Med.* 2006;17(6):10.

97. Rush R, Kumbhare D. Spasticity. *CMAJ.* 2015;187(6):436. doi:10.1503/cmaj.140405.

98. Lundström E, Smits A, Terént A, et al. Time-course and determinants of spasticity during the first six months following first-ever stroke. *J Rehabil Med.* 2010;42(4):296–301. doi:10.2340/16501977-0509.

99. Pathak MS, Brashear A. Spasticity. In: Truong D, Dressler D, Hallett M, eds. *Manual of Botulinum Toxin THerapy.* Cambridge, UK: Cambridge University Press; 2009.

100. Sangelaji B, Estebsari F, Nabavi SM, et al. The effect of exercise therapy on cognitive functions in multiple sclerosis patients: a pilot study. *Med J Islam Repub Iran.* 2015;29:205.

101. Haselkorn JK, Loomis S. Multiple sclerosis and spasticity. *Phys Med Rehabil Clin N Am.* 2005;16(2):467–481. doi:10.1016/j.pmr.2005.01.006.

102. Christiansen CH, Baum CM, eds. *Occupational Therapy: Enabling Function and Well-Being.* 2nd ed. 1997. http://ovidsp.ovid.com/ovidweb.cgi?T=JS&PAGE=reference&D=psyc3&NEWS=N&AN=1997-30090-000. Accessed June 13, 2016.

103. Foley PL, Vesterinen HM, Laird BJ, et al. Prevalence and natural history of pain in adults with multiple sclerosis: systematic review and meta-analysis. *Pain.* 2013;154(5):632–642. doi:10.1016/j.pain.2012.12.002.

104. Moulin DE, Foley KM, Ebers GC. Pain syndromes in multiple sclerosis. *Neurology.* 1988;38(12):1830–1834. http://www.ncbi.nlm.nih.gov/pubmed/2973568.

INDEX